The Standard Normal (z) Distribution

z	.00	.01	.02	.03	.04	.05	.06	.07	.08	.09
0.0	.0000	.0040	.0080	.0120	.0160	.0199	.0239	.0279	.0319	.0359
0.1	.0398	.0438	.0478	.0517	.0557	.0596	.0636	.0675	.0714	.0753
0.2	.0793	.0832	.0871	.0910	.0948	.0987	.1026	.1064	.1103	.1141
0.3	.1179	.1217	.1255	.1293	.1331	.1368	.1406	.1443	.1480	.1517
0.4	.1554	.1591	.1628	.1664	.1700	.1736	.1772	.1808	.1844	.1879
0.5	.1915	.1950	.1985	.2019	.2054	.2088	.2123	.2157	.2190	.2224
0.6	.2257	.2291	.2324	.2357	.2389	.2422	.2454	.2486	.2517	.2549
0.7	.2580	.2611	.2642	.2673	.2704	.2734	.2764	.2794	.2823	.2852
0.8	.2881	.2910	.2939	.2967	.2995	.3023	.3051	.3078	.3106	.3133
0.9	.3159	.3186	.3212	.3238	.3264	.3289	.3315	.3340	.3365	.3389
1.0	.3413	.3438	.3461	.3485	.3508	.3531	.3554	.3577	.3599	.3621
1.1	.3643	.3665	.3686	.3708	.3729	.3749	.3770	.3790	.3810	.3830
1.2	.3849	.3869	.3888	.3907	.3925	.3944	.3962	.3980	.3997	.4015
1.3	.4032	.4049	.4066	.4082	.4099	.4115	.4131	.4147	.4162	.4177
1.4	.4192	.4207	.4222	.4236	.4251	.4265	.4279	.4292	.4306	.4319
1.5	.4332	.4345	.4357	.4370	.4382	.4394	.4406	.4418	.4429	.4441
1.6	.4452	.4463	.4474	.4484	.4495	.4505	.4515	.4525	.4535	.4545
1.7	.4554	.4564	.4573	.4582	.4591	.4599	.4608	.4616	.4625	.4633
1.8	.4641	.4649	.4656	.4664	.4671	.4678	.4686	.4693	.4699	.4706
1.9	.4713	.4719	.4726	.4732	.4738	.4744	.4750	.4756	.4761	.4767
2.0	.4772	.4778	.4783	.4788	.4793	.4798	.4803	.4808	.4812	.4817
2.1	.4821	.4826	.4830	.4834	.4838	.4842	.4846	.4850	.4854	.4857
2.2	.4861	.4864	.4868	.4871	.4875	.4878	.4881	.4884	.4887	.4890
2.3	.4893	.4896	.4898	.4901	.4904	.4906	.4909	.4911	.4913	.4916
2.4	.4918	.4920	.4922	.4925	.4927	.4929	.4931	.4932	.4934	.4936
2.5	.4938	.4940	.4941	.4943	.4945	.4946	.4948	.4949	.4951	.4952
2.6	.4953	.4955	.4956	.4957	.4959	.4960	.4961	.4962	.4963	.4964
2.7	.4965	.4966	.4967	.4968	.4969	.4970	.4971	.4972	.4973	.4974
2.8	.4974	.4975	.4976	.4977	.4977	.4978	.4979	.4979	.4980	.4981
2.9	.4981	.4982	.4982	.4983	.4984	.4984	.4985	.4985	.4986	.4986
3.0	.4987	.4987	.4987	.4988	.4988	.4989	.4989	.4989	.4990	.4990

Research in Nursing

RESEARCH IN NURSING

Holly Skodol Wilson
RN, PhD, FAAN

 Addison-Wesley Publishing Company

Nursing Division, Menlo Park, California
Reading, Massachusetts • Don Mills, Ontario • Wokingham, U.K.
Amsterdam • Sydney • Singapore • Tokyo • Mexico City
Bogota • Santiago • San Juan

Sponsoring editor: Thomas Eoyang
Production coordinator: Julie Kranhold □ Ex Libris
Book designer: Wendy Calmenson
Manuscript editor: William Waller
Illustrations: Carl Brown

Portions of the text have appeared in substantially
altered form in *The Journal of Nursing
Administration* as "Research Reflections." The
author and publisher thank *The Journal of Nursing
Administration* and the J. B. Lippincott Company for
their permission to adapt material for this text.

Library of Congress Cataloging in Publication Data

Wilson, Holly Skodol.
  Research in nursing.

  Includes bibliographies and index.
  1. Nursing—Research—Methodology.   I. Title.
DNLM: 1. Nursing. 2. Research. WY 20.5 W748r
RT81.5.W55 1985   610.73′072   84-28439
ISBN 0-201-09737-0

 cdefghijk-HA-898765

Addison-Wesley Publishing Company
Nursing Division
2725 Sand Hill Road   Menlo Park, California 94025

PHOTO CREDITS

Suzanne Arms: Part 1
Gabrielle Beasley: Chapter 14
Jeffry Collins: Part 2; Chapter 5
George Fry: Part 4; Chapters 4, 8, 11
© **Bruce Kliewe/Jeroboam:** Chapter 15
Wayland Lee: Chapters 7, 16
L. A. Takats: Chapter 10
William Thompson: Chapters 1, 9, 12, 17
Mark Tuschman: Part 3; Chapter 2
Holly Wilson: Chapters 3, 13

For my three daughters . . . Molly, Hillary, and Emily

Preface

This textbook and its accompanying supplements rest on a straight-forward but potentially revolutionary premise: *If nursing is to build a scientific body of knowledge and if nursing practice is to be shaped by research findings rather than tradition, intuition, or habit, then the investigative skills of all nurses, regardless of their educational level, must be as integral to their repertoire as communication skills and sterile technique.* All nurses must be prepared to know something, if not a good deal, about how to read, comprehend, evaluate, apply, participate in, and conduct research in nursing. Nursing science and nursing research must become as interesting and accessible to every nurse clinician as they are to a career nurse scientist.

Content and Features

The premise of this text may be revolutionary, but it is not original. As discussed in Chapter 1 and reflected throughout this text, it is a goal stated formally and informally at every level of the profession. **Research in Nursing** addresses this goal by:

- Challenging *the traditional assumption* that to become an informed consumer of research in nursing a nurse must first be trained to conduct independent research. Appreciating a fine painting or a gourmet meal, after all, does not require you to become an artist or a chef. In our profession the research degree is earned at the doctoral level, but we cannot afford to rely solely on doctorally prepared nurses to bridge the research–practice gap. Research consumership can and must be learned early in a nursing student's educational career. This text, therefore, discusses the skills of intelligent research consumership after presenting an introduction to science and the research process that highlights the relevance to nursing practice and crucial ethical concerns.

- Demonstrating *the application of research to all aspects of the nursing profession*, but particularly to clinical nursing practice. Students usually choose nursing as a career because they want to help, care, support, and comfort, not because they want to analyze, conceptualize, theorize, or criticize. Failure to show the important relationship between the two sets of activities, however, has been a major stumbling block to the integration of research as a *value* for every practicing nurse. In specific chapters devoted to the topic of application, as well as through a kind of textual "role modeling" on virtually every page, **Research in Nursing** makes the case that *knowing how we know* is essential to *doing what we do.*

- Choosing *an informed, conversational tone and writing style.* By demystifying research terminology, the text presents scholarship not as the dry, esoteric, and pretentious exercise it is sometimes reputed to be, but as the lively, engaging, and sometimes humorous enterprise it often is.

- Emphasizing *the qualities of discovery and creativity,* as well as precision and rigor, that underlie the best in nursing research. Scientific imagination is given its proper place alongside scientific accuracy and technique.

- Presenting, in two chapters, *the methodologies of qualitative research.* In our early stage of scientific maturity, description and generating theory are as vital to our development as testing hypotheses and verifying theory. Numerous examples of field studies and qualitative analyses are therefore discussed to show the power and promise that these methodologies can offer research in nursing.

- Reinforcing information through *clear pedagogical devices.* Chapter outlines, objectives, lists, boxes, tables, figures, annotated examples, summaries of key ideas and terms, further readings, a research glossary, and appendices of research resources enrich the content, making it easier on the eye and more accessible to the mind.

- Offering *a package of supplements* that assist the instructor and motivate the student. The *Instructor's Manual* is keyed to the text chapter by chapter and includes topical lecture outlines, transparency masters, and activities for individual, small-group, and full-class learning. The extensive bank of test questions addresses the learning objectives for each chapter. *Applying Research in Nursing* is an innovative application and resource workbook for students and contains action-oriented assessment tools, exercises, and practice opportunities to use the skills of research consumership and methodology discussed in the text.

Audience

This comprehensive introductory text provides the nursing student with the knowledge and skills required of nurses in investigative roles, ranging from research consumer to scientific investigator. It is therefore appropriate as a reference for an issues or professionalism course in diploma or associate-degree curricula, where research in nursing is covered as a unit or topic; as a required text in an introductory course in nursing research, whether at the baccalaureate or beginning masters level; or as a resource for more advanced graduate students and practitioners seeking a book that conveys the fascination and scope of this growing field. Nurses employed in health-care settings, where research is emerging as a significant aspect of leadership, will find this text a worthwhile addition to their personal and institutional libraries.

Organization

Research in Nursing is organized into four parts. Part 1 introduces the reader to science as a way of knowing and the research process as the tool of science. It advances values and attitudes that foster an appreciation of the significance of science and research to nursing practice and patient care. It also addresses the nurse's role in respecting and advocating research ethics.

Part 2 focuses on the skills of research consumership, from acquiring a research vocabulary to preparing a complete, formal research critique.

Part 3 is devoted to the steps of actually conducting a scientific investigation. It gives equal attention both to qualitative data collection techniques such as observation and interviewing and to quantitative data collection using psychosocial and biological instrumentation. Analysis procedures for qualitative data and statistical procedures, along with a full chapter on the use of computers in nursing research, conclude this part.

Part 4 provides the developing scholar with specific guidelines and strategies for communicating the methods and findings of scientific work through journal articles, books, scientific papers, and talks at professional meetings.

All chapters need not be assigned, nor is adhering to a single sequence necessary to make the text a coherent learning tool. The extensive glossary of research terminology, research resources, and samples in the appendixes, and statistical tables and symbols included on the endpapers add to the reference utility of this text.

Building the scientific basis for clinical nursing practice is a top priority for nursing research in the 1980s. While each chapter of this text sustains the importance of this priority, the values of studies in nursing administration, nursing education, nursing history, and nursing philosophy are also underscored. Thus the title, **Research in Nursing**, reflects scientific diversity rather than an exclusive focus on clinical nursing research.

Acknowledgments

Writing this book reminded me that an author's work requires a long encounter with solitude. Sustaining my energy and enthusiasm for the project would have been impossible without the support, help, inspiration, and contributions of certain key people. I acknowledge them here with my warmest thanks.

- The nursing students at Sonoma State University and the University of California, San Francisco, to whom I've taught the required introductory nursing research courses since 1974, and whose responses convinced me of the worth of this book's contents. Also the doctoral students at UCSF who generously shared their in-progress work as examples and illustrations.

- My colleagues and friends Sally Hutchinson, Jane Norbeck, Ada Lindsey, and Nancy Stotts, who contributed their expertise by authoring chapters on "Getting Started," "The Theoretical Context," "Psychosocial Instruments," and "Biophysiologic Variables."

- A former graduate student and enduring friend, Geoff McEnany, who wrote the *Instructor's Manual* and made it the best and wittiest in nursing. And Sally Hutchinson again for making our collaboration on *Applying Research in Nursing* interesting and fun.

- My sponsoring editor at Addison-Wesley, Thomas Eoyang, whose commitment to this project and to the worth of nursing and nurses inspired involvement from us both that regularly exceeded the call of duty. He taught me that nursing is the best example of "applied humanities" as well as an applied science.

- My production coordinator, Julie Kranhold of Ex Libris, whose taste, competence, good humor, and calm in the face of deadlines and typical book-producing crises sustained a sense of graciousness, teamwork, and cooperation throughout the tedious phases of putting the ideas into print.

- The W. K. Kellogg Leadership Fellowship whose belief in the leadership of ideas for advancing social good provided important sources of support while I wrote this book.

- The following authorities who reviewed and critiqued chapters in this book during its development:

Sarah Lee Bleeks, DePaul University
Catherine Connelly, George Mason University

Arline Duvall, Clemson University
Elaine Dyer, Brigham Young University
William Fite, Tallahassee Medical Center
Deborah Frank, Florida State University
Sandra Funk, University of North Carolina, Chapel Hill
Ruth Harris, Adelphi University
Josephine Lutz, University of Wisconsin, Madison
Sharon McDonald, San Diego State University
Lillian Nail, University of Rochester
Natalie Pavlovich, Duquesne University

Chester Peachey, Goshen College
Michael Rice, University of Arizona
Mary Ann Schroeder, Medical College of George
Evelyn Stacy-Spencer, Castleton State College
Ingrid Swenson, University of North Carolina, Chapel Hill
Judith Wakim, Austin Peay State University
Jean Watson, University of Colorado

And to all those other family members, friends, students, and colleagues who in a small and big sense helped make it happen.

Holly Skodol Wilson

Biographical Notes

About the Author

Holly Skodol Wilson, RN, PhD, FAAN, is a professor in the Department of Mental Health and Community Nursing, School of Nursing, at the University of California, San Francisco, where she teaches the required introductory research course for registered nurse students in the articulated BS/MS program. It was for this course that she was awarded the Outstanding Teacher of the Year Award by students at their 1983 and 1984 commencements. Her clinical and research interests focus on the severely and chronically mentally disordered, psychogerontology, and psychiatric nursing diagnosis. She has authored and coauthored eight other books and contributed over 40 articles to scholarly journals. She contributes a regular feature entitled "Research Reflections . . . A Resource for Nurse Executives" to *The Journal of Nursing Administration* and is on the review boards of *Nursing Outlook*, *Nursing Research*, and *Advances in Nursing Science*. She is active nationally and internationally as a speaker and consultant and has taught in Japan, The People's Republic of China, and Kenya, East Africa. Her honors include Distinguished Alumni, Duke University, School of Nursing; Distinguished Dissertation of the Year, U.C. Berkeley; and the American Nurses' Foundation Scholar Citation. During the writing of this text and its supplements, she was awarded a Kellogg National Leadership Fellowship to study international models of care for the mentally disordered elderly.

About the Contributors

Sally A. Hutchinson, RN, PhD, is an assistant professor in the College of Nursing, University of Florida. She teaches qualitative research methods to masters and doctoral students and a course on cultural influences in nursing care. A recipient of Division of Nursing pre- and post-doctoral research fellowships, she presently is studying nurses who are chemically dependent. She has published in numerous nursing journals and contributed chapters to several nursing research texts. She was a seminar leader and a co-leader of Professional Seminar Consultants' study tours to China and Africa. Her scholarly interests are in anthropology, qualitative research methods, and psychiatric nursing.

Ada M. Lindsey, RN, PhD, FAAN, is a professor and chairperson, Department of Physiological Nursing, School of Nursing, at the University of California, San Francisco. Her more recent major contributions have been to graduate nursing education. She has been an active member of both the Oncology Nursing Society and the American Association of Critical Care Nurses, serving on the research committee of each organization. The focus of her clinical and research interests has included cachexia and anorexia in cancer patients and the influence of moderator variables, such as social support, on health outcomes. She has authored and coauthored a number of book chapters and journal articles and has presented her work at national and international meetings.

Jane S. Norbeck, RN, DNSc, FAAN, is an associate professor and department chairperson in the Department of Mental Health and Community Nursing, School of Nursing, at the University of California, San Francisco. Her Chapter 11, "Collecting Data with Psychosocial Instruments," is an outgrowth of her work in developing and refining instruments to measure social support and life stress. In addition to methodological research on instrumentation, her research efforts center around the role of social support in health and functioning outcomes. These studies have included psychosocial predictors of complications of pregnancy, the functioning of single parents, and coping with job stress in critical care nursing.

Nancy A. Stotts, RN, EdD, is an assistant professor and coordinator of the graduate specialty "Adult Nursing: Surgical," in the Department of Physiological Nursing, School of Nursing, at the University of California, San Francisco. Her clinical expertise and research are focused in the area of surgical nursing, including wound healing, nutrition, and nursing education. She has been active in the American Association of Critical Care Nurses and currently serves as a member of the Research Committee. She has authored and coauthored a number of journal articles and book chapters.

Contents

Research in Nursing

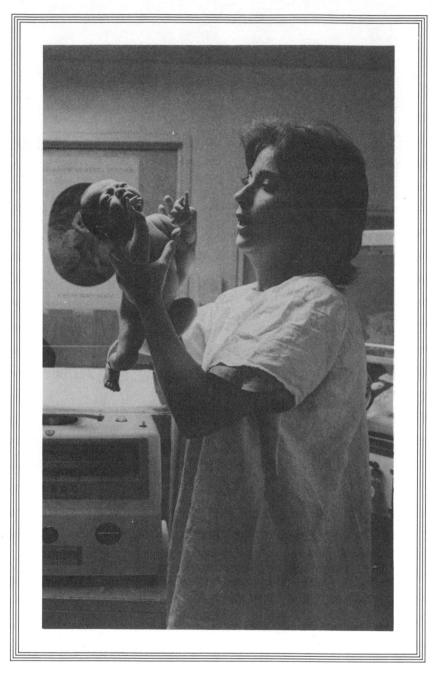

"The scientific approach is the systematic attempt
to understand and comprehend the world . . . , to
enter deeply into the world . . . to achieve a rational
expression . . . or the order and beauty of
operation that lies behind it."

A. Jacox (1974)

I

Scientific Research, the Nursing Profession, and You

Chapter 1

What Is Nursing Research?

Ways of Knowing

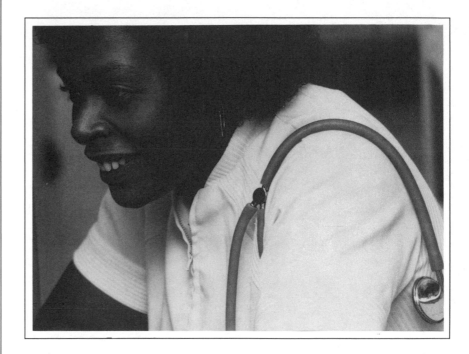

The scientific approach offers nurses a valuable resource for answering difficult clinical and health-related questions. The true scientist is not created by learning technical methods, but rather by mastering their use.

Chapter Outline

Chapter Objectives

After reading this chapter, the student should be able to:

- Appreciate the meaning and usefulness of the scientific method of problem solving and decision making in nursing practice
- Compare the scientific approach with (1) trial and error and common sense, (2) authority and tradition, (3) inspiration and intuition, and (4) logical reasoning
- Identify the assumptions, characteristics, and aims of the scientific approach
- Compare the positivist philosophy of science with the symbolic interactionist philosophy
- Locate a nursing study on a continuum based on its relevance to nursing practice
- Recognize types of nursing studies through identification of study purpose and design
- Explain ten typical steps in the research process
- Trace the major landmarks in the developmental history of nursing research, specifying one significant outcome for each
- Interpret the implications of past trends for the future of nursing research

In This Chapter . . .

The August night was hot and sticky despite the hum of the hospital's antiquated air conditioning system. The man tossed in his narrow bed as the other three figures in the ward lay sleeping. He groaned and opened his eyes to the darkness. His body felt prickly, and his heart was pounding harder than usual. He searched for the dab of light emanating from the nurses' station down the hall. The patient tried to settle back into his sleeping position, but a peculiar sensation inside his abdomen brought him wide awake, and he was overcome with the feeling that something terrible was about to happen. It felt like a mouse running up and down inside of him. His heart was swelling, filling his chest and forcing its way up into his throat. The mouse increased its frantic run and began to spin inside, scratching his guts with its claws. A wave of nausea swept over him, and a veil of sweat covered his face. Trying not to disturb the others, the man reached for his call bell and

rang for the nurse. "I'm sick, I'm sick as hell," he whispered to her. Two months later this man, who had been admitted to the hospital for cartilage repair associated with an old soccer injury, died of acute adult leukemia.*

That same August night, five floors higher in the hospital, an eager pair of mothers watched as a nurse walked into their room with two pink babies balanced carefully in her arms. The babies were yelling with open, hungry mouths. Their waiting mothers gathered them in, and the nurse moved between the sucking infants, gently adjusting a position here, offering a word of encouragement there, and feeling a sense of satisfaction and tenderness about her work.

*Panger, Daniel. *The Dance of the Wild Mouse*. Glen Ellen, Calif.: Entwhistle Books, 1979.

The realities of human suffering and joy challenge and enrich our practice of the scientific, professional discipline of nursing. Each day you may carry out tasks that are viewed by others as rewarding, frightening, or even distasteful. You will often have to rely on your own judgment in the absence of complete information. Your work may arouse in you feelings of compassion, outrage, guilt, pity, anxiety, confusion, or curiosity. Confronting these experiences requires both the *engaged* and the *analytic* ways of knowing (Ackerman 1969):

The Engaged style of knowing demands effective human contact between the individual and the object of his/her attention. The Analytic style gives the individual precision tools with which to manipulate the environment (p. 855).

The engaged study of humanities, according to Prior (1962), "includes types of learning that are directly concerned with human responses to all forms of experience" (p. 11). This conception strongly resembles the definition of nursing in the American Nurses' Association's social policy

statement (1980): "Nursing is the diagnosis and treatment of human responses to actual or potential health problems" (p. 9). From studies that emphasize the engaged style we derive our notions of freedom, justice, imagination, commitment, loyalty, beauty, and compassion. Yet professional nursing also requires nurses to have at their command:

a large body of knowledge that is theoretical as well as empirical, extends beyond practical and established nursing knowledge, [and] includes a large selection of alternative explanations and predictions for nursing problems . . . some of which are abstract, complex, and not clearly understood, and require nursing actions which may be innovative and probabilistic (Waters et al 1972 p. 5).

In short, nursing competence requires mastery of analytic knowing as well as engaged knowing.

Although some philosophers argue that the engaged style of knowing is dramatically different from the analytic style in its language, content, and goals, Bronowski (1956) sums up the approach to science that you will learn about in this chapter:

The discoveries of science and the works of art . . . are explorations of a hidden likeness or unity. . . . This is the act of creation in which an original thought is born and the act is the same in . . . science and in art (p. 30).

Science and research are indeed keystones in the edifice of professional nursing practice, but they do not stand alone. Nursing's goals of wisdom, vision, social significance, accountability, fulfillment, collegiality, and excellence can be achieved only when we synthesize the engaged with the analytic—the humanities with the sciences. Nursing research at its best captures this synthesis.

The scientific approach, when conceived of as a process of learning about patients of the sort whose stories began this chapter, has been defined by Jacox (1974) as:

The systematic attempt to understand and comprehend the world, . . . to enter deeply into the world, not just superficially, but to achieve a rational expression in language and mathematical symbolism of the order and beauty of operation that lies behind the external world (p. 6).

Not everyone writing about research shares my judgments and biases, which include the following ideas:

1. Scientific research does not pretend that the knowledge conveyed is literal and irrevocable truth. Many research textbooks and courses inhibit genuine inquiry by their dogmatic methodological pretensions and mechanical procedures. Such an approach simply obscures good ideas and fails to inspire students.

2. Science does, of course, involve a process of proof, but it also involves a spirit of *discovery*.

3. Knowledge won through research is not just knowledge of facts, but of *facts interpreted*; good scientists realize that such knowledge is fragile, open to doubt, and subject to change.

4. Most of the principles of scientific research are applied in thoughtful nursing practice, and the substance of much research exists in everyday nursing practice.

Read on if you are a nurse or nursing student who believes that research is more than the meticulous application of given procedures to relatively insignificant questions, and if you wish to penetrate the mystique of research methods so that you will know

- what to look for in research studies
- what meanings to assign their findings
- how to put findings into practice
- how to use your curiosity, imagination, and reasoning to adapt the technology of science to acquiring fresh knowledge and solutions to practical problems

The aim of Chapter 1 is to define the meaning of science and research for nurses who will be conducting studies themselves or applying study findings in their clinical practice. In this chapter you will learn about the scientific way of knowing as contrasted with the alternatives of common sense, tradition, intuition, and logical reasoning. We will also consider two major philosophies of science, several types of nursing study, the typical steps in the research process itself, and the historical evolution and the future directions of nursing research. Finally, the chapter aims to help you learn how nursing research can foster your own intellectual development, advance the nursing profession, and improve the quality of care given to patients.

Chapter 1 opens the door to a rich adventure in the world of discovery and scientific competence. Take a stand when you read it. Argue about the ideas. Be opinionated. Later, soften your attitude to one, in Kerlinger's (1966) terms, of "intelligent conviction and emotional commitment." Technical competence is empty without a basic understanding of the nature and promise of research in nursing.

Why Do Research?

Nurses make decisions and solve problems each and every day in the process of delivering care to patients. This section encourages you to pause and consider the basis on which you answer clinical questions. Imagine the following situation.

A mother-to-be was admitted to a California hospital at 3:40 A.M. in active labor. An external monitor was applied, and her membranes broke about 20 minutes later. When her physician's associate checked in at 5 A.M., the obstetrical nurse expressed concern about the monitor tracing and asked him to check it. After he did so and did a pelvic exam on the laboring mother, he *suggested* that the nurse call the patient's primary obstetrician. Unknown to him, however, was the fact that the obstetrician had left standing orders not to be disturbed between 10 P.M. and 7 A.M., "except in an emergency." Because the associate did not *declare* this case to be an emergency, the nurse followed the standing orders. By 7:30 the monitor was exhibiting a marked late deceleration, and by 10 the obstetrician had come to the hospital and performed an emergency Caesarean section. The newborn exhibited signs of brain damage. Now, at 3½ years of age, he is a spastic quadriplegic with mental retardation (Snyder 1983).

How does a nurse decide what to do in such a situation? Should he or she follow the standing instruction of an authority and abide by the institution's traditions? Or is there an independent accountability to the patient that requires the nurse to recognize the seriousness of the situation from the monitor tracings and make judgments on some other basis?

If you are inclined to favor the latter alternative, consider another situation. Imagine that you have taught prenatal classes to expectant parents for five years. One of your patients has been complaining of severe nausea and vomiting and is taking Bendectin (a combination of doxylamine and pyridoxin). She reads in the local paper that the drug's manufacturer is no longer making and distributing the drug but that it has not been withdrawn from the market and will continue to be available until supplies in the hands of drug distributors, wholesalers, and pharmacies are exhausted. She asks *you* whether it is true that taking this drug will cause pyloric stenosis in her infant. Or will nausea and vomiting, without treatment, themselves increase the same risk? Would she be better off taking a different drug, even though it has not been so well studied as Bendectin? The mother-to-be seeks your counsel. On what basis do you respond?

Questions in everyday nursing practice as well as health-care planning surround you. Is it true that hospital nurse vacancy and turnover rates have declined significantly since 1979 and that what used to be a severe nursing shortage has been succeeded by hiring freezes and mandatory dropoffs without pay each month to prevent layoffs (*Demand for Nurses* 1983, Aiken 1982)? Are old women "sicker" than men when it comes to the incidence of chronic diseases, or do they just outlive men and thus become more susceptible?

If you were planning a prevention program targeted to the reports that older women get osteoporosis three to five times more often than men and therefore have more bone fractures in later life, would you recommend calcium supplements, high-protein diets, exercise, or supplemental estrogen? On what bases would you decide? Should women over the age of 47 be taught breast self-examination for cancer despite the fact that the incidence peaks in women between

42 and 47 (McKeever 1983)? Should elderly women have a pelvic exam as part of a usual physical assessment? What is the risk to young children of electrically powered beds with automatic bed-lowering controls, or "walk-away switches"? Do most patients know the names of the drugs they take? their purpose? how and when to take them? when to stop? what food, drinks, and other drugs to avoid? what side effects can occur? The scientific approach as reflected in nursing research offers you important resources for answering difficult clinical and health-related questions.

Ways of Knowing

Although this text advocates the scientific method as the way to address the questions posed in the last section, there are alternative ways of knowing:

- *You can use trial and error combined with common sense.* If the other patients in your prenatal class who took Bendectin did not have babies with pyloric stenosis, then your common sense might compel you to say that the drug was safe.
- *You can use authority and tradition.* If following the stated rules in procedure books and standing orders is your choice, you will not feel obligated to make an independent interpretation of the fetal monitor's tracings for evidence of an emergency.
- *You can use inspiration and intuition.* If your engaged style of knowing compels you to predict that elderly women are disadvantaged by the level of care they receive, you will be inspired to become an advocate for better care for the aged, minorities, and other disadvantaged groups and support teaching them self-care.
- *You can use logical reasoning.* If your own sense of logic alerts you to the ideas that (1) children and some adults are particularly curious about how mechanical beds operate, (2) the metal underparts of such a bed can have a scissors, or guillotine, action, and (3) being caught between the stationary portion of the bed and its moving frame could crush a child to death, you will conclude that removing or deactivating the "walkaway" down switches on these beds, at least in pediatric and psychiatric wards, is definitely indicated.

What Is the Scientific Approach?

The way of knowing developed in this book is that of scientific research blended with what Diers (1983) has defined as "clinical scholarship"—a stretching of one's mind for new insights. Let's begin with some basic *assumptions* that underpin the scientific approach:

1. It is better to be knowledgeable about the world than to be ignorant of it.

2. Scientists can use their senses to apprehend an external reality.

3. Observers of the world are able to relate ob-

Table 1-1   Summary of Basic Points About the Scientific Approach to Knowing

Assumptions	Characteristics	Aims
The existence of underlying order in the universe	Built-in self correction for objectivity	Build a body of theories that describe, explain, and predict
The value of knowledge over ignorance	Reliance on empirical evidence	Solve practical problems
Use of empirical evidence		
Existence of causal relationships		
Conceptualizations are based on observation		

servations conceptually and make meaning out of them.

4. It is possible to discern an underlying order in the psychosocial as well as the physical world.

5. Cause and effect relationships exist in the social *and* physical orders.

Given these assumptions, we can define *scientific inquiry* as a process in which observable, verifiable data are systematically collected from the world we know through our senses to describe, explain, or predict events. The scientific approach has two *characteristics* that the other ways of knowing do not—(1) *self-correction*, or *objectivity*, and (2) *the use of sensory, or empirical, data*.

This approach to knowing has built-in checks throughout the investigative process. If a scientist finds that a particular hypothesis is supported in an experiment, he or she will also test alternative hypotheses, and this testing must be open to the criticism of others. The quality of objectivity is what some authorities call the checks that attempt to distance the way of knowing as much as possible from the scientist's personal beliefs, values, and attitudes.

The second key characteristic is that the scientific approach appeals to evidence (called empirical data) in a systematic way.

The basic *aims* of scientific inquiry are to (1) develop explanations of the world (these explanations are called *theories*—see Chapter 10) and (2) find solutions to problems (see Chapter 2). The key features of the scientific approach are summarized in Table 1-1. Although these two aims in nursing science are related, some research emphasizes the development of our general understanding of human beings in interacting with their environment, whereas others emphasize the determination of effectiveness of specific nursing interventions in practice situations.

Now that we have examined the assumptions, characteristics, and aims of the scientific approach, we can contrast it with the common-sense way of knowing, in Table 1-2.

In sum, if as a clinician you began to wonder why some myocardial infarction patients were allowed to drink ice water and others were not, you could draw on books of procedure, your past experiences, trial and error, and common sense to arrive at an explanation. *Or* you could try to use the tools of science to answer your question.

Despite the commonly accepted principles of the scientific approach just discussed, scientists themselves can differ in how they view this approach. To capture the subtle diversity here, we must think for a moment about the dominant perspectives on the philosophy of science.

Table 1-2   Scientific Knowing Versus Common Sense Knowing

Scientific Approach	Common Sense
uses conceptual schemes that have been empirically tested	may accept fanciful explanations
acquires evidence to test theories according to systematic methods	selects evidence on the basis of personal experiences or preferences, usually to verify a personal position
uses a controlled method for ruling out other variables that might explain a phenomenon	makes little or no attempt to control variables
tends not to deal with metaphysical explanations that cannot be empirically tested	may be highly metaphysical or spiritual
has a built-in mechanism for self-correction	allows explanations to persist even if incorrect

Two Perspectives on the Philosophy of Science

Two schools of thought, or intellectual traditions, provide the major philosophies of science reflected in nursing research questions and procedures. These schools of thought are sometimes called a researcher's *epistemology*. The first school of thought is called the *positivist* tradition, and the second, the *symbolic interactionist*, or *neo-idealist*, tradition. The positivists, according to Sjoberg and Nett (1968), adhere to the following opinions about science:

1. Scientists can and do attain objective knowledge of both the physical and the psychosocial worlds.
2. The logic of inquiry and research procedures should be the same whether one is studying plants or people.
3. Social order in the universe is relatively mechanistic.
4. Objectivity in research can be obtained by setting forth a formal research design.

The nonpositivists, or neo-idealists, subscribe to a different set of beliefs:

1. Fundamental differences exist between the natural, or physical, sciences and the psychosocial sciences that require different methods for each.
2. Research that studies the whole person must take into account both the historical dimension of human action and the subjective aspects of human experience.
3. There is no one objective reality waiting to be measured.
4. If scientists are to comprehend people, they must come to understand each person's own definition of his or her reality.
5. Social order is constantly in a state of becoming. Therefore, scientists cannot impose rigid categories on a social world that is constantly in the process of evolution.

For extensive illustrations of how the positivist philosophy is reflected in nursing research, see Chapter 15, on applying statistics to quantitative analysis. Likewise, see Chapter 13, on field methods, and Chapter 14, on the craft of qualitative analysis, to see how the symbolic-interactionist perspective influences research practices. The basic distinction is that positivists advocate methods dictated by rules of verification, whereas symbolic interactionists emphasize being pragmatic and seeking whatever is meaningful and useful.

Types of Nursing Research

Earlier in this chapter I specified the two aims of scientific inquiry: (1) to develop theories that increase the state of knowledge and (2) to solve problems or make decisions for what are considered practical purposes. Research conducted with the first aim is often called *basic*, or *pure*, *research*. It is often compared to building blocks, on which increments in knowledge and further research are based. Research directed to the second aim is usually called *applied research*. It includes not only studies directed toward solving practical problems and making nursing decisions but also clinical trials aimed at developing and evaluating a new program, product, method, or procedure.

This somewhat dated distinction becomes a bit fuzzy when used to categorize research conducted in a practice discipline such as nursing. Suppose you were to do a study of the health care needs of elderly Hispanic-American women. Your study's purpose and design might be limited to building a data base and thereby contributing to a body of knowledge in an area where there has been a paucity of research. In this sense, by the standard definition your research would be basic—knowledge for knowledge's sake. Someone else, however, might subsequently use your findings to alter aspects of nursing care for this population of patients, thus transforming a basic study into an applied study by using the findings to reform the ills of practice.

Diers (1979) equates virtually *all* nursing research with applied research when she enumerates three distinguishing properties of research problems in nursing:

1. The potential nursing research problem must involve "a difference that matters" in terms of its consequences for improving patient care.

2. The nursing research problem also has a relationship to more conceptual issues and therefore has the potential for contributing to theory development and our body of scientific nursing knowledge.

3. Finally, a research problem is a nursing research problem when nurses have access to and control over the phenomenon being studied.

According to these criteria, all nursing research is a blend of pure and applied research, and the critical point is its *clinical relevance* for nursing practice and our knowledge about that practice. Studying a topic that really makes no difference to patients, that is not an instance of a class of related problems, or that is not within nursing's domain all escape Diers's definition of nursing research.

In sum, according to Diers and many of her colleagues at the Yale University School of Nursing, as well as researchers at other centers, knowledge in practice professions is *for something*; specifically, in nursing, it is for improving the services given to the consumers of nursing services. If a nurse studies factors that contribute to the success of integrating the education and practice roles in nursing, by Diers's definition the study would probably be classified as research in administration! If another nurse studies how baccalaureate nursing students learn to care for terminally ill patients in the context of routine clinical instruction, the nurse is conducting a study in the field of education. But if you were to study the effects of rate of injection on intensity and duration of first and second pain of intramuscular injection, you would be a nurse conducting a nursing research study.

The Pure–Applied Continuum

An alternative to the old basic–applied distinction that is probably more useful in classifying types of nursing studies is a *pure–applied continuum* based on *how relevant* (1) the subjects, (2) the content, and (3) the conditions are to real-world nursing problems and decisions (Cooperative Graduate Education in Nursing 1975). (See Figure 1-1.) This continuum can be divided into five stages.

Stage 1—Not Directly Relevant   If you were a nurse physiologist interested in the mechanisms of skin healing and were studying the optimum time and temperature of wet soaks on guinea pigs' wounds in a laboratory, your research would be identified as a Stage 1 study on the pure–applied continuum in Figure 1-1. Such a study is not directly relevant to the practice of nursing.

Stage 2—Relevant Topic *or* Subjects   If you were interested in the concept of hunger and

were conducting a laboratory study with college students who drank Metrecal through a tube from behind a screen with no visual cues to how much they had consumed, your study, designed to determine if there is a natural factor that influences feeling satisfied, would be located at Stage 2 because your study is being conducted with people instead of animals—but the topic of hunger and satiation is not specifically related to a nursing activity.

Stage 3—Relevant Topic *and* Subjects   If you wanted to know whether premature infants placed in different body positions consumed different amounts of energy, you would be working at Stage 3 of the continuum because your study both involved people as subjects and compared different positioning choices, a topic of direct concern to nursing practice.

Stage 4—Relevant Topic, Subjects, and Trial Conditions   If you wanted to study whether it makes a difference to the recovery rate of hospitalized children when a nursing care plan also takes into account the needs of their parents, you would be testing nursing intervention under special conditions, a Stage 4 study. (Of course, one of the problems with a study under special conditions is that the conditions themselves may account for the results.)

Stage 5—Normal Field Conditions   Studying the quality of nursing care for chronically ill pa-

Figure 1-1   Pure-applied continuum based on relevance to nursing practice.

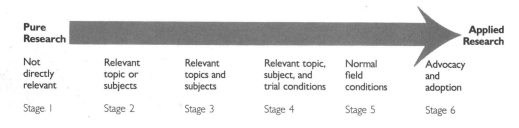

Pure Research					Applied Research
Not directly relevant	Relevant topic or subjects	Relevant topics and subjects	Relevant topic, subject, and trial conditions	Normal field conditions	Advocacy and adoption
Stage 1	Stage 2	Stage 3	Stage 4	Stage 5	Stage 6

tients with different staffing patterns under normal hospital conditions would qualify as a Stage 5 study.

Stage 6—Advocacy and Adoption Research that demonstrated the applicability of primary nursing—in which one nurse is totally responsible for a case load of patients—to a diverse array of practice settings would be at the extreme "applied" end of the continuum, or at Stage 6.

Classification by Purpose and Design

Nursing research can also be classified by its purposes and related study designs. Table 1-3 summarizes five of the major purposes of re-search—to explore, to describe, to explain, to experiment, and to test a method—and cites illustrative contemporary nursing studies for each.

Other Typologies of Research

Nursing studies can also be categorized as primarily inductive (moving from observation to explanation to general theory) or deductive (testing hypotheses deduced from theory). Or they can be described as *factor-isolating*, *factor-relating*, *situation-relating*, or *situation-producing*. These subjects are taken up in detail in subsequent chapters on design and theory (Chapters 6 and 10).

Table 1-3   Types of Nursing Study According to Purpose or Design

Type	Purpose	Methods	Examples
Exploratory	To obtain a richer familiarity with a phenomenon and clarify concepts as a basis for further research	Interviewing, participant observation, document analysis, case studies	Passage through hospitalization of severely burned, isolated school-age children (Kueffner 1976)
			An exploratory study of the meaning of current dance forms to adolescent girls (Wilson 1968)
Descriptive	To obtain complete and accurate information about a phenomenon	Interviews, questionnaires, direct observation, analysis of records	An epidemiologic study of psychiatric symptom pattern change (Nakagawa, Osborne, Hartmann 1972)
			Patient problems related to tube feeding (Walike et al 1975)
			Patient reaction to sound in an intensive coronary care unit (Marshall 1972) *(continued)*

Table 1-3   Types of Nursing Study According to Purpose or Design (continued)

Type	Purpose	Methods	Example
Explanatory	To provide conceptual analyses grounded in observation of human behavior	Interviews, participant observation, constant comparative analysis	Fairing: Control of staff work in a healing community for schizophrenics (Wilson 1978)
			Three phases in the development of father involvement in pregnancy (May 1982)
Experimental and quasi-experimental	To test hypotheses about relationships	Experiments, quasi-experiments	A physiological, behavioral approach to understanding the mechanisms of obesity and anorexia (Walike 1973)
			Effect on postoperative recovery rate and comfort of four approaches to nursing care of dogs: A Pilot Study (Hadley et al 1970)
			The effect of stimulation on the sleep behavior of the premature infant (Barnard 1973)
			Adjustment to widowhood after a sudden death: Suicide and nonsuicide survivors compared (Demi 1978)
Methodological	To develop or refine a new research technique or procedure	Validity and reliability tests	Developing a psychometric instrument for the use of children's drawings in cross-cultural research: Problems, procedures, and potentials (Schuster 1971)
			Development of a symptom distress scale (McCorkle, Young 1978)
			Quantification of self-report data from two-dimensional body diagrams (Voda et al 1980)

Steps in the Research Process

If the basic aim of science is to find general explanations of natural events so that we can describe and predict such events, scientific research is the systematic empirical investigation of presumed relations among these natural phenomena. *In other words, if developing theories and verifying them are the goals of science, the research process is the tool of science.* It represents one particular approach to coming to know that something is or is not true. The purpose of research is to discover solutions to problems and generate general principles and theory by applying scientific procedures designed to increase the chances that data collected will be reliable, relevant, and unbiased.

To increase the chance that any particular study meets the criteria of this definition, researchers customarily consider a sequence of phases, or steps, when planning the study. These steps may vary in their sequence and number depending on the purpose of the study and the style of the investigator. Abdellah and Levine (1965) list 12 major steps. Polit and Hungler (1983) describe 15 steps that "normally occur in sequence." Diers (1979) identifies nine "elements of all studies." Fox (1982) extends the list of stages to 20. Seaman and Verhonick (1982) cut the number of phases to four. Treece and Treece (1982) group them into a list of five, and Sweeney and Oliveri (1981) place the number of steps at 12. All this goes to show that whether they are called steps, phases, or elements, it is likely that they will be expressed in different forms and numbers depending on the level of inquiry and type of study. In some cases the steps are rearranged, and in others some may be omitted. Research, however, is a process, and by definition it has some number of steps that occur in relation to one another. This section is intended not to present a tour of steps set literally in concrete but rather to use the metaphor of steps to describe the general line of thinking that most investigators consider when planning a study. My list, for the purpose of clarity and comprehensiveness, has *ten* modular, mobile, and flexible steps. They are

1. stating a research problem
2. defining the purpose of the research
3. reviewing related literature
4. formulating hypotheses and defining variables
5. selecting the research design
6. selecting the population and sample
7. conducting a pilot study
8. collecting the data
9. analyzing the data
10. communicating conclusions

Each of these steps is taken up in comprehensive detail for the consumer of nursing research (in Part 2), and for the conductor of research (in Part 3). To give you a sense of the whole picture, however, each stage will be described briefly here.

Step 1—Stating a Research Problem

An investigator's task initially involves moving from a broad area of interest to a more circumscribed problem that specifies exactly what he or she intends to study. Most investigators try to define their research problems as precisely as possible. A problem is often stated in the form of a question. Here are some examples from published nursing research studies:

- How many different treatments for pressure sores are advocated by nurses, and what rationales are given for their use?
- Do mothers who are not given a prepartum enema have higher rates of contamination than mothers who are given an enema?

- Do different postoperative activity schedules affect the recovery of physical fitness among athletes?
- Is there a relationship between types of care of indwelling urethral catheters and the incidence of urinary tract infection?
- What is the optimal length of time needed to obtain an accurate oral temperature with a glass thermometer?
- What is the effect of low-frequency auditory and kinesthetic stimulation on neurological functioning of the premature infant?

If a study problem remains too broad or vague, proceeding to subsequent stages of the process becomes very confusing. This is true even in the instance of field research and qualitative analysis, where the study problem per se may "emerge" from the data after a researcher enters the field (see Chapters 13 and 14). A research question, according to Brink and Wood (1983, p. 2), *"is an explicit query about a problem or issue that can be challenged, examined, analyzed, and will yield useful new information."*

Step 2—Defining the Purpose of the Research

The second step is sometimes called defining the rationale of the study. It is the researcher's statement of *why* the question is important and what use the answer will serve. It lets the reader or funding agency know what to expect from the study. If the investigator's purpose is highly expedient—that is, just to fulfill requirements for a course or promotion—most of your colleagues in the scientific community will perceive it. The purpose of a study also influences its review by an institutional review board, (see Chapter 3). Many nursing studies are challenged on the basis that they seem to be exercises in methodology with no real or even conceivable benefit to anyone. A trivial purpose will influence judgments about the risk–benefit ratio if human subjects are involved. An excellent example of the statement of a study's purpose is the report of Kathryn Barnard's (1973) classic research on the effects of environmental stimulation on the sleep of premature infants:

Previous work with full term neonates and older infants supports the general notion that particular kinds of stimulation assist in the regulation of sleep and arousal status. Given this evidence and the increasing evidence that quiet sleep in the immature infant can improve neurological development . . . *the purpose of the current investigation was to study the effect of regular, controlled stimulation on the neurological functioning in the infant born prematurely* (p. 15).

Step 3—Reviewing Related Literature

If researchers want their study to build on, confirm, or even transcend the existing knowledge in a discipline and thereby qualify as a real contribution to science, they must know what has already been done. A review of the literature provides the researcher with ideas for defining concepts and instruments for their measurement (see Chapter 10). A theoretical framework is an essay in which the investigator relates the existing concepts and theories and research methods and findings to his or her study question and purpose (Brink and Wood 1983). At the least, constructing such a framework provides relevant concepts for the research; at best, it can give the researcher a full awareness of facts, issues, prior findings, theories, and instruments that might be related to the study question.

Step 4—Formulating Hypotheses and Defining Variables

Hypotheses are statements of the relationship between two or more concepts, or variables (see Chapter 4). Some studies are intended to *develop* hypotheses (exploratory, descriptive, and grounded theory designs), and others are intended to *test* hypotheses using the statistical principles in Chapter 15. Stating hypotheses requires not only that there be sufficient knowledge on a topic to make a prediction about the outcome of a study but also that the researcher can specify definitions for the variables under investigation in measurable terms. Finally, the investigator must articulate the relationship between or among the variables. Hypotheses can be explicitly stated, as Sitzman and her colleagues (1983) did in their study of biofeedback training:

HYPOTHESIS (H_I): Emphysema and chronic bronchitic patients who receive a biofeedback training program to decrease their respiratory rate will have a significantly decreased respiratory rate at the end of the training program and one-month follow-up.

HYPOTHESIS (H_{II}): Emphysema and chronic bronchitic patients who decreased their respiratory rate by the end of the biofeedback training program will have significantly increased their tidal volume at the end of the training program and at one-month follow-up (p. 219).

Hypotheses (H) may also be stated as null hypotheses (H_0) (see Chapter 9), which essentially test the idea that *there are no significant differences* in what is called the criterion, dependent, or outcome variable other than *what can be attributed to chance*. Because stating hypotheses requires the investigator to specify the concepts being studied, it is also important at this point to determine how these variables are going to be defined for the purpose of measuring them. For example, social support might be defined as a score on a written self-report scale, or inventory. This step is called *operationally defining* the variables. If you do a convincing job, your study is said to have construct, or concept, validity. The ideas of validity and measurement will be thoroughly discussed in subsequent chapters (see Chapters 4 and 11).

Step 5—Selecting the Research Design

A research design is a well-thought-out, systematic, and even controlled plan for finding answers to study questions. It offers a roadmap or blueprint for organizing a study, from methods of data collection through methods of data analysis. Chapter 6 covers the array of possibilities that are available for structuring the research plan.

Step 6—Selecting the Population and Sample

Once researchers have reduced a general idea of interest down to a specific study question, reviewed the related literature, and decided on a plan for designing their study, they must choose a study population and select a sample. A *population* refers to the group to be studied. To whom should the study's findings apply? Populations that have been the focus of recent nursing studies include divorced fathers, older persons, hospitalized children, disadvantaged minorities, depressed women, nursing mothers, patients with cancer, patients with AIDS, patients who have had surgery, and nursing students. The *sample* refers to those elements of a population from whom data will actually be collected and from whom generalizations to the population will be made. The details of various kinds of sample and procedures for selecting them are spelled out in Chapter 9.

Step 7—Conducting a Pilot Study

If you are an undergraduate student just venturing forth on your first attempt at using the method of scientific inquiry to solve a problem, answer a question, or make a decision, it may not be feasible or practical to do a small-scale practice run, called a *pilot study*. If you are working on a master's thesis, doctoral dissertation, or postgraduate research, however, you can learn a lot about the strengths and weaknesses of your larger project's intended design, sample size, and data-collection instrument by doing a pilot study. Such attempts have been so helpful in strengthening nursing studies by weeding out problems in advance that many funding agencies are not inclined to approve study proposals for which no pilot study has been conducted (see Chapter 8).

Step 8—Collecting the Data

The scientific method is characterized by a reliance on information collected from the empirical, or observable, world to make statements about what is true. Any study that goes beyond "armchair speculation" eventually requires the researcher to collect data. Data sources may be people, documents, or laboratory materials, and data-collection instruments may include interviews, questionnaires, physiological tests, and psychological tests. All of these possibilities are covered in depth in Chapters 11, 12, and 13. The basic point, however, is that by moving either from observation to idea (called *inductive theory*) or from idea to observation (called *deductive theory*), the scientific method relies on an *empirical* basis for discovering or testing knowledge. Data relevant to the variables being studied are collected using the researcher's senses and measurement tools. The amounts of time and energy required for this step in the process vary according to the research design. Field studies, historical research, surveys, and most experiments all demand a lot of both during this phase.

Step 9—Analyzing the Data

The next step in the research process involves taking the data that have been collected apart and reorganizing them so that the researcher can make some sense of them in relation to the study question, research objectives, or stated hypotheses. Analyses of numerical data can be accomplished using the statistical procedures discussed in Chapter 15. Qualitative data such as open-ended questionnaire responses, observational field notes, interview transcripts, case studies, documents, and the like can be analyzed according to a variety of approaches explained in Chapter 14. The most important part about this step is to *have a plan in mind, the requisite skills for doing it, and the realization that this work is the source of answers to the original research questions.*

Step 10—Communicating Conclusions

The researcher's challenge at the final stage is to explain the results of the investigation and link them with the existing body of knowledge in the discipline. Whether published articles or books, spoken presentations, or both are used, the study's real contribution cannot be judged unless the conclusions are communicated to colleagues and critics (see Chapter 17). As Polit and Hungler (1983) put it, "Even the most compelling hypothesis, the most careful and thorough study, and the most dramatic results are of no value to the scientific community if they are unknown" (p. 52). Communicating the conclusions, interpreting the real meaning and implications of the findings, recognizing the study's possible limitations, and suggesting directions for future lines of inquiry culminate the research process and provide the investigators with yet another chance to synthesize their imaginative, insightful, engaged style with their rigorous, systematic analytic one.

Most researchers acknowledge these steps as conventions, or recipes, and then with creativity, imagination, and pragmatism vary and adapt them to the unique situation they are addressing.

The History of Nursing Research

In 1983 two history-making announcements were made. The first involved the creation of a center for nursing research. As a result of the reorganization of the American Nurses' Association (ANA) headquarters, the first Center for Research for Nursing was established. It is responsible for developing a distinct and coordinated research program to serve as the source of national data for the profession. It encompasses the former ANA Department of Research and Policy Analysis, the American Academy of Nursing, and the American Nurses' Foundation. The principal function of the Center is to conduct studies and surveys to:

- support the work of policy bodies
- provide for administration of extramurally funded projects
- prepare grant applications to secure funding for research
- coordinate external fund-raising activities

The second announcement reported that legislation to create a National Institute of Nursing was introduced in Congress. The move was prompted by recommendations in a 1983 Institute of Medicine Report that called for a federally established entity *to place nursing research in the mainstream of scientific investigation.* Nursing research has a history, which provides the backdrop for these two steps forward. Earlier landmarks are summarized in Box 1-1.

Nursing Research in the 1980s

As Box 1-1 illustrates, since at least the early 1950s nursing research has received increased federal funding and professional support. Centers for research have been developed, the number of doctorally prepared nurses engaged in the

scientific enterprise has increased, and avenues for communicating research reports (journals, conferences, and meetings) have expanded. Nursing research is viewed as a legitimate field of interest not only for students at the entry level but also for *all nurses.* Spruck's 1980 National League For Nursing (NLN) survey of 286 accredited baccalaureate nursing programs revealed that research content was included as required coursework in 83% of the schools, and the remainder were moving toward incorporating a research component. A second survey, by Thomas and Price (1980), obtained usable responses from 205 of the 291 NLN-accredited baccalaureate nursing programs in the United States. Of them, 198 reported explicit provision for teaching nursing research in their programs; the remaining seven were in the process of developing research content. In sum, the question "Should nursing research be taught at all levels of nursing education?" has been replaced with the contemporary question "What should be taught about nursing research, at what level, and how?"

Evidence abounds that our profession has reached a consensus that some involvement in research at all levels of educational preparation is necessary for the advancement of the nursing profession and the welfare of patients. With such an overpowering agreement, one would expect that nursing research in the 1980s would be an unquestionable success story. Unfortunately, this is not the case. McClure (1981) summarizes the problem:

Far too few practitioners are genuinely concerned about research process or outcomes. . . . The vast majority of active nurses are concerned about the professionalization of nursing . . . but they have little knowledge of and even less interest in nursing research. . . . Our practice is almost entirely founded on personal wisdom rather than scientific conclusions (p. 66).

Box 1-1   Historic Landmarks in Nursing Research

Date	Event	Outcomes
1853–1856	Florence Nightingale records detailed observations about the impact of nursing care during the Crimean War	She fosters the idea that nursing practice should be based on disciplined inquiry.
1923	The Goldmark Report is published, after a comprehensive study of nursing education sponsored by the Committee for the Study of Nursing Education and funded by the Rockefeller Foundation	The report maintains that advanced preparation is essential for teachers, administrators, and public health nurses. It encourages the hiring of registered nurses for hospital care to free nursing students to study. Yale University's School of Nursing is established. The Vanderbilt University and Western Reserve University schools of nursing follow. The real pioneers had been Teachers' College, Columbia University (1899) and the University of Minnesota (1910), the first schools to emphasize the higher education of nurses.
1948	The Brown Report is published	The report recommends studies of in-service education, nursing functions, nursing teams, practical nurses, roles and attitudes, nurse–patient relationships, hospital environments, and the economic security of nurses. The National Accrediting Service is begun in 1950 under Dr. Helen Nahm to establish a sound method of accrediting nursing education programs
1952	*Nursing Research*, the first official journal for reporting studies related to nursing and health, is published	Nursing investigators are provided with a means for communicating the results of their research
1953	The Institute of Research and Service in Nursing Education is founded at Columbia University under the directorship of Dr. Helen Bunge	It becomes the first formal structure within a university for conducting nursing studies
1955	The American Nurses' Foundation, supported by the ANA, is established	It serves as a receiver, administrator, and donor of grants for research in nursing
1955	The nursing research grants and fellowship programs of the Division of Nursing of the U.S. Public Health Service are established	Grants for research into causes, diagnosis, treatment, control, and prevention of physical and mental diseases are authorized

Box 1-1   (continued)

Date	Event	Outcomes
1957	The Department of Nursing in The Walter Reed Army Institute of Research is established	It parallels research by physicians and dentists into patient care; develops a core of nurse practitioners–researchers
1963	The Surgeon General's Consultant Group on Nursing issues a report.	The report recommends a substantial increase in federal support for research in nursing and the training of nurse researchers
1963	Lydia Hall conducts a classic study of care of the chronically ill patients at the Loeb Rehabilitation Center in New York	Examples of research on patient care begin to influence the emergence of conceptual frameworks to define the nature of nursing practice
1966	A team of nurse researchers collaborates with social scientists at the University of California at San Francisco on studies of death and dying	Sociological methods and concepts begin to appear in the repertoire of nurse researchers
1968	The Mugar Library at Boston University establishes a nursing archive	It fosters nursing research and brings together a significant collection on the topic
1970	The Lysaught Report is published by the National Commission for the Study of Nursing	The report urges that research in both nursing education and practice be financed
1976	Elizabeth Carnegie reports a steady increase in the number of clinical investigations published in *Nursing Research*	The value of clinical, or practice-related, research emerges as dominant over studies of nurses themselves or of education and administration
1976	The Commission on Research of the ANA recommends that preparation for nursing research begin at the undergraduate level	Courses and integrated objectives requiring some level of research competence appear in nursing curricula
1968–present	The Western Interstate Commission for Higher Education in Nursing compiles data-collection instruments for practice and education; it sponsors conferences and workshops on conducting research and applying findings	The visibility of nursing's growing involvement in research increases
1970s	A number of refereed research journals for nursing are established, including *Advances in Nursing Science*, *Research in Nursing and Health*, and *The Western Journal of Research in Nursing* (see Chapter 17)	Nurse researchers have more vehicles for communicating their study findings to a growing community of nurse scientists

"To do," not "to study," sums up a prevailing attitude that day-to-day clinical problems are too far removed from nursing research and that research seems esoteric, dull, or even meaningless to the practicing nurse.

Accounting for the Discrepancy

What accounts for such a dramatic discrepancy between what nursing leaders espouse as a value and the negative attitudes and avoidance behaviors many clinicians and nursing students express? McClure (1981) cites the need to create an environment in the service arena that supports research by nurses. She also notes what she calls the "faculty withdrawal syndrome," which has resulted in:

1. lack of patient-focused research
2. lack of interdisciplinary research with other health-care professionals
3. estrangement of service from education
4. devaluing by nurses of academic preparation
5. devaluing by others, both inside and outside the health-care delivery system, of academic preparation for nurses
6. isolation of nursing faculty from service settings

Added to McClure's list are the following points:

7. lack of a cumulative knowledge base for nursing practice
8. lack of programmatically oriented research, as opposed to small, unimportant, independent studies
9. lack of replication of nursing studies

Finally, echoing authors who have lamented the substitution of "tenacity for inquiry" and an addiction to a "pseudotechnical mentality," Wilson (1982) cites the tendency to view research according to an overly dogmatic, "cook-book" approach as a block to nurses' full expression of their creative talent through scientific discoveries with relevance to practice.

Characteristics of the New Era of Nursing Research

The approach to science and research expounded in this text involves closing the gap between research and practice. Research does not become nursing research merely because it is done by a nurse. Many authors have distinguished between what they call nursing research and research in nursing. *Nursing research* on the one hand, is research into the process of care and the clinical problems encountered in the practice of nursing. *Research in nursing*, on the other hand, is the broader study of people and the nursing profession, including historical, ethical and policy studies. If we agree that the business of nursing is *practice* and also agree that the business of nursing research is answering questions and solving problems about that practice, then nursing practice and nursing research share the common goal of *improving nursing care*.

Carrying out this emphasis on nursing practice, the ANA Commission on Nursing Research (1980) has identified *priorities* for clinical nursing research during the 1980s. They include the areas of:

1. health care and prevention of illness
2. development of cost-efficient delivery systems for nursing care
3. development of strategies that provide effective nursing care to high-risk groups

Research does not have to be complicated to be good and useful. We must be wary of trying at all cost to rigidly adhere to methods that were developed in the natural, or "hard," sciences. They may well be inappropriate for studying nursing phenomena in a natural setting. Emerging alternative methods are increasingly interesting to nurses involved in clinical research.

The shift in recent years toward describing nursing phenomena, evaluating outcomes of nursing intervention, and building empirically based theories that will be the cornerstones of a nursing science does not preclude the value of what Diers (1983) has called "clinical scholarship":

Scholarship is different from research. It implies . . . contemplation [and] the stretching of the mind for new insights. . . . Good research reporting may well fall into the definition of scholarship; mechanical reports which provide data but not insight, do not (p. 3).

Tomorrow's nursing research will continue to emphasize studies of the interaction of physiological and psychosocial mechanisms in human experiences of stress and coping, evaluations of nursing interventions, the transfer of research findings into textbooks and practice, a focus on high-risk and underserved groups such as the elderly and minorities, and the creation of a body of scientific nursing knowledge. And today's student of research in nursing will be involved in its conduct and application.

Nursing Research and You

My own introductory course in nursing research is scheduled from 3 P.M. to 6 P.M. on Wednesdays in a huge, windowless lecture hall where the 52 RN students doze, having been in classes non-stop since 8 that morning. Almost without exception, students' initial reactions to the course are negative.

Student Reactions—Before

1. *Inadequacy*: "In every new nursing class, I'm ready to jump in and love it. But the thought of starting the research course evoked memories of my statistics instructor frantically scribbling statistical formulas and computations all over the blackboard that I just couldn't follow. I didn't understand all this validity and reliability language and, frankly, was afraid I might not even pass. Research is just not my level. Leave it to the scholars and nursing leaders."

2. *Resentment*: "I came back to get my degree because I want to be a head nurse in a CCU (critical care unit). I have absolutely no intention of becoming a teacher or of making research my career. I don't understand why our whole class is required to take the research course! My schedule is so packed that I can't take the elective in pharmacology that would really be practical to me in my clinical work."

3. *Boredom*: "I went into nursing because I find working with people exciting, interesting, and challenging. Research makes me think of cold, objective, eccentric scientists in laboratories, people who carried slide rules around in their pockets in high school, and pages of dull tables and charts full of numbers. My interests are music and play therapy for kids. Research with all its rigor, precision, and control sounds totally boring to me."

These unpleasant but normal feelings, if unchanged by teachers, textbooks, and experiences, probably account in part for why much of nursing practice relies on conventional wisdom instead of a scientific basis for direction and guidance. If, however, research can be translated into the fascinating, versatile, funny, and powerful tool that it often is, students' attitudes and reactions can be transformed.

Student Reactions—After

1. *Identification*: "Researchers are human, interesting, flexible, and creative. What a great

discovery! An intelligent, critical mind is a pleasure to behold, and to nurture. I think I'll be a better nurse because of it. I'd never thought of myself as a potential leader or writer. Now, I feel I've got the skills and motivation to try it. The pilot study I did for the research course has been accepted for publication in the *Western Journal for Research in Nursing*! I've made scholarliness and intellectual craftmanship part of my definition of a truly professional nurse."

2. *Competence*: "My professional skills of using the library, reading, and writing clearly developed more in the research course than in the entire rest of the program. I've learned an entirely new way of approaching clinical questions and I think the care and advice I give to patients will be better because of it."

3. *Demystification*: "Realizing that research isn't as rigid, structured, useless and dogmatic as some would say, decreased my anxieties about keeping up with it at least for applications to my practice. I'm no longer reluctant to pick up a copy of *Nursing Research* magazine."

4. *Enthusiasm*: "The subject of nursing research has become very important to me and I think it's critical to our profession's development. I have a new respect and enthusiasm about nursing's developing scientific basis and even hope to get my doctorate someday."

Learning about the scientific method and the research process is undoubtedly largely an intellectual task. But attitudes and values can be shaped as well. Nursing research allows you to bring the engaged and the analytic ways of knowing together in ways that make you a better nurse. A true scholar and scientist is not created by being taught technical methods, tools, or even a theoretical base. A true scholar and scientist transcends these tools and is the master of their use. You will learn the tools of research in the chapters that follow, and they will seem a lot less esoteric and formidable. But it is the wisdom acquired from using them in a spirit of inquiry that will make you a member of the scholarly and scientific community in nursing's future.

Summary of Key Ideas and Terms

✔ The value and usefulness of the scientific approach for making real-world decisions about nursing practice are clearer if you realize that:

- Science doesn't have to be dogmatic and mechanistic.

- Science involves a process of discovery as well as a process of proof.

- Science requires interpretation of facts, and these interpretations can change.

- Most of the principles and topics for nursing research exist in the practice of clinical nursing.

✔ The *scientific approach* offers an alternative tool for making decisions and solving practical problems that can substitute for or augment trial and error and common sense, authority and tradition, inspiration and intuition, and logical reasoning.

➤ *Scientific inquiry* is based on specific assumptions about the existence of a basic natural order in the world. It has the characteristics of self-correction and empiricism. And it aims to develop explanations, called theories.

➤ The positivist and symbolic interactionist traditions are two distinctly different perspectives on the philosophy of science that influence the kinds of study a nurse might conduct.

➤ It is possible to classify types of nursing studies along a pure—applied continuum based on their relevance to nursing practice. Studies can also be classified according to their purpose and study design.

➤ The *research process* is the tool of science. It involves a series of progressive steps that usually include some version of the following:

- stating the study problem
- defining the purpose of the research
- reviewing related literature
- formulating hypotheses and defining variables
- selecting the research design
- selecting a population and a sample
- conducting a pilot study
- collecting data
- analyzing data
- communicating conclusions

➤ The history of nursing research dates back only to the 1850s. Since then, landmark events have occurred to dramatically increase the amount, quality, and availability of nursing studies, particularly those dealing with nursing practice itself, rather than nurses or nursing education and administration.

➤ It is likely that at least understanding and using the results of nursing studies to improve practice will become an essential part of all nursing education programs.

➤ Bridging the gap between nursing research and nursing practice and avoiding an overly dogmatic approach can transform indifferent and negative attitudes toward research among clinicians and students.

References

Abdellah F, Levine E: *Better Patient Care Through Nursing Research*. New York: Macmillan, 1965.

Ackerman JS: Two styles: A challenge to higher education. *Daedalus* Summer 1969:855–868.

Aiken LH: The nurse labor market. *Health Aff* Fall 1982; 1:30.

American Nurses Association: *Nursing: A Social Policy Statement*. Kansas City, Mo.: 1980.

Barnard K: The effect of stimulation on the sleep behavior of the premature infant. *Commun Nurs Res* 1973; 6:12–33.

Brink J, Wood MJ: *Basic Steps in Planning Nursing Research*. Philadelphia: Lippincott, 1983.

Bronowski J: *Science and Human Values*. New York: Julian Messner, 1956.

Cooperative Graduate Education in Nursing: *Nursing Research Television Cassettes #1*. New York: American Journal of Nursing Co., 1975.

Demand for nurses does a drastic turnaround. *Miami Herald* January 2, 1983.

Demi AS: Adjustment to widowhood after a sudden death: Suicide and nonsuicide survivors compared. *Commun Nurs Res* 1978; 11:91–99.

Diers D: *Research in Nursing Practice*. Philadelphia: Lippincott, 1979.

Diers D: Clinical scholarship. *Image* Winter 1983; 15:3.

Fox DJ: *Fundamentals of Research in Nursing*, 4th ed. Norwalk, Conn.: Appleton-Century-Crofts, 1982.

Hadley BJ et al: Effect on postoperative recovery rate and comfort of four approaches to nursing care of dogs: A pilot study. *Commun Nurs Res* 1970; 3:121–137.

Jacox A: Theory construction in nursing: An overview. *Nurs Res* January/February 1974; 23:4–13.

Kerlinger FN: *Foundations of Behavioral Research*. New York: Holt, Rinehart & Winston, 1966.

Kueffner M: Passage through hospitalization of severely burned, isolated school-aged children. *Commun Nurs Res* 1976; 7:181–197.

Marshall LA: Patient reaction to sound in a coronary care unit. *Commun Nurs Res* 1972; 5:93–97.

May KA: Three phases in the development of father involvement in pregnancy. *Nurs Res* November/December 1982; 31:337–342.

McClure ML: Promoting practice-based research: A critical need. *J Nurs Adm* November/December 1981; 11:66–70.

McCorkle R, Young K: Development of a symptom distress scale. *Commun Nurs Res* 1978; 11:5–6.

McKeever LC: Equality and quality of care for older women. *Calif Nurse* September 1983:5.

Nakagawa H et al: An epidemiological study of psychiatric symptom pattern change. *Commun Nurs Res* 1972; 5:9–27.

Panger D: *The Dance of the Wild Mouse*. Glen Ellen, Calif: Entwhistle Books, 1979.

Polit D, Hungler B: *Nursing Research*, 2nd ed. Philadelphia: Lippincott, 1983.

Prior ME: *Science and the Humanities*. Evanston, Ill.: Northwestern University Press, 1962.

Schuster HH: Developing a psychometric instrument for the use of children's drawing in cross-cultural research: Problems, procedures, and potentials. *Commun Nurs Res* 1971; 4:151–158.

Seaman C, Verhonick PJ: *Research Methods for Undergraduate Students in Nursing*, 2nd ed. New York: Appleton-Century-Crofts, 1982.

Sitzman J et al: Biofeedback training for reduced respiratory rate in chronic obstructive pulmonary disease: A preliminary study. *Nurs Res* July/August 1983; 32:218–223.

Sjoberg G, Nett R: *A Methodology for Social Research*. New York: Harper & Row, 1968.

Snyder MC: *Calif Nurse* September 1983:2.

Spruck M: Teaching research at the undergraduate level. *Nurs Res* July/August 1980; 29:257–259.

Sweeney MA, Oliveri P: *An Introduction to Nursing Research*. Philadelphia: Lippincott, 1981.

Thomas B, Price M: Research preparation in baccalaureate nursing education. *Nurs Res* July/August 1980; 29:259–261.

Treece EW, Treece JW: *Elements of Research in Nursing*. St. Louis: Mosby, 1982.

Voda AM et al: Quantification of self-report data from two-dimensional body diagrams. *West J Nurs Res* Fall 1980; 2:707–729.

Walike B: A physiological and behavioral approach to understanding the mechanisms of obesity and anorexia. *Commun Nurs Res* 1973; 6:201–211.

Walike B et al: Patient problems related to tube feeding. *Commun Nurs Res* 1975; 7:89–112.

Waters VH et al: Technical and professional nursing. *Nurs Res* December/January 1972; 21:124–131.

Wilson HS: The meaning of current dance forms to adolescent girls: An exploratory study. *Nurs Res* November/December 1968; 17:513–519.

Wilson HS: Fairing: Control of staff work in a healing

community for schizophrenics. *J Psychiatr Nurs* March 1978; 16:24–38.

Wilson HS: Teaching research in nursing: Issues and strategies. *West J Nurs Res* 1982; 4:366–377.

Further Readings

Armiger Sr. S: Scholarship in nursing. *Nurs Outlook* 1977; 22:162–163.

Benoliel F: Scholarship—A women's perspective. *Image* 1975; 7:22–27.

Bernstein J: *Experiencing Science.* New York: Basic Books, 1978.

Brown JS et al: Nursing search for scientific knowledge. *Nurs Res* January/February 1984; 33:26–32.

Gortner SR: Research for a practice profession. *Nurs Res* May–June 1975; 24:193–197.

Kaplan A: *The Conduct of Inquiry.* San Francisco: Chandler, 1964.

Kuhn, TS: *The Structure of Scientific Revolutions.* Chicago: University of Chicago Press, 1970.

Meleis A et al: Toward scholarliness in doctoral dissertations: An analytic model. *Res Nurs Health* September 1980; 3:115–124.

Mills CW: *The Sociological Imagination.* London: Oxford University Press, 1959.

Roe A: *The Making of a Scientist.* New York: Dodd, Mead, 1963.

Schwab JJ, Brandween PF: *The Teaching of Science.* Cambridge, Mass.: Harvard University Press, 1966.

Chapter 2

Using Research to Improve Nursing Practice

Why, Where, and How?

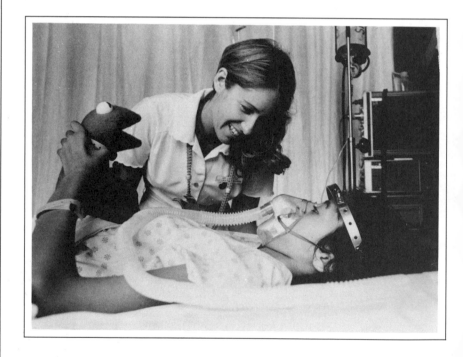

The time has come to close the gap between research and practice. The business of nursing is practice, and the business of nursing research is answering questions about that practice. Both share the common goal of improving patient care.

Chapter Outline

Chapter Objectives

After reading this chapter, the student should be able to:

- Delineate investigative roles for nurses at all levels of educational preparation
- Describe progress made toward building a scientific base for clinical nursing practice
- Formulate directions for the future of nursing research that will promote the goals of scientific inquiry
- Enumerate areas of consensus about research priorities for the 1980s
- Compare and contrast four levels of reading
- Apply useful reading techniques
- Demonstrate skills of systematic skimming and analytic reading levels to comprehend a report of research findings
- Use indices, periodical catalogs, and reference librarians to find research literature relevant to nursing
- Demonstrate familiarity with nursing's primary research journals
- Explain the significance of institutional and regional models for applying research findings to practice
- Realize the value and relevance of research in nursing to the development of the profession and to the quality of patient care

In This Chapter . . .

Voices in the vanguard of leadership in nursing call for bridging the gap between research and practice, a gap sometimes viewed as an abyss. This involves a two-way process: making nursing practice (rather than education or administration) a more frequent focus for research, and increasing the application of research findings to practice. Editorials in nursing journals, officers in professional associations, and probably your own teachers all assert that without an empirically grounded body of scientific knowledge on which to base clinical practice, nursing's stance as a profession is weak. Everybody seems to agree that it is critical that nursing develop a scientific base and that research is the way to get it. Florence Downs (1981), editor of *Nursing Research*, writes: "We are and for some time have been a profession in a hurry. Yet, research is not something that can be brewed over night and ingested the next morning" (p. 332). Downs goes on to remind us that "premature consumption of findings certainly might be hazardous to someone's health."

Applying research to practice would be a lot easier if:

- the scientific community were closer to bringing some sense of order to the proliferating nursing research literature
- all nursing students were better prepared to find, read, and understand it
- service organizations were structured to foster such applications

On the first point, Gortner (1980) writes: "An onlooker might characterize most nursing research as discrete, nonaggregated studies of isolated empirical phenomena for which the underlying science or explanatory theory is not known or not yet well-defined" (p. 205). She adds:

"Were we to dream about the vitality and credibility of our science 10 years hence, it would be that a number of well-defined, programmatic areas of research could be ongoing, each containing not one or two, but a dozen or more investigators" (p. 206). That leaves us, however, with the second and third points. Even if the quest to identify and build a scientific knowledge base that would replace traditions and habits is increasingly successful, practicing nurses, perhaps even you, will continue to experience frustration. For one thing, the knowledge base grounded in research findings that is needed to practice intelligently is hard to locate. For another, even when you do find it, its presentation in the traditional scientific format may be difficult for you to interpret. Finally, practice agencies are rarely structured to encourage change based on systematic appraisals of nursing research findings.

This chapter gives you some beginning tools essential to becoming an astute and unintimidated consumer of research findings that can actually shape your future clinical nursing practice. In it you will find support for an investigative role of some kind for all nurses. It introduces you to a system for "active reading" that can be used on everything you read, including the most esoteric research protocol. It discusses solutions to problems you might have in finding and then becoming familiar with research literature. It shows you step by step how to comprehend a report of study findings and how to draw clinical implications from these findings. Finally, it summarizes characteristics that foster a research orientation in practice settings and tells some success stories about recent projects that have advanced the profession's commitment at long last to make research every nurse's business.

Basing Nursing on Research

Past Progress

The idea that research findings should be used to improve patient care is an accepted one among contemporary nurses. For at least ten years, nurses have shared the eagerness, expectation, and hope that nursing is at last about to achieve professional status. The strongest force in that direction has been nurses' growing progress in building a scientific base for nursing practice. We have witnessed the study of research reserved in our not-so-distant past for the master's, doctoral, and postdoctoral levels, integrated into almost all basic entry-level programs in some form (see Box 2-1). Similarly, just as some degree of research competence is becoming part of every nurse's educational preparation, nursing research departments are springing up in hospitals and health care agencies. According to Parker and Labadie (1983), the functions of these departments include:

- providing leadership for nurses interested in designing and participating in a variety of scientific investigations
- providing consultation for nurses in investigative roles
- conducting seminars and workshops to help nurses learn research methods
- devising strategies to increase and intensify research activity within the agency
- participating in establishing guidelines for protection of the rights of human subjects (see Chapter 3)
- serving on research committees made up of staff nurses
- motivating nurses to become actively involved in seeking solutions to patient problems through scientific inquiry

- considering methods to share significant research findings
- coordinating research displays at appropriate occasions
- interacting with nurses employed in educational institutions to achieve shared goals
- seeking out available community resources for research

Likewise, at the level of the American Nurses' Association, the first national research center and clearinghouse was finally established in 1983. Its goals include:

- archival compilation of research findings related to nursing and the delivery of care to patients
- consultation services
- fund raising and administration to support nursing research
- publication and orderly dissemination of nursing research
- assembling lists of nursing problems that have a high priority for investigation

The Center for Nursing Research will serve to link together existing nursing research and scientific organizations, such as the American Nurses' Foundation (ANF) and the American Academy of Nursing (AAN).

Present Barriers

Despite this rather impressive past progress, problems still arise when the means for actually translating nursing research findings into practice decisions are explored. Unlike some disciplines, nursing has not yet systematically reviewed all of its important research reports and

---

Box 2-1   *Investigative Functions of a Nurse at Various Educational Levels*

Associate Degree in Nursing

1. Demonstrates awareness of the value or relevance of research in nursing.
2. Assists in identifying problem areas in nursing practice.
3. Assists in collection of data within an established structured format.

Baccalaureate in Nursing

1. Reads, interprets, and evaluates research for applicability to nursing practice.
2. Identifies nursing problems that need to be investigated and participates in the implementation of scientific studies.
3. Uses nursing practice as a means of gathering data for refining and extending practice.
4. Applies established findings of nursing and other health-related research to nursing practice.
5. Shares research findings with colleagues.

Master's Degree in Nursing

1. Analyzes and reformulates nursing practice problems so that scientific knowledge and scientific methods can be used to find solutions.
2. Enhances the quality and clinical relevance of nursing research by providing expertise in clinical problems and by providing knowledge about the way in which these clinical services are delivered.
3. Facilitates investigations of problems in clinical settings through such activities as contributing to a climate supportive of investigative activities, collaborating with others in investigations, and enhancing nursing's access to clients and data.
4. Conducts investigations for the purpose of monitoring the quality of the practice of nursing in a clinical setting.
5. Assists others to apply scientific knowledge in nursing practice.

Doctoral Degree in Nursing or a Related Discipline

1. Provides leadership for the integration of scientific knowledge with other sources of knowledge for the advancement of practice.
2. Conducts investigations to evaluate the contribution of nursing activities to the well-being of clients.
3. Develops methods to monitor the quality of the practice of nursing in a clinical setting and to evaluate contributions of nursing activities to the well-being of clients.

Graduate of a Research-Oriented Doctoral Program

1. Develops theoretical explanations of phenomena relevant to nursing by empirical research and analytic processes.
2. Uses analytical and empirical methods to discover ways to modify or extend existing scientific knowledge so that it is relevant to nursing.
3. Develops methods for scientific inquiry of phenomena relevant to nursing.

SOURCE: American Nurses' Association, Commission on Nursing Research, *Guidelines for the Investigative Function of Nurses*, Kansas City, Mo.: American Nurses' Association, 1981.

extracted the knowledge that is valid and relevant for practice. Perhaps the *Annual Review of Nursing Research*, edited by Harriet Werley and Joyce Fitzpatrick and published in its first issue by the Springer Company in late 1983, will among other efforts move nurses in the desired direction.

A second barrier derives from the fact that, despite repeated acknowledgments that a scientist's responsibility includes *replicating work to establish the limits of a study's findings*, few examples of repeating prior scientific work can be found in either nursing literature or nursing practice. Isolated studies seldom offer findings that can be a direct and valid basis for making changes in practice, because the real world rarely matches conditions in a single study design.

Because nursing is not just a profession and not just a scientific discipline but *a professional discipline*, nurses can also assume responsibility for going beyond the traditional scientific dissemination of research in publications or paper presentations. They can translate the information gathered through research into professional practice. In Barnard's (1980) words, "Emphasis should be placed on getting researchers and clinicians to interact. New technologies exist to improve our ability to communicate. We must take them" (p. 212). Futurists predict that communication about research in the next decade will be not only through libraries, bookstores, and periodicals on computer but also through video monitors in individual nurses' offices, homes, and work places. Teleconferencing among investigators and health care agencies will become common, and the problem of communication delay will be diminished. (The time lag in making new information available to clinicians is now estimated at two to three years for journals and up to ten years for books.)

Future Prospects

In June 1979 an invitational conference entitled "Knowledge for Practice: Directions for Re-

search in Nursing" was convened by the Division of Nursing, Bureau of Health Manpower, U.S. Department of Health, Education, and Welfare (now the Department of Health and Human Services). Its objective was to assess nursing research at the time and predict what it would be like in 1990. The conference participants attempted to delineate research topics that would have the greatest potential for improving nursing care. They also recommended strategies for applying nursing research to practice.

In considering the future, Gortner (1980) summarized the past by noting that most early research was commissioned by the nursing profession *to study itself*. Studies of nursing supply, distribution, job satisfaction, job turnover, and education seemed to be direct outgrowths of the need during World War II for an adequate number of nurses to serve both civilian and military demands. By 1970, however, the emphasis had shifted to practice-related nursing research (see Chapter 1). Federally funded studies were carried out at distinguished schools of nursing, including Case Western Reserve University, Ohio State, Wayne State, Yale, and the University of California at Los Angeles and at San Francisco. These studies dealt with topics such as maternal–infant attachment, death and dying, the care of patients with drug and psychiatric problems, and services for geriatric, maternity, pediatric, and surgical patients. Nursing research became a source of hope for establishing a science of health care through systematic inquiry into the problems encountered in nursing practice, the characteristics and health care needs of patients, and the interpersonal interaction between nurses and patients. *In less than 20 years nursing research shifted from the study of the profession itself to the study of phenomena with which nursing is concerned.*

When it comes to the future, Gortner predicts the emergence of multiple clinical trials of standardized protocols for stress reduction, medication adherence, and decubitus care, for example. As these shifts occur, participating in clinical research and using the findings as the basis for

Box 2-2   Results of WICHE Delphi Survey of Research Priorities

Rank   Item

1. Determine valid and reliable indicators of quality nursing care.

2. Determine and evaluate interventions by nurses that are most effective in reducing psychological stress of patients.

3. Find means of enhancing the quality of life for aged in institutions.

4. Determine factors that contribute to self-care education of patients with chronic disease.

5. Determine means for greater utilization of research in practice.

6. Determine effective means of communicating, evaluating, and implementing change in practice.

7. Discover effective nursing intervention for alleviating stress in patients with terminal disease.

8. Develop physical and psychological assessment procedures that provide information for improved patient care.

9. Study nursing intervention for the management of pain.

10. Clarify patients' rights and role as decision-makers in their own health care.

11. Explore ways to sensitize nurses to the needs of family members of critically ill patients.

12. Determine effective nursing intervention for reducing respiratory and circulatory complications for surgical patients.

13. Explore means of educating the public to optimize use of the health care system.

14. Establish relationship between clinical nursing research and quality care.

15. Find out which nursing behaviors and care settings are most likely to produce positive effects on individuals or families in a crisis-prone situation.

SOURCE: Delphi Survey of Clinical Research Priorities. Boulder, Colo.: WICHE, 1974.

modifications in practice will become an important aspect of every nurse's role.

Clinical Research Priorities

In 1974 the Western Council on Higher Education for Nursing (WCHEN) and the Regional Program for Nursing Research Development surveyed 328 nursing faculty members to try to determine the future research priorities in nursing. What has become known as the *Delphi Survey of Clinical Research Priorities* (1974) revealed 150 priority items in three areas:

1. priorities important to the nursing profession

2. priorities for which nurses should have responsibility

3. priorities that would have the most influence on patient welfare

Box 2-2 lists the top 15 research priorities from the *Delphi Survey* that relate to patient welfare.

In 1980 the Commission on Nursing Research of the ANA highlighted the research–practice link when it issued its definitions, directions, and examples for research in the 1980s; these are presented in Box 2-3.

The clinician and the researcher have an exchange of expertise to make and a profit to both patients and the profession to share. Many authorities, such as Jacox, writing in *Nursing Research* in 1980, believe that research programs that will receive funding in the next decade are most likely to be those that emphasize this collaboration because they:

1. focus on knowledge basic to providing clinical nursing care, such as pain assessment and alleviation or care of a specific population, for example, the frail elderly

2. involve nurses from both academic and practice settings working collaboratively

3. include testing or clinical trials of nursing interventions

---

Box 2-3   ANA Commission on Nursing Research

Directions for Research	Examples

Directions for Research

Priority should be given to nursing research that would generate knowledge to guide practice in:

1. promoting health, well-being, and competency for personal care among all age groups

2. preventing health problems throughout the life span that have the potential to reduce productivity and satisfaction

3. decreasing the negative impact of health problems on coping abilities, productivity, and life satisfaction of individuals and families

4. ensuring that the care needs of particularly vulnerable groups are met through appropriate strategies

5. designing and developing health care systems that are cost-effective in meeting the nursing needs of the population

6. promoting health, well-being, and competency for personal health in all age groups

Examples

Examples of research consistent with these priorities include the following:

1. Identification of determinants (personal and environmental, including social support networks) of wellness and health functioning in individuals and families, e.g., avoidance of abusive behavior such as alcoholism and drug use, successful adaptation to chronic illness, and coping with the last days of life

2. Identification of phenomena that negatively influence the course of recovery and that may be alleviated by nursing practice, such as, for example, anorexia, diarrhea, sleep deprivation, deficiencies in nutrients, electrolyte imbalances, and infections

3. Development and testing of care strategies to do the following:

   • Facilitate individuals' ability to adopt and maintain health enhancing behaviors (e.g., alterations in diet and exercise)

   • Enhance patients' ability to manage acute and chronic illness in such a way as to minimize or eliminate the necessity of institutionalization and to maximize well-being

   • Reduce stressful responses associated with the medical management of patients (e.g., surgical procedures, intrusive examination procedures or use of extensive monitoring devices)

   • Provide more effective care to high-risk populations (e.g., maternal and child care service to vulnerable mothers and infants, family planning services to young teenagers, services designed to enhance self-care in the chronically ill and the very old)

   • Enhance the care of clients culturally different from the majority (e.g., Black Americans, Mexican-Americans, Native Americans) and clients with special problems (e.g., teenagers, prisoners, mentally ill), and the underserved (the elderly, poor, and the rural)

   • Design and assess, in terms of effectiveness and cost, the models for delivering nursing care strategies found to be effective in clinical studies

SOURCE: American Nurses' Association, Commission on Nursing Research, *Research Priorities for the 1980's*, Kansas City, Mo.: American Nurses' Association, 1981.

---

4. are undertaken in settings or agencies where research is an integral part of every nurse's role

If you are among the growing number of nurses who are aware of the need to use research findings in your work but still find the idea somewhat intimidating because research reports are hard to find, the jargon is unfamiliar, and the benefits to practice not easy to determine, the next section of this chapter should help.

Understanding Research Findings

The Art of Active Reading

In 1940 Mortimer J. Adler and Charles Van Doren wrote a fantastic little volume called *How to Read a Book* (published by Simon & Schuster). It immediately became a best-seller and has since been translated into French, Swedish, German, Spanish, and Italian. The book hangs, as most good books do, on a single central idea: that *it is important for an intelligent reader to be able to read different things better* (not necessarily faster, but with more comprehension). The Adler and Van Doren volume proceeds to introduce the reader to "the basic rules of the fine art of intelligent reading"—an essential skill if you are to apply research results from studies conducted by others to your clinical work. Regrettably this book is now out of print, but the essentials of its method and insights follow.

A piece of scientific writing is usually complex. The amount of it that you comprehend often depends of the amount of active thinking that you put into the process of reading it and the skill with which you perform the separate acts involved in good reading. Active-reading skills enable you to go beyond mere reading for information to *reading for understanding*. This level of understanding is possible when you know not only what a writer has to say but also what he or she means and why. According to Adler and Van Doren, "Being informed is a prerequisite to being enlightened. The point is, however, not to stop at being informed" (p. 11). The lessons that follow are as relevant to active listening as they are to active reading and so can be put to work at conferences and symposia as well as on journal articles and books. Engaging in active reading is the opposite of passively dragging your way through seemingly endless pages of material that you don't understand. Instead, it is a process of actively questioning the material you read and of thinking about it according to an organized plan that allows you to make sense out of even the most difficult parts. Active reading lets you answer the question "What does this really say?" The effectiveness of your reading is determined by the amount of skill you put into it. Realizing the differences between levels of reading is basic to improving your reading skill. The four levels are elementary reading, systematic skimming, analytic reading, and comparative reading.

Elementary Reading   The first level of reading is also called initial, or rudimentary, reading. It refers to the kind of reading we do as children in passing from illiteracy to literacy. Because you are well into reading this text, we can assume that any problems you might have in reading nursing research literature are not at the elementary level.

Systematic Skimming   The second level of reading is called systematic skimming, or pre-reading. The aim of this level is to get the most out of a publication in a limited amount of time. When you read at this level, your aim is to examine the surface of the publication and learn everything that the surface can tell you, such as the structure, the qualifications of the author, the ingredients or parts, and the overall category of the article or book. Systematic skimming helps you decide what to read in a journal or book and in what sequence. Many of us become intimidated by research journals because we try to start at the beginning and plow through them from page one without even looking at the Table of Contents to see what might be relevant to our interests or work.

Analytic Reading   The third level of reading makes somewhat heavier demands on you. Here is where you ask questions of what you are reading so that you can truly understand it. These questions can be asked in any order, but together they form the framework for active reading.

1. *What is the book (journal or article) about as a whole?* You have to figure out what the fundamental theme or thesis of a piece is and how it is developed.

2. *What is being said in detail, and how?* Here you need to discover the author's main ideas, assertions, and arguments.

3. *Is the book, journal, or article true in whole or part?* If you have read something seriously, you must make up your own mind on this question. The strategies for conducting a formal research critique offer you an approach to doing this in the case of a report of research findings (see Chapter 7).

4. *What of it?* If what you have read provides information, you ought to ask yourself about its significance. Here is where you can use your own scholarly talents to perceive clinical implications of a study even if the investigators themselves haven't done so.

Comparative Reading The fourth and highest level of reading requires that you place what you are reading in relation to other things you have read that are related. With comparative reading you can construct an analysis of a subject that doesn't appear in any single article or book. In short, this fourth level of reading is the most reliable way of *keeping up to date* on a topic or subject. It requires that you keep either a real or mental file of new ideas or findings in your area of clinical interest and always assess each new work that you read in light of that file of ideas. Are you reading a really new idea? a credible replication of a previously published idea? a contradiction to a prominent idea? Although this is the most difficult of the reading levels, Adler and Van Doren say about it, "The benefits are so great that it is well worth the trouble of learning how to do it" (p. 20). Let us turn to a few more "how tos."

Reading Techniques Useful for All Levels

Active reading, as you can see, involves engaging in a mental dialogue with the authors of a book, article, or paper presentation. See Box 2-4 for some devices that can help you accomplish this fruitfully.

Guides to Systematic Skimming

1. Quickly read the title page and preface (or abstract, if it is a journal article). Get an idea of the subject, and place the article or book in the appropriate category in your mind. Is it a theoretical treatise, an article on methodology, or an actual report of findings? If you have answered yes to the last option, is the problem under investigation of conceivable clinical relevance to the patients you are working with or might work with in the future?

2. Look carefully at the table of contents in a book or the headings in an article to get a general sense of the structure of the piece. They ought to act as a road map by alerting you in advance of where you are headed.

3. Check the book's index. Make a quick estimate of the range of topics included to see which, if any, are relevant to your interests. You can use the index in this text to get some practice.

4. Read the publisher's blurb or any boldface excerpts. It is common for authors to try to summarize their main points in these spots.

5. From your knowledge of the general nature of the book's or article's contents, look more carefully at chapters or sections that seem pivotal. For example, in the case of a report of research, read the section with the heading Findings or Conclusions.

6. Finally, leaf through the whole piece, dipping in here and there for a paragraph. Re-

---

Box 2-4 *Helpful Guides for Reading Comprehension*

Underline or highlight. Get in the habit of underlining or highlighting points of major significance, particularly the central thesis of a book or article.

||| *Use vertical lines in the margin.* This is just another way of emphasizing a key paragraph or section of a page that might be too long to underline.

✳ *Put stars or asterisks in the margin* to let you quickly locate the most important ideas in the piece.

Write numbers in the margin to indicate a sequence of points in the unfolding logic of an argument or to designate any other list.

(cf p. 25) *Write page numbers in the margin* to indicate where else in the book or article the author makes relevant or even contradictory points. Some readers use the abbreviation *cf*, which means compare, or refer to. For example, in reading a research report you might want to compare its findings to the list of original hypotheses to be sure that an investigator had not drawn unreasonable conclusions.

I think I can use these techniques *Write questions and reactions* in the margins or at the top or bottom of a page. Here is where you can quickly summarize your own personal understanding of what you have read and how it relates to what else you have read.

---

member to read the last few lines, because most authors sum up what is important in their work at its conclusion.

Systematic skimming requires that you become a detective actively looking for clues about a book's or article's major theme so that you can decide whether it deserves any more of your time. You should be able to place it in your mental card catalog (or your real one) and return to it later if necessary. All of this should take anywhere from a few moments to less than an hour, even with a full-length book.

A final suggestion about systematic skimming is that you don't try to understand every page of a research report or theoretical paper the first time through, particularly if it contains unfamiliar jargon or complicated statistics. This is the most important rule. Don't be afraid to seem to be superficial at first. Read quickly through even the hardest parts. You will be much better prepared *to read it well the second time through*.

Guides to Analytic Reading

There are nine rules for analytic reading:

1. Try to discern whether a book or journal article is reporting findings that have been reached according to the canons of science or whether it is essentially based on personal trial and error, or what is often called "conventional clinical wisdom." Examples of the former are more likely to be found in journals that have research and nursing science as their stated editorial target. Nursing's four major research journals are examined later in this chapter.

2. Try to state in a sentence or two what an article or book's main theme is. Sociologists Glaser and Strauss, who have taught nurses, call this the "little logic" of a book or article. It is *little* because it can be expressed in a short space. It is *logic* because it is the hook, or central premise, that holds the piece to-

gether. In the case of a report of study findings, you often find the "little logic" in the statement of the study's purpose or the statement of the study problem.

3. Try to "X-ray" a book or article to uncover its structure and see how the major parts are organized. A study that is testing a hypothesis probably follows a fairly typical format for presentation (see Chapter 17). If you are reading an exploratory or descriptive study or one designed to develop rather than test hypotheses, or if you are reading a historical or case study report, you may encounter a wide variety of blueprints for the article or book's structure.

4. Find out what main questions or problems the article or book has set out to answer. Determine which of them are primary and which are secondary. In a research article you should be able to do this by reading the findings and conclusions and comparing them with the study purposes, objectives, or hypotheses.

5. Find the important and unfamiliar words and determine their meaning. There may be a whole new vocabulary to digest. Use Chapter 4 and the Glossary of research terms in this text to help.

6. Mark the most important sentences in an article or book, and uncover the propositions they contain. A good place to practice this step is when reading the conceptual framework for a study proposal or report (see Chapter 10).

7. Locate or construct the basic arguments or premises. This rule is more likely to apply to a theoretical analysis or an expository piece than to a report of empirical findings.

8. Find out what solutions or conclusions an author has come up with. Are there other solutions?

9. Be able to say with reasonable certainty, "I understand it" before you begin to criticize it. The specifics for how to critique

a research study are covered in detail in Chapter 7.

Guides to Comparative Reading

Comparative reading is designed to get a cumulative perspective on a question or topic. The five steps involved are used when you are comparing more than one source on a subject to establish their relationship to one another and to your own understanding of the subject.

1. Find the relevant passages that bear on your question, needs, or interests.

2. Translate the ideas of the various authors into your own terms.

3. Formulate your own set of questions, and read comparatively to determine how the respective authors do or do not address them.

4. Define any issues that emerge so that you can recognize, sort, and arrange controversies or contradictory findings in the literature.

5. Analyze the discussions you read by asking, "Are they true?" and "What of it?"

A Step-by-Step Example

The best way to learn the skills of systematic skimming and analytic reading is to practice them. As an example, let us try them out on an article from *Nursing Research* written by Lim-Levy.*

Systematic Skimming

1. Read the title and preface or abstract quickly to get an idea of what the article is about. In Lim-Levy's article the following information appears in italics at the very beginning:

*Lim-Levy, F. "The Effects of Oxygen Inhalation on Oral Temperature." *Nurs Res* May/June 1982; 131:150–152.

A study was conducted to determine the effect of oxygen inhalation by nasal cannula on oral temperature. One hundred healthy adult subjects were randomly assigned to a control and three experimental groups that received 2, 4, and 6 liters per minute of oxygen for 30 minutes. Oral temperatures were measured before and 30 minutes after oxygen treatment. The data analysis did not show any effect of the treatment (p. 150).

This is clearly a published report of an experimentally designed study. The report has implications for clinical practice—specifically, how to take the temperature of people who are getting oxygen.

2. What is the structure of the article? This article is relatively short. Its only headings are "Methods" and "Results and Discussion." We can assume that it roughly follows the typical format for presenting the results of research to test a hypothesis.

3. Because this article does not have an index, we will look instead at the references at the end (p. 152). They give us some ideas about what else we might want to read.

4. Read any boldface excerpts. We have already read an excerpt in italics.

5. Read the pivotal and final sections. In the next-to-last paragraph, the author sums up her study findings in straightforward clinical terms:

This study did not show a significant effect of oxygen inhalation on oral temperature (p. 152).

Analytical Reading   Having inspected the research report entitled "The Effect of Oxygen Inhalation on Oral Temperature" by Lim-Levy, we can now reread it more critically at the analytic level.

Rule 1 of analytic reading is to know what kind of piece you are reading. Because of its appearance in *Nursing Research* and its format, we know that we are reading the results of an empirical clinical study. We are further told that the study was conducted by a nurse clinical specialist in medical–surgical nursing.

Rule 2 is to locate the article's "little logic." We find it on page 150 in the fourth paragraph:

This study sought to determine how oxygen inhalation by nasal cannula affects oral temperature. If oral monitoring is not adversely affected, there is no need for rectal or axillary procedures.

Rule 3 is to identify the article's structure. We see by the format that it is a report of a hypothesis-testing study.

Rule 4 is to find out what the main problem or question was. We can see on page 150 that this study set out to test the following hypothesis: "Oxygen inhalation by nasal cannula of up to 6 LPM does not affect oral temperature taken with an electronic thermometer."

Rule 5 is to come to terms with the author's vocabulary. Some of the phrases that you would want to understand when reading this report would include:

- informed consent from subjects (see Chapter 3)
- random assignment to treatment groups (see Chapter 6)
- analysis of variance (see Chapter 15)
- statistical significance (see Chapter 15)

Rule 6 uncovers the basic premises, propositions, and arguments. In this study we can extract the following line of argument.

1. Oxygen inhalation by nasal cannula is believed to affect oral temperature; in many instances, therefore, body temperature is taken by the rectal or axillary method rather than orally.

2. Many patients find that having their temperature taken rectally is uncomfortable, and nurses find that taking either rectal or axillary temperature is more time-consuming than the oral method.

3. This study of 100 healthy adult male and female volunteers ranging in age from 18 to 56 years was designed to determine whether indeed oxygen inhalation by nasal cannula of up to 6 LPM does affect oral temperature measurement when taken with an electronic thermometer.

4. The study design controlled for some factors known to affect oral temperature and procedures for taking the temperature itself, in order to enhance the study's validity and reliability, respectively.

5. Findings indicated that there were no statistically significant changes between pre-oxygen temperatures and temperatures taken 30 minutes after the start of oxygen.

6. The clinical implication of this study is that changing from the oral method to the rectal or axillary method is unnecessary as well as being inconvenient and inaccurate when charting a patient's temperature graph.

Rule 7 is to figure out what conclusions the author has reached and make sure you understand them. Based on F and p values that were not statistically significant (see Chapter 15), the author concludes that oxygen inhalation does not significantly affect oral temperature. But she recommends that further research using higher oxygen concentrations and longer treatment and febrile patients be conducted (p. 152).

If you wished to move on to the level of comparative reading, you would consult the *Cumulative Nursing Index* (discussed later in this chapter) for additional studies on the clinical topic of oral temperature taking. Using the approach to reading research suggested above is one way of keeping up to date while using your reading time efficiently so that you really understand what you have read.

Finding Research Literature

Indexes, Abstracts, and Computer Searches

Literature that may be relevant to nursing practice often cuts across traditional disciplinary boundaries. Box 2-5 summarizes indexing and abstract resources that you may need to consult to locate literature in fields related to nursing.

Computerized searches also offer access to the literature on a designated subject (see Chapters 9 and 16). To use them, identify from one to several topics for a search analyst, to whom you probably have access through the computer terminal in your university library or hospital. Computer searches are not only quicker and more efficient, but you can often get more current information than that published in indices and abstracts. In most cases there is a fee for using these systems.* The primary computerized literature searches useful in nursing research are listed in Box 2-6.

Finally, the key sources for nursing literature itself are summarized in Box 2-7.

You now have a framework of questions for inspecting, analyzing, and accumulating ideas and conclusions from research that is published or presented. But in order to use these skills, of course, you must know where to start to find reports that are relevant to nursing practice.

---

* To find out more about how to use them, see the *Encyclopedia of Information Systems and Services*, Detroit: Gale Research Company, 1978.

A good place to begin is the *Cumulative Index to Nursing and Allied Health Literature* in your school of nursing or hospital library, or with your reference librarian. These resources will probably lead you to discover nursing's principal research-oriented journals. The next section of this chapter offers you an overview of each of them.

Nursing's Primary Research Journals

Locating reports of research that may be relevant to your clinical practice will become a lot easier once you are familiar with nursing's primary research journals. As of publication of this text there are four of them: *Nursing Research*, *Advances in Nursing Science*, the *Journal of Research in Nursing and Health*, and the *Western Journal of Nursing Research*. Research studies are sometimes published in the general-practice and specialty nursing journals, and social science and medical literature also often contains information that can be useful to nursing. The *Cumulative Index to Nursing and Allied Health Literature*, mentioned above, as well as the *International Nursing Index*, the *Cumulative*

Box 2-5   Indexing and Abstract Resources for Fields Related to Nursing

Abstracts for Social Workers

Bibliography of Reproduction (Cambridge, England)

Bibliography of Suicide and Suicide Prevention

Child Development Abstracts and Bibliographies

Dissertation Abstracts (microfilm from Ann Arbor, Michigan)

Excerpta Medica

Hospital Abstracts

Hospital Literature Index

Index Medicus

International Index

National Library of Medicine Catalogue (monthly holdings of the National Library of Medicine, Bethesda, Maryland)

Psychological Abstracts

Research Grants Index (U.S. Government Printing Office, Washington, D.C.)

Sociological Abstracts

Box 2-6   Primary Computerized Literature Searches

1. DATRIX (Direct Access to Reference Information)— Contains over 150,000 dissertation abstracts on University Microfilms
2. ERIC (Educational Resources Information Center)
3. HEIRS (Health Education Information Retrieval System)
4. MEDLINE/MEDLARS—Indexes over 2900 biomedical and nursing journals
5. National Clearing House for Mental Health Information of the National Institute of Mental Health
6. NEXUS—American Association for Higher Education's telephone information referral service
7. PAIS, PATELL, PADAT (Psychological Abstracts Information Services)—Available through tape leasing, direct access terminal, and printout
8. SSIE (Smithsonian Science Information Exchange)
9. U.S. Commerce Department's National Technical Information Service

---

Box 2-7   Abstracts, Indices, and Reviews of Nursing Literature

1. *Annual Review of Nursing Research*—Initiated in 1983 to critically review important work so that students, faculty, and other scholars can recognize the advances made, the existing gaps, and the areas that need further work. Volume 1 was *Human Development Through the Life Span*, Volume 2, *The Family*, and Volume 3, *The Community*.

2. *Cumulative Index to Nursing Literature*—Published quarterly with annual compilations since 1956 that draw from 54 journals in nursing and related fields.

3. *Facts About Nursing*—Published by the American Nurses' Association in Kansas City, Missouri. It includes information on numbers and distribution of nurses, their employment status, types of education programs, student characteristics, graduates, and the major nursing organizations.

4. *Indexes to Nursing Periodicals*—Published annually and in cumulative form.

5. *International Nursing Index to Periodical Literature*—Published by the American Journal of Nursing Company.

6. *Nursing Research Abstracts*—Between 1959 and 1978, a regular feature of *Nursing Research*.

7. *Nursing Studies Index*—Published by J. B. Lippincott, Philadelphia, it contains an annotated guide to reported studies and methodology papers from more than 200 sources.

Table 2-1   Characteristics of American Nursing Research Journals

Title	Circulation	Cost	Issues per Year	Length (words)
Nursing Research	8300	$20.00	6	3500
Advances in Nursing Science	3700	$32.75	4	4000
Research in Nursing and Health	1500	$25.00	4	2500–5000
Western Journal of Nursing Research	800	$20.00	4	6050

SOURCE: Adapted from McCloskey and Swanson (1982).

Medical Index, and computerized biographical literature searches such as MEDLINE, are methods for keeping up to date with these references.

Nursing Research *Nursing Research* is nursing's oldest and most widely circulated professional journal whose "preferred subject content" is research (McCloskey & Swanson 1982) (see Table 2-1). It is published six times a year by the American Journal of Nursing Company in New York City. There are about ten full-length articles per issue.

Despite the fact that *Nursing Research* is nursing's oldest and most widely read source of research findings, its circulation of 8500 as of a 1981 survey pales when compared with that of nursing's most popular general practice journals. In 1981 *Nursing 81* had 550,000 subscribers, *The American Journal of Nursing* had 385,000, and *RN* had 350,000. We can expect these statistics to change, though, as the value of nursing research to improving clinical practice is increasingly recognized. Investigators will be expected to make the practice implications of their research more explicit, service settings will benefit by developing systems for using research findings in practice, and nurses will need the skills required to read, understand, and interpret research-oriented literature.

Advances in Nursing Science (ANS) *Advances in Nursing Science* is published quarterly by Aspen Systems in Maryland. The primary purpose of this journal is "to stimulate the development of nursing science." *ANS* focuses on empirical research, theory construction, concept analysis, practical application of research and theory, and investigation of values and ethics that influence the practice and research activities of nursing science. Since the first issue was published in October 1978, it has targeted all of its issues to specific topics. The feature topics for each issue appear in Table 2-2. Each issue has approximately seven full-length articles. Notices of upcoming research or scientific conferences are included near the end.

Western Journal of Nursing Research (WJNR) The *Western Journal of Nursing Research* was begun in 1979 by Phillips-Allen Publishers of Anaheim, California, and its first editor, Pamela Brink. *WJNR* was initiated to serve the growing need of nurses in the western United States to share information about what they are doing. It has a three-pronged editorial philosophy:

1. The communication and dissemination of nursing research can be practical.
2. Nursing research is only good if it is used.
3. Talking about research makes it more useful.

To these ends *WJNR* serves three different functions:

1. It publishes completed research papers.
2. It disseminates information about research conferences, grants available, and developing research projects.
3. It provides "how to" comments on the research process and its functions.

The journal is correspondingly divided into three distinct sections:

1. Three or four feature articles, each followed by at least two commentaries and an author's response.
2. The Information Exchange, including meeting calendar, grant deadlines, brief news reports, brief conference reports, research briefs, requests for assistance, and book reviews.
3. Technical notes, problems in doing research, ethical issues, research utilization, and strategies for teaching research. Each is written by an expert in the area.

WJNR also publishes the proceedings of the annual conferences of the Western Society for Research in Nursing in its summer issue.

Research in Nursing and Health (RN&H) *Research in Nursing and Health* is published quarterly by John Wiley and Sons of New York City. The titles of articles in this journal are indexed in the *Cumulative Index to Nursing and Allied Health Literature, Social and Behavioral Science Index, Index Medicus, International Nursing Index, Public Health Reviews, Social Science Citation Index,* and *Sociological Abstracts.* The first issue of *RN&H* was published in April 1978.

This journal's intent is to publish nursing theory, nursing research, and scholarly and analytic works that lead to improvement and refinement of both theory and research. *RN&H* also publishes significant inquiries into nursing administration and education, as well as inquiries into the nature of health. The journal's goal has al-

Table 2-2   Feature Themes for Past Issues of
Advances in Nursing Science

Issue	Date	Topic
Vol. 1, No. 1	October 1978	Practice-Oriented Theory: Part 1
Vol. 1, No. 2	January 1979	Practice-Oriented Theory: Part 2
Vol. 1, No. 3	April 1979	Ethics and Values
Vol. 1, No. 4	July 1979	Stress and Adaptation
Vol. 2, No. 1	October 1979	Nursing Diagnosis
Vol. 2, No. 2	January 1980	Nursing Intervention
Vol. 2, No. 3	April 1980	Politics of Care
Vol. 2, No. 4	July 1980	Holistic Health
Vol. 3, No. 1	October 1980	Nursing Theories and Models
Vol. 3, No. 2	January 1981	Women's Health
Vol. 3, No. 3	April 1981	Nursing Education
Vol. 3, No. 4	July 1981	Attachment, Loss, and Change
Vol. 4, No. 1	October 1981	Accountability and Scholarship
Vol. 4, No. 2	January 1982	Accountability in Practice
Vol. 4, No. 3	April 1982	Nursing and Culture
Vol. 4, No. 4	July 1982	Physiological Variables
Vol. 5, No. 1	October 1982	Application of Theory
Vol. 5, No. 2	January 1983	Research Methods
Vol. 5, No. 3	April 1983	Community and Environmental Health
Vol. 5, No. 4	July 1983	Professional Issues
Vol. 6, No. 1	October 1983	Development and Aging
Vol. 6, No. 3	January 1984	Testing of Nursing Theory
Vol. 6, No. 3	April 1984	Patterns of Health Behavior
Vol. 6, No. 4	July 1984	Crisis Intervention
Vol. 7, No. 4	October 1984	Research Tools

ways been to publish what is "new, true, and important." Each issue includes approximately five feature-length articles.

As of September 1983, *RN&H* announced an experimental program in the submission and publication of manuscripts that allows authors who have access to personal computers or word processors to submit manuscripts either on computer diskettes or electronically by telephone using a modem (see Chapter 16). Text files need to be prepared using either Wordstar or Select software programs. (These are the two word-processing programs most frequently used by authors who write on the computer.)

Using Research Findings in Practice

An Institutional Model

The emphasis of this chapter has been on helping the individual practicing nurse overcome barriers to applying research findings to his or her practice. Morse and Conrad (1983) have developed an eight-step process by which hospitals and health agencies can put research into practice on the institutional level. These steps are:

1. Identify a clinical need or problem by checking data sources such as management reports, audit scores, incident reports, and patient charts.

2. Use indices to nursing literature and the help of a reference librarian to locate literature relevant to the problem or need identified in step 1.

3. Evaluate relevant research reports by critiquing them (see the questions in Chapter 7).

4. If the research study is relevant and scientifically sound, assess its applicability for achieving clinical objectives related to your original problem or need.

5. Prepare a written plan that includes:
   - a statement of the clinical problem
   - a list of clinical objectives for alleviating the problem
   - a description of the new procedures that will reduce or alleviate the problem
   - a detailed budget of labor and equipment costs
   - anticipation of any effects the change suggested in the research might have on hospital policy or procedure
   - a schedule that will help allocate time devoted to the project

6. Obtain cooperation and permission, which involves "selling" the plan to the hospital administration, the nursing staff, the physi-

cians, and the patients.

7. Carry out the plan in an atmosphere of open communication and support.

8. Evaluate the process according to the four possible outcomes that can follow implementation of an innovative technique:
   - The innovation may actually be harmful and therefore should be stopped.
   - The outcome may be neutral, reflecting no change.
   - The outcome may be to realize the clinical goals.
   - The outcome may be positive or negative but, in either case, unexpected. For example, a program to teach self wound care to the elderly may be so time-consuming that the stress of staff to complete other assignments may become overwhelming.

Whatever the outcome, the authors of this model urge clinicians who attempt to use it to communicate with the researcher who conducted the original study so that new problems can be identified and addressed. Interaction between clinicians and researchers is essential. Hinshaw and her associates (1981) acknowledge that research in the practice setting can bring forth major conflicts in the areas of risk taking, vested interests, the rights of research subjects, and the need to produce both scientific and practical knowledge. But they add that collaboration and negotiation between nursing staff and researchers can make it work.

A Regional Model: The WICHE Project

Under the auspices of WICHE (the Western Interstate Commission for Higher Education), the U.S. Department of Health, Education, and

Welfare funded a six-year project that had as its original goal investigating the feasibility of increasing nursing research activities through a regional effort. An underlying assumption of the project was that research is necessary to develop a body of validated nursing knowledge on which to base improvements in the quality of nursing given to the public. Many believed that this project was the first large-scale attempt to link the knowledge producers with the practitioners in practice settings.

Part III of the final report of this project (Krueger et al 1978) is devoted to what its author called "research utilization." During the course of the project the participating nurses had an opportunity to identify problems that needed research-based solutions; this activity was not unlike the first step of the institutional model we just examined. The nurses then developed skills in reading and evaluating research for use in practice, learned more about how to locate usable research findings, and developed detailed plans for introducing change into their settings. Although its authors reported that the project was ultimately effective in helping nurses use research in clinical practice, the major problem was the difficulty experienced in finding valid, reliable nursing studies with clearly written implications for nursing care. The categories of clinical problem for which research findings were sought are summarized in Table 2-3.

The implications of the WICHE project were not only that nurses have the skills for evaluating research for possible application in the clinical area but also that *nurse researchers themselves need to write implications for nursing practice into their reports of findings*. Some responsibility must be taken for bringing the research report into a form that can be easily used by nurses in the practice setting (see Chapter 17).

Project participants offered a number of other recommendations based on their experiences. They expressed a need for a centralized index on nursing research (a research hot line), or "Index Nursicus," that would be similar to *Index Medicus* but specifically targeted to research literature. They agreed that research should be taught as

Table 2-3   Categories of Nursing Problems Selected by Nurses in the WICHE Nursing Research Development, Collaboration and Utilization Project

Nursing Problem	Percentage of Nurses
Clinical nursing	
Patient teaching	29.0
Patient assessment	21.3
Psychosocial problems	3.2
Primary care	4.9
Other direct care	14.7
Problem-oriented records	16.5
Continuity of care	14.7
Nonclinical nursing	4.9

part of all basic nursing education and that it should be followed up through continuing education. They urged researchers, in the meantime, to simplify the language used in research reports and to conduct more clinical studies. Participants and project staff alike concluded that:

The use of research in nursing practice would be greatly accelerated by systematic identification, evaluation, and collation of generalizations in a form that is easily accessible to practitioners. Only then can the major difficulties of research utilization be diminished and valid research findings made available (Krueger et al 1978, p. 299).

In the final recommendation the following conclusions were drawn:

Institutions must value and be committed to research in order to develop resources for its conduct. The value is institutionalized through its stated philosophy and goals. It is operationalized through job descriptions, recruitment policies, [and] retention and promotion criteria that reward nurses with research skills (p. 332).

It seems that the WICHE project's message is that nursing research will move forward only if skilled researchers collaborate with others who have clinical competency and ideas for clinically useful research problems.

A State Model

A more recent effort to apply research in practice was the five-year Conduct and Use of Research in Nursing (CURN) project, sponsored by the Michigan State Nurses' Association. This project attempted to stimulate the conduct of research in clinical settings and help nurses learn new ways of using research findings in their practice. It resulted in a set of nine volumes (Horsley 1981–1982), which earned the 1983 Book of the Year Award presented by *The American Journal of Nursing*. The volume titles give a sense of the range of clinical research that was involved:

- *Mutual Goal Setting in Patient Care*
- *Closed Urinary Drainage Systems*
- *Distress Reduction Through Sensory Preparation*
- *Pain*
- *Intravenous Cannula Change*
- *Preventing Decubitus Ulcers*
- *Preoperative Sensory Preparation to Promote Recovery*
- *Reducing Diarrhea in Tube-Fed Patients*
- *Structured Preoperative Teaching*

The project's principal investigator, Jo Anne Horsley, concluded from the project that research will be accepted by practicing nurses if it is relevant to practice and is communicated broadly through journals and conferences.

The Sigma Theta Tau Regional Research Conferences

Yet another prototype to explore the dissemination and utilization of research in nursing practice were the Sigma Theta Tau Regional Research Conferences. The primary goal of these conferences was to promote research-based nursing practice by identifying study findings that were ready to be used in practice. A second goal was to suggest further steps to be taken in research areas where the findings were not yet ready for clinical application.

Shaping Practice Through Nursing Studies

Part 2 of this text is devoted to reading, understanding, and evaluating nursing studies in depth. Chapter 7 of that part offers you precise guidelines for conducting a formal study critique. In the meantime, however, it is crucial that you recognize that nursing research published to date has indeed shaped nursing practice and that you have the tools to make a preliminary assessment of a study's clinical potential. Here are two illustrations of the first point.

- As a result of a group of studies done in 1977–1978 by Barbara W. Hanson and her colleagues (Walike & Walike 1977), the undesirable effects of lactose intolerance in patients receiving tube feedings have been eliminated by the removal of lactose from these formulations. Concurrently, the nausea, abdominal cramps, and distention caused by the inability to digest milk sugar need no longer be experienced by tube-fed patients who have lactose intolerance.

- Because of work done by Martinson et al (1977) with families of leukemic children in Minnesota, hundreds of children are now able to remain at home with their families during the terminal phase of their illness.

As far as the second point is concerned, you can begin your assessment of research by noting that good clinical studies, according to Fuller (1980), have the following characteristics in common:

1. They study a problem that occurs frequently in a definable population of patients.
2. The standard way the problem has been dealt with is unsatisfactory.
3. Some index of the problem can be measured.
4. The proposed solution alters patient care.

When you read or hear reports of clinical studies, use the following preliminary set of questions to help you consider their scientific merit and possible utility (Fawcett 1982):

1. Has the original study been replicated?
2. If so, are the findings similar in a variety of situations?
3. Is corroboration of findings in clinical situations done with actual patients who receive nursing care?
4. What were the risks and benefits of the nursing action tested in the study?
5. Does the study focus on a significant problem in clinical practice?
6. Do nurses have clinical control over the study variables?

7. Is it feasible to carry out the nursing action in the real world?
8. What is the cost of implementing the nursing action?
9. What contribution to client health status does the nursing action make?
10. What overall contribution to nursing knowledge does the study make?

Nursing research that meets these criteria will help you improve the quality of life for patients in your care regardless of their health status. From nursing research, for example, we will learn better ways of intervening with the frail elderly, the chronically ill, and the terminally ill. Research done by nurses includes both laboratory and clinical studies and may cut across traditional disciplines and methods. In the past, research-based nursing practice was more a litany being preached than a reality. But you are part of the tension and excitement of a new era for nursing research. In this era all nurses, whether they make research a central part of their career or not, will need the skills to read, understand, and apply the expanding body of findings to their practice, to participate in the clinical studies of others, and to safeguard the rights of human research subjects under their care. If practitioners collaborate in the entire research process, the outcomes will be used. Remember, the clinician and the researcher have an exchange to make and a profit to share.

Summary of Key Ideas and Terms

✔ Applying the growing number of findings from clinical nursing research to practice would be easier if (1) the scientific community were further along in bringing some order to the proliferating research literature; (2) all nursing students were better prepared to find, read, understand, and appreciate these findings; and (3) service organizations were structured to foster such applications.

✔ Evidence of progress toward establishing a *scientific basis* for nursing practice includes (1) an agreed-upon consensus about investigative roles for nurses at all levels of educational preparation, (2) the emergence of research departments in service agencies, and (3) the establishment of a national research center to coordinate, support, and disseminate nursing research.

✔ Although research conducted by nurses includes various types of study and cuts across traditional disciplines, priority for the 1980s is given to clinical research directly related to developing the knowledge and information needed for the improvement of nursing practice.

✔ The art of *active reading* is one set of strategies to help nurses assimilate research reports.

✔ Reading occurs at four major levels: (1) elementary, (2) systematic skimming, (3) analytic, and (4) comparative. Each level has specific steps or rules to help nurses read for understanding.

✔ Searching cumulative indexes and your library's periodical catalog or consulting with a reference librarian will reveal that nursing currently has four journals that have research and nursing science as their preferred subject matter: *Advances in Nursing Science*, the *Journal of Research in Nursing and Health*, the *Western Journal of Research in Nursing*, and *Nursing Research*, the oldest and most widely circulated of them.

✔ Systematic skimming of a journal such as *Nursing Research* will make its scientific style less intimidating and more accessible for the clinician.

✔ Systematically skimming and analytically reading a sample research report with clinical relevance can increase your ability to read and understand others like it.

✔ Applying research findings to clinical practice requires that investigators make their work more accessible to practitioners, that practitioners develop their skills of active reading and listening and keep up with research developments, and that service agencies adopt philosophies and strategies that reward putting research findings into practice.

References

Adler M, Van Doren C: *How to Read a Book*. New York: Simon & Schuster, 1940.

Barnard KE: Knowledge for practice: Directions for the future. *Nurs Res* July 1980; 29:208–212.

Delphi Survey of Clinical Research Priorities. Boulder, Colo.: WICHE, 1974.

Downs F: Editorial. *Nurs Res* November/December 1981; 30:332.

Fawcett J: Utilization of nursing research findings. *Image* June 1982; 14:57–59.

Fuller E: Selecting a clinical nursing problem for research. *Image* June 1982; 14:60–61.

Gortner S: Out of the past and into the future. *Nurs Res* July/August 1980; 29:204–207.

Hinshaw AS et al: Research in practice: A process of collaboration and negotiation. *J Nurs Adm* February 1981: 33–38.

Horsley JA: *Using Research to Improve Nursing Practice* (Series of Clinical Protocols 9 vols). New York: Grune and Stratton, 1981.

Jacox A: Strategies to promote nursing research. *Nurs Res* July/August 1980; 29:213–217.

Krueger J et al: *Nursing Research: Development, Collaboration and Utilization.* Germantown, Md.: Aspen Systems, 1978.

Lim-Levy F: The effect of oxygen inhalation on oral temperature. *Nurs Res* May/June 1982; 31: 150–152.

Martinson IM et al: When the patient is dying: Home care for the child. *Am J Nurs* November 1977; 77: 1815–1817.

McCloskey JC, Swanson E: Publishing opportunities for nurses: A comparison of 100 journals. *Image* June 1982; 14:50–56.

Morse JM, Conrad A: Putting research into practice. *Can Nurs* September 1983; 79:40–43.

Parker M, Labadie G: Demystifying research mystique. *Nurs Health Care* September 1983:383–386.

Walike BC, Walike JW: Relative lactose intolerance: A clinical study of tube-fed patients. *JAMA* 1977; 238:948–951.

Further Readings

Diers D: Application of research to nursing practice. *Image* 1982; 14:62–64.

Gortner SR, Phillips TP: Contributions of nursing research to patient care. *J Nurs Adm* 1976; 6:28–31.

Jacox A, Prescott P: Determining a study's relevance for clinical practice. *Am J Nurs* November 1978; 78:1882–1889.

Ludeman R: The paradoxical nature of nursing research. *Image* 1979; 11:2–8.

Martinson IM: Nursing research: Obstacles and challenges. *Image* 1976; 8:3–5.

Newman MA: What differentiates clinical research? *Image* 1982; 14:86.

O'Connell KA, Duffey M: Research on nursing practice: Its nature and direction. *Image* 1976; 8:6–12.

Paletta JL: Nursing research: An integral part of professional nursing. *Image* 1980; 12:3–6.

Smoyak S: Is practice responding to research? *Am J Nurs* July 1976; 76:1146–1150.

Spross JA et al: Committee evolution in a medical center. *Nurs Res* January/February 1981; 30:30–31.

Chapter 3

Ethics and the Rights of Research Subjects

Keeping Science Ethical

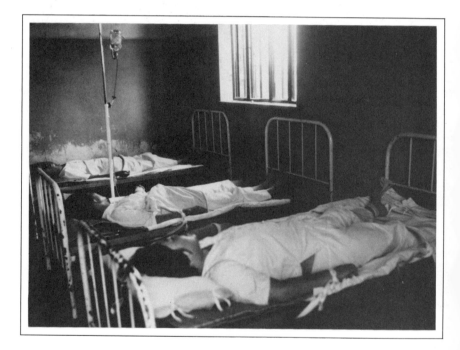

In the not-so-distant past, violations of human rights under the guise of scientific advancement took place with shocking frequency. Nurses are in key positions to assert and maintain the protective values of their profession.

Chapter Outline

Chapter Objectives

After reading this chapter, the student should be able to:

- Describe examples of historic cases of abuse of human subjects' rights
- Demonstrate awareness of the characteristics of ethical scientific research
- Compare the similarities between two existing codes of research ethics
- Recognize human subjects who are particularly vulnerable to risk in nursing research
- Analyze five categories of risk associated with research procedures
- Evaluate a research study's provisions for the protection of human rights: (1) to be free from harm, (2) to be given full disclosure, (3) to have self-determination, and (4) to have privacy, anonymity, and confidentiality
- Define *ethics, risk–benefit ratio, minimal risk, debriefing, informed consent,* and *institutional review board*
- Formulate a human subjects protocol and an informed consent form that comply with principles of research ethics and protect the rights of human subjects
- Appreciate the complexity involved in balancing individual rights with society's rights to the development of scientific knowledge
- Advocate the protection of human rights and the principles of ethical research in clinical and scientific activities according to a personal and professional ethical framework

In This Chapter . . .

A young teacher of bioethics in nursing once said: "Reasoning in ethics means bringing all one's faculties in a balanced way to bear on the sincere concern for human well-being in general and the meaning of human experience. . . . Being reasonable in ethics is more like having integrity than like being smart." *Ethics* is that branch of philosophy concerned with two basic questions: (1) "What is right or good?" and (2) "What should I do?" The moral judgments involved in answering such questions are most highly developed when the process of arriving at them and the reasons for believing in them are clear and convincing. At the heart of ethical judgments are the reasons for them. The goal of this chapter is to help participants in and consumers of nursing research develop a way of thinking about the complex ethical issues and dilemmas that are often associated with human science.

The ethics of research are the product of recent years, although they rest on long-honored moral traditions. In the not-so-distant past, violations of human rights under the guise of scientific advancement took place with shocking frequency. From 1932 to 1972 more than 400 black Alabama sharecroppers and day laborers were subjects in a government study designed to deliberately withhold treatment for syphilis to study the untreated disease. James H. Jones has recounted this sad tale in his book *Bad Blood: The Tuskegee Syphilis Experiment* (1981). In the early 1960s Timothy Leary and Richard Alpert (a lecturer and an assistant professor at Harvard University) stretched the tolerance of the scientific community with their use of human subjects in studying the effects of psilocybin and LSD. In 1963 a physician injected hospitalized elderly patients at the Jewish Chronic Disease Hospital in Brooklyn with live cancer cells without informing them. Yet another abuse of experimentation took place in the pneumonia, flu, and meningitis experiments conducted on incarcerated residents of two state mental hospitals in Pennsylvania. Accounts of research using the poor, destitute, and mentally retarded crowd the history books. Some of the most tragic and profoundly troubling violations were the Nazi "medical" experiments conducted by highly qualified scientists and physicians with appalling disregard for the rights of their captive subjects.

This chapter helps you to answer the question "How ethical is my research project?" It also provides you with a list of characteristics of ethical research and codes formulated to increase the likelihood that nursing's desire for scientific knowledge is compatible with the dignity and rights of individuals and social groups. It acquaints you with four fundamental rights of human research subjects and assists you step by step in developing a consent form and a protocol that might be required by your institutional review board. Such a board must conclude that the process of *informed consent* is adequately provided for in a research plan and that *an appropriate balance exists between potential benefits of the research and the risks assumed by the subjects.*

Making Science Ethical

Doctors regularly conduct research studies to identify a particular pathological process or to find out how effective an experimental medical regimen or surgical treatment is when compared with the "standard treatment." Examples of such studies include "Protein Utilization in Females With Glucose Intolerance During Pregnancy" or "Phase I/II Study of Hyperthermia Treatment Technique and Tolerance of Skin and Subcutaneous Tissues to a Temperature of 50-45°C," or "Experimental Fetal Therapy." Pharmacologists collaborate with others in drug trial studies in which the agents being investigated have names such as "BCNU-FU-HU-6MP" (used for the treatment of malignant brain tumors) and research questions include "What is the optimal dose?" "Is it most effective when used alone or in combination with other treatment?" "What are the side effects?" "By what biochemical mechanisms does it work?" "Can less be given?" "For which patients is it most useful?" Dentists study procedures for improving dental hygiene, for dental surgery, or for the use of investigational oral devices. All of the above studies may be conducted with animals or with human subjects.

Nursing research, however, tends to focus more consistently on people—their health attitudes, experiences associated with illness, values, coping behaviors, support systems, community networks, and environmental stressors. Consequently, human subjects are almost always involved in nursing research. Being aware of their rights is a major part of a nurse's responsibility when planning a research project, assisting in someone else's research, or evaluating a research article.

Characteristics of Ethical Research

Ethical research includes protecting the rights of human subjects but encompasses a broader list of characteristics (see Figure 3-1):

• *Scientific objectivity* means that you (or any other investigator) include all data points, including those that are unsupportive, try to be aware of personal values and biases, and don't preconceive a study's outcome or engage in any misconduct, fraud, or acts of bad faith in connection with the research.

• *Cooperation* with duly authorized review groups, agencies, and institutional review boards. This means that you submit your proposed research to the appropriate committee in charge of reviewing provisions for the protection of subjects' rights and are willing to comply with their recommendations. Many journals require that study reports contain a statement that the research was approved from an ethical standpoint by the appropriate institutional committee.

• *Integrity* in representing the research enterprise. This means that you do not withhold information about your study's possible risks, discomforts, or benefits, nor do you intentionally deceive study subjects on these matters.

• *Equitability* in acknowledging the contributions of others. This means that you give credit where credit is due in publications, by listing coauthors, or in speeches and presentations, by acknowledging the work of others.

• *Nobility* in the application of processes and procedures to protect the rights of human subjects. This means that you actively assume responsibility for protecting subjects from harm, deceit, coercion, and invasions of privacy, even when your own study may be inconvenienced.

• *Truthfulness* about a study's purpose, procedure, methods, and findings. You do not attempt to disguise your research or conduct it "under cover."

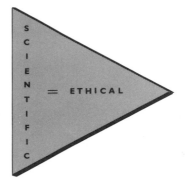

Figure 3-1 Making the scientific ethical.

- *Impeccability* in use of any privileges that may be associated with the researcher's role. You keep data anonymous and confidential. You are discrete about what you learn about people.
- *Forthrightness* about a study's funding sources and sponsorship. You disclose all sources of financial support as well as any special relationship between a study and its sponsors in publications and presentations of research findings.
- *Illuminating* to your discipline's body of scientific knowledge through your publications and presentations of research findings. Research should yield fruitful results.

- *Courage* to publicly clarify any distortions that others make of your research findings.

Codes of Research Ethics

The preceding characteristics of ethical research are reflected in most professional codes of ethics for research. Box 3-1 presents the Code of Professional Ethics of the American Sociological Association, and Box 3-2 presents a summary of the American Nurses' Association's Human Rights Guidelines for Nursing in Clinical and Other Research. Conducting your research based on such codes will help you keep the *scientific, ethical*.

The Rights of Human Research Subjects

Protecting the rights of human subjects who are involved in research has become a high priority throughout all the professional and scientific communities. Nurse researchers are often among the most responsible and conscientious investigators when it comes to respecting the rights of subjects. The responsibility for assuring that a study is ethical is no longer exclusively the investigator's. Recent guidelines such as those in Boxes 3-1 and 3-2 have been established to ensure an unbiased review. They rely on two historical documents.

The Nuremberg Code

The first internationally accepted effort to set up formal ethical standards governing human research subjects is now known as the Nuremberg Code, or Nuremberg Articles. When the U.S. secretary of state and secretary of war learned that the defense of the Nazi doctors during the trials of war criminals after World War II would center on justifying their atrocities on the ground that the doctors were "engaged in im-

portant research," the American Medical Association was asked to appoint a group to develop a code of ethics for research against which sadistic experiments on concentration camp prisoners would be judged. Box 3-3 contains the historic articles of the Nuremberg Tribunal.

The code requires informed consent in *all* cases and makes no provision for any special treatment of children, the elderly, or the mentally incompetent. Thus, its definitions of the terms *voluntary*, *legal capacity*, *sufficient understanding*, and the *enlightened decision* have been the subjects of numerous court cases and the focus for several presidential commissions engaged in standard setting. The code itself disallowed any research on subjects who were not capable of giving consent.

The Declaration of Helsinki

The Declaration of Helsinki was issued in 1964 by the World Medical Association as a guide for physicians engaged in clinical research. Revised

Box 3-1   *Code of Ethics of Sociological Research and Practice*

A. Objectivity and Integrity

Sociologists should strive to maintain objectivity and integrity in the conduct of sociological and research practice.

1. Sociologists should adhere to the highest possible technical standards in their research. When findings may have direct implications for public policy or for the well-being of subjects, research should not be undertaken unless the requisite skills and resources are available to accomplish the research adequately.

2. Since individual sociologists vary in their research modes, skills and experience, sociologists should always set forth *ex ante* the disciplinary and personal limitations that condition whether or not a research project can be successfully completed and condition the validity of findings.

3. Regardless of work settings, sociologists are obligated to report findings fully and without omission of significant data. Sociologists should also disclose details of their theories, methods and research designs that might bear upon interpretation of research findings.

4. Sociologists must report fully all sources of financial support in their publications and must note any special relations to any sponsor.

5. Sociologists should not make any guarantees to subjects—individuals, groups or organizations—unless there is full intention and ability to honor such commitments. All such guarantees, once made, must be honored unless there is a clear, compelling and overriding reason not to do so.

6. Consistent with the spirit of full disclosure of method and analysis, sociologists should make their data available to other qualified social scientists, at reasonable cost, after they have completed their own analyses, except in cases where confidentiality or the claims of a fieldworker to the privacy of personal notes necessarily would be violated in doing so. The timeliness of this obligation is especially critical where the research is perceived to have policy implications.

7. Sociologists must not accept grants, contracts or research assignments that appear likely to require violation of the principles above, and should dissociate themselves from research when they discover a violation and are unable to achieve its correction.

8. When financial support for a project has been accepted, sociologists must make every reasonable effort to complete the proposed work, including reports to the funding source.

9. When several sociologists, including students, are involved in joint projects, there should be mutually accepted explicit agreements, preferably written, at the outset with respect to division of work, compensation, access to data, rights of authorship, and

continued

Box 3-1 (continued)

other rights and responsibilities. Of course, such agreements may need to be modified as the project evolves.

10. When it is likely that research findings will bear on public policy or debate, sociologists should take particular care to state all significant qualifications on the findings and interpretations of their research.

B. Sociologists must not knowingly use their disciplinary roles as covers to obtain information for other than disciplinary purposes.

C. Cross-National Research

Research conducted in foreign countries raises special ethical issues for the investigator and the professional. Disparities in wealth, power, and political systems between the researcher's country and the host country may create problems of equity in research collaboration and conflicts of interest for the visiting scholar. Also, to follow the precepts of the scientific method—such as those requiring full disclosure—may entail adverse consequences or personal risks for individuals and groups in the host country. Finally, irresponsible actions by a single researcher or research team can eliminate or reduce future access to a country by the entire profession and its allied fields.

1. Sociologists should not use their research or consulting roles as covers to gather intelligence for any government.

2. Sociologists should not act as agents for any organization or government without disclosing that role.

3. Research should take culturally appropriate steps to secure informed consent and to avoid invasions of privacy. Special actions may be necessary where the individuals studied are illiterate, of very low social status, and/or unfamiliar with social research.

4. While generally adhering to the norm of acknowledging the contributions of all collaborators, sociologists working in foreign areas should be sensitive to harm that may arise from disclosure, and respect a collaborator's wish/or need for anonymity. Full disclosure may be made later if circumstances permit.

5. All research findings, except those likely to cause harm to collaborators and participants, should be made available in the host country, ideally in the language of that country. Where feasible, raw data stripped of identifiers should also be made available. With repressive governments and in situations of armed conflict, researchers should take particular care to avoid inflicting harm.

6. Because research and/or findings may have important political repercussions, sociologists must weigh carefully the political effects of conducting research or disclosure of findings on international tensions or domestic conflicts. It can be anticipated that there are some circumstances where disclosure would be desirable despite possible adverse effects; however, ordinarily research

Box 3-1 (continued)

should not be undertaken or findings released when they can be expected to exacerbate international tensions or domestic conflicts.

D. Work Outside of Academic Settings

Sociologists who work in organizations providing a lesser degree of autonomy than academic settings may face special problems. In satisfying their obligations to employers, sociologists in such settings must make every effort to adhere to the professional obligations contained in the code. Those accepting employment as sociologists in business, government, and other non-academic settings should be aware of possible constraints on research and publication in those settings and should negotiate clear understandings about such conditions accompanying their research and scholarly activity.

E. Respect for the Rights of Research Populations

1. Individuals, families, households, kin and friendship groups that are subjects of research are entitled to rights of biographical anonymity. Organizations, large collectivities such as neighborhoods, ethnic groups, or religious denominations, corporations, governments, public agencies, public officials, persons in the public eye, are not entitled automatically to privacy and need not be extended routinely guarantees of privacy and confidentiality. However, if any guarantees are made, they must be honored unless there are clear and compelling reasons not to do so.

2. Information about persons obtained from records that are open to public scrutiny cannot be protected by guarantees of privacy or confidentiality.

3. The process of conducting sociological research must not expose subjects to substantial risk of personal harm. Where modest risk or harm is anticipated, informed consent must be obtained.

4. To the extent possible in a given study, researchers should anticipate potential threats to confidentiality. Such means as the removal of identifiers, the use of randomized responses, and other statistical solutions to problems of privacy should be used where appropriate.

5. Confidential information provided by research participants must be treated as such by sociologists, even when this information enjoys no legal protection or privilege and legal force is applied. The obligation to respect confidentiality also applies to members of research organizations (interviewers, coders, clerical staff, etc.) who have access to the information. It is the responsibility of the chief investigator to instruct staff members on this point.

SOURCE: Excerpted from "Toward a Code of Ethics for Sociologists," *The American Sociologist*, July 1984. Reprinted with permission of the American Sociological Society.

Box 3-2 *American Nurses' Association Human Rights Guidelines for Nurses in Clinical and Other Research*

The guidelines in this table attempt to specify several important entities: (1) the type of activities that are involved, (2) the rights that are to be protected, (3) the persons to be safeguarded, and (4) the mechanisms necessary to ensure that protection is adequate.

Guideline 1: Employment in Settings Where Research Is Conducted

Conditions of employment in settings in which clinical or other research is in progress need to be spelled out in detail for all potential workers. . . . Anyone employed in work that carries the potential of risk to others needs to be advised as to the types of risks involved, the ways of recognizing when risk is present, and the proper actions to take to counteract harmful effects and unnecessary danger.

Guideline 2: Nurses' Responsibilities for Vigilant Protection of Human Subjects' Rights

In all instances the prospective subject must be given all relevant information prior to participation in activities that go beyond established and accepted procedures necessary to meet his personal needs. . . . Nurses must be increasingly vigilant in their concern for subjects and patients who by reason of their situation and/or illness are not able to protect themselves effectively from externally imposed threat or injury. They must be sensitive to the tendency toward exploitation of "captive" populations such as students, patients, and inmates in institutions and prisons. All proposals to be used need to be discussed with the prospective subject and with any workers who are expected to participate as a subject or data collector or both. Special mechanisms must be developed to safeguard the confidentiality of information and protect human dignity.

Guideline 3: Scope of Application

The persons for whom these human rights guidelines apply include all individuals involved in research activities and include the following groups: patients, donors of organs and tissue, informants, normal volunteers including students, vulnerable populations that are "captive" audiences such as the mentally disordered, mentally retarded, and prisoners.

---

in 1974, the declaration differentiates between two major types of research: (1) that which is essentially therapeutic and (2) that which is essentially directed toward developing scientific knowledge and has no therapeutic value for the subject. The contemporary application of this document in nursing research emphasizes the re-quirement to inform research subjects when a clinical or nonclinical study will have no personal benefit to them and to avoid any subtle suggestion to the contrary. Both the Nuremberg Code and the Declaration of Helsinki served as the basis for the U.S. policies and regulations issued in 1966.

Box 3-2 (continued)

Guideline 4: Nurses' Responsibility to Support the Accrual of Knowledge

Just as nurses have an obligation to protect the human rights of patients, so do they also have an obligation to support the accrual of knowledge that broadens the scientific underpinnings of nursing practice and the delivery of nursing services.

Guideline 5: Informed Consent

To safeguard the basic rights of self-determination, consent to participate in research or unusual clinical activities must be obtained from the prospective subject or his legal representative. The subject needs to receive:

- A description of any benefit to the subject or to the development of new knowledge that might be expected
- An offer to discuss or answer any questions about the study
- A clear statement to the subject that he is free to discontinue participation at any time he wishes to do so
- Full freedom from direct or indirect coercion and deception

Guideline 6: Representation on Human Subjects Committees

There is increasing public support for systematic accountability to ensure that individual rights are not denied human subjects who participate in research studies. In most instances, the protective mechanism takes place through a committee judged competent to review studies and other investigative activities that involve human subjects. The profession of nursing has an obligation to publicly support the inclusion of nurses as regular members of Institutional Review Committees of this kind.

SOURCE: Adapted and summarized with permission from the American Nurses' Association, *Human Rights Guidelines for Nurses in Clinical and Other Research* (ANA Publication No. D-46 5M 7/75), 1975. Also found in ANA, *Guidelines in Nursing Research*, Kansas City, Mo.: 1975.

U.S. Policies and Procedures

The ethical protection of the rights of human subjects in research studies is no longer left solely to the judgment of the individual investigator, nor is the researcher's need to know something or even the benefit of society consid-ered adequate justification for any and all research practices. The previous abuses of human beings in the interest of science have resulted in insistence by the government agencies that support nursing, medical, biological, and social research that ethical standards be followed if a project is to be funded. In fact, the U.S. surgeon

---

Box 3-3 Articles of the Nuremberg Tribunal

1. The voluntary consent of the human subject is absolutely essential. . . .

2. The experiment should be such as to yield fruitful results for the good of society, unprocurable by other means of study, and not random and unnecessary in nature. . . .

3. The experiment should be so designed and based on the results of animal experimentation and knowledge of the natural history of the disease or other problems under study that the anticipated results will justify the performance of the experiment. . . .

4. The experiment should be conducted to avoid all unnecessary physical and mental suffering and injury. . . .

5. No experiment should be conducted where there is a prior reason to believe that death or disabling injury will occur. . . .

6. The degree of risk to be taken should never exceed that determined by the humanitarian importance of the problem to be solved by the experiment. . . .

7. Proper preparations should be made and adequate facilities provided to protect the subject against . . . injury, disability, or death.

8. The experiment should be conducted only by scientifically qualified persons. . . .

9. The human subject should be at liberty to bring the experiment to an end. . . .

10. During the experiment the scientist . . . if he has probable cause to believe that a continuation of the experiment is likely to result in injury, disability, or death to the experimental subject . . . will bring it to a close.

SOURCE: From J. Katz, *Experimentation with Human Beings*, New York: Russell Sage Foundation, 1972, pp. 289–290.

---

general, in 1966, and subsequent secretaries of the Department of Health, Education, and Welfare (1971) issued regulations governing the use of human subjects in research funded by the National Institutes of Health. The rules require that before research proceeds, an institutional review board functioning in accordance with specifications of the department must review and approve all studies. In 1981 two regulations were added. One excepted several categories of research from the review requirement. The other provided the option of an expedited review in instances where risks were presumed to be minimal (see Box 3-4).

Four Basic Rights

Balancing the obligation to conduct the most valuable study with the obligation to safeguard the rights of human subjects is not an easy task and embroils researchers and reviewers alike in stormy ethical issues. In all instances, however, from a moral point of view, the following list of four rights of research subjects must be protected.

The Right Not to Be Harmed   The regulations of the Department of Health, Education, and Welfare (now the Department of Health and Human Services) defined risk of harm to a research subject as exposure to the possibility of injury going beyond everyday situations. They included physical, emotional, legal, financial, and social harm. Directly withholding treatment in order to study the course of a disease is clearly a physiological danger. But risks to human subjects in a nursing study may also be more subtle. For example, subjects who are asked to complete a questionnaire, ostensibly dealing with "health issues," after the death of a child in their family may experience undue anxiety and the awakening of guilt if sensitive items are included that could evoke disturbing feelings associated with a devastating experience. This is particularly true if no *debriefing* (a process of disclosing to the subject all information that was previously withheld) is conducted afterward and no provision for referral to counseling is included in the study protocol. Merely agreeing to be confined for an extended period in a hospital for research purposes exposes a subject to an increased risk of hospital infections, boredom, and missed opportunities. The risk associated with participating in a randomized treatment study (see Chapter 6)

places the subject at a 50% risk of receiving care or treatment that may not be as effective as the standard or control treatment with which the experimental treatment is being compared. Simple procedures such as venipuncture performed for research purposes involve risks that range from a small bruise to death. Other risks include:

- Loss of confidentiality, which could occur if a nursing faculty member required that students

---

Box 3-4 *Research Activities Eligible for Expedited Review Under United States Rules*

1. Collection of hair and nail clippings, in a nondisfiguring manner; deciduous teeth; and permanent teeth if patient care indicates a need for extraction.

2. Collection of excreta and external secretions, including sweat, uncannulated saliva, placenta removed at delivery, and amniotic fluid at the time of rupture of the membrane prior to or during labor.

3. Recording of data from subjects 18 years of age or older using noninvasive procedures routinely employed in clinical practice. This includes the use of physical sensors that are applied either to the surface of the body or at a distance and do not involve input of matter or significant amounts of energy into the subject or an invasion of the subject's privacy. It also includes such procedures as weighing, testing sensory

acuity, electrocardiography, electroencephalography, thermography, detection of naturally occurring radioactivity, diagnostic echography, and electroretinography. It does not include exposure to electromagnetic radiation outside the visible range (for example, X rays or microwaves).

4. Collection of blood samples by venipuncture, in amounts not exceeding 450 milliliters in an eight-week period and no more often than two times per week, from subjects 18 years of age or older and who are in good health and not pregnant.

5. Collection of both supra- and subgingival dental plaque and calculus, provided the procedure is not more invasive than routine prophylactic scaling of the teeth and the process is accomplished in accordance with accepted prophylactic techniques.

6. Voice recordings made for research purposes such as investigations of speech defects.

7. Moderate exercise by healthy volunteers.

8. The study of existing data, documents, records, pathological specimens, or diagnostic specimens.

9. Research on individual or group behavior or characteristics of individuals, such as studies of perception, cognition, game theory, or test development, where the investigator does not manipulate subjects' behavior and the research will not involve stress to subjects.

10. Research on drugs or devices for which an investigational new drug exemption or an investigational device exemption is not required.

SOURCE: Committee on Human Subjects, *University of California, San Francisco Handbook*, San Francisco: University of California, 1980.

enrolled in a course complete a questionnaire about personal experiences with recreational drugs.

- Loss of privacy by becoming a subject in multiple studies because of one's serious illness or condition (for example, a cancer patient who is terminally ill may be willing to agree to anything to sustain hope for recovery).
- Being subject to additional procedures and tests as a consequence of participating in clinical research and then being charged for them. Most institutions require that investigators assume costs for tests done for research purposes.
- Being duped into thinking that participating in a study will positively affect one's care or condition directly, when in fact the advancement of knowledge or the development of a new commercial product may be the only benefit.
- Exploitation by commercial sponsors who ask patients to donate extra blood or endure discomfort or inconvenience so that the firm can develop a new, marketable product.

In summarizing the risks associated with research procedures, Reynolds (1972) identified *five categories*:

1. No positive or negative effects expected on the research subjects. These studies include chart reviews and tissue studies, and formal consent procedures and forms may be waived by some review boards in such cases.

2. Temporary discomfort, anxiety, or physical pain. Here the discomfort is no more than would be encountered in day-to-day living and ceases with the termination of the experiment. Simple venipuncture for taking a blood sample would fit into this category.

3. Unusual levels of temporary discomfort that may last beyond the end of the study and that may require a debriefing interview or conference to return a subject's anxiety to normal. An interview or questionnaire that evokes strong feelings or upsets the subjects

might fall into this category, as would research in which subjects are not told from the start the authentic question under investigation.

4. Risk of permanent damage, such as might result from the use of an investigational drug or device.

5. Certainty of permanent damage. Examples of this fifth category exist among the abuses of human subjects cited earlier in this chapter—the Nazi war experiments, the Tuskegee syphilis study, and the like.

Concern for protecting human research subjects has been extended beyond research that threatens bodily harm, such as drug toxicity or discomfort, to include research that threatens a subject's self-esteem, self-worth, values, composure, privacy, and even such abstract principles as religious freedom. The risks of anxiety, embarrassment, or other stressors must be weighted against the benefits in any study, and the *risk–benefit ratio* must be clearly disclosed to all research subjects before they agree to participate. Consider this ratio in the example of research involving human subjects on the next page. The preceding case illustrates the two key considerations that evolve when attempting to apply the right not to be harmed: (1) Certain subjects are vulnerable and may not be able to evaluate risks involved in a study (for example, unconscious patients). (2) The risk–benefit ratio of a research project may not justify exposure of subjects to the risks.

In the first instance, children, fetuses, the mentally disabled, the elderly, captives, the dying, and the sedated or unconscious are vulnerable groups of subjects (see Chapter 9). In such cases a guardian or advocate should be identified to provide special consideration and protection. Even here, however, there seem to be no simple answers, only complicated ones. For example, can a mother who has volunteered for an abortion have the interest of the fetus in mind when evaluating the risks associated with an untested intrauterine fetal research procedure? The

Example: The Prayer Experiment

In a study entitled "Positive Therapeutic Effect of Intercessary Prayer on an Intensive Care Population" the subjects were unknowingly to be assigned to one of two groups, experimental or control. If they were assigned to the first group, their bed number, diagnosis, and prognosis would be given to a group of Christians who would then pray for them for the entire time they were in the hospital. The purpose of the study was to "evaluate some of the various ways in which prayer helps critically ill patients."

Study problem

Experimental design
Treatment or independent variable
Study purpose

Discussion of the Prayer Experiment

Although the study seems simple and innocuous on the surface, the institutional review board of the university hospital that reviewed it found that it contained myriad problems and issues that needed to be unraveled. These problems were in the areas of protection of patients' autonomy and in the transmission of private information. The review board acknowledged that although many people would be happy to have someone praying for them, others might not feel so positively and might, in fact, hold serious objections. The criticism was felt by some members to raise the constitutional issue of freedom of religion, by others, the issue of privacy, and by still others, the simple risk of upsetting very ill patients. Upon reading the results, were they to be published in the lay press, some subjects might be quite angry to learn that they had unknowingly participated in such a study. The Belmont Report (U.S. National Commission 1978) identifies "respect for persons" as one key ethical principle used in research. What if a subject were a deeply committed non-Judeo-Christian or an atheist? Treating the intensive-care patients as if they were uninvolved persons with no feelings about whether a group of Christians who had been given private information about them should be praying for them would not be consistent with this principle. Thus, there appeared to be no adequate semblance of informed consent. Finally, the board raised questions about the risk–benefit ratio in this study. It noted that benefit to society is often dependent upon the strength of the research design. In this study it is very difficult to determine if one can ever be empirically "proved" right or wrong on the power of prayer. The committee questioned how the investigator would control for confounding variables, such as someone else, in or out of the prayer group, also praying for the control group members. How would the researcher distinguish spiritual help from physical help? (See Chapter 6.)

Risks

Risks
Risks

No consent procedure

Low benefit

The prayer experiment ultimately earned approval from the board once a simple consent form with full disclosure about the risks to human subjects became part of the protocol and the hospital chaplain (not the patient's primary nurse) was designated as the person to approach patients about participating in the study. Even then, its endorsement by the full committee was weak, illustrating that radiation, withdrawal of care, surgery, and chemotherapy in no way embrace the full range of risks to subjects.

fundamental rule here is that the less able a subject is to give informed consent, the greater the burden on the investigator to protect the subject's rights.

The second issue in calculating the risk–benefit ratio requires that risks to research subjects be justified by potential benefit to them in the case of clinical research or to society in the knowledge produced. The benefits, in short, should exceed the risks. Even then, the risks to a cancer patient of increased side effects from combining near-toxic levels of multiple chemotherapeutic agents with reported adverse effects, including susceptibility to infection, bleeding, increased fatigue, nausea, vomiting, kidney damage, hair loss, hearing loss, and abnormal liver function, may not always be justified by advancing society's knowledge of cancer treatment. This risk–benefit ratio continues as a primary objective standard by which we can judge the ethics of certain research procedures. The calculation of it involves naming the benefits and weighing them as well as considering the following two questions: (1) "How important is the research?" and (2) "How serious are the risks to human subjects?" Some critics, however, cite this standard as "typically American" in its pragmatism, in that it judges the morality of research practices by the results produced. Often the benefits of "basic" research (see Chapter 1) are difficult to identify. In any case, if harm, be it physiological or psychological, is involved, the investigator must explain how these risks will be minimized. The subjects must be fully aware of them, and the nature of the benefits expected from the study must be convincing. *Minimal risk* means that the risks of harm anticipated in the proposed research are not greater than those ordinarily encountered in daily life or during the performance of routine examinations or tests.

The Right to Full Disclosure Nurses who become involved in clinical research are in particularly tempting positions with respect to the ethical requirement for full disclosure of the purpose, procedures, and risks of an investigation.

This is true because of the ease with which research data about patients can be collected as part of clinical nursing practice without patients' knowledge or consent. In such situations a potential conflict also exists between the roles of clinician and investigator, arising from the inclination to adhere to the study plan against the best interests of the patient's care. Full disclosure involves informing subjects about the following aspects of any study:

- the nature, duration, and purposes of a study
- the methods, procedures, and processes by which data will be collected, expressed in straightforward lay terminology—for example, teaspoons or ounces of blood to be drawn, rather than cc's—in short, what will happen to them
- the use to which findings will be put and any personal or societal benefits that could derive from the research
- any and all inconveniences, potential harms, or discomforts that might be expected, including becoming a target for inclusion in future studies, risking loss of privacy or confidentiality, and commitment of personal unreimbursed time.
- any results or side effects that might follow from participation in a study, including follow-up interviews or questionnaires
- alternatives to participating in the study that are available to the subject
- the right to refuse to participate or to withdraw at any time
- the identities of the investigators and how to contact them

Full disclosure means that deception, either by withholding information about a study in the interest of protecting its validity or by giving a subject false information about the study, is unethical. Researchers have taken undercover jobs in mental institutions as nursing aides or attendants while engaging in observational research.

Patients have been told that a study was focusing on child development rather than on their own attitudes and behavior toward their battered children. The scientific rationale for deception is that knowing the point of the research would either influence the natural behavior of the subjects or their willingness to consent to participate or both. Researchers may argue, for example, that informing staff nurses that they are studying the amount of time the nurses spend on paperwork as compared with patient care might alter usual behavior. Furthermore, they may contend that in even the most extreme examples some experimental subjects, when looking back on their experiences, will report that the decep-

tion imposed on them was justified by the scientific knowledge gained and that they do not perceive the lack of full disclosure as unethical.

The Right of Self-Determination Research subjects who have the right of self-determination will feel free from constraint, coercion, or undue influence of any kind. This means that researchers will avoid coercive or seductive language in introduction letters and consent forms. Instead of referring to a study as the investigation of "a promising new relaxation technique for the pain experienced by cancer patients," for example, investigators will use a more neutral expression, such as "an experimental pain control technique

---

Example: The Obedience Experiment

One of the best-known studies in which deceit about the purpose of the research and the procedures involved resulted in upsetting the subjects was Milgram's famous 1963 research on obedience to authority. The study tried to determine how far subjects would go in obeying the commands of an authority figure, even when they knew they were harming another person. The study procedures required the research subjects to give what they understood to be increasingly strong electrical shocks to another person, who was acting the part of a victim. Of the 40 subjects, 65% continued to administer the shocks to the end of the required series, even though they were led to believe that they might be endangering the life of a powerless person. The investigators in the process urged them to go on despite instances of trembling, sweating, stuttering, and other indications of severe discomfort and outright anguish experienced by the subjects.

Study purpose

Methods involving deception

Risks

Discussion of the Obedience Experiment

Many experts say that it is preferable for researchers to tell subjects that they cannot let them know the exact nature of the research question until their participation is completed because of the likelihood that the data would be affected. This approach certainly seems less humiliating and embarrassing than lying to them. If you are afraid that full disclosure would make your potential subjects angry or cause them not to participate in your study, you should probably reconsider the design of the research. Under the right of full disclosure, subjects can refuse to participate, participate selectively, or withdraw from current participation without fear or endangering the quality of their care, even if their withdrawal damages your research. It is the nurse's responsibility to be sure that they are aware of this right. Anytime a subject withdraws from or declines participation in a research project, the investigator must be prepared to accept the decision graciously.

involving meditation." Similarly, any promises of getting special attention or of becoming famous by making a contribution to science or other masked inducements are strictly avoided. A nursing study investigating the effects of injection rates on the intensity of first and second pain of intramuscular injection stated forthrightly that (1) there were no known additional risks from being in the study, other than that the injection a subject received might be more or less painful than an injection given by another method, and (2) that there were no personal benefits to the study subjects, because the purpose of the study was to learn about intramuscular injection pain. If financial compensation is being offered to all or some subjects, the investigator will so state from the onset in matter-of-fact terms, including arrangements for prorated payments should subjects withdraw from the study before its completion. Financial compensation is intended to make up for inconvenience, not act as an inducement to participate in a study. Many research subjects feel pressured to participate in studies if they are in powerless, dependent positions, such as being a patient in a nursing home, or if they feel they must please nurses who are responsible for their treatment and care. Repeated follow-up letters, phone calls, or home visits to prospective respondents who have not returned mailed consent forms may be experienced as "pressuring" subjects to participate in research when they would really prefer not to do so.

The Right of Privacy, Anonymity, and Confidentiality　*Privacy* enables a person to behave and think without interference or the possibility that private behavior or thoughts may be used to embarrass or demean the person later. A study is considered truly *anonymous* if even the investigator cannot link a subject with information reported. *Confidentiality* means that any information that a subject divulges will not be made public or available to others. Even with the apparent clarity of such definitions, review boards

debate issues such as whether biomedical research using normal postcircumcision foreskins of infants should be treated like research on hospital records in a university teaching hospital, for which permission is not required, or should require informed consent from the infants' parents or guardians. Different definitions of these concepts result in different outcomes. The use of instruments such as hidden tape recorders, cameras, or one-way mirrors without a subject's knowledge or permission is an invasion of privacy. Personal activities, opinions, attitudes, beliefs, letters, diaries, and records are generally private property and may not be used as sources for research data without a subject's permission. Even certain records such as school or health records are released only with a person's consent. Invasion of privacy occurs when the subject is not aware of the information being elicited and the use to which it will be put.

If private information is to be collected, at a minimum the investigator will:

1. Maintain the anonymity of subjects by avoiding personally identifiable information on data-collection forms, substituting code numbers instead of names and keeping a master list under lock and key in a separate place.
2. Preserve the confidentiality of data sources by limiting people other than the principal investigator from access to the raw data. If a loss of confidentiality is threatened, all records and links to identity will be destroyed.

The investigator informs research subjects of the measures that will be used to maintain confidentiality and anonymity and to protect their privacy. In a study of stress and role strain in RN baccalaureate nursing students, subjects were told: "There is no identifier attached to the questionnaire, and once the data are pooled, they cannot be used to identify respondents in any way except for school attended." When publishing your research, you should use pseudonyms or general descriptions or report aggregate data only. Remember, however, that agreeing not to mention participants by name also means not identifying them by a combination of characteristics. For example, reporting the personality in-ventory data of a female full professor under the age of 40 in the department of psychiatric nursing of a university school of nursing that offers a doctoral program in California is tantamount to naming the data source.

Ensuring That Research Is Ethical

Although it is the responsibility of investigators to examine their own projects with all the conscience and candor they can summon, federal regulations require that institutions, including universities, hospitals, nursing homes, and health agencies, establish review committees on human research subjects, often called institutional review boards, or IRBs.

The Institutional Review Board

The activities that fall under the jurisdiction of board review were succinctly set forth in the 1974 Code of Federal Regulations:

. . . any research, development, or related activities which depart from the application of those established and accepted methods necessary to meet the subject's needs or which increase the risk of daily life.
(*Federal Register*, May 30, 1974)

Thus, an established nursing procedure with therapeutic benefit to patients does not fall under board jurisdiction, because it is not research. Yet a federally funded evaluation study of teaching strategies in a nursing course in which students are randomly assigned to one of two types of teaching will require that the investigator obtain informed consent from the student subjects and undergo board review.

Review boards are formed in any institution that receives significant federal funding or that does a significant amount of drug or device research regulated by the Federal Drug Administration (FDA). Many smaller hospitals and institutions have no board per se but have a research advisory committee that could substitute.

Most boards have instructions for investigators that include steps to be taken to receive approval, forms for a human-subjects protocol, guidelines for writing a standard consent form, and criteria for qualifying for an expedited rather than a full committee review. Each of these essential points for acquiring clearance for a proposed study is taken up in subsequent sections of this chapter.

Institutional review boards make final decisions on all federally funded research protocols involving human subjects. Their duty is to protect subjects from undue risk and deprivation of personal rights and dignity. This protection is achieved by reviewing the study's protocol to ensure that it meets the major requirements of ethical research, as summarized in Box 3-5.

Informed Consent

Most review boards use the *Code of Federal Regulations* (pp. 9–10) to define the meaning of informed consent:

. . . the knowing consent of an individual or his/her legally authorized representative, under circumstances that provide the prospective subject or representative sufficient opportunity to consider whether or not to participate without undue inducement or

Box 3-5   Federal Ethics Requirements for Research

In order to approve research covered by these regulations the IRB shall determine that all of the following requirements are satisfied:

1. Risks to subjects are minimized: (i) By using procedures which are consistent with sound research design and which do not unnecessarily expose subjects to risk, and (ii) whenever appropriate, by using procedures already being performed on the subjects for diagnostic purposes.

2. Risks to subjects are reasonable in relation to anticipated benefits, if any, to subjects, and the importance of the knowledge that may reasonably be expected to result. In evaluating risks and benefits, the IRB should consider only those risks and benefits that may result from the research (as distinguished from risks and benefits of therapies subjects would receive even if not participating in research). The IRB should not consider

possible long-range effects of applying knowledge gained in the research (for example, the possible effects of the research on public policy) as among those research risks that fall within the purview of its responsibility.

3. Selection of subjects is equitable. In making this assessment the IRB should take into account the purposes of the research and the setting in which the research will be conducted.

4. Informed consent will be sought from each prospective subject or the subject's legally authorized representative, in accordance with, and to the extent required by §46.116.

5. Informed consent will be appropriately documented, in accordance with, and to the extent required by §46.117.

6. Where appropriate, the research plan makes adequate provision for monitoring the data collected to insure the safety of subjects.

7. Where appropriate, there are adequate provisions to protect the privacy of subjects and to maintain the confidentiality of data.

8. Where some or all of the subjects are likely to be vulnerable to coercion or undue influence, such as persons with acute or severe physical or mental illness, or persons who are economically or educationally disadvantaged, appropriate additional safeguards have been included in the study to protect the rights and welfare of these subjects.

SOURCE: Committee on Human Subjects, *University of California at San Francisco Handbook*, San Francisco: University of California, 1980.

---

any element of force, fraud, deceit, duress, or other forms of constraint or coercion.

Documentation that research meets the criterion of informed consent relies heavily on the board's review of a signed consent form for subjects to be involved in research. The wording of this form features prominently in most reviews, because the board must verify that it is suitable for promoting the free self-determination of potential subjects, and otherwise it is difficult to actually verify the consent process.

Vulnerable Subjects   You can expect the board reviewing your protocol to exercise special care if your research involves subjects with *diminished capacity* to give free and informed consent. Prisoners, minors, fetuses, unconscious persons, psychiatric patients, the mentally retarded, students, fellows, and employees are all categories of subjects whom many boards will not approve if the desired research data can be obtained from the study of other adult or normal subjects. *Prisoners* are vulnerable because (1) no prisoner is truly a free agent, (2) financial compensation that might seem like a modest sum may constitute an excessive inducement in prison, where earning opportunities are minimal, and (3) prisoners may believe that participation in an experiment will shorten their sentence. *Minors, unconscious patients, psychiatric patients, and the mentally retarded* may be unable to evaluate the risks involved, and you will therefore need to seek consent from parents, guardians, or close relatives. *Students* should preferably be recruited from classes other than an instructor's own and must never have their participation, or lack of it, influence their grades or future recommendations from the faculty member conducting research. Similarly, *fellows* and *employees* must be clear that their job, promotion, salary, and status are in no way dependent on serving as a research subject.

Some nurse scientists argue that review boards devised to protect the rights of human subjects in research can sometimes obstruct the efforts of nurse researchers who study certain populations (see Chapter 9). Robb (1983) believes that researchers who strictly adhere to board conditions for obtaining written informed consent from the elderly in institutional settings risk losing entire study populations, because many elderly people prefer being interviewed or observed to signing a consent form. She cites a study designed to evaluate perspiration patches for estimating digoxin levels as an illustration of one that failed to recruit a single participant despite the fact that of 312 institutionalized elderly patients, 107 of them were taking digoxin. She urges researchers to find creative solutions to the burdens of written consent based on the urgent need for research into this population. Careful ethical reflectiveness requires that Robb's position be reconciled with the duty to protect the rights of vulnerable subjects. Consent should be conceived of as an agreement between two parties, investigator and subject, who have different degrees of power. Investigators are responsible for clarifying to a board what their approach to the patient was. The official consent form is only one way of putting the agreement into written form. Letters of agreement or verbal agreements made after reading an information sheet are alternative ways to document it (see Appendix A).

Elements of informed consent under federal guidelines are summarized in Box 3-6.

Writing a Standard Consent Form

Most investigators obtain consent through personal discussion. This process is recommended, because it allows questions to be answered on the spot. Consent documents, added to oral consent, may appear to be an unnecessary and quasi-legal burden. In addition to the legal requirements, however, there are two practical uses for a consent form: (1) It can aid the investigator by providing a checklist of discussion items. (2) It can aid the subject as a memory tool to be used at a later time; this suggests that a consent form should be readable and even engaging.

A consent form should tell a reasonable person from the proposed population the information he or she would wish to know in order to make an informed decision, in language that he or she is likely to understand. The suggested formats and language that follow are meant to replace previous, often stilted, language. (See Boxes 3-7, 3-8, and 3-9.) The organization is adaptable; it can be put in narrative, letter, or outline form as desired. Short paragraphs with good margins are easy for most people to read. Investigators should consult with their review board in the cases of special populations (children, pregnant women, the mentally disabled).

Guidelines

1. The title should mention research in some way—for example, "Consent to Be a Research Subject."
2. The form should be consistent in person and verb tense.

Box 3-6   Elements of Informed Consent

A. Basic elements of informed consent. . . .

1. A statement that the study involves research, an explanation of the purposes of the research and the expected duration of the subject's participation, a description of the procedures to be followed, and identification of any procedures which are experimental;

2. A description of any reasonably foreseeable risks or discomforts to the subject;

3. A description of any benefits to the subject or to others which may be reasonably expected from the research;

4. A disclosure of appropriate alternative procedures or courses of treatment, if any, that might be advantageous to the subject;

5. A statement describing the extent, if any, to which confidentiality of records identifying the subject will be maintained;

6. For research involving more than minimal risk, an explanation as to whether any compensation and an explanation as to whether any medical treatments are available if injury occurs and, if so, what they consist of, or where further information may be obtained;

7. An explanation of whom to contact for answers to pertinent questions about the research and research subject's rights, and whom to contact in the event of a research-related injury to the subject; and

8. A statement that participation is voluntary, refusal to participate will involve no penalty or loss of benefits to which the subject is otherwise entitled, and the subject may discontinue participation at any time without penalty or loss of benefits to which the subject is otherwise entitled.

B. Additional elements of informed consent. When appropriate, one or more of the following elements of information shall also be provided to each subject:

1. A statement that the particular treatment or procedure may involve risks to the subject (or to the embryo or fetus, if the subject is or may become pregnant) which are currently unforeseeable;

2. Anticipated circumstances under which the subject's participation may be terminated by the investigator without regard to the subject's consent;

3. Any additional costs to the subject that may result from participation in the research;

4. The consequences of a subject's decision to withdraw from the research and procedures for orderly termination of participation to the subject;

5. A statement that significant new findings developed during the course of the research may relate to the subject's willingness to continue participation will be provided to the subject; and

6. The approximate number of subjects involved in the study.

SOURCE: From *Code of Federal Regulations*, Title 45, Part 46, Washington, D.C.: U.S. Government Printing Office, January 26, 1981.

Box 3-7   *Sample Experimental Subject's Bill of Rights*

The rights below are the rights of every person who is asked to be in a research study.

As an experimental subject I have the following rights:

1. to be told what the study is trying to find out

2. to be told what will happen to me and whether any of the procedures, drugs, or devices is different from what would be used in standard practice

3. to be told about the frequent or important risks, side effects or discomforts of the things that will happen to me for research purposes

4. to be told if I can expect any benefit from participating, and, if so, what the benefits might be

5. to be told the other choices I have and how they may be better or worse than being in the study

6. to be allowed to ask any questions concerning the study both before agreeing to be involved and during the course of the study

7. to be told what sort of treatment is available if any complications arise

8. to refuse to participate at all or to change my mind about participation after the study is started. This decision will not affect my right to receive the care I would receive if I were not in the study.

9. to receive a copy of the signed and dated consent form

10. to be free of pressure when considering whether I wish to agree to be in the study

If I have other questions, I should ask the researcher or the research assistant. In addition, I may contact the institutional review board, which is concerned with protection of volunteers in research projects. I may reach the board office by calling 123-4567 from 8:00 A.M. to 5:00 P.M., Monday to Friday, or by writing to the Committee on Human Research, State University.

Participation in research is voluntary. I have the right to refuse to participate and the right to withdraw later without any jeopardy to my nursing care [my grades, my employment].

---

3. The date of typing and page number should appear in the lower left corner.

4. Legal language should not be used. There is no reason to use *herewith* or *hereby*, for example. "I understand that . . ." also tends to place words that might not be true in the subject's mouth. A consent form is at most a piece of evidence, not a legal document.

5. The name and phone number of the investigator should be clear and explicit.

Box 3-8   Sample Form: Consent to be a Research Subject

Ms. Nightingale is a nurse studying the way a certain blood component, called XYZ, works. To do the study, she needs blood from healthy people and from people with colds. If I agree to be in the study, a technician will draw a maximum of 100 cc's (approximately 3 ounces) of blood from my arm vein. This will be done in her lab at 1842 Clinics. Drawing blood may be uncomfortable and could produce a bruise or, rarely, an infection. There will be no benefit to me, though the study may produce information of use to nurses in the future.

I have had the opportunity to talk with Ms. Nightingale about the study. I may reach her at 123-4567 if I have questions later.

I will be paid $5.00 for this donation of blood. (If I am an employee, I agree not to participate during my work hours.)

I have received a copy of this form and the Experimental Subject's Bill of Rights to keep. I have the right to refuse to participate or to withdraw at any time without any jeopardy to my employment, my grades, or my care at this clinic.

_____	_____
Date	Subject's Signature
_____	_____
Date	Investigator's Signature

Investigators not subject to a review board should consult the state law for the elements of informed consent required by their state. The easiest organization is as follows:

Organization

1. Statement of Purpose and Introduction: This section should answer the questions "What is being studied? why?" "Why me?" "Who are the investigators?" "What is going on that is different from normal?" This part should set the stage for the remainder of the form and provide a quick review.

A study is being done by F. Nightingale, RN, Ph.D., to learn more about the causes of [whatever the condition is]. She has asked me to be in the study.

A diet called XX is currently the standard treatment for my condition. It is known that a percentage of people do not respond to XX. An experimental diet called YY is being tested in people who have not responded to XX. Because I have not responded to XX, I have been invited to be in the study.

Note: The word *new* connotes *better* to many people. *Experimental* is a more descriptive word for use in applications.

---

2. Procedures: Subjects need to know "What will happen to me if I participate that would not otherwise happen to me?" Standard or new procedures that would not ordinarily be done to these patients should be included. They should be described in terms of the subjects' experience (blood drawing) rather than laboratory terms (CBC). Procedures affecting the selection of care (random allocation) or others that a subject

---

Box 3-9   *Sample Consent Letter*

Dear X:

B. Smith, RN, and L. Jones, RN, are educational researchers who are interested in learning about how students choose their nursing career. They have completed an initial study of people who have no idea what they are going to do, and now they wish to compare this group with people who have a very definite idea about their goals. They have asked me to contact a few of my nursing students to see if they would be interested in responding.

If you agree to participate, please return the questionnaire I have enclosed to them at the address listed. There is identifying information on the form. If you would agree to a further interview, please fill that in at the same time. If you would not agree, then leave the information blank to help protect your own privacy.

You might be interested in further information from them before agreeing to participate. You may call them at 123-4567. Of course, no one must participate in any research if he or she does not wish to do so.

Sincerely,

Professor X, RN, Ph.D.

---

might wish to know about (for example, contacting a relative) are included. The form must be complete enough to allow a subject to make plans (baby-sitting, transportation).

- Group A will have the standard treatment for 6 weeks instead of the usual 3 weeks.
- Group B will have the usual treatment time (3 weeks but at twice the usual amount).

If I agree, I will return to see the nurse practitioner in the clinic for ten additional monthly visits of one hour each. At each visit I will have the following tests that will not be for my diagnosis or treatment . . .

If I agree to participate, I will be interviewed for one hour. The questions will concern my background and how I feel about the treatment my family has received in the clinic. This will take place in my home or another place we agree on. If I agree, the interview will be tape-recorded.

In the study I would be randomly assigned to one of two groups. I would have a 50/50 chance of assignment to either group. Neither my nurse nor I would make the choice. The two groups are:

3. Risks and Discomforts: Subjects should be able to gain a fair idea of the risks they will be taking and of the discomforts they might experience as a result of consenting. These include potential legal, economic, and psychological risks as well as physical risks. In some behavioral or social science studies, the term *disadvantages* might be more useful. A rule of thumb is that a side effect that is "relatively" frequent or that is "relatively" serious or permanent should be included. A side effect a reasonable person would wish to know about (sterility, scarring) should obviously be mentioned.

This drug may cause an allergic reaction such as skin rashes or hives. It can also cause a rare allergic reaction, similar to an allergic reaction to penicillin, which can be life threatening.

Taking blood from a vein may cause a bruise or, rarely, an infection.

I may be assigned to a group that is later shown to have had more side effects or less effective treatment. This information will not be known until the study data are analyzed.

As a result of answering this questionnaire, there is a possible loss of my privacy. The investigators will separate names from responses and will keep the names coded and locked so my confidentiality will be protected as much as possible under the law.

Participation in this study may involve the risk of arousing concerns about my family members or the oncology unit that are upsetting to me. Counseling references will be available to me.

The amount of radiation I will be exposed to is relatively small. Small doses may have potential harm, but the risk is difficult to measure with any precision. If I have many X-ray exams or if I am, or might be, pregnant, I should discuss this with the investigator.

Do not forget to include the statement on treatment and compensation for harm if there is any real or foreseeable risk of physical harm that exceeds what is considered "minimal." Each institution has its own particular compensation statement. An example might look like this:

If I am physically injured as a result of being in this study, treatment will be available. The costs of such treatment may be covered by the university, depending upon a number of factors. For information I may call 123-4567.

4. Benefits: An unbiased statement should be included discussing personal and societal benefits. It should not be overstated or read like an advertisement.

There will be no direct benefit to me from participating. The investigators hope to learn more about diets XX and YY, which may help care for patients like me more effectively in the future.

The additional tests I will have done are not needed for my diagnosis or care. The information will be put in my record and could be of interest to my primary nurse.

Note: Most review boards do not consider money paid to subjects to be a benefit.

5. Alternatives: This section should describe the therapeutic or treatment options open in lieu of participation in this study. If the only alternative is simple refusal (for example, to throw away the questionnaire) this section may be omitted.

Instead of having my care chosen by the study, I may ask my own nurse to make the decision. The treatments available are diets XX and ZZ, but not YY.

6. Questions: Few subjects comprehend all details immediately or without some discussion. It is essential to offer a way to find an investigator for a later discussion. If there is a possibility of emergency reactions, a 24-hour number should be used.

I have talked with Ms. Nightingale and her assistant about this study and have had my questions answered. If I have other questions, I may call her at 123-4567.

7. Bill of Rights: The experimental subject's bill of rights (see Box 3-7) must be used when physically invasive procedures are involved. Studies that do not use a bill of rights ought to include the final paragraph from the Bill of Rights on any consent form.

Participation in this research is voluntary. I have the right to refuse to participate and the right to withdraw later without any jeopardy to my nursing care [my grades, my employment].

---

8. Payment: Money is offered to pay for expenses, inconvenience, time, and trouble. It should not provide "undue influence" or reflect payment for acceptance of risk.

I will be paid $10.00 for each visit plus an added $5.00 whenever blood is drawn. This will total $XX.00 if I complete all the visits.

---

9. Signatures: The subject's signature should always be placed first. Other signatures may be requested. When children are involved, they should be asked to sign if they are old enough (over 7) to consider the questions, and their parents should generally be asked to give "permission" for their participation. The investigator's signature should also be included. A witness is not necessary for most studies but may be desired by the investigator or sponsor.

Sample consent forms can be found in Boxes 3-8 and 3-9.

The letter in Box 3-9 could be used in conjunction with a more formal consent form to be presented at the time of the interview. That consent form would cover the interview and tape recording. It might talk more about the advantages (such as receiving a copy of the published report) and the disadvantages (such as loss of time and inconvenience) of participation.

Preparing a Protocol for a Review Board

An institutional review board, once having established that informed-consent procedures are being followed, is also charged with disapproving any activity that falls under its jurisdiction whose risks are not outweighed by the sum of the benefit to subjects and the importance of the knowledge to be gained. Most committees have difficulty approving protocols entailing high personal risks to subjects if the benefit is purely social or if the research design raises questions about whether it is possible to gain any benefits at all. The committee will look for evidence that you have built precautions for minimizing risks into your procedures and will examine the strength of the research design in the protocol you submit. Making this determination requires that you prepare a full "human subjects protocol" and submit it to the board along with your consent form. The example on the next page will guide you in this task.

Checklist for a Human Research Application

The following material is not an outline. Use it as a checklist against which to review your protocol. (See also Chapter 8 and Appendix A.) Does your submission include the following?

A. *Cover Sheet*: Fill this out completely each year.

B. *Protocol*: This usually should be a maximum of ten pages of text, and it should generally not be a copy of your grant application. Instead it covers:

  1. background
    (a) context of work
    (b) competence of investigator—previous work done by others and self
    (c) justification for current study in humans
  2. specific aims of the study
    (a) hypotheses, questions to be an-

Example: Procedure for Submitting a Protocol to a Review Board

1. In most institutions, no federally funded study involving human subjects may begin until IRB approval is obtained.

2. Investigators should usually allow a minimum of 6 weeks for IRB review of any moderately complicated study, although some institutions require 6 months.

    The Committee must usually receive multiple copies of the protocol (complete with all required information). These protocols are then circulated and are discussed during the meeting following their receipt or are considered without a full meeting of the Committee.

    Each IRB has its own specific guidelines

3. IRB review usually proceeds in the following way:

    (a) The Committee may decide that the proposal does *not* involve subjects at risk. For the purposes of DHEW, this Committee action is equivalent to approval.

    (b) The committee may decide that the proposal does involve subjects at risk. If this is the case, the Committee must review the proposal for the risk–benefit balance, the protection of rights of subjects, and the adequacy of informed consent. After doing so the Committee may:

    · approve the protocol as submitted;
    · approve the protocol contingent on minor revisions;
    · request outside review of the protocol and then reconsider;
    · require significant modification of the protocol before approval;
    · request the investigator to discuss problems with the Committee;
    · reject the protocol.

    Possible outcomes of an IRB's deliberations

4. Notice of the Committee's decision will be sent to the Principal Investigator following the Committee consideration. In the event of a rejected protocol the following applies:

    The decisions of the Committee on Human Experimentation made on the basis of technical and ethical judgments are final, and may not be appealed. However, it appears that occasionally during Committee consideration of a proposed protocol the investigator feels the Committee is showing bias, or that an inordinate amount of time is being taken in reaching a decision. Mechanisms usually exist within an institution to review complaints about bias or delay.

    Bias or extraordinary delay can be grounds for a complaint against an IRB

SOURCE: Adapted from *Committee on Human Subjects Handbook*, University of California at San Francisco, 1980.

swered, data to be gathered or tested, description to be made

(b) relevance to continuing work in this field

3. significance

    (a) benefits to individual subject or patient, if any

(b) benefits to the class from which the subject is drawn

(c) benefits to science, society, or humanity in general

4. methods

    (a) general study design

    (b) methods of data analysis

(c) subjects
   (1) number and number per group (Why this number?)
   (2) source and access to subjects (If subjects are recruited from an agency other than that represented by the IRB, permission should be obtained from them)
   (3) criteria for inclusion and exclusion
   (4) discussion of risks (physical, social, economic, other)
   (5) methods used to minimize the risks
   (6) consent process
   (7) vulnerable population? why? (see special regulations)
(d) duration of the study
5. procedures
   (a) detailed explanation of what will be done to each subject and how that compares with what would be done were it not for the study
   (b) risks of each procedure (added time? physical? psychological?)
   (c) precautions to minimize risks (such as coding of records, debriefing of subjects, erasing of audiotapes)
   (d) frequency and duration of each procedure or test
   (e) location of studies
6. compensation of subjects
   (a) amount (Why that amount? Will all subjects receive the same?)
   (b) amount, if any, to be withheld until the end (Why?)

7. records: Where will they be stored? Where will consent forms be stored?
C. *Consent form(s)*: This should be in lay language and in consistent person and tense.
   1. background: What is this study about? What are the investigators hoping to show?
   2. procedures: What will happen or change as a result of agreeing to participate?
      (a) extension of time, if any
      (b) return visits, if any
      (c) randomization or placebo
   3. risk, discomforts, disadvantages: obvious and subtle points that the subject should be aware of before agreeing
   4. benefits: a balanced presentation of benefits to self or others
   5. alternatives, if any, including that of refusing to be in the study and having standard care
   6. questions: assurance of investigator's readiness to answer questions and a phone number to use to contact investigator
   7. money: terms of payment where applicable
   8. refusal or withdrawal: assurance of right to refuse or withdraw without jeopardy to whatever is applicable
   9. receipt: Notice that the consent form and Experimental Subject's Bill of Rights (for health care experiments) are to be given to the subject

Nursing and the Ethics of Research

This chapter began with questions about how to make your own scientific research ethical and how to tell if someone else's studies are ethically sound. Advocates for research subjects, your own conscience, and review committees whose members have no particular investment in a particular study all are methods of safeguarding the rights of human subjects. Nurses who are research investigators themselves or who assist in the research projects of others are in a position to assert and maintain the protective values of the profession. A study design that deprived one group of patients of relaxation techniques for labor pain or preoperative teaching, for example, would be unethical unless provisions were made for alternatively effective care. Projective psychological tests like the Rorschach inkblot test may represent an invasion of privacy if patients do not know that such tests may measure traits that the patients wish to conceal. Furthermore, patients are vulnerable to requests to participate in research when the person approaching them with the request is the nurse whom the patient depends on for care.

As Walker (1983) points out, obtaining approval for clinical investigations can be time-consuming and cumbersome, making it difficult for some nurses to conduct research in hospitals. But it is difficult for *anyone* to conduct clinical research unless he or she has demonstrated scientific rigor, sophistication, political savvy, and concern for the ethics of research on human subjects.

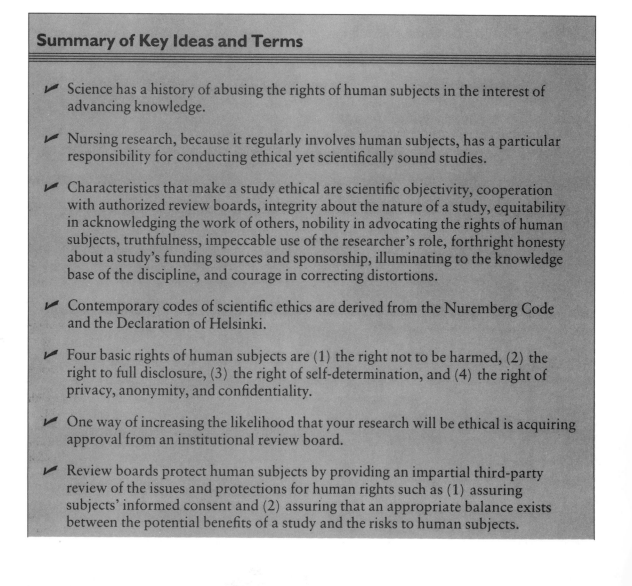

Summary of Key Ideas and Terms

- Science has a history of abusing the rights of human subjects in the interest of advancing knowledge.

- Nursing research, because it regularly involves human subjects, has a particular responsibility for conducting ethical yet scientifically sound studies.

- Characteristics that make a study ethical are scientific objectivity, cooperation with authorized review boards, integrity about the nature of a study, equitability in acknowledging the work of others, nobility in advocating the rights of human subjects, truthfulness, impeccable use of the researcher's role, forthright honesty about a study's funding sources and sponsorship, illuminating to the knowledge base of the discipline, and courage in correcting distortions.

- Contemporary codes of scientific ethics are derived from the Nuremberg Code and the Declaration of Helsinki.

- Four basic rights of human subjects are (1) the right not to be harmed, (2) the right to full disclosure, (3) the right of self-determination, and (4) the right of privacy, anonymity, and confidentiality.

- One way of increasing the likelihood that your research will be ethical is acquiring approval from an institutional review board.

- Review boards protect human subjects by providing an impartial third-party review of the issues and protections for human rights such as (1) assuring subjects' informed consent and (2) assuring that an appropriate balance exists between the potential benefits of a study and the risks to human subjects.

✔ Board approval is required for federal and much other funding of research.

✔ Particular care must be exercised in gaining informed consent from vulnerable subjects such as children, the mentally disabled, prisoners, and the like.

✔ It is important to follow your institution's board guidelines when writing a study protocol and consent form.

References

American Nurses' Association. *Human Rights Guidelines for Nurses in Clinical and Other Research.* Kansas City, Mo.: American Nurses' Association, 1975.

American Sociological Society. Toward a code of ethics for sociologists, *Am Sociol*, July 1984: 1–4.

Code of Federal Regulations. Title 45, Part 46. Washington, D.C., January 26, 1981.

Committee on Human Subjects. *University of California at San Francisco Handbook.* San Francisco: University of California, 1980.

Jones JH: *Bad Blood: The Tuskegee Syphilis Experiment.* New York: Free Press, 1981.

Katz J: *Experimentation With Human Beings: The Authority of the Investigator, Subject, Professions and State in the Human Experimentation Process.* New York: Russell Sage Foundation, 1972.

Reynolds PD: On the protection of human subjects and social science. *Int Soc Sci J* 1972; 24:694–695.

Robb SS: Beware of the informed consent. *Nurs Res* May/June 1983; 32:132.

US Department of Health, Education, and Welfare. *The Institutional Guide to DHEW Policy on Protection of Human Subjects.* Washington, D.C.: US Government Printing Office, 1971.

US National Commission for the Protection of Human Subjects of Biomedical and Behavioral Research. *The Belmont Report: Ethical Principles and Guidelines for the Protection of Human Subjects of Research.* DHEW Publication No. (05) 78-0012. Washington, D.C.: US Government Printing Office, 1978.

Walker M: As I see it . . . Research with patients requires commitment, savvy. *Am Nurse* July/August 1983:5.

Further Readings

Abdellah F: Approaches to protecting the rights of human subjects. *Nurs Res* 1967; 16:316–320.

Arminger B Sr: Ethics of nursing research: Profile, principles, perspective. *Nurs Res* 1977; 26:330–336.

Barber B: The ethics of experimentation with human subjects. *Scientific American* 1975; 234:25–31.

Beecher HK: Ethics and clinical research. *N Engl J Med* 1966; 274:1314.

Berthold JS: Advancement of science and technology while maintaining human rights and values. *Nurs Res* 1969; 18:514–522.

Creighton H: Legal concerns of nursing research. *Nurs Res* 1977; 26:337–341.

Davis DJ, Aroskar MA: *Ethical Dilemma and Nursing Practice.* New York: Appleton-Century-Crofts, 1983.

Downs F: Ethical inquiry in nursing research. *Nurs Forum* 1967; 6:12–20.

Gortner SR et al: The institutional review board: A case study of no-risk decisions in health-related research. *Nurs Res* January–February 1981; 30:21–24.

Gray B: An assessment of institutional review committees in human experimentation. *Nurs Digest* 1976; 4.

Holden C: Ethics in social science research. *Science* 1979; 206:537–538.

Jacobson SF: Ethical issues in experimentation with human subjects. *Nurs Forum* 1973; 12:58–71.

Jonas H: Philosophical reflections on experimenting with human subjects. Pages 209–235 in: *Bioethics.* Shannon TA (editor). New York: Paulist Press, 1976.

Krueger J, Davis A: *Patients, Nurses and Ethics.* New York: American Journal of Nursing, 1981.

May KA: The nurse as researcher: Impediment to informed consent? *Nurs Outlook* 1979; 27:36–40.

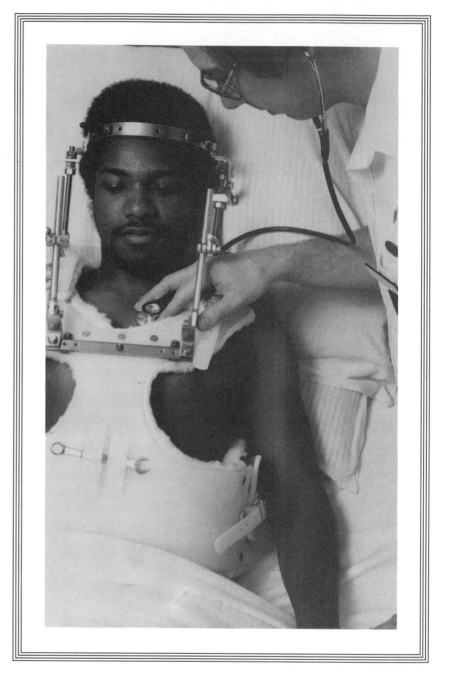

"Research in nursing has as its aim improving clinical judgment—the artful and scientific processes nurses use to arrive at decisions about how, when, where, with what means, why and toward what end any nursing act is done."

D. Diers (1979)

2 A Consumer's Guide to Nursing Research

Chapter 4

The Language of Science

How to Read Research

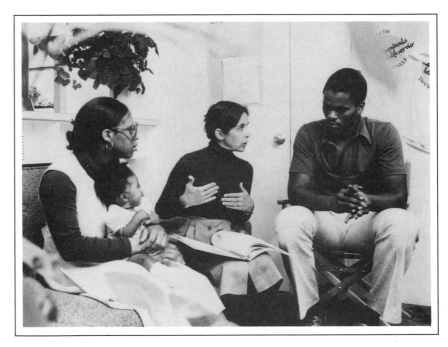

Before you can evaluate the worth of a scientific article and interpret it to your clients, you have to understand it. Learning a new vocabulary is only part of the solution.

Chapter Outline

Chapter Objectives

After reading this chapter, the student should be able to:

- Explain why typical research articles are often low on readability
- Recognize when long or impersonal words and sentences can be translated into plain, conversational language
- Describe the arrangement of headings and subheadings in a typical research journal article
- Interpret presentations of information in each section of a journal article
- Define the meaning of some commonly used research terms
- Critically analyze information usually disseminated in graphs and tables
- Overcome attitudinal obstacles to reading nursing research reports effectively

In This Chapter . . .

Have you ever felt the frustration of not being able to understand what the author of a scientific article means? Did you ever become bogged down in what seemed to be heavy, stale, cliché-ridden jargon that lost sight of direct and possibly forceful ideas? Did the research report you read catch and hold your attention, or did you find yourself eager to move on to a more interesting popular piece of clinical writing in the *American Journal of Nursing*, *Nursing '85*, or *RN*? Did you conclude that it's no wonder that practitioners of the past have avoided participating in and implementing nursing research as part of their professional role?

In this chapter you will be given step-by-step lessons for building the language repertoire and mental processes that will result in clear "translation" of and thinking about the research-oriented writing you read. In the framework of analytic reading, *you will come to terms with research terminology*. Naturally, the arts of

reading and thinking can be learned only by constant practice. This chapter encourages you to set up a training program for yourself so that reading even highly complex research literature will become second nature to you. Don't stop practicing till you reach that point. The student applications and resource book that accompanies this text (see *Applying Research in Nursing: A Resource Book*) can provide you with a wealth of guided opportunities. You can also find them in the nursing research literature resources outlined in Chapter 2.

Topics covered in *this* chapter include (1) understanding the format of a research journal article, (2) translating the language of science, and (3) strategies for interpreting visual presentations of data in tables and graphs. You don't have to be a career researcher to decipher nursing research, evaluate it, and use research findings as a basis for your clinical practice.

Readability

In most dictionaries, "readable" is defined as "easy" *or* "interesting" to read. Actually, to most people, readability means ease of reading *plus* interest. Most of us want to make as little effort as possible while we are reading and want something to carry us forward like an escalator. We want to be inspired or interested as well as informed. Flesch (1960) has created a formula for successful communication in 25 rules for effective writing listed in Box 4-1.

Flesch adds that for most of us, graph and chart reading is *not* one of the three Rs! *People need training to learn from visual presentations*. In view of the preceding points, it should come as no big surprise that nursing research reports, protocols, and methodology at first seem low in readability according to Flesch's conception of it.

The plain-talk style of writing that makes for popular magazine articles is decidedly absent in most reports of scientific research. The problem of reading research literature effectively becomes partly a matter of language translation and partly a matter of context translation. We will be considering both in the pages that follow.

In Pursuit of Translation

One of the promises that you were made in this chapter's introduction was that you would emerge from reading this chapter with a stronger grasp of the language and vocabulary of nursing's scientific enterprise. You will undoubtedly encounter multisyllable words, jargon-ridden paragraphs, and technical terminology in re-

---

Box 4-1   25 Rules for Effective Writing

1. Write about people, things, and facts.
2. Write the way you talk.
3. Use contractions.
4. Use the first person.
5. Quote what you said.
6. Quote what was written.
7. Put yourself in the reader's place.
8. Don't hurt the reader's feelings.
9. Forestall misunderstandings.
10. Don't be too brief.
11. Plan a beginning, middle, and end.
12. Go from the rule to the exception, from the familiar to the new.
13. Use short names and abbreviations.
14. Use pronouns rather than repeating nouns.
15. Use verbs rather than nouns.
16. Use the active voice and a personal subject.
17. Use small, round figures.
18. Specify! Use illustrations, cases, examples.
19. Start a new sentence for each new idea.
20. Keep your sentences short.
21. Keep your paragraphs short.
22. Use direct questions.
23. Underline for emphasis.
24. Use parentheses for casual mention.
25. Make your writing interesting to look at.

SOURCE: From R. Flesch, *How to Write, Speak, and Think More Effectively*, New York: Harper & Row Publishing Company, 1960.

---

search articles you read. Here are, however, a couple of preliminary strategies for understanding them when and if you meet up with them:

1. Give yourself time to understand different and unfamiliar words and expressions.
2. Pause between reading heavy sentences.
3. Mentally fill in the spaces between ideas with your own reasoning about them.
4. Think of illustrations or personal rephrasings that help you reach a personal understanding of an author's ideas.
5. Try to translate them into your own mental, conversational talk.

Some Plain Talk About Research in Nursing

In 1976 the American Nurses' Association's Commission on Nursing Research, with the co-operation of a distinguished list of nurse researchers, published a document called *Research in Nursing: Toward a Science of Health Care*. In it, using conversational, popular language and a lot of photographs, the authors explain what research in nursing is and give some superb examples of clinical discoveries made through scientific inquiry. They describe research in nursing as

investigating . . . the area of knowledge where the physical and behavioral sciences meet and influence one another, in an effort to study how health problems relate to human behavior and how behavior relates to health and illness. . . . Research in nursing addresses the human and behavioral questions that arise in the treatment of diseases and the prevention of illness and maintenance of health (p. 1).

The document goes on to introduce the reader to some selected projects conducted by nurses that represent important advances in health care knowledge and the study of people with health

Example 1: Alleviating Pain

A series of relaxation exercises carried out once or twice a day may relieve the intensity of pain or relax patients so that they are better able to cope with pain according to results of tests by a nurse researcher. Working with three groups of patients—those having elective surgery such as gall bladder removal or hernia repairs, those having rheumatoid arthritis and cancer patients—the nurse researcher was able to validate that pain can be relieved by methods other than medication (p. 3).

Example 2: Understanding Obesity

Although the cause of obesity is not known and its treatment is notably unsuccessful, a nurse researcher believes that the answer to treatment of the obesity problems lies in understanding more about the mechanisms which underlie feeding behavior and control appetite. Her research project, which is directed at understanding hunger and satiety, is exploring the role of many different hormones and substrates contained in the blood and their influence on appetite and regulation of body weight. These studies are being carried out on monkeys whose anatomy and physiology is similar to that of humans (p. 7).

Example 3: Screening for Cystic Fibrosis

A nurse research project has provided a breakthrough in effectively screening victims and carriers of cystic fibrosis, a process that has been impeded by lack of an efficient test system that could be readily made available to clinical laboratories (p. 9).

Example 4: Womb Simulation for Premature Infants

Premature babies given special treatment and conditions to simulate prenatal womb life achieve a greater degree of development than similar infants provided standard conditions according to information compiled by a nurse researcher. Normal, full-term infants can usually sleep for 60 minutes at a time, while a baby who normally would be in the womb for another eight weeks lacks the nervous system development that controls sleep behavior, which in turn affects weight gain and physical development. . . . The nurse and her research team simulated womb conditions by playing a tape-recording of a heart beat for 15 minutes every hour, and rocking the mattresses of the isolettes in which the babies were placed. Those infants living in the womb-simulated situations slept more quietly and gained more weight than a group of similar babies of the same age used in comparison studies. The nursing research team is continuing efforts to determine the best time in an infant's life to begin simulation, how loud a heart beat is advantageous, the intensity of rocking that is most productive and at what point visual stimulation might be used (pp. 10–11).

Example 5: Coping with Home Dialysis

Patients using an artificial kidney machine at home have advantages over those who continue treatment in hospitals according to a nurse researcher studying the relationships in home dialysis triads and patient outcomes. The study, which investigates how cooperation among patient, spouse, and doctor makes a difference for the patient using home dialysis, indicated that home treatment resulted in better physical health, closer adherence to medical regimen, greater amounts of work and leisure time activities, fewer hospitalized days and fewer emergencies for the patient. . . . The study of families successfully coping with dialysis is yielding information about the ways they make adaptations which maximize the quality of life for the patient and minimize the disruption of other family members (p. 13).

SOURCE: From American Nurses' Association, Commission on Nursing Research, *Research in Nursing: Toward a Science of Health Care*, Kansas City, Mo.: American Nurses' Association, 1976.

problems. The project descriptions are excellent examples of how technical writing styles and esoteric language can be translated into highly readable material. After reading a few of these illustrations (Examples 1–5 on pp. 91 and 92), use the strategies in the rest of this chapter to translate some published research reports into plain talk yourself.

Speaking the Language of Science

Meaning and Context

Before you can evaluate the worth of a scientific article, you have to understand it. Learning what may be a new vocabulary is part of the solution. But vocabulary alone isn't all of it. We understand the meaning of even unfamiliar words when we first understand their context. What this means is that you can use terms such as *vitamin deficiency* or *wound infection* when teaching patients who may never have heard them if you put them in a context that the patients can use to interpret what they mean. Likewise, you understand unfamiliar research terminology once you grasp its context in the research process. Unfortunately, building a research vocabulary isn't as easy as merely looking up words in a resource such as the glossary at the end of this book. Even the term *science* has

somewhat different meanings under different conditions. If you look it up in a glossary, you will probably find a definition like this:

Science: A branch of study . . . concerned with the observation and classification of facts, esp. with the establishment of verifiable general laws.

If, on the other hand, you asked a nurse theorist what he or she meant when speaking of nursing science, the response might be more like this:

Science is an interconnected series of concepts and conceptual schemes that have developed as a result of empirical observation and guide future observations, descriptions, and prediction.

Clearly, these two definitions of science are different. The first emphasizes facts, and the second emphasizes concepts. Having advanced an argument for placing the meaning of scientific language in the appropriate context as one way of making it easier to understand, I will move on to consider the language of science *within the context of* the format of a typical scientific article.

Typical Format of a Research Journal Article

Almost all research journal articles are divided into sections with headings and subheadings. The arrangement of these headings usually follows a somewhat standardized format. If you are familiar with it, you can get the most out of the time you spend reading, because you understand the context that each section intends to establish. You will also have a better chance of getting your own articles published in scientific journals if you should decide to conduct your own research (see Chapter 17). Huck, Cormier, and Bounds (1974), in a handy little book called *Reading Statistics and Research*, outline the typical sections of a research article with the headings arranged as follows (pp. 3–4):

1. Abstract
2. Introduction
   - Review of the literature
   - Statement of purpose
3. Method
   - Subjects
   - Design
   - Materials (data collection)
   - Procedure (data analysis)
4. Results (conclusions)
5. Discussion
6. References

Let us examine each of these sections with a bit more care.

   Abstract   An abstract is located at the beginning of a research article. Its purpose is to sum-

marize the entire piece as briefly as possible. An abstract usually provides the following information about the study:

1. its purpose, objectives, or hypotheses
2. a description of the participants or sample members
3. a brief explanation of data-collection and analysis procedures
4. a summary of important findings (Huck, Cormier, & Bounds 1974, p. 4)

   The accompanying example is an illustration of an abstract. It offers you an overview of what you will find in the article that follows. Because it is *located at the beginning* of an article, you can read it in a minute or two and then decide whether to systematically skim or analytically read the whole article. Because it helps you use your reading time wisely, an abstract serves a very useful purpose. It also is your first encounter with what may be some unfamiliar words. If the study is one that relates to your interest areas, you will have a chance to read about the subjects in more depth and get a fuller grasp of the meaning of terms as you go on with the article.

Sample Abstract

A national survey of a stratified random sample (n = 240) of accredited hospitals with critical care units (CCUs) was conducted in order to describe the current practice of restrictions imposed upon myocardial infarction (MI) patients. A cross-sectional correlation survey with a two-stage mailing was used.

The first-stage mailing at the institutional level was sent to the head nurses of the CCUs (n = 600). Nurses were requested to give: (a) importance and frequency ratings of selected coronary care nursing practices; (b) information about the use of discontinuance of two specific restrictions: ice water and rectal temperature measurements. Follow-ups by mail and/or telephone yielded response rates for about 87%.

The conceptual framework, "Diffusion of Innovations," was used to assess the diffusion of the results of studies published in clinical journals. Despite findings that cast doubt on the practices of restricting ice water and rectal temperature measurement, coronary precautions are commonly practiced.

Hours spent reading and the number of journals read correlate (p less than .001) with greater levels of awareness in nurses that such restrictions are in question. Levels of awareness are *not* related to the importance and frequency ratings for those restrictions. Differences among nurses do not explain differences in ratings. If research is to be used, nurse researchers and managers need to actively intervene in care. Passive diffusion of research results is inadequate, unsure, and slow.

SOURCE: From K. T. Kirchoff, "A Diffusion Survey of Coronary Precautions," *Nursing Research*, July/August 1982, vol. 31, p. 196.

Let's go back to the components of an abstract and figure out what we've just read. First, an abstract provides the purpose, objectives, or hypotheses of the study. In this example the purpose is "to describe the current practice of restrictions imposed on myocardial infarction (MI) patients" in CCUs throughout the United States. We'd probably add in view of the conclusions that another descriptive purpose of the study was to determine if practicing these restrictions had any relationship with whether nurses read about the latest research on the subject in professional journals.

Second, the sample abstract tells us that the participants in the study were a sample of 600 randomly selected nurses and head nurses from a stratified random sample of 240 CCUs in accredited hospitals throughout the country. The selection of random sampling tells us (as do the large sizes of the samples) that the investigator wanted to increase the possibilities of generalizing her findings to the total population of accredited CCUs by obtaining a representative sample, and not just to a case study of one institution or even a particular region's practices. (See Chapters 7, 9, and 15.)

As far as procedures are concerned, the researcher mailed some instruments to head nurses and randomly selected staff nurses in accredited settings who were willing to participate. She asked them to provide information about the awareness and use or nonuse of coronary precautions and their typical journal reading habits as well as some additional information. She used a statistical technique to correlate these categories of information that yielded a number called a p value that she compared with values in a statistical table (see Chapter 15).

Fourth, the abstract gives us a summary of important findings. Although the researcher found that nurses who spent more hours reading had greater levels of *awareness* that coronary restrictions were in question, being aware didn't seem to alter clinical practice. This finding led the author to argue for the importance of active programs to get research findings into practice.

Introduction The introduction of a research article usually contains two parts, (1) a review of the literature and (2) a statement of the study's purpose. Most authors begin with a discussion of previous relevant studies that they or others have conducted. This background of information is important to figure out how the study being reported relates to previous knowledge in a field. It is important to ask yourself if the study at hand is so unique and original that little or nothing of any importance has preceded it, or if the investigator just didn't bother to look up the prior research or theoretical literature on his or her topic. The discussion of previous research can be as short as one or two sentences or as long as several pages. The following three paragraphs constitute the literature review in our sample study report.

Sample Literature Review

The term "coronary precautions" covers a list of restrictions imposed upon myocardial infarction patients, including restriction of: hot and cold beverages, rectal temperature measurement, stimulant beverages, and sometimes vigorous back rubs (Kirchoff 1981).

Several clinical and laboratory studies of cardiac changes following the ingestion of ice water have been conducted (Cohen, Alpert, Francis, Vieweg, and Hagan 1977; Fitzmaurice and Simon 1974; Houser, 1976; Pratte, Padilla, and Baker 1973). The general conclusions were that a normally consumed amount of hot or ice water (200 cc) was *not harmful* to a recent myocardial infarction patient, although Pratte, Padilla, and Baker (1973) found that ingestion of 600 cc of ice water by normal males in the supine position was related to changes in electrical activity in the heart.

Two studies of the cardiac changes following the measurement of rectal temperature were found (Gruber, 1974; McNeal, 1978). Measurement of rectal temperatures *did not* cause bradycardia or arrhythmias. No studies were found that discounted the restriction of stimulant beverages, none were found that mentioned vigorous back rubs. Except for the findings of Fitzmaurice and Simon, and Pratte and colleagues, the results of the studies were rarely available to critical care nurses [Kirchoff, p. 196].

Having summarized the relevant literature leading up to a current study, the author usually states the specific goals or purposes of the study. In our sample article the researcher says:

Sample Purpose

A survey of current practice was designed to assess the impact of the published studies on the practices of restricting ice water and the measurement of rectal temperature. Nurses who read these publications might have reduced the frequency of or even eliminated these practices, rendering further research meaningless [Kirchoff, p. 196].

Translating the paragraph above, the author means, "Because published studies have dem-

onstrated that restricting ice water and rectal temperature-taking with coronary patients isn't necessary, one would expect nurses who read to have abandoned these restrictions. I decided to do a survey to find out if in fact they have." When you look for the literature review and study purpose in a research report, be prepared to find them either as separate headings or grouped together under the heading "Background" or "Introduction."

Method   This is the section of a research article where the author explains in detail exactly how he or she conducted the study. The reason for going into such elaborate detail is so that a reader could replicate the study. According to Huck and his colleagues (1974, p. 6), the author addresses four main questions in the method section of a research article:

1. Who participated in the study?
2. What type of research design was used?
3. What materials (data) were needed?
4. What procedures were the participants required to do?

A full description of the subjects who participated in the study and the process by which they were selected (sampling procedure) is important for the reader to know, because the conclusions of most studies are valid only for people who are similar to the subjects in the study. In our sample article the author does a good job of telling us the criteria for including nurses in the sample to receive survey instruments and of the number ($n = 524$) who actually completed the data collection forms. She also tells us how she selected the head and then staff nurses, using a random sampling procedure from a list provided by the head nurse of settings who met study criteria.

For any study purpose, several designs can be used. Chapter 6 is devoted to a discussion of these in detail. The design gives you an idea of the overall plan for organizing the study and some predictions about how data might be statistically treated. Our sample article informs us that this particular study used "a cross-sectional national descriptive/correlational survey of critical-care nurses employed in acute medical-surgical hospitals." We understand that instead of a design in which two or more groups are compared on some characteristic or another (an experimental design), this study mailed a survey to a national sample of critical-care nurses and then correlated certain responses with other responses.

Materials are the measurement devices used to collect data from the subjects. One might use a questionnaire, a thermometer, or an interview, but whatever the instrument, the researcher should tell you whether he or she used a new instrument constructed especially for this study or an older instrument developed by somebody else (see Chapter 11). The author should describe exactly how the measurements were done and particularly report on a self-developed instrument's *validity* and *reliability* (see Glossary). If the instrument comes from somewhere else but is modified for use in the study being reported, the author should explain how the original was modified. In our sample article the instruments were described like this:

Sample Description of Instruments

A one-page questionnaire, printed on two sides called the *Unit Form*, contained closed-ended items. The questions were designed to elicit information about the institution (hospital) and the unit (CCU). Face validity of the items was assumed on the basis of the demographic nature of the items and simplicity of the format. Pretesting of the instrument on a small national sample of hospitals ($n = 24$) revealed no omitted responses and no apparent inconsistencies in the data.

The *Staff Nurse Selection Sheet* consisted of a one-page grid, which required the head nurse to list full-time registered nurses working the day or evening shift. . . . No changes in this instrument were needed on the basis of pretesting during the pilot study.

The *Nurse Form* was designed to obtain a national picture of current coronary care practices and to provide data for the analysis of the diffusion of the results of published research relating to two specific practices; the restriction of ice water and the restriction of rectal temperature measurement. The form consisted of a five-page questionnaire, divided into three parts. The first page contained explicit directions and described the clinical situation of an uncomplicated MI patient. . . . All the forms and the method were pretested in the pilot study. After the completion of the pilot study and preliminary analysis, the revised instruments were submitted to a nationally recognized cardiovascular nurse clinician for review [Kirchoff, pp. 197–198].

The procedure section describes how the study was conducted. Remember, it is supposed to include enough detail so that a reader could replicate the study. Here's an excerpt from our sample article to give you a sense of how detailed the procedure discussion was:

Sample Procedure

A letter addressed to the director of nursing was mailed to each of the randomly selected institutions. At the sample time, a cover letter, Unit Form, Staff Nurse Selection Sheet, and a return stamped envelope were sent to the "Head Nurse, CCU" at each of the selected hospitals. A second letter and an additional copy of the Unit Form and Staff Nurse Selection Sheet along with another return envelope were sent to all head nurses who had not responded within three weeks. After another three and a half weeks, a third similar follow-up was sent to those nurses. . . . Attempts were made to contact the remaining head nurses by phone. About two months after the beginning of the first-stage mailing, with a majority of the responses from the CCU's received, the second-stage mailing was initiated [Kirchoff, p. 198].

You can either skim through the specifics of the write-up of a study's procedure quickly to move to the results, or you can use it as a step-by-step road map to critique or replicate a study.

Results   The results of a study tend to be reported in the text, summarized in tables, or presented visually in a graph or figure (see Chapter 17). It is absolutely critical that you be able to understand and evaluate the results of any study that you read. Sometimes researchers have used a statistical test incorrectly (see Chapter 15), sometimes they have drawn conclusions that go far beyond what can be justified by the sample and study design, and sometimes the tables are inconsistent with what the authors explain in the text. The results of our sample study were reported in the text like this:

Sample Results

Avoiding the use of rectal thermometer and restricting ice water received moderate importance and frequency ratings but large standard deviations, indicating high variability among the sample of nurses. . . . The most common origin for practice of both these restrictions is unit policy. . . . The most important nurse variable in a multiple regression is the number of years since most recent graduation, but the total explained variance despite the inclusion of 10 significant variables was only 6%. . . . Reading the *American Journal of Nursing*, the number of journals read and the hours spent reading per week were significantly correlated with level of awareness that the coronary care precautions were being questioned. But the effect of awareness (reading) on persuasion (the importance ratings) and on adoption (the frequency ratings) showed no significant differences. . . . *Being aware did not affect how important the nurses thought the restrictions were or how frequently they reported practicing the restrictions* [Kirchoff, p. 200].

Discussion   The preceding section on results presents a report of how the statistical analysis turned out. The discussion section explains what the results mean with regard to the study's purposes and relates them to a theoretical context (see Chapter 10). Many authors also use this part of a research article to tell us why they think their results turned out the way they did and to suggest new types of study for future research. Sometimes the discussion section is called "Conclusions." Our sample study conveys the nontechnical interpretation of the study findings this way:

Sample Discussion

Coronary precautions are widely practiced. The awareness of published studies has not changed practice. Although the passive diffusion [of research results] process has some effect on awareness, it has little effect on persuasion or adoption. . . . Some studies require a translation process before they are put to use. . . . Passive diffusion of research results is inadequate, unsure, and slow. A process of active intervention on the part of those nurses qualified to evaluate completed studies is needed [Kirchoff, p. 201].

Our sample study also presents some of the results in tables. The final section of this chapter is devoted to overcoming some of the obstacles to interpreting visual representations of study findings.

References   A research article ends with a list of books and articles to which the author referred during the study report. This list can be a useful resource if you want to tackle a comparative reading of the major ideas associated with a topic. Reading the references cited at the end of a study report can also familiarize you with the findings and logic that led the author up to the study being reported. The reference list at the conclusion of our sample article includes articles and books on research utilization and communication of findings as well as on coronary care precautions.

Now that we have at least an initial idea of what the article is about and have decided that it is of interest to us, we are in a position to read it at an analytic level with a particular eye toward coming to terms with the research terminology in context (see Chapter 2).

Coming to Terms with Research Terminology

Concepts, Constructs, Conceptual Frameworks, and Theory

Concepts are abstractions that allow us to categorize observations based on certain commonalities and differences. For example, nurses study a diverse array of concepts including *infection, bonding, activity level, elimination, stress, coping, loss, pain, self-esteem, accountability, self-care, rhymicity, locus of control, limiting intrusion,* and *institutionalization,* among others. Some concepts are names for concrete observations that can be measured directly, and others rely on what are called "proxy measures," because they cannot be directly measured by counting pulse rate or respirations or some other directly observable phenomenon. (See Chapter 15 for more on measurement scales and measuring.)

Certain more abstract concepts are called *constructs,* because they have been created (constructed) by scientists for a research purpose. Examples of constructs include *positive reinforcement* from learning theory, *learned helplessness* from psychology, *bureaucratization* and *social class* from sociology, and in the case of our example study, *diffusion of innovation,* probably from social psychology and communication theory. Science is concerned with explaining and refining the concepts that classify and make sense of the order in the world and with generalizing from the specific or particular to the abstract, that is, with generating and testing theories. (See Chapter 10 for more on theory and theoretical frameworks.) In our example, concepts included in the study were not only the major one, *diffusion of innovation,* but also *coronary precautions,* and *communication channels.* We are introduced to these concepts and the process of mental relations (awareness, persuasion, decision, and confirmation of decision) in a section of the early part of the article headed "Conceptual Framework." Here we learn that others (Rogers & Shoemaker 1971) formulated relationships between and among the concepts and constructs in this study in a model that included a source (researchers), an innovation (the discontinuance of two coronary precaution restrictions), communication channels (research publications), and communication receivers (staff nurses in coronary care units).

Operationally Defining a Concept

Although many of us can function adequately with a highly personal or even vague idea of what a concept means in day-to-day practice, a researcher must translate the concepts in his or her study into variables that can validly represent the concept under investigation and reliably be measured (see Chapter 9). An *operational definition* of a concept specifies what a researcher does to make the concept measurable. It defines a concept so that someone else will measure it in the same way. When concepts have been operationalized, they are called *variables*—meaning something that varies and has different values that can be measured. For something to be called a variable, therefore, it must be able to have at least two values. *Sex* is a variable; *female* is not a variable, but rather a value for the variable sex. Many studies are criticized primarily on the approach the researcher has used to operationalize concepts that are being studied. It is the researcher's job to try to make his or her operational definitions plausible in the eyes of critical readers. (We'll talk about how one accomplishes this goal in Chapters 7 and 8.) In order to replicate someone's study, we have to know how the concepts and other terms were defined. They are usually defined according to their relationship to the problem being studied in a particular investigation. In our sample study the study *settings* were coronary care units, selected using a stratified random sampling procedure, in accredited hospitals that were willing to participate. The *individual nurses* were randomly selected staff nurses (every possible sample member had an equal chance of being selected) identified by head nurses as "registered nurses with at least one year of experience in the unit, at least 75% of time spent in patient care, full-time employment, and assignment to the day or evening shift." In addition, the head nurses from participating units were included in the mailing. If you want to use research results from this or any other study in your own work, you have to look to operational definitions that are closest to your own definitions of concepts and other terms.

Distinguishing Independent and Dependent Variables

Variables are often labeled as *dependent* or *independent*. The *dependent variable* (DV), also called the output or criterion variable, is the study variable that is under investigation. It's the one that the researcher determines *as a result* of conducting the study. In some cases it is the *effect* or *outcome* of an experimental procedure. The variability in the dependent variable presumably *depends* on the cause or conditions that may be manipulated by the researcher in the study. The dependent variables in our ex-

ample study were the persuasion about and adoption of research findings about coronary precautions. In most studies the dependent variables are the ones that the researcher is intending to understand, explain, or predict. The dependent variables in our example are measures of the outcome of innovation diffusion. They constitute what the researcher measures about the subjects *after* they have experienced or been exposed to the independent variable.

Independent variables (IVs), on the other hand, are the causes or conditions that the investigator manipulates or identifies to determine the effects or outcomes. Their values are established independently by the investigator ahead of time. They constitute the *input* of an experiment and precede the measurement of the dependent variable.

It is usually not too hard to spot the difference between the independent variables and the dependent variable(s) in a research study. Sometimes they are alluded to in the study title: "A Diffusion Survey of Coronary Precautions" means that the study is about the impact of the diffusion of research knowledge about coronary precautions on the practice arena. The statement of study purpose sometimes reveals that an investigator has set out to establish the effects of something (IV) on something else (DV) (for example, the effects of preoperative teaching on postoperative recovery or of therapeutic touch on perception of pain). The same statement is sometimes made in reverse order: "This study was conducted to see whether a client's self-esteem [DV] was affected by changes in levels of physical exercise [IV]." In both cases, though, the investigator is doing the same thing: manipulating or selecting an IV or several of them to determine whether it (they) affects or changes measurements in the DV(s).

It is possible to have both multiple dependent variables and multiple independent variables, but all must be operationally defined. In our study example the investigator correlated nurse variables that included *11* independent variable measures with two important coronary

Table 4-1   Correlation of Two Importance Ratings with Nurse Variables [a]

Nurse Variable		Ice Water (n)	Restrictions Rectal Temperature Measurement (r)	(n)
Years since basic education	.13 [d]	513	.04	518
Years since most recent education	.13 [c]	512	.08 [b]	517
Years of nursing experience	.12 [c]	516	.06	521
Years of CCU experience	.07 [b]	516	−.01	521
Years of experience in unit	.03	513	−.01	518
AACN membership	.00	515	−.03	520
ANA membership	.06	515	.08 [b]	520
Reads AJN	.00	519	.08 [b]	513
Reads Heart & Lung	.00	519	−.11 [c]	513
Number of journals read	.06	519	−.01	513
Hours week reading journals	.01	506	−.05	510

[a] Pearson Product-Moment Correlation

[b] p < .05

[c] p < .01

[d] p < .001

SOURCE: K. T. Kirchoff, "A Diffusion Survey of Coronary Precautions," *Nursing Research*, July/August 1982, vol. 31, p. 199.

care restrictions—on ice water and on rectal temperature-taking (see Table 4-1). Together, these independent and dependent variables allowed her to reach conclusions about research knowledge diffusion, at least when it came to CCU nurses and patients and the practice of coronary precautions.

Uncontrolled, or Confounding, Variables

So far everything seems straightforward in our sample article's new vocabulary. The investigator has decided on what the independent and dependent variables are to be and operationally defined them. She has obtained a sufficiently large sample, using a stratified random sampling procedure of accredited hospitals that have CCUs and nurses doing patient care on them who meet certain criteria. She has collected data

about them, using a series of survey forms that allow her to classify them along 11 "nurse variables" related to her study question about innovation diffusion. She has obtained dependent variable data from her subjects by asking about awareness and persuasion ratings on two important coronary-care precautions, restrictions on ice water and rectal temperature measurement. Finally, based on our outline of the typical format for a scientific article, you would expect her to interpret her statistical results and draw conclusions. But it isn't always that simple. The researcher has to take into consideration other relevant variables that might have effects on the DV other than or in addition to the IVs. If these other variables are not taken into account, they can confuse the interpretation of a study's results, because they confound the effects of the IV. Not surprisingly, they are therefore called *confounding variables*, which, if they are not controlled in the study design or procedure, may be called *uncontrolled variables. Extraneous variables* is yet another term that may be used to refer to these factors.

In our sample study report the researcher concluded that the effect of awareness (reading) on persuasion (the importance ratings for both restrictions) and on adoption (the frequency ratings) as determined by a statistical test called analysis of variance (ANOVA—see Chapter 15) was not significant or meaningful. That is, reading or being aware of research that challenged the value of the coronary-care precautions did not affect how important the nurses thought the precautions were or how frequently they practiced them. The investigator decided to take a look at any possible confounding variables that might account for her study findings. In doing so, her statistical analysis allowed her to add the following information about potential confounding variables:

1. Larger medical centers in urban locations, with educational programs for nurses, had significant but weak relationships to lower ratings on the frequency and importance of the two questioned coronary-care precautions.

2. Federal and nonprofit institutions had lower importance and frequency ratings for the rectal temperature measurement.

3. Nurses employed in units that used special procedures for measuring cardiac output (thermodilution technique) had lower ratings for restriction of ice water.

Including both head nurses and staff nurses and reporting these additional findings about practices on the unit that were not among the independent variable measurement list was one way that this researcher attempted to "control" for potentially confounding variables.

Hypotheses

A *hypothesis* is the statement of relationships the researcher expects to find between a study's independent and dependent variables (see Chapter 9). This statement might be in the form of a question, but more often the question is called the study problem, and the hypothesis is a declarative sentence. This statement may be designated by the symbol H, or H_0 if the researcher is going to test the reverse of his or her hypotheses. In the latter case, H_0 is called the "null hypothesis" (see Chapter 9). If there are several hypotheses in any single study, a number might follow the letter H (H_1, H_2, H_3). Some studies are designed to *generate rather than test* preconceived hypotheses (see Chapters 9, 10, and 14) and thus don't begin with any formally stated hunches, let alone hypotheses about expected relationships. In our sample study's survey design, formal hypotheses weren't stated from the outset. But one might assume that the researcher had an informal hunch that being aware of the research literature would indeed influence practice decisions about coronary precautions—a hunch that was *not* substantiated in the study data.

Data

Data are the information the investigator collects from the subjects or participants in the research study. The values for variables or concerns in a study constitute its data. The data on importance and frequency (and difference) for selected CCU nursing actions collected in the course of our example study are summarized in Table 4-2. (Note that when referring to *data*, because it is a plural noun, the proper verb is *are* or *were*, not *is* or *was*.)

Instruments

Instruments are the devices used to record the data obtained from subjects. Many instruments are used in nursing studies, including interview transcripts, questionnaires, intelligence tests, rating scales, performance checklists, pencil and paper tests, and biological measurement devices (see Chapters 11, 12 and 13). Among the most

Table 4-2   Importance and Frequency Ratings and Difference Scores for Selected CCU Nursing Actions (*n* = 524 Nurses)

CCU Nursing Action	Importance (I)		Frequency (F)		Difference (I − F)	
	M	s	M	s	M	s
Insure EKG monitoring	6.98	.14	6.92	.37	.06	.37
Assess chest pain quality	6.88	.41	6.55	.82	.33	.73
Relieve anxiety	6.75	.53	6.17	1.00	.58	.93
Maintain IV	6.74	.90	6.74	.91	−.01	.53
Provide quiet	6.43	.84	5.53	1.25	.90	1.23
Teach Valsalva avoidance	6.30	1.12	5.68	1.58	.60	1.30
Restrict coffee[a]	6.00	1.46	6.16	1.52	−.16	1.29
Restrict visiting time	5.89	1.24	5.32	1.38	.36	1.26
Check temperature/4 hours	5.62	1.46	6.09	1.35	−.47	1.16
Bathe the patient	5.46	1.64	5.75	1.48	−.28	1.23
Avoid rectal thermometer use[a]	5.37	1.85	5.96	1.91	−.09	1.63
Restrict cola[a]	5.32	1.72	5.13	2.06	.19	1.60
Provide sedative at night	5.28	1.24	5.09	1.16	.19	1.02
Restrict ice water only[a]	4.90	2.15	5.15	2.22	−.22	1.68
Restrict tea[a]	4.76	1.96	4.28	2.31	.47	1.74
Restrict fluid intake	4.63	1.83	4.30	1.80	.33	1.19
Restrict cold fluids[a]	4.35	2.04	4.32	2.15	.04	1.51
Avoid vigorous back rub[a]	4.08	2.07	4.26	1.97	−.18	1.67
Restrict hot fluids[a]	3.81	2.07	3.70	2.17	.12	1.51
Feed the patient	2.92	1.91	3.10	1.84	−.20	1.46
Give bedpan for defecation	2.78	1.87	3.32	1.84	−.55	1.54

[a]Coronary precaution item

SOURCE: K. T. Kirchoff, "A Diffusion Survey of Coronary Precautions," *Nursing Research*, July/August 1982, vol 31, p. 199.

important questions to evaluate when sizing up the worth of any instruments used to measure variables in a nursing study are their *reliability* and *validity*. A reliable instrument will produce consistent results, or data, on repeated use, usually because the investigator has standardized the procedure for administering it. Taking a blood pressure several times and obtaining the same readings given unchanged conditions is an example of a reliable measure. A valid instrument is one that measures what it is supposed to measure. A paper and pencil test of a client's knowledge about his or her diabetic diet may measure reading skill rather than grasp of nutritional information. Obviously this issue is a lot more complicated when you are measuring an abstract variable such as professional commitment or social network than when you are measuring a more direct and concrete one such as weight, height, or temperature (see also Chapters 11 and 12).

Population and Sample

The *population* for a study (symbolized by a capital N) is the total possible membership of the group being studied. But because it is not always feasible to study everybody, a microcosm of the population, called a *sample* (designated by a lower-case *n*) of participants or respondents is usually selected. In the instance of our sample study, the *n* was 600 staff nurses and 235 eligible hospitals. Of these, 524 nurses returned usable questionnaires after three mailings, yielding a *response rate* of 87.3%. Completed questionnaires were received from head nurses from 202, or 86%, of the eligible sample. When a sample is representative, the investigator is in a better position to conclude that the study results are generalizable to the entire population of nurses and settings that make up the universe applicable to the study.

Hawthorne and Halo Effects

The Hawthorne and the Halo effects are two other terms that are often used when talking about research studies. The *Hawthorne effect* refers to the change in people's observed behavior that occurs merely because they know they are being studied. (It was first observed in the Hawthorne plant of the Western Electric Company.) Subsequent studies have discovered that productivity or job satisfaction can change temporarily when management makes a change of any kind, purportedly due to the extra attention workers believe they are receiving. The Hawthorne effect can occur in all kinds of study situations when data reflect the effects of the study itself.

The *halo effect* refers to an observer's tendency to rate certain subjects as consistently high or low on everything because of the overall impression that the subject gives the rater. Strategies to lessen the effects of inaccurate responses include the *double-blind* method of studying a particular care or treatment approach. In this procedure neither the care givers nor the patients know whether the experimental or control treatment procedure is being administered (see Chapter 6).

Interpreting Visual Presentations

You'll have to be the one who discovers the sometimes obscure trend hidden in a research article's table or chart. Take, for example, Table 4-3 from our sample article and use the following guidelines to help you understand it and others:

- Try to spot trends. You must see in this table that the most frequent *source* of both coronary care restrictions cited by nurses in the study sample was "unit policy."

- Decide whether the author has picked the right measure of central tendency (see Chapter 15). There are three statistical averages: the mean (the sum total divided by the number of cases); the median (the midpoint between the upper and lower halves); and the mode (the case that is most common). It's important for you to evaluate which is the *best* way to describe the central tendency for any study question.

- Pay attention to the range of numbers in charts or graphs (see Chapter 15). In reporting "Importance" and "Frequency" scores the authors of the sample article write: "Avoiding the use of rectal temperatures and restricting ice water received moderate importance and frequency ratings, but large standard deviations indicated high variability among the sample nurses" (p. 199) (see Table 4-4).

- Look for exceptions. In Table 4-3 we can see that the category "missing data" accounted for only 8 and 12 of the 524 sample members.

Table 4-3 Type of Restriction by Reported Frequencies for Origins of Restrictions ($n = 524$ Nurses)

Origins of the Restrictions	Type of Restriction	
	Ice Water	Rectal Temperature Measurement
Not ordered	117	180
Physician	34	20
Unit policy	312	252
Nurses	30	35
Combinations of above	15	16
Other	8	9
Missing data	8	12
Total	524	524

SOURCE: K. T. Kirchoff, "A Diffusion Survey of Coronary Precautions," *Nursing Research*, July/August 1982, vol. 31, p. 199.

Had the number of exceptions been large, we would evaluate the apparent trends differently.

- Compare figures presented in the text with those in the charts and tables, keeping alert for contradictions or inconsistencies.

- Read the captions that accompany tables and figures carefully and compare them with the results and discussion presented in the text. Together they will tell you a great deal about any study that you read.

- Look up unfamiliar statistics to determine if they were used correctly. Chapter 15 in this text offers resources. A good basic statistics book is another source.

Know Their Data

In the methodology corner of *Nursing Research*'s July/August 1981 issue, Dr. Barbara S. Jacobsen wrote a guest essay entitled "Know Thy Data." She commented that inferential and confirmatory data analyses were rapidly becoming more widespread in nursing studies, perhaps because nurse researchers have greater access to and skill in using computers to analyze their data. An unfortunate side effect, according

to the author, is that "researchers know their F ratio and p values (statistics), but do not know their data. . . . Confirmatory design and analyses may be easier to teach and computerize, but all too often it is learned in a mechanistic way and performed as a ritual" (p. 254).

The consequence of this is that you may be forced to make false interpretations of statistics. Jacobsen reports an incident in which an excited researcher raved that the computer had isolated a "key variable" in her questionnaire that correlated with everything! (Correlation shows the extent to which values of one variable are related to values of another variable.) Often these correlations were difficult to explain. An illustration of the latter case was that "number of people living in the household correlated with a measure of depression." It took a scatter diagram printout that looked like Figure 4-1 to illuminate the mystery. The two outliers (subjects who were very different from the rest of the group) simply lived in large institutions and also happened coincidentally to be depressed. When their scores were removed, the positive correlations between numbers of people in the household and depression score changed to reveal the *absence* of any correlation. The

Table 4-4   Factor Loadings for Importance Ratings of Selected CCU Nursing Actions with Rotated Factor Matrix (*n* = 524)

Nursing Action	Factor 1 Temperature	Factor 2 Caffeine	Factor 3 Rest	Factor 4 Psychological	Factor 5 Cardiac Stimulants
Restrict cold fluids[a]	.85	.21	.23	−.01	.09
Restrict ice water only[a]	.46	.18	.04	.12	.10
Restrict hot fluids[a]	.75	.20	.13	.01	.11
Restrict coffee[a]	.22	.63	.00	.15	.21
Restrict tea[a]	.20	.65	.12	.03	.05
Restrict cola[a]	.17	.84	.12	.06	.09
Feed the patient	.16	.11	.58	.01	.10
Give bedpan for defecation	−.01	.01	.61	.03	.05
Avoid vigorous back rub[a]	.31	.12	.33	.02	.25
Relieve anxiety	.00	.03	−.01	.60	.07
Provide quiet	.12	.09	.16	.64	.12
Avoid rectal thermometer use[a]	.22	.17	.11	.08	.50
Teach Valsalva avoidance	.08	.12	.13	.25	.45
Eigenvalue	4.46	1.80	1.51	1.15	1.10
% Total variance	21.3	8.60	7.2	5.5	5.2
Cumulative % total variance	21.3	29.8	37.0	42.5	47.7

[a]Coronary precaution item

SOURCE: K. T. Kirchoff, "A Diffusion Survey of Coronary Precautions," *Nursing Research*, July/August 1982, vol. 31, p. 198.

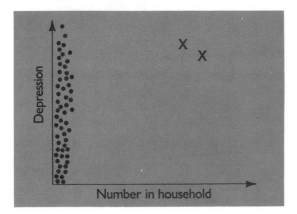

Figure 4-1 Scatter diagram

visual diagram of score frequencies solved the mystery.

Extreme scores in a data set can likewise make it appear that no relationship exists between two variables. A single outlier (extreme score) can invalidate means, standard deviations, regression coefficients, and *t* tests. Jacobsen maintains that visual presentations (see Figure 4-2) can help a researcher know when to question the validity of statistical analyses. They can help you uncover patterns in the data that offer suggestions and cues for future research and enable you to better "know *their* data" (see also Chapter 17).

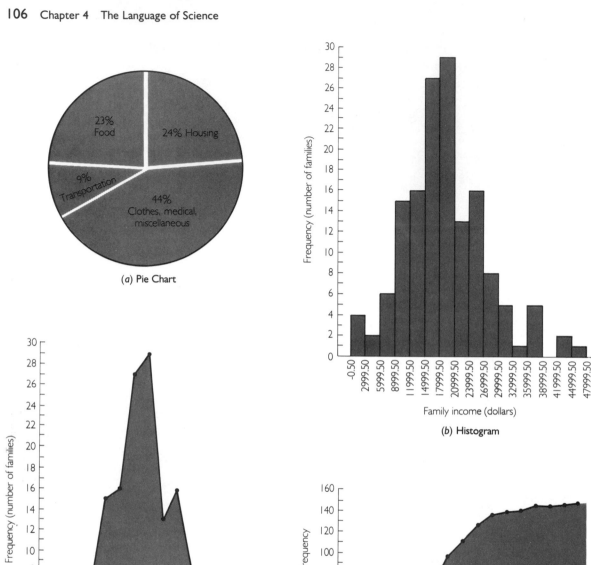

(a) Pie Chart

(b) Histogram

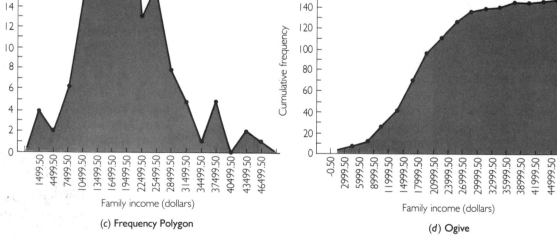

(c) Frequency Polygon

(d) Ogive

Figure 4-2 Types of graphs.

Summary of Key Ideas and Terms

✔ You can popularize a piece of scientific writing *for yourself* and make it more readable by *mentally* translating long or impersonal sentences and words into your own plain, conversational talk.

✔ The format for a typical research journal article usually follows these headings: (1) abstract, (2) introduction, (3) method, (4) results, (5) discussion, and (6) references. Each has a standard location and purpose that you can anticipate.

✔ Concepts, constructs, conceptual frameworks, and theories are abstractions that are used to classify observations of patterns in the world.

✔ An operational definition of a concept or construct specifies what a researcher does to measure it so as to be sure others will interpret its meaning in the same way.

✔ Independent variables (IVs) are the causes, conditions, and inputs that are established or manipulated before measuring the dependent variable(s).

✔ Dependent variables (DVs) are measures of outcome and consequences that depend on exposure to the independent variable.

✔ Confounding, extraneous, or uncontrolled variables are all those variables that might also affect the dependent variable and confuse your interpretation of the effects of a study's independent variable(s).

✔ Hypotheses are statements of relationship that the investigator expects to find between a study's independent and dependent variables.

✔ Data are the information collected from a study's subjects or participants.

✔ Instruments are the tools or devices used to collect data or information from study subjects.

✔ The population is the total possible membership of the group being studied.

✔ The sample is a microcosm of the population selected as actual participants or respondents.

➤ The Hawthorne effect refers to the tendency of people's behavior to change just because they know they are being studied.

➤ The halo effect refers to a person's inclination to respond to an entire set of items or questions in the same way or to an observer's tendency to rate subjects based on the overall impression that they have made.

➤ You can increase your ability to correctly interpret visual presentations of data in tables and graphs by (1) trying to spot trends, (2) deciding whether the author has used the best measure of central tendency, (3) paying attention to the variability in a data set, (4) looking for exceptions and outliers in the data, (5) comparing figures presented in tables with those in the text, (6) reading captions for figures and tables, and (7) looking up unfamiliar statistics in a basic statistics book.

References

Campbell DT, Stanley JC: *Experimental and Quasi-Experimental Designs for Research.* Chicago: Rand McNally, 1966.

Flesch R: *How to Write, Speak, and Think More Effectively.* New York: Harper & Row, 1960.

Hays WL: *Statistics for the Social Sciences.* New York: Holt, Rinehart & Winston, 1973.

Huck S, Cormier W, Bounds W: *Reading Statistics and Research.* New York: Harper & Row, 1974.

Jacobsen B: Know thy data. *Nurs Res* July/August 1981; 30:254–255.

Kaplan A: *The Conduct of Inquiry: Methodology for Behavioral Sciences.* San Francisco: Chandler, 1964.

Kirchoff KT: A diffusion survey of coronary precautions. *Nurs Res* July/August 1982; 31:196–201.

American Nurses' Association, Commission on Nursing Research: *Research in Nursing: Toward a Science of Health Care.* Kansas City, Mo.: American Nurses' Association, 1976.

Rogers EM, Shoemaker F: *Communication of Innovations*, 2nd ed. New York: Free Press, 1971.

Further Readings

Fawcett J: Editorial: On development of a scientific community in nursing. *Image* 1980; 12:51–52.

Notter L: Editorial: The research attitude begins on the undergraduate level. *Nurs Res* March/April 1974; 23:99.

Newman MA: What differentiates clinical research? *Image* 1982; 14:86.

Parker ML, Labadie GC: Demystifying research mystique. *Nurs Health Care* September 1983:383–386.

Spector NC, Bleeks SL: Strategies to improve students' attitudes to research. *Nurs Outlook* May 1980:300–304.

Chapter 5

Discovering Research Problems in Clinical Practice

Nurses' Investigative Role

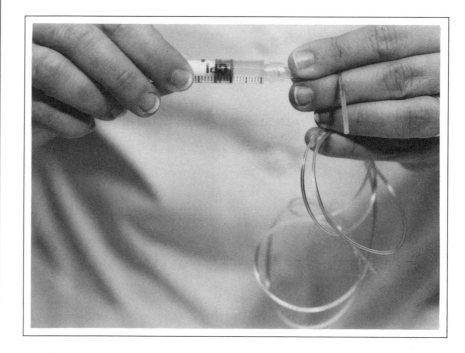

Theoretical and clinical sensitivity begin with your ability to raise important and meaningful questions in the course of giving nursing care.

Chapter Objectives

After reading this chapter, the student should be able to:

- Recognize sources of research problems
- Distinguish between researchable and nonresearchable clinical questions
- Describe why "value" questions and "yes or no" questions are not amenable to answering with the scientific method
- Compare and contrast types of research problems, including factor-isolating, factor-relating, situation-describing, and situation-predicting questions
- Formulate a researchable problem from a general topic area of interest
- Evaluate problem statements in published research reports according to the criteria of significance, researchability, and feasibility
- Appreciate problem identification as an investigative role for all nurses regardless of their level of preparation

In This Chapter . . .

Building a scientific basis for nursing practice requires a wide variety of investigative skills on the part of nurses. One of the most important ones is being able to ask sensitive, astute, and potentially *researchable* questions in practice situations. Clinicians are in the best possible position to converse with colleagues and patients and learn about how they interpret their experiences. A nurse who sees research as inquiry, not just technical instrumentation, will watch and listen for the underlying reality of the practice world. A nurse with an inquiring mind will develop skills in observing and analyzing that help him or her *discover* important questions and problems in the course of giving nursing care. Each dressing change, catheterization, and bed bath becomes an opportunity not only to care for other human beings but also to learn about topics that demand research-based explanations. Theoretical and clinical sensitivity begin with your ability to raise the important and meaningful questions in your nursing practice. In fact, the American Nurses' Association's Commission on Nursing Research agreed that (1) demonstrating awareness of the value and relevance of research in nursing, (2) assisting in

identifying problem areas in nursing practice, and (3) assisting in collecting data within a structured format have become investigative functions that *all nurses*, including those prepared in diploma and associate degree programs, should be able to perform (ANA 1981a). In the language of the commission:

Building a scientific base for clinical practice is the priority for nursing research in the 1980's. To maximize the benefits of developing a scientific base for use in practice, mechanisms are required that ensure that scientific knowledge contributes to practice and in turn that the problems encountered in practice have an impact on the focus of the knowledge generated. Nurses performing different roles in nursing contribute to the interplay between practice and research (ANA 1981b).

This chapter gives you strategies for thinking about sources of research questions and ways to differentiate between clinical problems that can be researched and those that cannot. It discusses kinds of research problem, an approach to writing them, and criteria for evaluating those that served as the basis for studies that you read or hear about.

Finding Research Problems

Research begins with a study question, or what is called a *researchable problem*. This problem may concern nursing education, nursing administration, history, ethics, or a social or natural science question related to health that interests a nurse researcher. But if it is to address the priorities cited by leaders in the profession and if it is to meet the strictest definition of nursing research, it stems most likely from nursing practice or patient care. Patient-care problems have generally been defined as difficulties or concerns experienced by patients or the nurses caring for

them. These are often situations in which there is a *discrepancy* between nursing practice as it is and what would be desirable.

Even though every clinical situation is replete with possible study questions, deciding on a specific one can be difficult for a beginning investigator. It is sometimes hard to settle on one problem when so many seem to demand attention. In other cases we are so accustomed to explaining things automatically to ourselves

Table 5-1   Experience As a Source of Research Problems

Type of Reaction	Illustration
Wishes and desires	"I wish these children wouldn't get so upset when I come in to change the dressings on their burns."
Gripes	"There's never enough time for discharge planning with these postmastectomy patients."
Questions	"I wonder if it's feasible to start a cardiac rehab program for post-MI patients here?"

based on common sense or conventional wisdom that we fail to see the possible light that could be shed through scientific inquiry. Sometimes the stress, hectic schedule, or even boring routine of our work has suffocated our tendency to be curious about connections, trends, patterns, and ideas. At other times low morale, rapid turnover, fatigue, or habit obstructs our ability to bring curiosity, imagination, and critical sensibilities to bear on our practice. But once, as Diers says (1979, p. 12), "you are in the right frame of mind, researchable problems in nursing will probably find you!"

Sources of Research Problems

Valid sources of research problems in nursing include your own experience, patterns or trends, somebody else's completed research, and your intellectual and scientific interests.

Your Own Experience   The best source of clinical research topics is probably your own experience. All of the personal reactions listed in Table 5-1 can be turned around into researchable questions.

Patterns or Trends   A second major source of research problems can be tapped when a practitioner makes the imaginative leap that transforms an undifferentiated accumulation of individual cases into a reasoned pattern. It takes an inventive mind to notice the way a particular

phenomenon occurs and to become involved in asking why. Such a nurse becomes an observer and interpreter of reality. One curious nurse working with patients in a nursing home noted certain incidents over a three-month period (see example).

Example: Trends in Using Psychotropic Medication Among Elderly Clients

Hazel S. came to the nursing home when her husband Sam of over 60 years was admitted because of a bout with pneumonia. Since no one else was available to look after her, she was admitted with him. Her anxiety and confusion over Sam's illness resulted in a prescription for regular Mellaril. She subsequently became stuporous and combative. She lost control of bowel and bladder function and was confined to bed. Weeks later when her husband took her home and she was no longer over-sedated, her orientation returned completely to normal.

Mary M., an 80-year-old woman with dementia, was admitted to a nursing home screaming. Thorazine was prescribed to "quiet her down." A week later we discovered that she had a fractured femur.

Jerry C., a 74-year-old man, became confused and agitated following loss of consciousness after a fall. He was given Thorazine but became more disruptive, so Haldol and Mellaril were added. He finally developed a severe parkinsonian syndrome that led to discontinuation of his drug therapy. From then on his mental status improved dramatically.

This nurse's list of anecdotes and case studies extended beyond the few examples described above. She eventually began to wonder whether *as a pattern* nursing home staff members tended to use psychotropic agents continuously to ease their burden rather than episodically to ease the temporary distress of the elderly patients. Her observations of a pattern resulted in a national survey that addressed questions of misuse of psychotropic drugs in nursing homes with elderly patients. Her findings had a direct impact on changing patient care for the better.

Somebody Else's Completed Research Research problems that don't develop from your own first-hand experience are often suggested by literature that reports the work of others. Sometimes specific recommendations that a study be replicated with another group of patients or in another setting prompt research. At other times an author's suggestions for further research in the discussion section of his or her report of findings can be a source of a study question. Most often, however, study questions are stimulated when you read about contradictory results or controversial nursing issues that have limited or no empirical findings on which to base a conclusion or decision. For example, recent research on the relationship between holding and touching newborns in the delivery room and subsequent parental bonding has yielded mixed results.

Similarly, questions about the advisability of a 25-pound weight gain during pregnancy, seven-day-a-week jogging, and the growing array of diets pour out of contradictory "hospital studies." Not only can a review of others' published research help you formulate a researchable question, but it can also guide you in deciding whether replicating the work of others is useful or unnecessary. You need not confine your reading to the formal research reports of others. Case studies and clinical descriptions often yield valuable nuggets of what Diers (1979, p. 25) calls "clinical nursing wisdom." In using this kind of literature you can build up a rich accu-

mulation of common events and experiences and compare them with your own to discover themes and patterns that lead to research questions.

Your Intellectual and Scientific Interests The major difference between research topics that grow out of real-world practical concerns and those that are primarily dictated by scientific interest is that the latter are less likely to involve study of a particular clinical situation for the sake of knowledge that can be used in *that situation*. Research topics generated from scientific interests usually concern themselves with more general and abstract explanations of phenomena. Questions that derive from this source are directed toward developing an organized accounting of the universe by discovering systematic relatedness out of what seems at times to be a bewildering collection of unconnected statements and descriptions of facts and events.

Despite continuous polemics about nursing's focus, mission, responsibilities, and scope of practice, much of nursing science remains a grab-bag collection of data, unverified assumptions, ritualized practices, and vague hunches. Some research questions are expressly directed toward developing a grand theory of nursing that would fit together nursing concepts into logical and systematic relationships (see Chapter 10). The accompanying example on p. 114 illustrates such a study.

Gill and Atwood's question illustrates research intended to test the applicability of a nursing theory under real-world conditions. Box 5-1 summarizes the priorities for clinical research and selected examples identified by the ANA's Commission on Nursing Research.

Identifying Research Problems

Identifying a research question is one of the earliest steps in the research process (see Chapter 1), and the subsequent procedures depend on its being clear and explicit. There are unfortunately

Example: An Experiment in Healing

Nurse researchers Barbara Gill and Jan Atwood published a report in *Nursing Research* (March/April, 1981) entitled "Reciprocy and Helicy Used to Relate mE6F and Wound Healing." The concepts *reciprocy* and *helicy* are drawn from the homeo-dynamics principles of Martha Rogers's theory of nursing. They deal with "the integration between human and environmental fields, and the unidirectionality of their curvilinear progression along the space–time dimension" (p. 68). Their research asked if these two concepts adequately organize and explain the healing and/or reepithelialization of a small epidermal wound made on the back of a young Yorkshire-mix pig.

A grand theory of nursing

Test of Rogers' theory in a clinical situation

no foolproof rules to guide a researcher in formulating truly significant questions about a topic. He or she can only try to create the conditions that some experts believe are conducive to formulating important problems. These conditions are:

- systematic immersion in the subject by first-hand observation
- study of existing literature and discussion with people who have accumulated practical experience in the field
- maintaining a critical, curious and imaginative frame of mind in order to be alert to the new and unexpected

Whenever you find yourself surprised, frustrated, or puzzled, or whenever you express a complaint, a wish, a question, or a hope, you have the basis for a research problem that can be refined under the conditions above.

Nonresearchable Questions   By this time you must be convinced that a constant parade of research questions is passing before your eyes each day in your clinical work. But all questions that are personally interesting to you or even clinically relevant are not necessarily researchable ones. If you are going to participate in research yourself or evaluate the usefulness of research

that you read, you must be able to make the distinction. *A researchable problem is one that can be investigated using the process of scientific inquiry set out in Chapter 1.* Two major types of nonresearchable question need to be differentiated from questions that can direct scientific inquiry. These are (1) "value" questions and (2) "yes or no" questions. Let's look briefly at each to see why they don't qualify as sound researchable questions.

Questions of value are "should" questions. They seek information that reflects the values that people have or the policies that institutions have. You can recognize them because they either start with the word *should* or include it in the question. For example:

- Should all mothers be encouraged to breast-feed?
- Should all fathers participate in the experience of labor?
- Should nurses on pediatric units wear white uniforms?
- Should hospital shifts be 8 hours or 12 hours in length?
- What should be the nurse's role in hospice care?
- What should be the educational level for entry to professional practice?

Box 5-1 ANA Priorities for Clinical Research

Topic priority should be given to nursing research that would generate knowledge to guide practice in:

1. Promoting health, well-being, and competency for personal care among all age groups;

2. Preventing health problems throughout the life span that have the potential to reduce productivity and satisfaction;

3. Decreasing the negative impact of health problems on coping abilities, productivity, and life satisfaction of individuals and families;

4. Ensuring that the care needs of particularly vulnerable groups are met through appropriate strategies;

5. Designing and developing health care systems that are cost-effective in meeting the nursing needs of the population; and

6. Promoting health, well-being, and competency for personal health in all age groups.

Examples of research consistent with these priorities include the following:

- Identification of determinants (personal and environmental, including social support networks) of wellness and health functioning in individuals and families, e.g., avoidance of abusive behaviors such as alcoholism and drug use, successful adaptation to chronic illness, and coping with the last days of life.

- Identification of phenomena that negatively influence the course of recovery and that may be alleviated by nursing practice, such as anorexia, diarrhea, sleep deprivation, deficiencies in nutrients, electrolyte imbalances, and infections.

- Development and testing of care strategies to do the following:

  Facilitate individuals' ability to adopt and maintain health-enhancing behaviors (e.g., alterations in diet and exercise).

  Enhance patients' ability to manage acute and chronic illness in such a way as to minimize or eliminate the necessity of institutionalization and maximize well-being.

  Reduce stressful responses associated with the medical management of patients (e.g., surgical procedures, intrusive examination procedures, or use of extensive monitoring devices).

  Provide more effective care to high-risk populations (e.g., maternal and child care service to vulnerable mothers and infants, family planning services to young teenagers, services designed to enhance self-care in the chronically ill and the very old).

  Enhance the care of clients culturally different from the majority (e.g., Black Americans, Mexican Americans, Native Americans) and clients with special problems (e.g., teenagers, prisoners, and the mentally ill), and the underserved (the elderly, the poor, and the rural).

- Design and assessment, in terms of effectiveness and cost, of models for delivering nursing care strategies found to be effective in clinical studies.

All of the foregoing are directly related to the priority of developing the knowledge and information needed for improvement of the practice of nursing.

While priority should be given to this form of clinical research, there is no intent to discourage other forms of nursing research. These would include such investigations as those utilizing historical and philosophical modes of inquiry, and studies of manpower for nursing education, practice, and research, as well as studies of quality assurance for nursing and those for establishment of criterion measures for practice and education.

SOURCE: American Nurses' Association, Commission on Nursing Research, *Research Priorities for the 1980's*, Kansas City, Mo.: American Nurses' Association, 1981.

As stated, none of these questions would qualify as a truly researchable one. These are questions of value. Questions that are designed to discover what values people hold can be researchable, but these are not the same as questions about what values people should hold. To transform the preceding list into researchable questions about values held, it would have to read something like this:

• What percentage of newly employed staff nurses in postpartum-care settings believe that all new mothers should be encouraged to breast-feed?

• What is the extent of agreement among first-time fathers that they should participate in the experience of labor and delivery?

• What are the opinions of pediatric nurses about the advisability of wearing white uniforms?

• What is the preferred shift length among hospital nurses?

• What definitions of the role of hospice nurse are advanced by nursing leaders in this movement?

• What do members of the ANA believe is the basic educational preparation for entry into professional nursing practice?

Translating the first list of value questions into researchable questions has involved editing out the *shoulds*. The revised list deals with statements of fact, of *what is* or of *how things compare*. In summary, as long as a proposed research question is really a matter of opinion or philosophy, it can't be answered by conventional research methods without transforming it. Research can provide a basis of facts addressing the consequences or outcomes of holding one value or policy position or another, but "should" questions are better answered by logic or persuasion than by empirical investigation.

The second category of question that does not meet the requirements of researchability comprises those that can be answered with a simple

yes or no (or even maybe). Such questions may prompt collection of facts or data, but they don't really link up to a broader theoretical problem and offer explanations or predictions. What makes research, research is its obligation to go beyond data collecting to influence theory. Examples of static "yes or no" questions are:

• Do most nurses in city hospitals have a baccalaureate degree?

• Are patients kept waiting for pain medication after they request it?

• Do patients rest well in ICUs?

• Do most prostate surgery patients become confused after surgery?

In order to qualify as researchable, these questions would have to be transformed so as to suggest a reason for bothering to collect the information needed to answer them. For example:

• What is the relationship between educational preparation of nurses and quality of care at city hospitals?

• What are the consequences of keeping patients waiting for pain medication after they request it?

• What conditions in ICUs contribute to diminished rest patterns for patients?

• What behavioral cues can nurses use to predict that a patient will become confused after prostate surgery?

These changes involved asking a question about the relationship of two variables associated with the topic of interest.

Researchable Questions Questions of value, opinion, or policy and accumulations of data can be immensely valuable in clinical problem solving. But it takes questions that produce generalizable information for guiding practice under other conditions to make a nursing problem a nursing *research* problem. Good research problems reduce a complex area of interest or topic to

Table 5-2 Types of Researchable Question

Type	Illustration
Why are things this way?	Why do some settings use primary nursing?
	Why do cancer patients without hope participate in painful experiments?
What would happen if . . . ?	What would happen if third-party payers were reimbursed specifically for nursing care?
	What would happen if all nurses were doctorally prepared?
	What would happen if sex education were taught in all the schools?
Which approach would work better?	Is group or individual counseling more effective with clients who abuse alcohol?
	Does a back rub with conversation or a back rub without conversation result in greater relaxation?
Who might benefit from this?	Would laboring mothers benefit from being encouraged to choose their own position in the delivery room?
	Would hospitalized children have faster recoveries if parents were taught to participate in their care?
	Would infant mortality rates in developing countries be influenced by a prenatal teaching program?

a set of simple questions that demand answers, answers that can be found by taking some action. The question "Should mothers bathe newborns daily?" must be transformed into "What is the relationship between daily baths for newborns, maternal bonding, and infant infections?"

Asking a clear, significant, researchable question becomes a key to subsequent decisions about research design, data collection, and data analysis. An overly complex, fuzzy, or non-researchable question bogs a study down in confusion and inconsistency. Table 5-2 summarizes some sample types of researchable question and offers an illustration of each.

As you search for your own researchable questions or advise others about doing so, remember that many of the conventional routines ingrained as "standard nursing practice" have never been scientifically studied.

Asking Research Questions

Basic Question Forms

Research questions or problems ultimately involve the use of terms that can be measured on one of the scales described in Chapter 15. These basic stem words are:

- *Who?*
- *What?*
- *When?*
- *Where?*
- *Why?*

When the stem question that is attached to a

substantive topic changes, the entire direction of the study changes. "Who" questions require that you describe and categorize such information about populations as ethnicity, sex, age, social class, race, health status, and so on. "What" questions are either specific descriptive questions or more complex "what if" questions, in which you must describe relationships. "When" and "where" questions again include specific descriptive answers, including a time frame and a location. "Why" questions seek an explanation, as do "how" questions. I began my own doctoral dissertation many years ago by asking, "How is social order possible under conditions of espoused freedom in an anti-psychiatric community?" My master's thesis several years earlier asked a "what" question—"What is the meaning of current dance forms to adolescent girls?"

Some researchers have sorted these kinds of question into what are called *levels*, suggesting that different questions are appropriate when our level of existing knowledge is at a lower or higher level. For example, if we already know a great deal about a certain topic, asking lower-level "what" or "who" questions would not be appropriate. Likewise, if we don't even know the exploratory and descriptive "whats," "whos," and "wheres," asking "how" or "why" explanation questions is premature.

Types of Research Question

One system for distinguishing among the major types of research question (and the types of answer they yield) has been advanced by nurse researchers and philosophers originally associated with the school of nursing at Yale University. According to Dickoff et al (1968a,b), these types are:

1. factor-isolating
2. factor-relating
3. situation-relating
4. situation-producing

Factor-isolating questions ask, "What is this?" They are sometimes called factor-naming questions. They isolate, describe, categorize, or name factors or situations and provide descriptive definitions. In such studies the researcher doesn't attempt to introduce a change or to test hypotheses about theory. Instead, factor-isolating questions require that the investigator characterize as fully as possible a particular phenomenon. Sample factor- or situation-isolating questions are:

- What are the properties of parental bonding?
- What are the stages of the grieving process?
- What features characterize hospitals that have low turnover and high morale and function as magnets in recruiting nurses?

Factor-relating questions can be raised after factor-isolating studies have provided at least names for the important factors operating in a situation. Factor-relating questions ask, "What is happening here?" The goal is to determine how the factors that have been identified relate to one another. In some cases a factor-relating study question has not been preceded by formal factor-isolating studies. Instead, the researcher draws on his or her own experiential knowledge or published literature to determine what the relevant factors in a given situation might be. A question such as "What is the relationship of parents' own childhood experiences to engaging in subsequent child abuse or neglect?" is a factor-relating question. Studies of drug interaction or correlates of uncomplicated postsurgical recovery are examples of others.

Situation-relating questions ask, "What will happen if . . . ?" These questions usually yield hypothesis-testing or experimental study designs in which the investigator manipulates variables to see what will happen. Two examples are "Will reinforcement in the form of a token economy program decrease phobic behavior in a particular group of psychiatric patients?" and "Will biofeedback training decrease suffering among chronic pain patients?" These questions require answers that allow the researcher to make situation-relating and explanatory statements that specify both the direction and strength of relationships (see Chapter 15).

Situation-producing questions ask, "How can I make it happen?" These questions establish explicit goals for nursing actions, develop plans or prescriptions to achieve the goals, and specify the conditions under which the goals will be accomplished. Most researchers agree that situation-producing questions are the most complicated ones to answer. Example questions might include:

- How can I intervene to prevent postoperative vomiting?

- How can I best prepare a woman for labor and delivery?

- How can nursing services be organized to promote job satisfaction and quality of care?

Many experts believe that situation-producing research questions occur at the highest level of inquiry and must be based on the other three types of study. Situation-producing, or prescribing, questions are used eventually to conduct studies that will guide activity in the empirical environment of the practice setting. They are goal based and concerned with more than what is. They ask, "What must be done in order to achieve what is desired?" Situation-producing questions are based on what Johnson terms "knowledge of control" (1968). This is knowledge of action that can change a sequence of events toward specified desirable outcomes. The task is to discover the sequence of steps that will produce the goal state from the initial state.

Writing Research Problems

A Four-Step Approach

Writing a research problem can begin with any of the sources of questions discussed earlier in this chapter. Let's take the nurse's *wish* that the burned children she took care of wouldn't get so upset when she came in to change their dressings.* To transform her wish into a researchable problem, all she need do to begin is to turn that wish around and ask, "Why can't I get my wish?" In other words, Step 1 is to *clearly state the discrepancy.* Step 2 is to simply identify the *constraints that contribute to the discrepancy between what is going on now and what ideally should occur.* This involves thoughtful periods of brainstorming and consultation with others that might yield the following list of constraints:

* Adapted with permission from Cogen Television Cassettes, University of Nevada, Reno, 1975.

1. fear
2. prior experience of pain
3. lack of familiarity with the nurse
4. lack of trust in the nurse
5. fatigue
6. separation from parents
7. lack of information about what to expect
8. being caught off guard
9. low pain threshold
10. emotionally expressive personal style

Constructing a list like this one is, in effect, specifying the possible variables that might be studied. Once the list of constraints has been completed, a researchable problem can be formulated in Step 3 by *focusing on the most likely explanation.* Step 4 involves *rephrasing the problem in conceptual terms* to determine the impact of different approaches on burned children's levels of "being upset." So the hope that began as "I wish they wouldn't get so upset when I come in to change their dressings" becomes the researchable problem:

Will prior introduction of the nurse and explanation of the dressing change procedure result in a less upset response by burned children who are anticipating a dressing change when compared with children who have not had a prebriefing meeting with the nurse?

The steps involved in refining a general concern or area of clinical interest into a research problem, then, are:

1. Clearly state the discrepancy.
2. Brainstorm all the plausible obstacles or constraints or explanations.
3. Narrow the focus by selecting a few specific high-priority variables.
4. Rephrase the problem in conceptual terms.

This is only one of a long list of possible study questions that range from altering nurse activities to looking for a relationship between personality variables, developmental level, or cultural background and children's reactions to anticipated trauma. Researchers must choose from all of them the ones that will be most fruitful, eliminating those that are trivial or difficult to study, and then refine them into a question that can direct a study design.

A Two-Stage Approach

If you decide to conduct your own research or to participate with a research team, you will probably have a central role in specifying the details of the research question. Lindeman and Schantz (1982) offer an alternative system for moving from interest in several broad topics to a narrowed, formal problem statement or question

that will guide the conduct of the study: Stage 1 is formulating the question, and Stage 2 is refining the question.

Stage 1: Formulating the question   Most authors agree that research questions have two components, a stem and a topic. Stems can be simple or complex. For example, you might ask, "What are the effects of several types of oral hygiene on the dental health of leukemic patients?" (This is a simple stem that asks "what.") Or you might ask, "What causes postoperative infections, and when do they occur?" (This question asks about causes and occurrence; that is, it is a complex question that asks both "what" and "when.") The way you ask a question will influence the way you will answer it, so that it is important to choose the stem of your research question carefully. Reread the section of this chapter that tells you what kinds of answer different kinds of stem question will produce.

The *topic* is the other part of a research question. In nursing it may be attitudes, behaviors, feelings, beliefs, people, families, communities, health care problems, and so on. The important point about your topic is that you will need to specify how you intend to measure it through working, or operational, definitions. Some of the phenomena of interest to nursing are easier to measure than others. The further away a topic is from some observable indicator for it, the harder it is to operationally define. It's a good idea to write out all the topics that interest you in one column on a piece of paper and all the significant stem questions in another and then ask yourself: "Which of these questions is the one I really want to ask about the topic?" and "Which of the aspects of the topic best expresses what I really want to know about?" See the example in Table 5-3.

Once you have narrowed your focus to a specific stem and a topic of interest, *write an unedited statement of the question*. Free yourself from the self-imposed tyranny of correct grammar for the moment and think about satisfying only two criteria:

Table 5-3   Aid to Writing a Research Question

Stem Question	Topic
What?	Swallowing problems
What kinds?	Aspiration precautions in poststroke patients
How many?	
How often?	
How intense are . . . ?	
When do . . . ?	
Where do . . . ?	
Why do . . . ?	
How do . . . ?	

1. Your question has to be answerable by empirical evidence or data.

2. Your question involves a relationship between two or more variables.

Questions that meet both criteria include: "Does imaging affect patients' ability to cope with health crises?" "Does nursing monitoring increase compliance with a diabetic diet?" and "What is the relationship between massage therapy and pain relief?" In contrast, "Is imaging any good?" and "Should nurses use massage therapy?" are questions of value rather than questions that can be answered through empirical observation.

Having written a rough statement of your question, it is useful to *set up a simple three-column table of variables*. In the first column, write the variable that is being manipulated or examined (the IV). In the last column, write the variable you intend to measure to evaluate the impact of the first variable (the DV). In the middle column, write the variables other than the ones you wish to test that could influence the one you intend to measure. These are called extraneous variables (see Chapter 4), and a list of them can become fairly long. So our sample question, "Does imaging affect patients' ability to cope with health crises?" might look like this:

Independent Variable(s)	Other Factors	Dependent Variable(s)
Imaging	Type of crisis	Coping with
	Support system	health crises
	of patient	
	Relationships	
	with therapist	
	Past life	
	experiences	
	And so on	

Once your three-column table is complete, you may want to request critiques from peers to determine whether you should add, modify, or delete variables from any of the columns. The edited table provides a skeleton conceptualization of your research problem and is ready for refinement in Stage 2.

Stage 2: Refining the Question The second stage of writing a good research question, according to Lindeman and Schantz (1982), is refining it. In the refinement stage you must build a bridge between the current research-based knowledge related to your topic and the step you intend to undertake. Lindeman and Schantz suggest using a matrix, or building block, approach to sort through related studies that you have discovered in the course of reviewing the literature. On the *y* axis of the matrix, put types of

Table 5-4   Literature Review Matrix

Types of Literature	Effects of Imaging	Timing	Patient Characteristics/Nurse Characteristics
Theory			
Replication			
Experimental			Doe, 1985
Exploratory	Smith, 1983		
Descriptive			
Survey		Jones, 1984	

study, and on the *x* axis, put categories of variables related to your study question. Table 5-4 offers a hypothetical matrix for our proposed question about the use of imaging to help patients cope with health crises.

Organizing existing literature and integrating it helps you decide whether to formulate your research question as an experiment or as a nonexperimental study. This process can also help you to make decisions about instruments and about methods for controlling extraneous variables.

Evaluating Research Problems

Deciding which research studies are worth trying to carry out at an individual or institutional level in practice requires that you be able to evaluate the adequacy of the research question or questions on which the study was based (see Chapter 2). Some studies that you read clearly look as if they were done as exercises in methodology for a course or program requirement. They give the impression that the investigator chose the question because he or she thought it would make for an *easy* study. The topic may be trivial, the instruments self-made or imported, and the sample a one-shot captive population of "volunteers" in a single setting. Study questions sometimes grow out of a researcher's idiosyncratic interests but may make little or no conceivable contribution to either practical problems or nursing theory. Finally, keep an eye open for study questions that are so ambiguous, vague, or difficult to define that variables can't be measured. To evaluate the potential useful-

ness of any particular study's question, consider using the following criteria:

- significance
- researchability
- feasibility

Significance

Kaplan (1964) recalls an anecdote involving a drunkard searching under a street lamp for his house key, which he dropped some distance away. Asked why he isn't looking for it where he dropped it, he replies, "It's lighter here." Much research, according to Kaplan, is conducted in much the same way as the drunkard's search. Really important problems are not always those that are most interesting to the researcher or easiest to study.

The problem studied should advance knowledge of phenomena that are objects of inquiry in the field. Even though a question may reflect an individual researcher's thoughts and imagination, it must be articulated in a conceptual system that is understandable to others in the scientific community. Significant research problems yield contributions to the science or the discipline of nursing in a meaningful way. Insignificant study questions are trivial, obvious, or expedient.

Researchability

Researchability demands that a study problem imply the possibility of empirical testing. This means not only that a question about the possibility of a relationship between variables is asked but also that the variables under scrutiny must somehow be measurable (see Chapter 15). As we saw earlier in this chapter, certain questions of value or policy may be important to philosophers and administrators but cannot be studied using empirical testing procedures.

Within nursing, according to Donaldson and Crowley (1978), there is a need to know and to work from descriptive theories as well as prescriptive ones. As Gortner and Nahm (1977) have also pointed out, some studies are basic, in that they are applicable to a general understanding of human behavior or responses to illness, and other studies are applied. Both are needed and significant in a professional discipline, because each discipline has a principal aim that influences the perspective of that field, the way it conceptualizes the relevant world, and the questions it poses for investigation. Because of the uniqueness of each discipline's perspective, it is not possible to simply borrow theory or knowledge from other disciplines. Viewing phenomena from the perspective of healthy functioning of individuals in interaction with their environments will generate distinctive research at all levels and a defined structured body of knowledge.

In addition to studies that raise significant clinical questions, which constitute the emphasis of this text and contemporary priorities in nursing, *the need persists for philosophical, historical and other types of inquiry within the discipline of nursing*, not only to build the knowledge base but also to refine the social relevance and value orientations of the discipline itself. Important research questions are those raised in the context of theoretical considerations that have meaning to the discipline *and* the practice of nursing.

A researchable problem is stated clearly and unambiguously as either a question or a statement. For example, an investigator can ask, "What are the effects of group meetings on locus of control among in-patient psychiatric clients?" Other ideas can be best stated in a declarative sentence: "The problem in this research is to identify nursing functions that help patients achieve behaviors necessary for control of their hypertension" or "The study problem is to determine the effect of episodic apnea on sleeping patterns in chronic respiratory patients." Questions have the advantage of putting study problems in a simple and direct way. For that reason I recommend asking a question. A problem put in statement form is also easier to confuse with the statement of a study's purpose, and the two are not the same.

A researchable problem or question follows logically and consistently from a review of what is already known about a topic. It is the next logical question to pursue given what has been learned in the past (Lindeman & Schantz 1982).

Feasibility

Polit and Hungler (1983) remind us that a good study problem should also be feasible in terms of:

• Time. The problem should be sufficiently restricted that enough time will be available to study it.

- Availability of subjects. There must be enough participants with the desired characteristics who will be willing to cooperate.
- Cooperation of others. The problem must be one that host settings and approval boards (see Chapter 3) are likely to endorse.
- Facilities and equipment. Research problems must be framed in such a way as to be possible given the space, office equipment, transportation, consultation, and computer facilities available.
- Money. Study questions must not only be proposed in the context of sufficient budget but must also be sufficiently worthwhile to justify the anticipated cost of studying them.
- Experience of the researcher. The problem "should be chosen from a field about which the investigator has some prior knowledge or experience" (p. 70). Furthermore, the investigator should either possess the requisite skills to collect and analyze data or have access to those who do.
- Ethical considerations. A research problem may not be feasible if it poses unfair or unethical demands upon potential subjects (see Chapter 3).

Having considered the significance, researchability, and feasibility of a study problem in general, you can then use the following set of questions to evaluate the problem in a piece of research:

1. Is the statement of the problem clearly presented early in the report?
2. Have the investigators placed the study problem within the context of existing knowledge and prior work on the topic?
3. Are the concepts or variables that are included in the study problem measurable?
4. Is the problem significant to the development of knowledge about the discipline or the practice of nursing?
5. Can a feasible study design be developed to address the question?

To sum up, knowledge of the characteristics of a good research question helps researchers formulate valid problem sttements for their own research and helps research consumers select study findings that have scientific merit to put into practice.

Your Role

Whether you are evaluating the research of others to decide whether to use their findings in your clinical practice or are engaging in your own research enterprise, you need to know what characterizes a good question, where to find one, and how to articulate your question to others in proposals, presentations, or reports of findings. This chapter has presented you with some tools and strategies useful in accomplishing all three. No matter how technically correct a research question is, however, nothing can substitute for being genuinely interested in and curious about the topic or area you elect to study. You may be spending a long time on it, and your future career may be shaped by your research interests, so choose a research topic that really matters to you and to the goals of the profession.

Summary of Key Ideas and Terms

✔ All nurses, regardless of their educational preparation, share the investigatory role of discovering and evaluating research problems.

✔ Most clinical research problems exist where there is a discrepancy between what is desirable and what is actual in nursing practice.

✔ Important sources of research problems include (1) your own experience, (2) patterns or trends, (3) somebody else's completed research, and (4) your intellectual and scientific interests.

✔ The ANA's Commission on Nursing Research has identified research that would guide practice as having the highest priority for the 1980s.

✔ A researchable problem can be differentiated from a "value" question or a "yes or no" question by its ability to be solved using the process of scientific inquiry.

✔ Most research questions in nursing fall into the categories of factor-isolating questions, factor-relating questions, situation-relating questions, and situation-producing questions.

✔ The following steps will help you move from a topic of interest to a research question:

- Step 1 State a discrepancy between what exists and what is ideal or desired.
- Step 2 Identify the constraints that contribute to a discrepancy between what goes on and what should occur.
- Step 3 Focus on the most likely explanation.
- Step 4 Rephrase it to interpret the problem in conceptual terms.

✔ A well-stated research question should:

- be answerable by empirical evidence
- involve a relationship between two or more variables

✔ A table of variables and literature review matrix are additional tools useful in formulating and refining research questions.

✔ The criteria for evaluating your own or somebody else's research problem are significance, researchability, and feasibility.

References

American Nurses' Association, Commission on Nursing Research: *Guidelines for the Investigative Function of Nurses*. Kansas City, Mo.: American Nurses' Association, 1981(a).

American Nurses' Association, Commission on Nursing Research: *Research Priorities for the 1980's*. Kansas City, Mo.: American Nurses' Association, 1981(b).

Cogen Television Cassettes, Reno: University of Nevada, 1975.

Dickoff J, et al: Theory in a practice discipline part I: Practice oriented theory. *Nurs Res* September/October 1968(a); 17:415–435.

Dickoff J, et al: Theory in a practice discipline part II: Practice oriented research. *Nurs Res* November/December 1968(b); 17:545–554.

Diers D: *Research in Nursing Practice*. Philadelphia: Lippincott, 1979.

Donaldson SK, Crowley DM: The discipline of nursing. *Nurs Outlook* February 1978; pp. 113–120.

Gill B, Atwood J: Reciprocy and helicy used to relate mE6F and wound healing. *Nurs Res* March/April 1981; 30:68–72.

Gortner SR, Nahm H: An overview of nursing research in the United States. *Nurs Res* January/February 1977; 26:10–33.

Johnson D: Theory in nursing: Borrowed and unique. *Nurs Res* November/December 1968; 17:545–554.

Kaplan A: *The Conduct of Inquiry*. San Francisco: Chandler, 1964.

Lindeman CA, Schantz D: The research question. *J Nurs Admin* January 1982; 6–10.

Polit D, Hungler BP: *Nursing Research*, 2nd ed. Philadelphia: Lippincott, 1983.

Further Readings

Fuller EO: Selecting a clinical nursing problem for research. *Image* 1982; 14:60–61.

Hodgman EC: Closing the gap between research and practice: Changing the answers to the 'who,' the 'where' and the 'how' of nursing research. *Int J Nurs Stud* September 1979; 16:105–110.

Kalisch B: Creativity and nursing research. *Nurs Outlook* May 1975; 23:314–319.

McHugh NG, Johnson JE: Clinical nursing research: Beyond the methods books. *Nurs Outlook* June 1980; 352–356.

Notter L: Nursing research is every nurse's business. *Nurs Res* January 1963; 2:49–51.

Chapter 6

Recognizing and Evaluating Study Designs

Blueprints for Research in Nursing

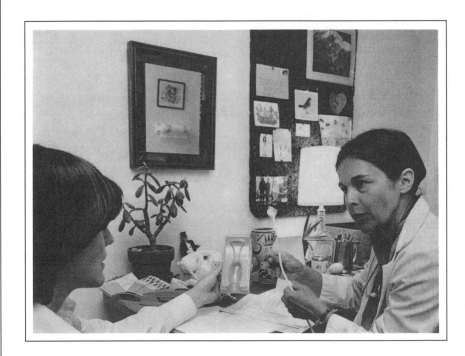

You as a research consumer must be prepared to evaluate study designs for their scientific merit and your wisdom in selecting them.

Chapter Outline

Chapter Objectives

After reading this chapter, the student should be able to:

- Determine whether a study includes the six generic elements of a research design
- Evaluate the match between a study's overall purpose and the type of design employed
- Classify study designs according to whether their major emphasis is on discovery or on accuracy and control
- Differentiate between external and internal criticism in historical study designs
- Specify the major steps in each type of study design
- Compare the advantages and disadvantages of each major type of study design
- Recognize correctly the type of study design used in reports of nursing research
- Explain the three hallmarks of true experimental study designs
- Discuss the concepts of reliability and validity in relation to experimental study designs
- Formulate design remedies to counter potential threats to the internal and external validity of experimental designs
- Describe the major types of experimental design
- Compare and contrast quasi-experimental designs with experimental designs
- Account for the major disadvantages of ex post facto study designs
- Discuss the purpose of methodological research

In This Chapter . . .

Suppose you are responsible for providing nursing care to a 50-year-old woman during her postoperative recovery from gallbladder surgery. What do you do first? What do you avoid? How much of anything is going to be enough to prevent postoperative complications? What strategies will work? To help you answer these questions and accomplish the clinical goals set for this patient, you need to devise a *workable plan*. The plan is customarily called a nursing care plan. It offers you and the other clinicians working with this patient a blueprint, or organized design, for achieving certain specified objectives, such as the prevention of wound infection, pneumonia, thrombosis, and other complications that can follow such surgical procedures. The plan would take on quite different configurations if it were intended to accomplish an alternate purpose, such as decreasing a patient's anxiety or teaching someone about a diabetic diet.

Designs accomplish much the same thing for scientific research. They are the plans used to get answers to research questions that are valid and reliable according to scientific canons (see Chapter 4 and Glossary). The design is the overriding program, or protocol, for the research. It includes strategies for sample selection, data collection, and data analysis and a timetable. Strategies refer specifically to the methods and procedures that will be used to:

1. answer the research questions empirically as validly, objectively, accurately, and economically as possible
2. control the experimental, extraneous, and error variances that might be associated with the particular phenomena being studied (see Chapters 4 and 15).

Research designs suggest what observations or measurements to make, how to make them, and what to make *of* them. In effect, *research designs imply a set of instructions that tells an investigator how data should be collected and analyzed in order to answer a specified research problem.* There are almost as many designs as there are possible approaches for attempting to establish that something is or is not true. But as is the case with nursing care plans, certain designs are better suited to certain levels of inquiry, research purposes, and types of problem than are others. Kerlinger (1973) wrote:

All man's disciplined creations have form. Architecture, poetry, music, painting, mathematics, scientific research—all have form. Man puts great stress on the content of his creations, often not realizing that without strong structure, no matter how rich and how significant the content, the creations may be weak and sterile. So it is with scientific research. Without content . . . good theory, good hypotheses, good problems—the design of research is empty. But without good form . . . adequately conceived and created . . . little of value can be accomplished. . . . Many of the failures of research have been failures of disciplined and imaginative form (p. 290).

Thus, researchers can choose from a wide variety of plans for addressing their study problems, but you as a reader must be prepared to evaluate critically not only the type of design that was used but also *the wisdom of selecting it*.

What follows in this chapter is an overview of the range and diversity of study designs. Specific sampling, data-collection, and data-analysis operations are discussed in detail in Part III. Here, we will consider the elements of a study design, the purposes for which research is done, and the design options best suited to each. We will compare and contrast nonexperimental, quasi-experimental, and true experimental designs and examine examples of nursing studies that have used various approaches. We will take a look at the advantages and disadvantages of each type of design within the framework of the key concepts of *validity* and *reliability*. After all, the scientific method is important to us insofar as it is really a process for knowing what is true (see Chapter 1), even though we believe that truth is less a static set of external laws than a representation of an episode in evolving history.

Elements of a Good Research Design

Some authorities on nursing research would have you believe that the more highly rigorous experimental and quasi-experimental study designs, in which phenomena of interest are isolated and controlled in laboratory settings, are by their very nature more elegant and therefore better than other designs. This view is associated with the logical positivist view of science (Silva & Rothhart 1984). Listening in on an institutional review board's meeting, a funding agency's grant proposal review, or even an editorial board's discussion of research manuscripts would undoubtedly reveal further supporters of such a position. After all, the nineteenth and twentieth centuries have witnessed the awesome achievements in the physical and biological sciences that the experimental approach to research questions generated. Furthermore, members of this camp suggest that researchers who use qualitative designs try too often to squirm out of describing the precise details of their methodology, expecting instead that their findings will be accepted on faith (Downs 1983).

Other authorities, representing an alternate point of view sometimes called historicism (Laudan 1977), caution us to reflect on the philosophical congruence of nursing's commitment to belief in the whole person, individual uniqueness, personal autonomy, and experiential relativism with the scientific reductionism and instrumentalism that characterize experimental designs. Munhall (1982) points out that under the direction of an experimental design and a logical positivist or empiricist philosophy, the scientist chooses an observable, measurable part of a person's human response or environmental context, becomes distant from the problem in order to be objective, places individuals into groups to eliminate the influence of confounding variables, and applies results to the mean, or average, of all cases stated. In her appraisal, the basic premises of the experimental design are that individuals are alike according to categories and that experience is all quantifiable and measurable; the result is a mechanistic, reductionist world view in which people's human responses are viewed as reactions to a predetermined stimulus selected to produce a desired outcome (p. 177). Munhall asks, "Is nursing practice philosophy and nursing research philosophy in apposition or opposition?" She concludes by advocating the congruence of approaches outlined in this book's chapter on qualitative analysis and associated with a symbolic interactionist philosophy of science (see Chapters 13 and 14).

The position you take on the issue of *which* research design has the most heuristic potential for the advancement of nursing knowledge ultimately depends on *your* philosophy of science. Whatever stance you elect, it is important that you be able to recognize the type of design employed in any study you read or hear about and to evaluate its soundness on its own terms as well. The following list contains what Schantz and Lindeman (1982) isolated as the six generic elements of all research designs, whatever the type:

1. setting—where the research will take place
2. subjects, who will be the recipients of an experimental treatment or will be observed
3. sample—a reasonable number of subjects, so that the researcher can make compari-

sons or describe a phenomenon, and the procedure for obtaining them

4. treatment—what the research intervention will be, in an experimental design, or conditions under which data will be collected, in a nonexperimental design

5. measurement, observation, or data-collection methods

6. plan for communication of results, including the way the data will be analyzed and interpreted

Spelling out each of these decisions in detail, so that the purpose of the research is served and the research question answered, increases the likelihood of creating a tight and logical study design. A correct experimental design, for instance, is intended to isolate variables of particular concern or interest so they can be examined under known conditions, to eliminate bias, and to reduce the margin of error, enabling the researcher to have confidence in the truth of his or her conclusions.

Matching Research Design and Research Purpose

Every study, of course, has its own specific substantive purpose. You might find, for instance, that a study is designed to find out whether structured preoperative teaching will significantly increase a postsurgical patient's ability to cough and deep breathe. Or a study might be designed to identify the mental health care needs of the deinstitutionalized elderly or to describe the influence of religion on nursing in western civilization. Most investigators think of research purposes as falling into several main groups, or categories. Diers (1979) uses the following categories of research studies in nursing:

1. Factor-naming, or factor-searching, studies describe, name, or characterize a phenomenon, situation, or event in order to gain familiarity with it or achieve new insights. In more traditional sources this research is called exploratory and descriptive. It answers "what" questions and "who" questions (see Chapter 5).

2. Factor-relating, or relation-searching, studies are done to develop links among variables and describe the relationships that are found. These studies go on at the second level of inquiry after a phenomenon has been explored, named, and described. Many

qualitative and grounded theory studies fall into this category (see Chapter 14). These studies address "how" questions (see Chapter 5).

3. Association-testing studies, also called explanatory or correlational studies, seek to determine what factors occur or vary together without either changing the natural situation (manipulating it) or attempting to reach conclusions about whether one causes another. They address "if, then" questions (see Chapter 5).

4. Causal hypothesis-testing studies test a causal relationship between variables and are also called true experiments, or explanatory studies and attempt to answer "why" questions (see Chapter 5).

In the first two types of study the major emphasis is on *discovery*, and the research design must be *flexible* enough to permit the investigator to use any strategy that might be helpful in obtaining rich and broad-ranging data on a phenomenon. In studies that are aimed at the third and fourth purposes, the prime issue is one of *control* and *accuracy*. Thus, the design must minimize bias, control variance, and enhance the reliability and validity of the evidence obtained. The fourth category of study seeks in addition to allow inferences to be made about cause and effect in the very particular scientific sense (see Glossary). When reading a report or proposal for a study, you may not always find its purposes as clear-cut as the preceding discussion might have led you to believe. In actual practice a study may have some overlap of purpose. But the distinctions made by sorting studies into four types by purpose are helpful as we turn our attention to understanding the various types of study design.

Historical Study Designs

Most scholars agree that history is an activity engaged in for the purpose of learning the truth about the past. History is also a discipline of study that has established methods for collecting and evaluating evidence about the past. In fact, the clearest characteristic of the historical research method is that its data already exist. The purpose of historical research is to explain the present or to anticipate the future based on a systematic collection and critical evaluation of data pertaining to past occurrences. Historical study designs call for a prescribed approach to examining and interpreting data contained in historical sources such as diaries, letters, documents, and journals. Hockett (1955) emphasized the importance of efforts to establish the validity and reliability of historical research when he wrote:

The aim of historical research is to ascertain facts, as they must be made the basis of all conclusions. . . . Statements are the raw materials with which the historian works and the first lesson he must learn is that they must not be mistaken for facts. They may be facts but that cannot be taken for granted. . . . In view of the possibilities for error, it becomes the duty of the historian to doubt every statement until it has been critically tested (p. 13).

Christy (1975) echoed this warning by reminding us that "the danger lies in the fact that we tend to believe anything in print, especially if it is found in an old document." Use of a historical design, therefore, requires that the researcher employ two separate processes to estab-

lish the validity and reliability of the data before using them to reach a conclusion: external criticism and internal criticism. These processes are hallmarks of sound historical research.

External Criticism

External criticism refers to examination of the historical data sources (maps, letters, books, documents, inscriptions, artifacts, and the like) for their validity, genuineness, or authenticity. Documents cannot be taken to reflect the truth unless they are really what they appear to be rather than forgeries or frauds. Techniques that historical researchers use to establish the authenticity of their data sources include consideration of the age of the paper, the kind of ink used, the appearance of watermarks, the match with other samples of handwriting, the congruity with other evidence of the author's or originator's ideas, or the use of a variety of laboratory procedures that determine characteristics (age, composition, and so on) of materials. In the case of book or article manuscripts, the historian must determine who the true author was. Questions that help establish authorship include:

- Is the manuscript an original or a copy?
- Is it dated?
- Could it have been written by anyone else?
- Might it be a forgery?

Other problems with which a historian must deal in the process of evaluating data for their validity include the possibility that a previous historian misidentified a document, the chance of errors due to translations or even transcriptions from other languages, and the likelihood that documents have been altered or changed. Canons of historical research require that the historian get to original, primary sources in order to minimize the chance of distortion and error.

Internal Criticism

Once the validity of data sources is established, the historical researcher turns his or her attention to determining the *accuracy of the statements contained within the documents or historical material*. The process involved in making such a determination is called *internal criticism*. It requires the following steps:

- The researcher must be certain that he or she understands the information contained in the documents. As with all other designs discussed in this chapter, being aware of one's own biases and expectations is a basic requirement to avoid interpreting statements so that they provide false support for one's own hypotheses or pet notions.
- The investigator must be knowledgeable about the meaning of terms and statements in their historical and cultural context. Consultation with translators and linguists can sometimes help in this area. Munhall and Oiler (1985) remind us that words take on different meanings in different cultures, eras, and social settings. *Goodynurse*, for example, at the time of the Salem witch trials referred *not* to nurses but to married, middle-class women in the Puritan community.
- The researcher must subject the statements to a phase of negative criticism in which efforts are made to corroborate the truth reflected in them. Most authorities believe that the further

an author moves from reporting an eyewitness account, the less reliable are the statements. Establishing the reliability of a rendition of what occurred usually requires *two independent primary sources that corroborate* each other. Comparing accounts of the same events and finding agreement increases confidence in the data. Evidence is considered "probable" when the researcher has information from *one primary source that passes the tests of authenticity* and *finds no substantial evidence to the contrary*. If neither of these routes to confidence in the truth of the data is available, the historian is dealing from the substantially weaker position of "possibility." Historical research requires the ability to find evidence, group it, evaluate it, interpret it, and communicate it in relation to important questions, themes, or hypotheses.

Steps in a Historical Research Design

The historical researcher begins a study with a clearly stated research problem that has resulted from narrowing down a broader, more general area of interest (see Chapter 5). Christy (1969), a nurse historian, studied "the impact of the leadership of the Nursing Department at Teachers' College, Columbia University, on changes and major events in American nursing during the first half of the twentieth century." Data in historical research such as Christy's study consist of evidence about events, people, situations, and so on that were created in the past. Instead of manipulating variables or designing data-collection tools, the historian must rely on documents from the past. Such documents are considered either *primary sources* (firsthand information) or *secondary sources* (second- or thirdhand accounts). Examples of primary sources include letters, eyewitness accounts, diaries, photographs, and legal or public documents. These are materials that existed at the time of the event. Secondary sources might be newspaper articles, reference books, and hearsay. These are the end products of studying primary data. Once the problems of data availability, data gaps, and evaluation of data validity and reliability are surmounted, the final step in a historical research design is synthesis, analysis, and articulation of the findings. This last step involves the historian in building into a related whole the facts that have been verified. Determining the meaning of facts, discovering relationships among them, and presenting them in a way that is interesting to the reader are among the challenges. Obviously, documentation in the form of footnotes and references is critical to verifying sources used by a historian to reach his or her conclusions. The steps implicit in the process of historical research described above are:

1. Formulate a researchable problem that is best approached with a historical research design.
2. Specify the data needed to address the research question.
3. Determine that sufficient data are available.
4. Collect known data, new data, and previously unknown data sources (primary and secondary).
5. Evaluate data sources through external and internal criticism.
6. Initiate the descriptive synthesis of findings in a written report while continuing to collect data.
7. Draw interpretive conclusions with respect to the original research question.

Advantages and Disadvantages of Historical Research

The value of historical research to nursing has only recently been recognized. Some of the archives established for the preservation of nursing's documents and other related material are listed in Box 6-1. Table 6-1 summarizes important general sources of information for the historian. The orientation to the past of historical

research has as its major advantage the potential for illuminating a current question through the intensive study of carefully selected material that already exists.

Disadvantages of the historical research design include the following:

- The investigator must rely on finding data that already exist and cannot develop new data.

Box 6-1   Archives of Historical Nursing Documents

- Archives of the Department of Nursing Education, Teachers' College, Columbia University, New York
- Historical Book Collection, Sophia Palmer Library, American Journal of Nursing Company, New York
- Historical Collection, Reference Room, National League for Nursing, New York
- Lillian Wald Collection, Special Collections, Butler Library, Columbia University, New York
- Adelaide Nutting Historical Collection, Russell Library, Teachers' College, Columbia University, New York
- Elizabeth Carnegie Nursing Archive, Schlesinger Library, Radcliffe College, Cambridge, Massachusetts
- Mary S. Gardner Papers, Women's Archive, Schlesinger Library, Radcliffe College, Cambridge, Massachusetts
- Maternity Center Association Archives, Maternity Center Association, New York
- Nursing Archive, Mugar Library, Boston University, Boston
- Nursing Historical Collection, Welch Memorial Library, Johns Hopkins University, Baltimore
- Nursing History Collection, National Library of Medicine, Bethesda, Maryland
- Nursing Museum, Pennsylvania Hospital, Philadelphia

Table 6-1   General Sources of Information for Historical Research

Reviews	Journals	Bibliographies	Newspapers and Journalism
American Historical Review	Journal of American History	Historical Bibliographies	Journalism Quarterly
Canadian Historical Review	Journal of Modern History	A Guide to Historical Literature	American Journalism
Catholic Historical Review	Journal of the History of Medicine and Allied Sciences	A Bibliography of the Negro in Africa and America	Quill
Economic History Review	Journal of Southern History	Bibliographic Index	Columbia Journalism Review
Book Review Digest	Past and Present	Biography Index	New York Times Index
Index to Book Reviews in the Humanities	Social Sciences and Humanities Index	Guide to Periodical Literature	Journalism Educator

- The investigator cannot alter the form in which data appear but must attempt to understand them in the form in which they are found.

- The investigator must analyze and interpret the meaning of data without the advantage of being able to ask clarifying questions.

- The data may be incomplete and have gaps in crucial areas.

- The investigator must be able to translate concepts, terms, and ideas in light of their historical period and context.

- The investigator must overcome obstacles of time, resources, freedom of movement, and language to search for and evaluate data resources.

- The investigator cannot predict an accurate timetable for completion of a historical study. Not only must data be located and evaluated, but insights that tie together these masses of data must ultimately be reached.

Two historical studies are noted in the example below. Such studies can serve to interpret the past and supply perspective to contemporary

Examples: Historical Designs in Nursing Research

In a study entitled "Social Characteristics of Death as a Recorded Hospital Event" Jeanne Benoliel (1977) attempted to discover these characteristics in teaching hospitals in the decade 1961–1971 through a retrospective analysis of 4380 patient medical records.

The study question
Existing medical recording as a data source
The time period for the study was 10 years

Helen Nakagawa and Oliver Osborne (1972) conducted a historical epidemiological investigation over a 26-year span of "presenting complaints" from records of first-admission state hospital patients in King County, Washington. Their purpose was to discover dominant trends in these complaints in the context of changing sociocultural, environmental, and treatment practices.

Hospital records data source
The study question
The time period for the study was 26 years

problems and issues by suggesting parallels, differences, and trends. For example, the emergence of specific nursing leaders, the establishment of nursing education in hospitals or institutions of higher learning, and the proliferation of nursing functions are all studied against a background of social needs, economic constraints, and the political climates of given periods.

Case Study Designs

Case studies provide an in-depth analysis of a subject for investigation such as an individual patient, a family, a hospital ward, a health care agency, a professional organization, or a group such as Recovery Incorporated or Alcoholics Anonymous (see Chapters 13 and 14). A case study is customarily done under natural conditions. It examines only a single subject or a small number of subjects with respect to a number of variables pertaining to history, current characteristics, and interactions. The case study design is useful in accomplishing the following purposes:

• gaining insight into little-known problems
• providing background data for the planning of broader studies
• developing explanations of social-psychological and social-structural processes
• offering rich descriptive anecdotes or examples to illustrate generalized statistical findings

Steps in a Case Study Design

Case studies, by definition, are both more flexible and more vulnerable to bias than many other designs, in that the investigator must make judgments about sources, amounts, and credibility of data without many rules or guidelines. In general, however, the steps involved in a sound case study design are as follows:

1. Determine the purpose of conducting a case study.
2. Identify the unit of analysis (individual, family, group, aggregate, organization, community).
3. Determine how data sources will be selected.
4. Specify the data-collection plan and methods.
5. Collect, analyze, and interpret data.
6. Write a report of findings.
7. Suggest directions for further research on the basis of these findings.

Advantages and Disadvantages of the Case Study

Nurse scientists who are working in a relatively unstudied area of investigation where there are few prior studies on which to base design decisions have often acknowledged the value of intensely studying selected case examples in order to stimulate insight and suggest hypotheses or even directions for future research. Much that is known in anthropology and medicine has depended for its start on the case study method. Psychoanalytic theory is based for the most part on Sigmund Freud's carefully documented case studies of psychiatric patients. Case studies can often provide information that is rich and otherwise difficult to come by. They are also well suited for studying a process over time. The use of this approach to develop conceptual explanations in field research is covered in detail in Chapter 13. Some believe that case study designs are virtually synonymous with descriptive research.

Descriptive single-subject research has indeed made valuable contributions to knowledge in psychopharmacology, psychotherapy, and medicine. Behavior modification studies are cited by Holm (1983) in the areas of weight control and childhood eating disorders as bringing research and practice closer together. Other descriptive case studies report how particular patients respond to specific situations or nursing approaches.

Holm argues that experimental approaches can also be used in case studies by modifying experimental design principles so that a subject's baseline data are compared with his or her data after an experimental intervention. A *single-subject experimental design* can also include what is called a *reversal phase*, during which the intervention must be withheld while measures of the dependent variable continue. Holm uses a hypothetical study designed to determine if the 2g sodium diet results in a significant decrease in blood pressure in a 25- to 35-year-old newly diagnosed hypertensive who is otherwise normal as an example of a study that could use a single-subject experimental design. Other topics that lend themselves to this design might be study of the effectiveness of a program of breathing exercises as measured by tidal volume, vital capacity, and respiratory rate; skin care interventions as measured by pre- and postintervention decubitus ulcer size and stage; or a stress reduction program as measured through blood pressure, pulse rate, weight, and sense of well-being. Replication of such studies should be encouraged, because they can generate confidence in findings and foster generalizability and are practical and realistic research approaches in most clinical studies. After all, if a process or effect is documented in one person, it might reasonably recur in others.

The major disadvantages of the case study design are still its problems with generalizability. It is difficult to argue with certainty that what is learned from a single case is representative of patterns or trends in the entire population. Furthermore, the methods for compiling case study data are not as rigorously prescribed as those for data collection under alternate study designs, resulting in what to critics may appear to be outright ambiguity. Considered from the other side of the coin, however, this very ambiguity may provide the flexibility necessary to bring inventive approaches to gathering a rich array of data and arriving at insightful interpretations of them. The other disadvantages of a case study design are those associated with its flexibility and lack of rigor and control. To elaborate:

- Investigators have no guidelines to help them decide how many data are enough.

- Because most of the data collected in case studies are based on interviews and observations

---

Example: A Case Study Design in Nursing Research

A research monograph entitled *Deinstitutionalized Residential Care for the Mentally Disordered: The Soteria House Approach* (Wilson 1982) used the case study design. It is a story of a community-based, residential care facility for severely mentally disordered, young diagnosed schizophrenics that professed a nonmedical approach. The book portrays a scene, a time in history, and a way of being in intimate detail: a locale is sketched, analyzed, and conceptualized. It is described by the authors of the book's Foreword as "documentation of a true social experiment told in the words of the participants" (Wilson 1982, p. xi). It stands alongside an array of descriptive and conceptual case studies published by nurses and social scientists on topics related to delivery of health care.

A case study of one health care setting

Institutions as well as people can be subjects for a case study
Involved generating a description and a grounded theory

obtained by the investigator and the circumstance is often one of a relatively long-term and close association between the investigator and the subject or subjects, the possibility of researcher bias influencing the findings and conclusions is always present.

- The cost effectiveness of case studies is open to criticism, because some authorities believe that the costs in terms of money and time are high relative to the relatively low value of the information obtained.

- A case study design is not adequate for testing causal hypotheses and definitely unsuited for trying to establish scientific cause and effect.

Survey Research Designs

Survey research designs involve studying populations or universes based on the data gathered from a sample drawn from them. The data are often gathered using a questionnaire completed by the study subjects. Survey research generally serves the purpose of *describing characteristics, opinions, attitudes, or behaviors as they currently exist in a population*, although other purposes are possible. The word *survey* means that information is being collected from a variety of subjects who resemble the total population on the characteristic(s) of interest to the researcher. For example, a nurse working in the field of psychogerontology might conduct a national survey of factors that affect access to health care resources among elderly women with Alzheimer's disease. When a survey studies a sample of the total possible population, it is technically called a *sample survey*. If the entire population is studied—for example, all doctorally prepared nurses in the United States—the survey may be called a *census*.

Types of Survey

Survey designs can be classified by the subjects from whom data are collected (*sample survey* versus *census* or *group survey* versus *mass survey*); by the methods used to collect the data (*mailed questionnaire survey, face-to-face interview survey*, or *telephone survey*); by the study's time orientation (*retrospective survey, cross-sectional survey*, or *longitudinal survey*); or by the study's purpose or objective (*descriptive*,

comparative, correlational, developmental, or *evaluative*.) A quick review of issues published in the last several years by *Nursing Research* would reveal the kinds of problem investigated using different types of survey. Although types of surveys may overlap and interact, let's consider each of them separately.

Mass Survey   Mass surveys involve collecting a relatively limited amount of superficial information from a large population or universe. The survey of all nursing education programs in the United States conducted every ten years by the National League for Nursing is one example. The kind of information collected in this instance is often demographic (age, sex, occupation, income, social class, educational level). Although identifying characteristics of the entire population or universe may be the study objective, a survey can be based on information collected from a sample carefully drawn from that population using a systematic sampling procedure (see Chapter 9).

Group Survey   A group survey may have a smaller sample size than a mass survey but usually incorporates a search for considerably more depth and scope of information. First, almost all surveys of this type ask respondents some identifying or descriptive information about their personal background and current situation. These preliminary questions often include age, sex, ethnicity, marital status, education, religious affiliation, political preference, income, parents' educational level, number of people living in the household, siblings, and occupation. See Figure 6-1 for an example of typical survey questions coded for computer processing (Chapter 16). The value of collecting these data along with data that bear on the actual research question is that knowing the characteristics of the sample allows an investigator to feel more confident about generalizing findings from the sample to a population. Occasionally, even a sample selected using random sampling procedures (see Chapter 9) turns out by chance not to represent the population from which it was drawn.

A second category of data often covered in typical group surveys involves the subject's social context, be it home or work environment. A study of stress experienced by nurses who work in intensive care or critical care units may include questions about the noise level, the frequency with which people die on the unit, the staff–patient ratio, the provisions for avoiding burn-out, and so on.

Yet a third category of questions addresses behaviors. A study of kidney transplant recipients, for example, might include questions such as:

1. What two foods that are high in salt do you avoid?
2. What two things do you do every morning at home to monitor your kidney function?
3. What do you do to decrease fluid retention in your tissues caused by the Prednisone you take?
4. What do you do to prevent muscle weakness that can be related to taking Prednisone?
5. What do you do when you miss a dose of Imuran or Prednisone?
6. What have you done when you notice you are having undesirable effects from your Prednisone or Imuran?

A fourth category of questions addressed in group surveys involves how much information about a topic the sample members have. The same survey of kidney transplant patients might also contain the following items.*

---

1. Circle the five things in the following list of symptoms that might indicate a rejection:
   a. pain over my kidney
   b. yellowish skin or eyes
   c. smelly urine
   d. weight increase
   e. flulike feeling
   f. decreased urine output
   g. nausea
   h. elevated temperature
   i. increased urine

2. If you were to wake up at home at 2:00 A.M. with pain over your kidney, what should you do? (Circle two answers.)
   a. Go to the hospital immediately.
   b. Call the transplant unit.
   c. Go back to sleep and see how you feel in the morning.
   d. Take your temperature and weigh yourself.

Yet another category of questions includes those that deal with psychological variables—subjects, opinions, feelings, attitudes, and values. A study designed to answer the question "What are the attitudes of adolescent diabetics who fail to comply with their diet regimen?" for example, would contain such psychological items or scales (see Chapter 11).

Face-to-Face Interview   In-person surveys can be used to address any of the possible content areas mentioned above, as can telephone interviews or mailed questionnaires. Certain topics, however, are best studied when trained interviewers meet with subjects in person and use a structured or semistructured interview schedule to collect data from them (see Chapters 11 and 13). Certainly, a study that aspired to look at a highly personal and sensitive question such as

*SOURCE: Questions related to kidney transplants taken from Wirth P, Barton C: Barton-Wirth kidney transplant knowledge questionnaire. (Unpublished instrument.) Kidney Transplant Unit, Moffit Hospital, University of California, San Francisco, 1983.

STUDENT SURVEY

ID (1-5) 1. Code Number: /_____/_____/_____/_____/_____/ (to be assigned)

2. Name (print): /_____ /_____ /_____/
            First   Mid. Init.   Last

MOEDUC (7) 3. Mother's level of education (Check one):

_____ Elementary school or less

_____ Some high school

_____ High school graduate

_____ Some college

_____ College graduate

_____ Post-graduate degree

_____ Other: _____

DEGHOPE (8) 4. What is the highest degree you expect to receive in your educational career? (Check one):

_____ Master's in nursing

_____ Master's in another field

_____ Doctorate in nursing

_____ Doctorate in another field

_____ Other (Identify) _____

_____ Don't know

5. What are the sources of financial support for your education this year? (Check all that apply).

SUPSELF (9)	_____ Self-support	SUPSCSHP (13)	_____ Scholarship	
SUPSAVNG (10)	_____ Savings	SUPGRANT (14)	_____ Grant	0 = No
SUPPARNT (11)	_____ Parents or relatives	SUPTRSHP (15)	_____ Traineeship	1 = Yes
SUPSPOUS (12)	_____ Spouse	SUPOTHER (16)	_____ Other	

EMPSTATS (17) 6. Which of the following describes your employment status while in school? (Check one):

_____ Full-time employment

_____ Part-time employment

EMPHOURS
(18-19)

_____ Hours per week, if part time

_____ Armed Forces, reserve or active

_____ Traineeship

_____ Fellowship

_____ Research Assistantship

_____ Other: _____

_____ More than one check

EMPHOURS #	Frequency
0	13
8	2
11	1
12	1
16	5
20	5
24	6
26	1
27	1
32	1

Figure 6-1 Student survey for program research and development in a nursing school.

"What are the personal, physical, cognitive, and psychological needs of young paraplegic men in the first six months after diagnosis?" would be difficult to approach through an impersonal mailed questionnaire. Sensitive subjects and sensitive questions usually should be studied through interviews. So should questions whose answers may need clarification or elaboration. But interviews, especially face-to-face ones, are very costly. They require planning, interviewer training, travel, and so on. They obviously have the distinct advantages of allowing for clarification and elaboration of a topic and high subject participation (see Chapter 9).

Telephone Interview Surveys over the telephone are less costly than face-to-face interviews, but they are also potentially less effective as a data-collection approach. They may be perceived as intrusive or annoying by respondents, and they certainly don't allow for the development of rapport needed to explore highly personal or sensitive topics. Interviewers must be trained for telephone interviews, an interview schedule must be developed, and telephone bills must be paid. The costs associated with travel, however, are avoided, and thus telephone interview surveys may represent a necessary compromise when face-to-face interviews are too costly. They may also be preferable to relying exclusively on mailed questionnaires.

Mailed Questionnaire Mailed surveys require that the subject be able to read, understand, and administer the questionnaire and be sufficiently motivated to return it to the investigator. Although mailed questionnaires generally have considerably lower response rates (sometimes as low as 15% or 20%, even if stamped, self-addressed envelope and engaging cover letter are included), they are often the only option available to a researcher who wants to collect data from a population spread over a great distance—for example, a multinational sample of executives in schools of nursing throughout the world (see Chapter 11).

Cross-Sectional Survey. Most of the examples discussed thus far take a single snapshot of certain variables in a sample, that is, collect data at a single point in time. If, however, a research question asks about change or development (or stability) over time, the investigator usually uses either a cross-sectional survey or a longitudinal survey. The former involves subjects who are at different points in the process of moving through an experience; they are surveyed at the same time and assumed to represent data collected from different times. For example, oncology patients who have recently begun radiation treatments and chemotherapy might be asked to respond to a set of interview questions or questionnaire items at the same time that other patients who have experienced at least one remission and exacerbation are asked to do so. The two groups are assumed to reflect different stages of the same process. One of the major limitations of this kind of time sampling (see Chapter 9) is that the researcher is always really talking about *different* people in the different phases, and a lot of intervening and confounding variables can affect the findings. Yet collecting data about change with this approach eliminates the possibility that respondents become "test-wise," and it is economical.

Longitudinal Survey As opposed to the cross-sectional survey, the longitudinal survey collects data from the *same* people at different times. At several major American university hospitals major studies on normal aging have actually followed adults for more than 20 years to uncover heretofore unknown aspects of the aging process. The primary strength of the longitudinal design is that the researcher does not have to assume that different groups are sufficiently comparable to designate them as representing different points of the same process. Its disadvantages are the amount of time it takes to complete even a short-term longitudinal study (less than five years) and the influence of studying subjects who become test-wise from repeated completion of similar data-collection instruments. Unless some dramatic shift has taken place in the study setting (a change of institutional mission, composition, or policy), most authorities agree that the cross-sectional design functions reasonably well as an approximation to at least a short-term longitudinal study.

Descriptive Survey   Surveys done for the purpose of providing an accurate portrayal of a population that has been targeted because of some specific characteristics are called descriptive surveys. They are often used to determine the extent or direction of attitudes or behaviors. A survey sponsored by the University of Miami collected interview and questionnaire data from 50 midwestern couples who were in their 70s or older and had been married for 50 years or more to describe the quality of a long-lasting marriage (Secrets of making marriages last [San Francisco Chronicle 1984], according to the study findings, were spending time together and sharing household chores.) Clearly, most descriptive survey data are analyzed with statistics, as covered in Chapter 15.

Comparative Survey   Some surveys are used to compare or contrast representative samples from two or more groups of subjects in relation to certain designated variables. A national survey of attitudes toward "professionalism" or "leadership aspirations" among graduates of baccalaureate and associate degree nursing programs would constitute an example of a comparative design. Sampling procedures must be carefully followed so that the groups to be compared will be as similar as possible on all variables that are not the focus of the study and to ensure that the sample is as representative as possible of the population from which it is drawn.

Correlational Survey   Surveys designed to discover the direction and magnitude of relationships among variables in a particular population of subjects are called correlational surveys. Another way of saying this is that in correlational

study designs the investigator studies the extent to which changes in one characteristic or phenomenon correspond with changes in another. One might investigate, for example, whether adaptive functioning in the year before the onset of an illness is related to coping with the stresses of illness and hospitalization. Discovering that factors that are of interest to nursing practice and health care are related through the use of correlational survey can often provide the basis for designing a more precisely controlled experiment that addresses cause and effect.

Evaluative Survey   Surveys conducted for the specific purpose of making judgments of worth or value are called evaluative surveys. More precisely, evaluation surveys allow the investigator to delineate, obtain, and provide information that is useful for judging decision alternatives when conducting a program or service. Evaluation studies can focus on *formative* (process) or *summative* (outcome) questions. In the former, the purpose is to *provide ongoing feedback* to people who are responsible for carrying out a plan or programs. In the latter case, the study is designed to focus on the *effectiveness of the outcome of the plan or program*. The purposes that an evaluation study can serve are as follows:

1. identifying goals or objectives to be evaluated
2. discovering how well objectives are met
3. determining the reasons for specific successes and failures
4. analyzing the problems with which a program must cope
5. ascertaining how long the effects of a program last
6. studying the success of alternative techniques
7. redefining the means for attaining objectives or the objectives themselves
8. interpreting the meaning of changes found
9. identifying unexpected outcomes of a program

The survey format is viewed by evaluators as a relatively effective and efficient way to gather information about achievement of a program's goals or objectives. Some authorities argue that unanticipated consequences should also be examined, and they advocate what are called *goal-free* evaluation plans. A survey should establish the variables to be measured, the sample population and sampling plan, what scales exist and what must be developed, and in the case of evaluation based on program goals, the yardsticks used to make judgments about the meaning of data that are collected.

A good evaluation survey design has the following ingredients (Wilson 1976):

- consideration of why one is evaluating and how the results will be used

- decisions and choices about what the objectives of data collection are or what questions require answers

- decisions about the nature of the sampling plan—from whom information will be needed and at what times

- formulation of a system for recording and storing data

- plans for checking out the objectivity, reliability, comprehensiveness, validity, and relevance of data

- plans for comparing groups if possible

- strategies for summarizing and reporting findings so they can be used for decision making and program improvement

- task assignments and time schedules

A poorly designed survey can produce masses of irrelevant information that make drawing conclusions difficult, and in the case of mailed survey instruments the problem of low return rate must be expected.

Criteria for judging the merit of evaluation study designs include familiar ones: internal and external validity, reliability, objectivity, relevance, significance, scope, credibility, timeliness, pervasiveness, and efficiency.

Example: A Context Evaluation Study

Steele and associates (1978) conducted three surveys to determine the need for a program to prepare clinical nurse specialists in child health nursing in a northeastern state. They considered their work to be an example of context evaluation, which looks outside a program or procedure to gather evidence that will be helpful in the planning process. Their first survey attempted to determine whether graduates of the proposed master's program in child health nursing would have opportunities for employment. Some authors would equate this type of evaluation with *needs assessment research*. Their second survey focused on the functions and tasks performed by clinical specialists in child health nursing. And the third survey was a modified *focus Delphi* technique, a special type of survey used for forecasting. This final survey was designed to try to identify the events that a large number of people felt would influence the field of child health nursing in the future. Data compiled from this survey were later used in determining content in the curriculum. The authors concluded retrospectively about their initial effort: "The survey attempted to elicit too much information and fell victim to one of the ills of survey research—loss of a great deal of data" (p. 8).

Context evaluation

Needs assessment research

Authors' self-critique

Steps in Survey Research

There is clearly overlapping in the types of survey we have just considered. They are not mutually exclusive. An evaluation survey can also be a mailed questionnaire and longitudinal survey. In general, all survey designs require that these steps be addressed:

1. State the research question.
2. Ascertain that the research question can be addressed with a survey design.
3. Decide on the type of survey to be used.
4. Translate the objectives of the survey into categories of question or item.
5. Identify the population of respondents or settings.
6. Use sampling procedures to identify a representative sample.
7. Design data-collection procedures.
8. Plan for analysis of data (see Chapter 15).
9. Pilot test data-collection and analysis approach.
10. Modify as indicated.
11. Collect and analyze data.
12. Write descriptive, comparative, or evaluative findings and draw conclusions (see Chapter 17).

Advantages and Disadvantages of Surveys

It is probably obvious in light of the diversity of types of survey that the strength of the survey design lies in its ability to combine flexibility of content and purpose with elements of precision and control. It can be used to gather information from a large number of subjects with comparatively minimal expenditure of time and money. Its methodology can be explicitly stated, making it easier to evaluate and to replicate in comparison with alternative designs that are high in flexibility. It can take advantage of existing standardized scales and questionnaires and can be structured so that data analysis can be accomplished using a computer (see Chapter 16).

Limitations of survey designs include:

1. the possibility of a low return rate due to the impersonal approach that often characterizes survey research

Example: A Survey Design in Nursing Research

Maria O'Rourke (1981) conducted a cross-sectional correlational survey of 633 healthy women between the ages of 21 and 44 to address the study question of *whether women's subjective appraisal of their psychological well-being differed in relation to the presence of menstrual and nonmenstrual symptoms.* Her study data were collected using a structured mailed questionnaire that included the General Well-Being Schedule and the Moss Menstrual Distress Questionnaire. Her results after statistical analysis indicated that although women experienced specific menstrual symptoms that were distressful, this did not negatively affect their assessment of their psychological well-being. She viewed the implications of her findings as important in clarifying misconceptions about the effect of menstrual cycle symptoms on women's mental health.

Cross-sectional correlation survey

Study question

Mailed questionnaires used to collect data

Study findings

Conclusions

2. the possibility that preconceived questions are irrelevant or confusing to the respondents and therefore yield meaningless data

3. the necessity of developing a system for storing and keeping track of a vast amount of data

4. the tendency of data obtained to be relatively superficial

5. the fact that survey data do not allow an investigator to answer cause-and-effect questions about related variables

Experimental Study Designs

The term *experiment* is sometimes used interchangeably in everyday conversation with *study* or *research project*. In the language of science, however, an experiment or experimentally designed study has a very specific meaning. It refers to a kind of study in which the researcher *manipulates* and thus controls one or more independent variables and observes the dependent variable or variables for the consequences, change, outcome, or effect. Furthermore, in a true experiment the investigator has the *power to assign subjects to either an experimental or control group* and ideally has the *power to use random sampling procedures to select them* in the first place. Summarizing, then, true experiments are characterized by the following features:

1. control over at least one dependent variable and manipulation of at least one independent variable by the investigator

2. random selection of sample members

3. random assignment of sample members to experimental and control groups

In the opinion of many philosophers of science, the true experiment is the ideal study design, because it measures relationships among variables with the most precision, rigor, and control. The control accomplished with an experimental design is best understood in terms of the idea of *control over variance*. The experimental study design can:

1. maximize systematically introduced experimental variance

2. control extraneous variance

3. minimize error variance

Let's look at each of these notions in a bit more detail, because they represent the assets of a true experimental design.

Strengths of Experimental Designs

Maximizing Experimental Variance A typical experiment begins with a hypothesis about the existence of a relationship between an independent variable and a dependent variable. The hypothesis, for example, may be that holding a newborn at time of delivery (IV) will be related to postpartum bonding behaviors in first-time fathers during the first three days after a baby's birth (DV) (Toney 1983). The investigator then randomly selects a sample of first-time fathers who meet specific inclusion criteria—for example, married, aged 20 to 32, father of a baby without deformities, delivery uncomplicated, and the like. At delivery the fathers who meet the sample criteria are randomly assigned to two groups by the investigator. The fathers in the experimental group are offered their newborn infant to hold for 10 minutes during the first hour after delivery. The fathers in the control group don't hold their babies until 8 to 12 hours after delivery. The null hypothesis tested in the study is H_0. There will be no significant difference in the frequencies of father–infant bonding behaviors between fathers who have early contact and those who do not. An experimental study design is selected because it can most accurately determine how much variance in the dependent variable (father–infant bonding behavior) can presumably be due to manipulation of the independent variable (holding or not holding an infant at birth). An experimental design is set up to allow the variance in the dependent variable due to the independent variable to show itself by being separated from the total variance in the dependent variable, which can be due to a lot of things, including chance. The means by which an experiment maximizes the experimental variance is by operating according to a precept of *planning and conducting the research so that the experimental and control conditions are as different as possible*. In the case of our example study, holding the newborn for 10 full minutes was contrasted to not holding the infant at all. Every effort was made to avoid introducing the ambiguity of holding for a few seconds or even touching for a moment.

Controlling Extraneous Variables   What controlling extraneous variables means is that variance in the dependent variable that might be due to something other than the influence of the independent variable is nullified or eliminated. This goal is accomplished in an experimental design in five ways:

1. A researcher can eliminate extraneous variables altogether as variables in the study. For example, if the researcher studying bonding had suspected that years of college education might have an effect on the dependent variable of father–infant bonding, she might have selected sample members for both her experimental and control groups who had zero years of college. In short, to eliminate the variance that might be due to some ex-

traneous factor, the investigator can select sample members so that they are homogeneous for that particular factor or variable.

2. The investigator can control the influence of extraneous variance through random selection of sample members and random assignment of subjects to the experimental and control groups. Proper randomization allows the investigator to assume that the experimental and control-group members are statistically equal on all possible extraneous variables.

3. The researcher can build an extraneous variable into the design of the experiment as yet another independent variable and collect data about its effect on the dependent variable (and its interaction with other independent variables).

4. The experimenter can match subjects in the control and experimental groups on the variable in question. Because matching can also have some disadvantages (including the possible loss of subjects from the study group), randomization and analysis of covariance are sometimes considered better controls.

5. Finally, certain statistical methods can isolate and quantify the amount of variance due to extraneous variance (see Chapter 15).

Minimizing Error Variance   Error variance can be associated with individual differences among subjects and what are commonly called measurement errors, such as those due to test fatigue, lapse of memory, fleeting feelings, and other unpredictable phenomena. The primary precept that experimental designs reflect to reduce error variance is that *to increase the reliability of measures is to reduce error variance*. This means that the less scores are allowed to fluctuate randomly on subsequent administrations of an instrument but rather are repeatable and consistent, the more reliable and free of error variance are the scores or values The visual representation of the meaning of measurement is:

$$M = \text{Actual Value} + \text{ or } - \text{Error}$$

Because the more reliable and accurate the measures are, the easier it is to identify systematic variance in the dependent variable, systematically controlled testing circumstances and procedures are also a requisite in an experimental design. In our sample study the researcher's trained observers observed both the experimental and control-group fathers for the same amount of time (10 minutes) while the father changed the infant's shirt and diaper. They assessed the father–infant bonding using an instrument for interaction assessment that had been tested in a number of prior studies.

Internal and External Validity in an Experiment

The ability of an experimental design to control variance contributes to what is called its *internal validity*. Internal validity refers to whether or not the manipulation of the independent variable really makes a significant difference on the dependent variable. The study we have used as an illustration found no statistically significant differences in bonding behaviors between fathers who had contact for 10 minutes with their newborn infants in the first hour after delivery and those who did not. The author explained this finding by reflecting on the possibility that certain demographic and situational factors that were not controlled in her design may have detracted from the study's internal validity.

External validity refers to the representativeness or generalizability of a study's results. In our study the author acknowledged that without cross-cultural replication her study findings were limited to predominantly middle-class Caucasian fathers who are married and have some college education. She acknowledged that

cross-cultural sampling would be indicated to increase her study's external validity, because different subcultures have different beliefs and methods of expressing affection and attachment. The basic experimental study design with control and experimental groups and pre- and posttests (often called a 2×2 design), and its variables are structured as they are to increase the experiment's internal and external validity.

Campbell and Stanley (1966), in their classic resource on experimental and quasi-experimental designs, list seven classes of extraneous variable that can represent threats to an experiment's internal validity. These are presented in Table 6-2.

The seven threats to internal validity are not only the ones that occur in the conduct of an experimental design, but most authorities agree with Waltz and Bausell (1981) that they occur as the most common extraneous variables. Many of the strategies in true experimental designs are intended to control or prevent their influence or the influence of yet another set of factors that act as threats to *external* validity. Most researchers deal with the threats to internal validity first because altering features of experimental designs makes them easier to control than are many of the threats to external validity.

External validity, as you recall, is defined as the extent to which the results of an experiment can be generalized to different subjects, populations, settings, treatments, and dependent variables. The primary threats to external validity derive from (1) population validity problems, (2) ecological validity problems, and (3) pretest sensitization.

Population Validity The concept of population validity means that the researcher can reasonably generalize from his or her actual sample to all possible sample members and likewise to the total population of interest to the investigator. If, for example, a nurse researcher were to conduct an experimental study to determine the effects of touch as a means of communication

Table 6-2   Extraneous Variables That Can Threaten Internal Validity

Classes of Extraneous Variables	Remedy and Rationale
1. *history*, which is defined as the influence of events that occur during the course of the experiment that might affect the dependent variable	1. Randomly assign subjects to experimental and control groups, because both groups could be assumed to have had exposure to the events that occur
2. *maturation*, which refers to processes that go on within the respondents themselves as a function of the passage of time	2. Complete the experiment in as short a time as possible to minimize developmental changes. Random assignment to control groups for the same reason as #1
3. *testing*, which is defined as the effect of having taken the test on retest scores	3. Don't test the same subjects. Build in a second control group that is tested the same number of times as the experimental group so as to be able to account for amount of change due to subjects becoming test-wise
4. *instrumentation*, which refers to lack of reliability or consistency in the way scores are assigned to a dependent variable	4. Keep scorers "blind" to which subjects are experimental-group and control-group members. Use standardized procedures and protocols for rating or scoring, to avoid biases. Give scorers as much practice as possible before they work with actual research data
5. *statistical regression*, which means that there is a tendency for subjects who score at extremes of a distribution to have less extreme scores when they are retested	5. This is only a factor when subjects are chosen for a study *because* of their extreme scores and can be taken care of through random assignment to control and experimental groups
6. *selection*, which refers to a tendency for certain types of subject to be alike if they are not randomly assigned to experimental and control groups	6. Avoid volunteers, and randomly assign to treatment groups to try to make groups as much alike as possible
7. *differential loss of subjects* from treatment groups during the course of an experiment	7. Little can be done about this factor except to document it as a potential limitation of the study when it occurs and try to prevent it by making every ethical effort to enable willing subjects to continue participating in the study.

SOURCE: From D. T. Campbell and J. C. Stanley, *Experimental and Quasi-Experimental Designs for Research*. Copyright © 1963 by Houghton Mifflin Company. Adapted with permission from Houghton Mifflin Company and American Educational Research Association.

with profoundly retarded children, he or she would want to be sure that:

- the responses obtained from sample members would be representative of potential responses from the target population
- results for subsets in the sample (for example, different sexes or age groups) would occur similarly in the population

Two strategies designed to minimize problems with population validity are to (1) define the accessible population as broadly as possible and then randomly sample as many subjects as is feasible and (2) use sampling procedures to increase the likelihood that the sample has the same constituencies (or characteristics) as the target population. If a researcher designs an experiment without employing these two sampling strategies and instead simply grabs subjects in a single setting as they become available, it is likely that the sample will be systematically biased or different from the population to whom he or she hopes to generalize the findings, and the study's external validity is compromised.

Ecological Validity   A study is ecologically valid if the experimental environment in which it is conducted is sufficiently explicit, clear, and consistent that it could be replicated by another investigator. In practical terms, avoiding problems with ecological validity requires that the researcher operationalize both the independent and dependent variables in detail and prevent the occurrence of the Hawthorne effect (see Chapter 4). Replication is said to be the final arbiter of all external validity questions (Waltz & Bausell 1981). In the study of touch with profoundly retarded children, the investigator would need to spell out in detail the nature of the touching (IV) and the indicators of responsiveness (DV), so that another researcher could replicate the study with different subjects or under different circumstances. Furthermore, effects that might be due just to knowing about participating in a study (the Hawthorne effect) would need to be counteracted by keeping caregivers blind as to the exact indicators being recorded (without, of course, violating ethical research conduct).

Pretest Sensitization   The final threat to external validity occurs when subjects are pretested (for example, on an attitude scale) and the taking of the pretest itself sensitizes the subjects to the experimental intervention that follows. If, for example, nurse practitioners were being studied for their attitudes toward caring for homosexuals before and after a series of workshops designed to clear up misconceptions and decrease prejudice, there could be a tendency for the test taken before the workshops to tip the subjects off about the researcher's interests or even the desired responses. The design strategy used to counter this tendency is to include a second control group that does not receive the workshops but receives only the posttest. Comparing this second control group's posttest scores with the posttest scores of the first control group—which was both pre- and posttested (but also didn't attend the workshops) should allow the researcher to estimate how much change in the dependent variable (attitudes) could be attributed to the pretesting itself. See Figure 6-2. Subtracting for the pretest influence allows the researcher to compare the posttest scores of the control and experimental groups and assume that any difference found is due to the workshops (IV).

Types of Experimental Design

All true experimental designs contain four strategies in one configuration or another. These typical experimental design strategies are:

1. manipulation of the IV(s)
2. an experimental group, which is exposed to the IV, and at least one control group that is not exposed to the IV

	Pretest	Workshop	Post test
Control group 1	Score = 50	No	Score = 60
Control group 2	No	No	Score = 55
Experimental group	Score = 50	Yes	Score = 65

Figure 6-2   A design to control for pretest sensitization.

3. random selection of sample members and random assignment of them to control or experimental groups
4. measurement of the effects of the IV(s) on the DV(s)

The logic of experimental designs is to structure the situation so that you have a sound basis for determining how much of the effect on a dependent variable is related to the independent variable and how much is due to chance.

After-Only Experimental Design   The "after-only," or "posttest-only," design is the simplest experimental design. In it the investigator assigns subjects to an experimental group and control group but *collects data only at the end of the treatment or exposure to the independent variable.* The soundness of the design relies on being able to assume that the two groups are comparable. Its weakness is that one must make this assumption at the beginning of the study without testing for it. From what we've seen earlier in this chapter, random sampling and random assignment to the two groups helps the investigator to have confidence in this assumption.

An example of an after-only experimental design appeared in Toney's 1983 study of the effects of holding the newborn on paternal bonding, mentioned earlier in this chapter. She randomly assigned 37 married, first-time fathers attending uncomplicated deliveries of normal infants to experimental and control groups (those who held and did not hold their infants at delivery). From 12 to 36 hours after the babies were born, bonding behavior frequencies were recorded during 10 minutes of father–infant interaction. Her findings revealed that early contact (IV) did not appear to enhance bonding behaviors (DV) in this study. Her study necessitated, by virtue of the nature of her question, an after-only design (see Figure 6-3).

Before–After Design   In the next design, subjects are measured before the experimental treatment on the same variables as after the treatment. The following example, published in *Nursing Research,* illustrates the most familiar and classic version of an experimental design (see Figure 6-4), called by some "the true experiment."

Randomized Block Posttest Design   A variation on the after-only design involves assigning subjects to experimental and control groups *after they have been ranked* with respect to some variable that is important to the dependent variable. For example, in a study of preoperative teaching methods and their respective effect on patient recovery rates, subjects might be matched according to the extensiveness of their surgical procedure before being assigned, one to the experimental group and one to the control group, by the flip of a coin (see Figure 6-5).

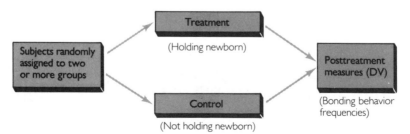

Figure 6-3 An after-only study design.

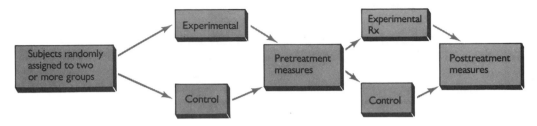

Figure 6-4   A before–after study design.

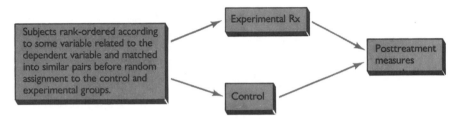

Figure 6-5   A randomized block posttest design.

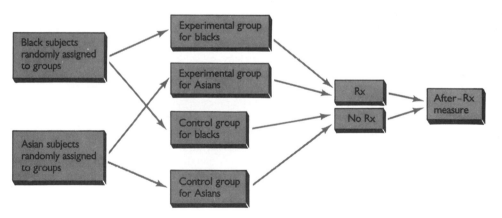

Figure 6-6   A 2 × 2 factorial design.

Factorial Posttest Design   When matching is done based on a nominal variable that can't be rank-ordered, for example, sex or race, but that is still assumed to have an effect on the dependent variable or to interact with the independent variable, a factorial design is used. Factorial designs can be constructed using three or four variables, which results in increased numbers of cells and the need for larger samples. The basic 2 × 2 factorial posttest design appears in Figures 6-6.

The types of experimental design we have examined generally reflect a comparison of the ex-

Example: An Experimental Design in Nursing Research

Slavinsky and Krauss (1982) tested the hypotheses that chronically ill psychiatric outpatients who received nursing services explicitly designed to meet patient needs for both support and growth in regard to both dependency and social competence over a two-year period would

Hypotheses tested

1. show a lower rehospitalization rate
2. spend more days outside of the hospital annually
3. have less treatment dropout
4. show a greater average decrease in symptom ratings
5. have fewer medication increases
6. show a greater average increase in socialization ratings
7. have a greater average increase in satisfaction with life situation ratings
8. have a greater average increase in satisfaction with care
9. show a better overall clinical adjustment in the group

These nurse researchers used a before–after design with an experimental group and a control group. Forty-seven medication-maintained patients were assigned to the treatment condition by starting randomly and then alternating assignment to the groups. Measures of the dependent variables were obtained, using home interviews, at three points: before treatment, after one year of treatment, and after two years of treatment. The sample was drawn from a population of long-term outpatients who spoke English and were stabilized on maintenance dosages of psychotropic medication. The experimental and control-group patients were not different on age, sex, race, social class, number of previous hospitalizations, years of illness, psychopathology ratings, and other indices. The 25 patients assigned to the nursing group received "nursing services designed to meet needs for growth and support in regard to social competence." Services included group therapy, on-call crisis intervention, and medication maintenance. Control-group patients ($n = 22$) attended medication clinics that did not use group or individual therapy. Both groups had similar care insofar as they had the same number of contacts each month and were assigned to one "therapist." Data were collected by trained raters, and the validity and reliability of the ratings were demonstrated. Analysis of variance (ANOVA) was used where possible to explore the interrelationship of baseline ratings, demographic data, and outcomes.

Experimental before–after study design

Interviews were the data collection method

Sample inclusion criteria

Study procedures

Ratings after one year of treatment were of limited value as predictors of final (two-year) outcome. And finally, to the surprise of the nurse researchers, their findings reflected that the individually oriented medical clinic model of care appeared more effective than the nurse-run clinic aimed at improving social adjustment. Flaws in the study design were cited as a possible explanation for findings that failed to support their initial hypotheses, but the investigators questioned whether it was reasonable to find that all three independent raters could have consistently introduced a systematic bias against the research hypotheses. In fact, the more likely bias would probably have been in support of the experimental intervention's outcomes. They did acknowledge, however, that "when an intervention is complex,

Findings

Study limitations

demanding, tedious, extended in time, involving multiple participants, and so on, there can be serious problems in maintaining treatment integrity." All of these characterized their independent variable, and thus their findings may have been influenced by problems of internal and external validity. Figure 6-4 visually depicts a classic pretest–posttest experimental design.

SOURCE: A. Slavinsky and J. B. Krauss, "Two Approaches to the Management of Long-Term Psychiatric Outpatients in the Community," *Nursing Research*, September/October 1982, 31:284–289.

perimental treatment or intervention with *no* treatment or intervention. Sometimes, control groups receive an alternative treatment or intervention (for example, "standard practice"), because receiving no treatment or a placebo would not be ethical. In this case, what is typically called the control group may be called the comparative group. As long as two groups are randomly assigned to experiences that differ from each other in an important way, the conditions for an experimental design have been met. This is true even when a second independent variable such as race or sex is not randomly assigned to subjects, as occurs in a factorial design. Study designs with posttest only and no control group have neither pretesting nor the potential for comparison and as such are considered weak, or *preexperimental*, designs. The design with pretest, posttest, and no control group is considered the second weakest. It has a few advantages over the former model in that changes in the DV can be identified, but without a control or comparative group, of course, it's impossible to determine which of all the possible extraneous or error variances they might be due to. This design is also called preexperimental by some authorities (Waltz & Bausell 1981).

Steps in Experimental Designs

Students wishing to study varieties of experimental design in more depth are encouraged to consult what is considered the most widely used classic resource on the subject, Campbell and Stanley's book *Experimental and Quasi-Experimental Designs for Research* (1966). In general terms, however, the array of experimental designs introduced in this chapter involve these steps:

1. State the research problem.
2. Determine that an experimental design is well matched to the problem.
3. Operationalize the independent and dependent variables.
4. Formulate the hypotheses to be tested.
5. Identify measures for the dependent variable.
6. Specify the full range of potential intervening variables and decide which should be controlled, which can be permitted to vary, and which can be ignored.
7. Design the experiment to test the hypotheses, including selecting the sample.
8. Collect data on "before" measures.
9. Implement experimental and control conditions.
10. Collect data on "after" measures.
11. Analyze data.
12. Present findings in relationship to hypotheses being tested.
13. Prepare discussion of conclusions, limitations, and implications for further study.

Example: An Experimental Design in Nursing Research

Levin (1982) sampled 138 preoperative adult patients and randomly assigned them to choice (experimental) and no-choice (control) conditions to answer the question of whether the choice of site for an injection and locus of control affect the perception of pain. Her experimental study tested four hypotheses:

Random assignment

Study question

1. Individuals given a choice in determining their preoperative injection site report less pain from an injection than individuals not given a choice.

Hypotheses

2. There is no relationship between locus of control (as measured by Rotter's Internal versus External Control Scale) and perception of momentary pain from injection when no choice in site is given.

3. When choice in site is given, persons with internal locus of control report less pain from injection than persons with external locus of control.

4. The addition of "locus of control" to "choice" accounts for more of the variance in perception of momentary pain than "choice" alone.

Levin's sample consisted of 54 male and 84 female preoperative patients who met specified criteria for inclusion, including being between the ages of 21 and 65, awaiting elective surgery, and having no history of neurologic dysfunction, chronic pain, drug addiction, or psychiatric history. Furthermore, all participants were able to read and speak English.

Sample size
Inclusion criteria

Pretreatment measures were obtained from both experimental and control patients when they were asked to rate the amount of injection discomfort from previous intramuscular injections (using graphic rating and visual analog scales). Participants were then randomly assigned to choice and no-choice groups. Those in the choice group were asked *where* (hip or thigh) they would prefer to receive their preoperative medications. Participants in the no-choice group were given their preoperative medicines without asking them to decide upon the site. Injection procedures were standardized, and nurses administering them were blind as to which group a patient was in, because the investigator told the nurse which site to use before she entered the patient's room. After receiving the preoperative injections, patients rated on pain scales the degree of pain they felt from the injection. Data were analyzed using the SPSS program for statistical analysis (see Chapter 15). Hypotheses 1, 3, and 4 were not supported. Hypothesis 2, which predicted no relationship between locus of control and perception of pain, was the only one supported. Unanticipated findings were that the pain of injection was apparently more closely related to the background and experience of the nurse who gave the injection and, among the female patients, their age. Younger women experienced injections as more painful than did older women.

Pretesting

Data collection tools

Study procedures

Posttesting

Statistical analysis done with a computer program
Findings are related to hypotheses
Additional unanticipated findings are reported

Advantages and Disadvantages of Experimental Designs

The rigor, precision, and control properties of experimental designs enable them to be the most powerful way for scientists to establish cause-and-effect relationships, or test causal hypotheses. Causal relationships are important to science because they allow us to predict and explain. For example, an experimental design could tell us if using a dry-abraded skin preparation caused poor quality EKG signals. Or it could tell us if using sterile saline solution and KY jelly caused an increase in the number of pathogens at the meatal introitus of male patients with an indwelling urinary catheter. *Causation* in the scientific sense requires three criteria:

1. *A cause must precede an effect in time.*
2. *There must be evidence that the causal variable (IV) and the dependent variable are associated.*
3. *There must be evidence ruling out other factors as possible determining conditions for the dependent variable.*

The scientific notion of causality acknowledges that in most cases it is a multiplicity of determining conditions that together make up the necessary and sufficient conditions for an event. A *necessary condition* is one that must occur if an effect is to occur. For example, trying drugs is necessary for drug addiction to occur (except, of course, with newborns). A *sufficient condition* is one that is always followed by the effect. For example, destruction of the optic nerve is a sufficient condition for blindness. Some phenomena are both necessary and sufficient, but these are rare (Sellitz et al 1976). The experimental design's strategies of (1) manipulation, (2) comparison, and (3) randomization help the investigator to rule out alternative causal explanations for changes in dependent variables.

Disadvantages of experimental designs also exist:

- Some variables are not feasible or ethical to manipulate. For example, assigning pregnant women to take a new drug found to be dangerous to fetal development in animal studies would not be ethically possible.
- Randomization and otherwise equal treatment of control and experimental groups can occur in a laboratory, but these conditions do not resemble what goes on under real-world conditions, and experimental findings can therefore be based on rather artificial circumstances.
- Experimental designs attempt to reduce variables to measurable terms. Many of the phenomena that are of importance to science in nursing are complex, multidimensional, and holistic and defy the reductionism that has worked reasonably well in the physical or natural sciences.

Despite these limitations, however, the evolution of nursing's research and theory base will probably yield increasing numbers of studies that employ experimental designs in the years to come.

Quasi-Experimental Designs

When it is not feasible for a researcher to implement all of the characteristics of an experimental design—for example, random assignment to control and experimental groups—alternative designs usually called quasi-experimental designs are selected. We will now take up several of the most familiar quasi-experimental options.

The Nonequivalent Pretest–Posttest Control Group Design

The most basic quasi-experimental design uses nonequivalent pretest and posttest and a control group. Huckaby (1978) used it in her study of cognitive and affective consequences of formative evaluation in graduate nursing students. One group of nursing students was taught the first quarter of the graduate program using formative evaluation as a mastery strategy. The students enrolled in the second quarter of the program were taught using conventional lecture and discussion. Pretreatment and posttreatment measures were compared for the groups. (They found that the innovative teaching strategy was associated with more positive affective behavior.) This type of quasi-experimental design is useful when a researcher cannot randomly assign subjects to different treatments but must rely instead on comparative groups. Collection of the pretreatment data allows the investigator to determine how similar the groups are on the variable of interest even though one cannot assume that the experimental and comparison groups are equal.

The Time Series Design

The time series design is used when the investigator can study only one group but uses "before" measures to establish a baseline against which to compare the posttreatment measure of the dependent variable. If, for example, a psychiatric inpatient unit policy shifted to include a system for implementing Joint Commission on Accrediting Hospitals (JCAH) standard compliant treatment plans, the nurse executive could design a study to compare observations associated with the quality of patient care in the setting before and after the treatment planning system. The time series design can be used either when a comparable group is not available or when it is not feasible to do other than use experimental subjects as "their own control" because of limited resources. Even though some authors include the time series design as a quasi-experimental design, Campbell and Stanley (1966) consider it to be preexperimental, because it fails to control so many confounding or extraneous variables. Expanding the design so that it includes a more extended time series and multiple data collection points both before and after introduction of the independent variable is an adaptation that they say qualifies as a quasi-experimental design with considerable integrity, because it strengthens the researcher's ability to attribute change in the dependent variable to the experimental treatment or manipulation.

Example: A Quasi-Experimental Design

Pamela Mitchell and her colleagues (1981) employed a quasi-experimental design to determine intracranial pressure (ICP) as measured by ventricular fluid pressure (VFP) with eight selected nursing-care activities in each of 20 patients. VFP was measured before and after turning the body to four positions, after passive range of motion (arm extension and hip flexion), and after rotation of the head to the right and to the left. Mean ICP increased for at least 5 minutes in all patients after one of the four turns and in 88% after half of the turns. Large increases in ICP occurred in the five patients for whom head rotation was done, but there was minimal change in ICP for passive range of motion procedures. A cumulative increase in ICP occurred with activities spaced 15 minutes apart regardless of what the activity was. No cumulative increase in ICP was found if procedures were spaced at least 1 hour apart.

Study question

Sample size

Study procedures

Findings

Advantages and Disadvantages of Quasi-Experimental Designs

From the point of view of controls for internal validity, quasi-experimental designs are thought to be superior to the preexperimental designs. Their disadvantages, however, include:

- They cannot test causal hypotheses.
- They do little to ensure external generalizability.

- They are more susceptible to the effects of both testing and experimental settings because of the frequent testing schedules.

These disadvantages can be mitigated by adding a nonequivalent comparative group, thus combining the features of the two major types of quasi-experiment presented on p. 156.

Ex Post Facto Study Designs

An ex post facto study is one that attempts to study something after the fact. Instead of introducing or manipulating an independent variable, the investigator selects subjects who have undergone some life experience. He or she then attempts to describe or explain it and, often, its possible relationships to some variable. Such correlations might be the presumed causes, but these cannot be confirmed, only tentatively suggested. Without the control that is possible in an experiment, the investigator must take things as they have already occurred and try to untangle them. Many nursing studies use ex post facto study designs. Andreoli (1981) attempted to determine if there were differences among diagnosed hypertensives who were compliant versus those who were not compliant on their prescribed therapy, at least with respect to measures of self-concept and health beliefs. Other investigators might wish to study the health habits of people who have early heart attacks, or drug use after the birth of a deformed baby, or cigarette-smoking patterns of men who develop lung cancer. In ex post facto studies the researcher selects and studies preexisting groups that have not been randomly selected but, in Kerlinger's (1973) terms, have been "self-selected" in that they have shared a common experience or characteristic.

The major disadvantage of ex post facto studies is that the investigator cannot establish cause-and-effect relationships, only correlational ones. This disadvantage is due to three weaknesses in the ex post facto design: (1) the researcher cannot actively manipulate the independent variable, (2) the researcher cannot randomly assign subjects to experimental treatments, and (3) the possibility for misinterpretation of study results is keen. Suggesting the plausibility of cause-and-effect links when strong correlations are found can be very tempting when an investigator discusses conclusions in an ex post facto study. It takes a sharp and critical reader to recognize that a researcher has gone beyond the data when writing up a study's interpretations.

Methodological Studies

One of the most difficult and challenging aspects of nursing research is the development of tools or instruments that are suited to answering nursing questions. Almost all published nursing studies use existing tools, modify existing tools, or require that the investigators develop their own data-collection instruments (see Chapters 11 and 12). For the most part, nursing research has tended to rely on psychometrics, biological measures, and sociometrics. Many authorities believe that nursing science needs to develop measurements that are specific to the interests of nursing research. Generally speaking, *methodological studies are those that are designed to develop, validate, or evaluate research tools or techniques.* Hurley, at New York University, is pioneering the use of the Psychological Stress Evaluator (PSE), a machine that translates the inaudible microtremors of focal muscles from a recording onto a paper tape in patterns that resemble electrocardiograms. Hurley has used the PSE in a study of communication between marriage partners and in a study of a family whose child had cancer. Winstead-Fry, also of NYU, is developing a statistical technique called multidimensional scaling to look at intergenerational patterns in family systems. Ketefian has developed a scale called Judgments About Nursing Decisions (JAND) to study the moral behavior of nurses. Kreuger developed the Subjective Experience of Therapeutic Touch measure as part of a study on touching during childbirth. Other examples of attempts to address methodological problems in nursing studies include a Nurse Practitioner Rating Form (Prescott et al 1981), an adaptation of the Organizational Climate Description Questionnaire so that it could be used to study neonatal intensive care units (Duxbury et al 1982), and Hinshaw and Atwood's work (1982), originally devised to develop strategies for evaluating the impact of change in staffing patterns on both nursing staff and clients.

Of particular interest to nurse researchers engaged in methodological studies has been the effort devoted to constructing approaches to measuring the *quality of nursing care.* Some have focused on structural variables, that is, the organization of the patient-care system; others have emphasized the actual process of giving care; and yet others have examined outcome as reflected in patient welfare. Some of the instruments developed for this purpose are the Slater Nursing Competencies Rating Scale (Wandelt & Steward 1975), which measures the competencies displayed by a nurse; the Quality Patient Care Scale (QUALPAC) (Wandelt & Ager 1974) for measuring the quality of nursing care received by a patient while care is being given; and the Nursing Audit (Phaneuf 1972) for measuring the quality of nursing care received by a patient after a cycle of care has been completed and the patient has been discharged.

The contemporary trends toward prospective payment for hospital care and consumer requirements for accountability from health professionals add to the importance of advancing the methodology and instrumentation for nursing science. Until nursing science moves from a preparadigmatic to a paradigmatic state in its evolution, both its legitimate problems and the corresponding methods for studying them are still in the state of becoming (see Chapter 10). "Acquiring a paradigm and the subsequent research it permits are signs of maturity in any scientific discipline . . . maturity not yet characteristic of nursing science. Students conducting research within existing paradigms learn the basis of their fields from similar models and usually agree about the fundamentals of methodology or acceptable evidence" (Meleis et al 1980, p. 119).

Nursing science—its philosophy, theories, and methods—is in transition. The informed clinician can become a highly valued and integral part of the development and testing of nursing theory by critically evaluating whether or to what degree the varieties of nursing study described in this chapter contribute to the actual solution of patient-care problems. In the opinion of many, herein will lie the criteria for assessing nursing's scientific progress as a professional discipline.

Designs Fit Study Problems

Earlier chapters in this text considered questions such as "What do nurses study?" and "Why are such topics important?" The emphasis in this chapter has been on *"How are nursing research questions studied?"* If you as a research consumer or as a participant in research yourself expect to have confidence in the credibility of research findings, you must be convinced that the plan or blueprint for conducting the study itself is one that effectively fits the question being asked. The design must not only suit the study purposes, answer the question, but also control for unwanted variance. As you may surmise, research designs can be simple or quite complex. If you want to pursue the topic of study designs in greater depth, try consulting one of the classic resources listed as further readings for this chapter. By now, however, you should have a good sense of the range, diversity, advantages, and disadvantages of the ones that are used most frequently in nursing research.

Summary of Key Ideas and Terms

- *Study designs* are the overall plans, or blueprints, for collecting and analyzing data in order to answer research questions as validly and reliably as possible and control for unwanted variance.

- An intelligent reader of research findings should be able to recognize the design used in a study report and evaluate its suitability for addressing a study's purpose.

- Designs for *factor-naming* and *factor-relating studies* emphasize flexibility and discovery; designs for *association-testing* (explanatory) and *causal hypothesis-testing studies* rely on control and accuracy.

- *Historical study designs* explain the past and its implications for the present and future by systematically collecting, evaluating, and interpreting evidence—such as letters, maps, books, artifacts, diaries, and public documents—that already exists.

- Processes of external criticism, to establish the authenticity of data sources, and internal criticism, to establish the accuracy of the statements or information contained within the data sources, are the critical hallmarks of sound historical research.

- Establishing the reliability of renditions of what occurred usually requires two primary (firsthand) sources that corroborate. Secondary sources (products of studying primary data or secondhand accounts) must be carefully verified before a historian can base conclusions on them.

🖊 *Case study designs* provide in-depth analyses of a single subject of investigation such as an individual patient, a family, a hospital ward, a professional organization, or the like in order to gain insight, provide background information for broader studies, develop explanations of human processes, and provide rich, descriptive anecdotes.

🖊 Despite notable contributions that single-subject studies have made in a number of disciplines, many critics believe they are limited in their generalizability.

🖊 Surveys are also called *nonexperimental designs* by some authorities, because they lack the control associated with true experiments. They can be done with large or small groups, using mailed or distributed questionnaires or interviews, to serve descriptive, comparative, correlational, developmental, and evaluative purposes. In general, they involve collecting information from a variety of sample subjects and generalizing the findings to the population of interest to the investigator.

🖊 Survey items are well suited to the study of demographic information, social characteristics, behavioral patterns, and information bases, and they have been used in a variety of nursing research studies.

🖊 A *cross-sectional survey* samples subjects who are at different points in moving through an experience and assumes that data collected from them represent different points in time. A *longitudinal survey* collects data from the same people at actual different points. In the latter, one doesn't have to make the assumption that the two groups are sufficiently comparable to designate them as representing different points in the same process or experience.

🖊 *Evaluative surveys* are used to judge the value or effectiveness of a program or strategy by providing formative (in-process) or summative (outcome) data and measuring them against specified criteria (for example, the program's goals). Context evaluation is called needs assessment research by some authorities.

🖊 In a true *experimental design* one finds the following hallmarks: (1) control over at least one independent variable and/or manipulation of at least one independent variable, (2) random selection of sample members, and (3) random assignment of sample members to control and experimental groups.

🖊 The strengths of an experimental design are that it can (1) maximize systematically introduced experimental variance, (2) control extraneous variance, and (3) minimize error variance.

✔ The ability of an experimental design to control variance contributes to its internal validity, that is, whether or not manipulation of the IV really made a difference on the DV. External validity refers to the representativeness, or generalizability, of a study's results. The experimental study design's use of randomization, control groups, and experimental groups; manipulation of the IV; and pre- and posttests, or measures of the DV, are all remedies to ward off threats to internal and external validity.

✔ Experimental designs are the only ones that can establish scientific causality. Causality requires three criteria: (1) A cause must precede an effect in time. (2) Evidence must indicate that the IV and DV are associated. (3) Evidence must as far as possible rule out other factors as determining conditions for the DV.

✔ *Quasi-experimental designs* are used when the investigator cannot randomly assign subjects to control and experimental groups but instead uses some form of comparative group.

✔ *Ex post facto designs* study something after the fact. Instead of introducing or manipulating an IV, the researcher selects subjects who have undergone some life experience and attempts to relate it to other variables. Such correlations, when they are found, should not be interpreted as cause and effect.

✔ *Methodological studies* aim to develop tools, instruments, or methods appropriate for answering nursing research questions. Of particular interest are instruments that measure quality of nursing care in terms of patient outcomes.

References

Andreoli KG: Self-concept and health beliefs in compliant and noncompliant hypertensive patients. *Nurs Res* November/December 1981; 30:323–328.

Benoliel JQ: Social characteristics of death as a recorded hospital event. In *Communicating Nursing Research*. Vol 10. Boulder, Colo.: WICHE, 1977.

Campbell DT, Stanley JC: *Experimental and Quasi-Experimental Designs for Research*. Chicago: Rand McNally, 1966.

Christy TE: *Cornerstone for Nursing Education*. New York: Teachers' College Press, Columbia University, 1969.

Christy TE: The methodology of historical research. *Nurs Res* May/June 1975; 24:189–192.

Diers D: *Research in Nursing Practice*. Philadelphia: Lippincott, 1979.

Downs F: One dark and stormy night. *Nurs Res* September/October 1983; 32:259.

Duxbury ML et al: Measurement of the nurse organizational climate of neonatal intensive care units. *Nurs Res* March/April 1982; 31:83–88.

Hinshaw AS, Atwood JR: A patient satisfaction instrument: Precision by replication. *Nurs Res* May/June 1982; 31:170–175.

Hockett HC: *Critical Method in Historical Research and Writing*. New York: Macmillan, 1955.

Holm K: Single subject research. *Nurs Res* July/August 1983; 32:253–255.

Huckaby LM: Cognitive and affective consequences of formative evaluation in graduate nursing students. *Nurs Res* 1978; 27:190.

Kerlinger FN: *Foundations of Behavioral Research.* New York: Holt, Rinehart & Winston, 1973.

Laudan L: *Progress and Its Problems: Toward a Theory of Scientific Growth.* Berkeley: University of California Press, 1977.

Levin RF: Choice of injection site, locus of control, and the perception of momentary pain. *Image* February/March 1982; 14:26–32.

Meleis AI et al: Toward scholarliness in doctoral dissertations: An analytical model. *Res Nurs Health* 1980; 3:115–124.

Mitchell P et al: Moving the patient in bed: Effects on intracranial pressure. *Nurs Res* July/August 1981; 30:212–218.

Munhall PL: Nursing philosophy and nursing research: In apposition or opposition? *Nurs Res* May/June 1982; 31.

Munhall P, Oiler C: *Nursing Research: A Qualitative Perspective.* Reston, Va.: Reston Publishing Co., 1985.

Nakagawa H, Osborne, O: An epidemiological study of psychiatric symptom pattern change: Pilot study findings. *Communicating Nursing Research.* Vol 5. Boulder Colo.: WICHE, 1972.

O'Rourke M: Psychological well-being and menstrual symptoms. *Communicating Nursing Research.* Vol 14. Boulder, Colo.: WICHE, 1981, p. 34.

Phaneuf MC: *The Nursing Audit: Profile for Excellence.* New York: Appleton-Century-Crofts, 1972.

Prescott P et al: The Nurse Practitioner Rating Form. *Nurs Res* July/August 1981; 30:223–228.

Schantz D, Lindeman CA: Reading a research article. *J Nurs Adm* March 1982; 30–33.

Secrets of making marriages last. *San Francisco Chronicle* February 3, 1984: 28–30.

Sellitz C et al: *Research Method in Social Relations.* New York: Holt, Rinehart & Winston, 1976.

Silva MC, Rothhart D: An analysis of changing trends and philosophies of science on nursing theory development and testing. *Advances in Nursing Science* January 1984; 6:2–13.

Slavinsky A, Krauss JB: Two approaches to the management of long-term psychiatric outpatients in the community. *Nurs Res* September/October 1982; 31:284–289.

Steele S et al: *Educational Evaluation in Nursing.* Thorofare, N.J.: Charles B Slack, 1978.

Toney L: The effects of holding the newborn at delivery on paternal bonding. *Nurs Res* January/February 1983; 32:16–19.

Waltz C, Bausell, RB: *Nursing Research: Design, Statistics, and Computer Analysis.* Philadelphia: FA Davis, 1981.

Wandelt MA, Ager JW: *Quality Patient Care Scale.* New York: Appleton-Century-Crofts, 1974.

Wandelt MA, Steward DS: *The Slater Nursing Competencies Rating Scale.* New York: Appleton-Century-Crofts, 1975.

Wilson HS: Curriculum evaluation research. In: *The Second Step.* Searight MW (editor). Philadelphia: FA Davis, 1976.

Wilson HS: *Deinstitutionalized Residential Care for the Mentally Disordered: The Soteria House Approach.* New York: Grune & Stratton, 1982.

Wirth P, Barton C: Barton-Wirth kidney transplant knowledge questionnaire. (Unpublished instrument.) Kidney Transplant Unit, Moffitt Hospital, University of California, San Francisco, 1983.

Further Readings

Babbie E: *Survey Research Methods.* Belmont, Calif.: Wadsworth, 1973.

Cook TD, Campbell DT: *Quasi-Experimental Design and Analysis Issues for Field Settings.* Chicago: Rand McNally, 1979.

McCoy FN: *Researching and Writing in History.* Berkeley: University of California Press, 1974.

Notter LE: The case for historical research in nursing. *Nurs Res* 1972; 21:483.

Shafer RJ (editor): *A Guide to Historical Method.* Homewood, Ill.: Dorsey Press, 1974.

Struening EL, Guttentag M (editors): *Handbook of Evaluation Research.* Beverly Hills, Calif.: Sage, 1975.

Suchman EA: *Evaluation Research: Principles and Practice in Public Service and Social Action Programs.* New York: Russell Sage, 1967.

Tuchman BW: *Practicing History.* New York: Knopf, 1981.

Weiss CH: *Evaluation Research.* Englewood Cliffs, N.J.: Prentice-Hall, 1972.

Chapter 7

Preparing a Formal Critique of Research

Judging Scientific Proposals and Reports

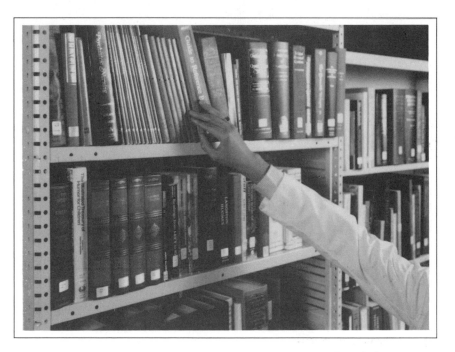

Leaders in nursing agree that all nurses, regardless of their educational level, should be armed with the necessary skills to conduct a thoughtful critique of research proposals and reports.

Chapter Outline

Chapter Objectives

After reading this chapter, the student should be able to:

- Recognize the value to nurses, as research consumers, of critiquing skills
- Distinguish between a research critique and a review
- Formulate strategies that contribute to making a critique constructive rather than destructive
- Comprehend seven basic criteria for critiquing and operationalize them in a framework of questions that the reader should raise
- Comprehend the rationale for asking the framework of critiquing questions and interpreting responses to them
- Discuss three major sources of error in research studies
- Explain 14 hallmarks of well-presented tables
- Analyze critical issues to the theoretical and logical basis of inquiry that underpin a thoughtful critique
- Apply the critiquing process to research proposals and reports of findings
- Appreciate the importance of preparing critiques that are concise, readable, rational, sensitive, accurate, and impartial

In This Chapter . . .

Criticism, in everyday parlance, is full of negative connotations. To criticize is "to censure, to blame, to reprove, to flay, to nitpick, to find fault, and to pan." But in particular literary, artistic, and scientific terms, criticism takes on an entirely different meaning—one associated with analyzing, reviewing, carefully dissecting, evaluating, or judging the merit of a piece of work. In this case, criticism refers to a finely sharpened skill for ascertaining an author or creator's meaning through an unbiased endeavor to examine the characteristics and qualities of his or her contribution to art or science. In fact, criticism as it was first introduced by Aristotle was meant to be a standard for "judging well."

Leaders in nursing all seem to agree that all nurses, regardless of their educational level, should be prepared with the skills that are essential to functioning in the role of research consumer (ANA 1976, Flemming 1980, Kramer et al 1981, Krampitz & Pavlovich 1981, Mallick 1983, Wilson 1982):

In this role practitioners read research reports of others, determine the scientific merit and clinical utility of the studies and apply findings where appropriate (Horsley & Crane 1982).

The ability to do all this depends ultimately on the nurse's skill in conducting a critique of the scientific merit of research proposals and reports. Unfortunately, most resources available to students don't do an adequate job of providing opportunities to learn the skills necessary for intelligent research consumership. Mallick (1983) and Krampitz and Pavlovich (1981) reviewed articles in nursing journals and existing textbooks to determine (1) whether the issue of teaching skills of criticism was addressed and (2) the methods for presenting the process of critical appraisal. They reflected a consensus in their conclusion that little has been written on the development of these critical evaluation skills.

The present chapter culminates Part II of this text, which has been devoted expressly to the skills of research consumership. In it, critiquing scientific proposals or reports is both described and illustrated in sufficient detail that students and practitioners can replicate the process themselves with confidence and credibility. A thoughtful critique of a research report requires more than merely knowing about a list of pertinent questions to ask, such as "Is the study question clearly stated?" or "Is the review of the literature sufficiently comprehensive?" Readers need standards against which to make such judgments, and perhaps equally important is a comprehension of the rationale for both asking and attempting to answer such questions when conducting a scientific critique. This chapter synthesizes the essential aspects of the preceding chapters in Part II on the qualities of good problem statements, the nature of evidence, the adequacy of explanation, the reliability and validity of a study's design, the handling of ideas, and the researcher's mind and virtues when generalizing from his or her findings. It presents a framework of fundamental questions and principles that underpin the process of critiquing a research proposal or report. Then it takes you the reader through a sample critiquing experience, focused on all aspects of a simulated proposal using the criteria, questions, and logic of scientific criticism.

What Is a Research Critique?

According to Leininger (1968), a *research critique* should be distinguished from a *research review*. A critique is "a critical estimate of a piece of research which has been carefully and systematically studied by a critic who has used specific criteria to appraise . . . the general features. . . . A research review on the other hand merely identifies and summarizes the major features and characteristics of a study" (p. 51). A research critique encompasses a descriptive account of what is in the study, but unlike a book report that merely summarizes the plot, the emphasis is on *making a judgment about the proposal or report's scientific merits and ultimate worth*. As must be evident from reading other chapters in this text, the scientific way of knowing is often far from flawless. Even the most conscientious researcher may have to compromise great ideas and inquiry strategies based on pragmatic and ethical considerations (see Chapters 3 and 9). The critic's challenge is to determine what the researcher has tried to do and to evaluate the strategies selected, given the overall constraints of the study. A critique presents both the criteria for and the evidence for the judgments that are made. These must be sufficient to allow another reader to form an opinion based on the critique. The art of scientific criticism can be demonstrated verbally or in a formal written document, but according to Leininger's classic article, "The most distinctive behavior of a research critic is to act in a judiciously critical but kind manner as he (or she) analyzes another person's work" (p. 53).

What Is the Purpose of a Research Critique?

The purpose of a research critique is to help an investigator refine and improve his or her program of inquiry and to help research consumers decide how to use findings from a study, based on a judicious appraisal of its strengths and limitations. Consider the example on p. 167.

Responding to such health-related questions is a regular part of a clinical nurse's role. Responding correctly requires that the nurse be skillful in critiquing studies like the one in this example.

Whether the research critique is undertaken so that scholarly colleagues can exchange information or perspectives that will advance a particular line of inquiry, or whether it is done to better inform health care consumers or other clinicians, a competent critique ought to represent a contribution to knowledge and be helpful.

Yet the critic must not confuse helpfulness with a lack of objectivity or be so earnest in his or her wish not to discourage or offend the investigator as to suppress or drastically disguise the critical points. Nurses who have practice in exercizing their critical sensibilities on the day-to-day problems of clinical practice can most certainly learn to bring the same inquiring, honest, benevolent mind to bear on the problems of research quality. Inculcating an involvement with the research enterprise in the role of research critic can foster identification and a sense of communality with the scientific community in nursing. Furthermore, it can integrate a research perspective into the evolving tapestry of each nurse's clinical interests. Preparing critiques of research proposals and reports that are objective, comprehensive, correct, respectful, and humane can work to the benefit of the nurse scientist, the nurse clinician, and the patients they serve.

Achieving these mutual goals requires that a

Example: Beer Therapy

Mr. H., a 65-year-old retired attorney with a history of hypertension and coronary heart disease, appeared for his regular blood pressure check and presented the nurse practitioner with an article he had clipped from his local newspaper. The headline read: "Beer or Jogging: A Hearty Choice." The article reported on a study, published in the *Journal of the American Medical Association* and conducted in Houston, which concluded that "drinking three beers a day is about as good as jogging when it comes to producing an effect that may decrease the risk of coronary heart disease." The researchers had found that volunteer runners and joggers registered about the same high-density lipoprotein (HDL), a type of cholesterol associated with heart disease, as did volunteer sedentary men who drank three cans of beer each day for the three-week period of the study. The rationale was that moderate drinking causes the liver to respond by producing the same or similar enzymes it produces in response to exercise. Mr. H.'s question to the nurse, of course, was whether he could now substitute three beers a day for the daily walking that he'd been encouraged to do, in view of these new scientific findings.

Clients seek health information from nurses

Partial reports of health research appear regularly in the popular press

Findings

Are the client's conclusions from the findings warranted?

---

critic and an investigator be able to differentiate between *constructive* and *destructive criticism.*

Constructive criticism is evident when the critic offers thoughtful comments which are given in such a way that they stimulate the researcher to use suggestions and motivate him (or her) to continue work on the study. In contrast, destructive criticism tends to thwart the researcher's interest in his (or her) work (Leininger 1968, p. 55).

The careful choice of words in a critique is often cited as one of the most important features of artful and sensitive criticism that the researcher being criticized will use rather than become defensive about. A few helpful do's and don'ts in dealing with the interpersonal aspects of critiquing research are summarized in Table 7-1. Research critiques that bear in mind their real purpose and attend to the potentially delicate social psychology of the researcher–critic relationship can provide valuable opportunities for scholarly and intellectual exchanges that can advance both the science and the professional practice of nursing.

What Are the Criteria for Good Research?

Recognizing the importance of upgrading standards of reporting clinical research, Field (1983) and Fleming and Hayter (1974) suggest that a combination of the following criteria be used when evaluating reports of nursing studies:

1. Clarity and relevance of the purpose.
2. Researchability of the problem.
3. Adequacy and relevance of the literature review.
4. Match between the purpose, design, and methods.
5. Suitability of the sampling procedure and the sample.
6. Correctness of the analytic procedures.
7. Clarity of the findings.

Table 7-1   Do's and Don'ts for Sensitive Critiques

Do	Don't
1. Try to convey a sincere interest in the study you are critiquing	1. Avoid excessive nit-picking and fault finding on trivial details
2. Be sure to emphasize the points of excellence that you discover	2. Never ridicule or demean an investigator personally
3. Choose clear, concise statements to communicate your observations rather than ambiguous ones	3. Don't try to include flattery that is designed merely to boost a researcher's self-esteem
4. When pointing out a study's weaknesses, include explanations that justify your comments about them	4. Don't base your summary and recommendations about the study on some loose and perhaps biased attitude toward the state of all science in a particular discipline or on a particular topic
5. Include supportive and encouraging statements where they are warranted	5. Don't write your critique in condescending, patronizing, or condemning language
6. Be aware of your own negative attitudes toward a particular approach to science or any personal hostilities that could distort your ability to judge a study on its own merits	6. Don't forget that your purpose is to advise the researcher and to improve the work
7. Offer practical suggestions that are not overly esoteric or unrealistic	
8. Remember that empathy for the researcher is often crucial to being an effective critic	

Clarity and Relevance of the Study's Purpose

All researchers should specifically state the aims of the study being evaluated. The author should clearly explain the reasons for doing the study and indicate why it is of any importance. Finally, the reader should be convinced that conducting the study is indeed worthwhile. A judgment about the potential value of a nursing study is easier to make if you ask three questions about it:

1. Will the study solve a problem relevant to nursing?

2. Will the facts collected be useful to nursing?

3. Will the study contribute to nursing knowledge?

Many authorities believe that in order to be classified as *nursing research*, studies have to make a first-order contribution to testing clinical nurs-ing interventions or patient responses to them (Field 1983). Others argue that contributions to nursing education and nursing administration, although termed *research in nursing*, are equally justifiable. The key point is to be sure that your critique does not condemn a researcher for failing to accomplish something that was not part of his or her purpose in the first place.

Researchability of the Study Problem

Chapter 5 goes into depth about how to state a researchable study problem. If you recall, a well-stated study problem should at least be able:

1. to be answered through measuring empirical evidence or data

2. to be stated as a question that involves the

existence of a relationship between two or more variables

Having established that the two most fundamental criteria are met in a study problem, other questions relevant to critiquing the quality of a study problem are:

3. Is the statement of the problem clearly and specifically articulated *early* in the proposal or report?

4. Have the investigators placed the study problem within the context of existing knowledge and prior work on the topic?

5. Are the hypotheses, or research questions, explicitly stated?

6. Are the concepts or variables operationally defined so that the methods for measuring them could be replicated?

7. Are the limitations and assumptions of the study included, and are they logically justifiable?

8. Does the problem statement accurately reflect the title of the study?

9. Are the study questions, or hypotheses, clear, specific, testable, and consistent with the study title, purpose, and subsequent literature review?

Adequacy and Relevance of the Literature Review

Whether it is called a "review of related literature" or "a theoretical framework" for the study, evidence that the researcher has a mastery of current knowledge on his or her topic of inquiry and has placed the proposed or reported study within its context is a third criterion for judging the scientific merit of research (see Chapter 9). Not only should you the critic find such a section in the material you read and the references listed at the document's end, but you must also be convinced that:

1. the investigator has selected references that logically pertain to the subject being studied and the methodology being used

2. the investigator has not merely presented a laundry list of sources but instead has integrated them into a background synthesis that suggests how the present study resolves controversies, fills gaps in knowledge, extends or refutes what is already known, and so on (see Chapter 10)

3. the literature review section is logically organized

4. the review does not omit classic or landmark sources (You may need to consult an expert in the substantive field of the investigation on this point if you are not familiar with the body of literature on a certain topic.)

5. the investigator has been open-minded enough to include references to prior work that may not be supportive

6. the literature review or theoretical framework makes sense as a rationale for framing the specific hypotheses or research questions being examined

7. the review provides justification for operational definitions of concepts or variables that have been advanced

8. the review supports the choices of data-collection tools and instruments in the present study

Agreement of Purpose, Design, and Methods

As you recall, the study design is the overall blueprint selected to answer the research question and enhance the study's validity and reliability, and the methodology is a description of the procedures for data collection and analysis to be used in a study (see Chapter 6). As a critic you should ask:

1. Does the investigator name and describe the study design, including its strengths

and weaknesses for the problem under scrutiny?

2. Is the study design well matched to the task of answering the specified study questions and controlling extraneous variables that could detract from the value of study findings? (See Box 7-1 for sources of error in research studies.)

3. Does the investigator provide evidence from pilot tests or published literature that the data-collection procedures are reliable and valid?

4. Does the investigator include a copy of the data-gathering instrument or other evidence that it is free from ambiguity, bias, or significant omissions?

5. Are the sources for and adaptations of non-original data-collection tools provided?

6. If the data-collection tools are self-developed, are the processes for developing them and reports for establishing their validity and reliability included?

7. Are the techniques for data collection logical and practical ways of acquiring empirical evidence on study variables?

8. Does the researcher include checks to guard against possible errors in collecting, recording, and tabulating data? (Such choices include card cleaning, if the data are on keypunched cards. See Chapter 16.)

9. If the design was experimental, do you find evidence of control of extraneous variables, manipulation of independent variables, randomization in both sample selection and assignment of sample members to treatment groups, and replicability?

10. What attempts were made to keep research conditions the same for all sample members?

11. Did the investigator try to keep subjects and researchers who were recording outcomes "blind" with regard to which intervention was being administered to whom?

Box 7-1   Potential Causes of Research Error

Data Characteristics

1. Inadequate sampling
2. Inaccurate measurement
3. Unrepresentative data
4. Careless observation
5. Intentionally distorted data

Analytical Characteristics

1. Mathematical errors
2. Incorrect choice of formulas
3. Comparison of nonanalogous data
4. Generalization based on insufficient data
5. Failure to acknowledge significant factors
6. Confusion of correlation with causation
7. Interpretation manipulated to support prejudice or preconception
8. Elimination of contrary evidence

Suitability of the Sampling Procedure and the Sample

Because it is usually not feasible to obtain data from every member or element in an entire population, the researcher should explain his or her approach to deciding which of all those possible study elements are to be used as sample members and data sources. When critiquing the study sample, you should be able to determine:

1. Did the investigator choose to use a probability or nonprobability sample? Why one or the other? (See Chapter 9.)

2. What strategies were incorporated to avoid collecting a biased sample about which one could not generalize to the target population?

3. Is the sample representative of the population to which findings are to be generalized?

4. Is the sample size large enough to meet the

assumptions of any statistical test that may be used in data analysis? (See Chapter 15.)

5. Is the sample size large enough to reduce the standard error?

6. What are the descriptive characteristics of the sample, particularly with respect to any variables that might influence study findings such as age, education, sex, or physical or psychological condition?

7. What criteria were used to enter eligible sample members into a study?

8. How was informed consent obtained and the rights of the human research subjects protected? For example did each subject get a complete and honest explanation of the purpose of the research, what was going to happen to him or her, and the use to which findings would be put?

9. Finally, were subject losses due to lack of follow-up or to dropping out detailed?

Correctness of Analytic Procedures

Data-analysis methods, including both statistical procedures and qualitative methods and appropriate references to them, should be clearly presented. Presentations of summary data should be clear enough to allow the reader to determine whether the statistical methods were the appropriate ones. Mention of the *power* of the test should be made, so that you and other readers can decide whether the study was conducted on a viable number of subjects and whether an increase or decrease in number of subjects could have affected the results and to what extent (see Chapter 9). Assumptions related to the use of statistics should all be made clear (see Chapter 15). In the case of qualitative analysis methods, sufficient detail about the analytic approach should be included so that another investigator could replicate the analytic operations (see Chapter 14). Specific questions that you should ask in the role of research critic include:

1. Does the author specifically name the statistical tests applied, along with the probability associated with significant values?

2. Does the author explain and provide references for analytic strategies for nonnumerical data?

3. Are the statistical tests used appropriate to the level of measurement (nominal, ordinal, interval, or ratio) represented by the data? (See Chapter 15.)

4. Is a distinction made between statistical and clinical significance?

5. Is the statistical procedure the right one to answer the specified research question?

Clarity of Findings

The results section of a research report normally contains a technical report of how the statistical or qualitative analyses turned out with respect to study questions or hypotheses to be tested. The discussion of results is usually devoted to a nontechnical interpretation of them. In addition to telling us what the results mean, some researchers use the discussion section to explain why they think the results turned out the way they did. Some authors will use the discussion section to suggest ideas for further research. Results themselves will usually appear in the text of the article, in one or more tables, or in graphs (technically called figures). As a research consumer, you must be able to read, understand, and critically evaluate the results in a research report to avoid uncritical acceptance of findings just because it's in print. You don't have to be a whiz in math to get the drift of a results section in a scientific article. Becoming familiar with research terminology (see Chapter 4) and the principles of scientific evidence that follow in this chapter will enable you to become much more comfortable with this task. Questions that you should ask in your role of research critiquer about reports and discussions of findings are given on the following page.

Box 7-2   Hallmarks of Well-Presented Tables

1. *Every table should have a title.* The title should represent a succinct description of the contents of the table and should help make it intelligible without reference to the text. The title should be clear, concise, and adequate and should answer the questions *What? Where?* and *When?* The title should always be placed above the body of the table.

2. Every table should be identified by a number to facilitate easy reference. *The number is in arabic numerals*, and it can be centered above the title or placed on the first line of the title.

3. The captions, or column headings, and the stubs, or row readings, of the table should be clear and brief.

4. Any explanatory footnotes concerning the table itself are placed directly beneath the table.

5. If the data in a series of tables have been obtained from different sources, it is ordinarily advisable to indicate the specific sources in an inconspicuous place just below the table.

6. In order to emphasize the relative importance of certain categories, different kinds of type, spacing, and indentation can be used.

7. It is important that all column figures be properly aligned. Decimal points and plus and minus signs also should be in perfect alignment.

8. Sometimes the columns are numbered to facilitate reference.

9. Miscellaneous and exceptional items are generally placed in the last row of the table.

10. Since it may be found very confusing to read a long table when all the rows or lines are single spaced, it is

a common practice to group the stubs or side-heads. Generally, grouping of stubs by fives or fours is very satisfactory.

11. Abbreviations should be avoided whenever possible, and ditto marks should not be used in a statistical table.

12. The actual arrangement of the major classes in the table depends on the facts and relationships that are to be emphasized. It should always be kept in mind, however, that a statistical table should be made as logical, clear, accurate, and simple as possible.

13. Columns and rows that are to be compared with one another should be brought close together.

14. Totals can be placed either at the top or at the bottom of the table. It might be pointed out in this connection that the *most conspicuous part of the table is the upper left-hand corner.*

---

1. Are interpretations of results clearly based on the data obtained?

2. Are reasons given for tabulating or presenting data in particular ways?

3. Can you detect error in any computations?

4. Are there any discrepancies between results presented in graphic form and results presented in the text of the report?

5. Do all the tables and graphs have titles?

6. Are the relationships of the variables in

tables clear and easy to figure out? (See Box 7-2 for additional characteristics of good tables and see Chapter 17.)

7. Has the researcher distinguished between actual findings, on the one hand, and interpretations made by the researcher, on the other?

8. Are the findings explicit enough for you the critic to decide if the interpretations are justified? (For example, some authorities agree that conclusions of any kind cannot

be drawn from data returns of less than 51% of the sample.)

9. Are minor or secondary findings overemphasized in the report and major or primary findings underplayed?

10. Are the findings clearly and logically organized?

11. Is the presentation of findings impartial and unbiased?

12. Do generalizations or conclusions go beyond the data collected or the population represented by the sample?

13. Are recommendations for further research offered?

14. Does the researcher include unsuccessful efforts and negative outcomes?

15. Are limitations that might have influenced the results noted?

What Are the Standards of Scientific Merit?

Good-quality research can use a variety of study designs (including descriptive and fieldwork techniques in which the investigator does not attempt to manipulate an independent variable). A sound research project can collect numerical or nonnumerical data. Research settings can be laboratories or natural conditions. The study can be based on a large number of subjects or a single case. A research project can be a one-shot study or an integral part of a continuing series of replicated studies. No one design or method is "best," and no one approach is scientifically most powerful. This attitude of flexibility and diversity also applies to techniques of analysis. *The critical point is that researchers always employ the study design and analytic procedure that answer the particular questions that are being studied.* Openness to experience can be seen as being fully as important a characteristic of the scientist as is the understanding of a research design. And the whole enterprise of science can be seen as but one portion of a larger field of knowledge in which truth is pursued in many equally meaningful ways, science being one of these ways.

Understanding the principles behind the framework of specific criteria and questions that are useful in the process of scientific criticism is as important to becoming a skilled research con-

sumer as is knowing which questions to ask. A clinician conducting a mental status examination of an 83-year-old woman in a psychiatric outpatient department knows to include interview questions about distant and recent memory. The clinician also knows that answers that indicate, for example, that the patient remembers the name of her high school principal but not the name of the current president of the United States or mayor of her city constitute evidence of memory impairment. But the most critical point is that this kind of memory impairment along with other specific evidence of diminished intellectual functioning signify the presence of dementia. In other words, the nurse must not only know what questions to ask, the areas in which to ask them, and what the answers may signify but must also comprehend why knowing all this is relevant in the first place. This idea is also true for the research critic and skillful research consumer. The rationale for asking the elaborate array of precise questions and considering the preceding seven specific criteria when appraising a research proposal or report of findings rests on principles or conventions associated with the logic of scientific work and the logic of inquiry.

Considering some of the more theoretical aspects of research critiques seems justified, if not essential, because they tend to be neglected in most books and articles on the subject of critiquing research in favor of a more "cookbookish" approach. Whereas pragmatic strategies for undertaking a critique of scientific research have consumed the first half of this chapter, we now turn our attention briefly to examining them in their relationship to broader logical and theoretical considerations about science. The goal here is to help the research consumer transcend a technician's role and attain the knowledge base appropriate for a true professional engaged in the application of scientific findings. Mere technical virtuosity without attention to rationale is unfortunately likely to lead to sterile results.

The Theoretical and Logical Bases of Inquiry

Certain theoretical assumptions about the nature of reality and the logic of scientific inquiry guide researchers in their choices of topics and their research procedures. They also offer a basis for evaluating or critiquing the research enterprise as reflected in study proposals and reports of findings. The principles set forth in this section, though not necessarily exhaustive, include those that strongly influence a critic's thinking when preparing a research critique. Sjoberg and Nett (1968), among others, believe that such principles influence the rules, procedures, and methods for conducting "good" science. Certain choices or actions are thereby judged as preferable to others in aiding the scientist's search for truth or empirically grounded knowledge. These rules have become the bases for the norms of science and the conventions on which scientists and scientific critics have reached some points of consensus. Even with agreement on conventions that reject the explanatory value of hunches, guesswork, or casual observation, methodological scrupulousness does not yield unquestionable, universal, or unalterable truths about reality. These principles should be used as keys to evaluating the merits of nursing research studies, not as methods for unlocking the doors to incontrovertible scientific laws. In Kaplan's words (1964, p. 5), "Standards governing the conduct of inquiry in any of its phases emerge from inquiry and are themselves subject to further inquiry." Because nurse executives and clinicians base the decisions that affect nurses' future on findings from nursing studies, however, we ought to be as well-informed as possible. Research consumers apply their skills and understanding of scientific criticism to help make that happen.

The Nature of Reality

A long-standing debate about whether reality is stable or fluid and whether humans respond to or create their environment underlies nursing studies (see Chapters 1 and 13). Scientists who argue that a fixed, stable order characterizes social as well as physical reality subscribe to canons of science directed toward accurately and precisely uncovering "what actually exists." Others, while conceding that there is a degree of order in the world, stress its ever-changing and complex nature and posit scientific methods that allow them to study this fluidity. Additionally, those who think of the environment as fluid tend to conceive of humans as interpreting and shaping their reality, whereas those who are committed to a conception of a fixed set of relations in the objective world tend to conceive of humans as responding, adapting, or coping with physical and social forces. Studies with the former orientation emphasize the value of the flexibility of field methods, and those with the latter assumptions require reliability and validity of measurement instruments that reflect the "actual value" of an operationally defined variable at a static point in time.

The Observer's Relationship to Observed Phenomena

Every nursing study indicates some assumption about the scientific observer vis-à-vis the variables being observed. The most marked divergence is between those associated with the logical positivist perspective, who assume that observers should be able to distance themselves and make unbiased observations, and the adherents of the *verstehen* approach, which contends that the observer always influences and is influenced by the reality under investigation. Obviously, the logical positivist values strategies or instruments designed to eliminate observer bias, and the *verstehen* scientist emphasizes the value of being aware of and reporting on the subjective, interpretive nature of the observer–observed interaction and his or her *attempts* to approach the ideal of objectivity (which many philosophers of science believe the logical positivist takes for granted but rarely achieves).

The Relationship Between Theory and Data

As Sjoberg and Nett (1968) point out, theory as a system of concepts or ideas is not unique to science but is basic to all systems of philosophy and religious thought (see Chapter 10). The essential difference lies in the use of empirical observation as the method of discovery or validation. Although scientists seem to agree that both theory and data are essential features of the scientific method, they disagree, as have philosophers since Kant and Hume, about the relationship between the two. Some nursing scientists define theory in rigorous terms that are applicable only to systems that involve sets of postulates from which testable hypotheses (proposi-

tions) can be derived. In the opinion of others, any logically related statements that explain an investigator's observations or make them meaningful can be considered as scientific theory in a broad sense. Nurse scientists and scholars sometimes disagree about whether theory or data have priority in the research process. The split between those researchers who stress theory and those who emphasize observation (data) in effect reflects the difference between adhering to a *deductive* theory-testing approach in science and more *inductive* inquiry that is oriented toward discovery (see Chapters 10 and 14). Clearly, evaluation criteria that address the quality of hypotheses, identification of independent and dependent variables, and the like are much more appropriate when the study under examination is in the deductive tradition.

The Value of Natural or Artificial Language

Natural language, on the one hand, is ordinary language. It may be vague, convey shades of emotion, and be somewhat ambiguous when used by different people. Artificial, or scientific, language systems, on the other hand, primarily try to free the scientific discourse from the perceived inadequacies of ordinary language. The ultimate artificial language is, of course, a mathematical formula. Many nursing studies should be judged on their adherence to a traditional "axiomatic" system of logic. That is, (1) a system of hypotheses is derived from previous research, (2) definition of key terms is advanced in "scientific" language, and (3) the hypotheses are subjected to test through empirical observation. Other studies reflect research procedures based on the notion that science is and should be *inductive*, in that it extracts out of nature (data) an order (a conceptual but "natural" explanation) to produce truth. A critic can't hope to resolve the controversy about the proper language and logical systems in nursing research, but he or she can be sensitive to the view about induction or inference that shapes the study problem and mode of analysis reflected in a particular study and resist evaluating it according to inappropriate criteria. Study designs and research procedures selected to maximize discovery and flexibility will necessarily require somewhat different yardsticks for measuring their quality and effectiveness than studies that emphasize accuracy, precision, exactness, and control (see Chapter 14).

Selection of Units of Analysis and Sources of Data

The way a nurse scientist elects to choose sample members and the kinds of data collected say a lot about his or her conception of the scientific method. Many of the technical procedures, particularly those involved in choosing a random sample, depart considerably from commonsense thinking. Before the investigator selects the sample members from whom data will be collected, he or she must have a clear conception of the ultimate range of generalizations from the study. Regardless of the type of sampling procedure (probability or nonprobability), most authorities alert us to the error of drawing generalizations from data that cannot be demonstrated to be typical, random, or representative in any sense. Even when one is studying the extremes of human action, where probability sampling would not be appropriate, one can expect to see careful, purposeful sampling and plans to discover whether the patterns that are discovered can be replicated with different groups.

The Nature and Adequacy of Proof

The nature and adequacy of proof engage the critic in the questions related to when data are considered adequate to support a given analytic scheme or set of hypotheses. The controversies surrounding this topic involve at least three related issues:

1. the necessity of quantifying data and the relative merits of tests of statistical significance versus multivariate analyses
2. the question whether prediction or understanding is the key criterion for judging the adequacy of one's data relative to one's theory or hypotheses
3. the most meaningful techniques for establishing the reliability and validity of evidence

The quantification of independent, dependent, and extraneous variables in any research situation is a function of the researcher's broader conception of the reality being studied. Many nurse researchers find it difficult to isolate and measure these variables precisely when they are investigating human problems that are amorphous and complex without imposing an artificiality or fictional nature on it. On one side of the debate are nurse scientists advocating the rigid adoption of measurement and statistical rules used so productively in many of the physical sciences. Others argue that the application of measurement and statistical rules and procedures to complex, interactional human systems still needs much more methodological research before all the issues associated with their use can be resolved. Proponents of the latter view point out that many of the proxy indicators used to "measure" nonunitary and abstract concepts or variables in nursing studies are often controversial, crude, or even meaningless. The problem is compounded further when nurse researchers apply powerful statistical procedures to nominal and ordinal scale measures. To manipulate nominal or ordinal data through the use of inappropriate statistics is viewed as imposing an artificial order on the nature of social reality.

Similarly, there is no firm consensus among nurse scientists about the criteria for judging the adequacy of an explanation or theory. Nurses who align themselves with the positivist scientific tradition contend that prediction is the key requirement. In this view nursing theory must ultimately be evaluated for its predictive power. From the symbolic-interactionist perspective, however, the function of nursing theory should be to promote understanding, thus rejecting the notion that human action can be predicted in mechanistic terms (see Chapters 1 and 10). Among advocates of this philosophy of science, understanding is the goal of inquiry, and coherence is the basis for judging truth. If the analysis or theory makes sense of the data under study in a coherent and internally consistent way, the explanation meets the criterion of adequacy.

Yet another point bearing on the nature and adequacy of proof is the matter of determining the reliability and validity of data. You will recall that reliability refers to the consistency among observers (or data-collection tools), and validity refers to the accuracy or adequacy of the data in view of the study question being asked (see Chapters 4 and 11). The test–retest and split-half techniques are procedures regularly used to determine whether data collected are consistent over time or across raters or observers. And the prediction or some variant thereof is basic to the means of validating measurement techniques. Critics of the standard techniques for establishing reliability charge that they tend to lead nurse researchers to sacrifice generality for specificity and reductionism. Critics of validity techniques based on predictability protest that nurse researchers require a fuller grasp of the conditions in which prediction can and cannot be effectively employed.

The preceding paragraphs merely highlight some of the issues related to an extremely complex matter. Blalock (1964) probably summarizes them best:

We would suggest flexibility as the guiding theme. In our haste to become 'scientific' we have perhaps overrigidly followed the few rules . . . which have been rigorously set forth (p. 185).

Norms that Govern the Dissemination of Research Findings

Advancement of nursing science must be built on prior achievements, and thus a body of nursing knowledge depends on rapid and widespread communication of research findings. When judging the effectiveness of dissemination of findings, a critic must consider evidence that the author has attended to:

- the nature of the audience or reference group (readership)
- the style employed in research reporting (see Chapter 17)
- the ethical norms that govern what should and should not be published (see Chapter 3)

The critic's task is to spot potentially significant contributions to knowledge in an expanding sea of research publications of variable quality. Conventions of form may dominate the questions a critic raises about a report of research, but true scientific advancement depends on creative ideas for both controversy and inspiration.

Critiquing a Sample Proposal

You will now have an opportunity to practice applying the critiquing criteria presented earlier in this chapter to a hypothetical sample research proposal (see Box 7-3). Doing so will help you extrapolate the knowledge and skills of critiquing research to other studies you encounter.

Having read the preceding simulated study proposal, you are now in a position to apply the criteria for a research critique, raise the set of questions related to each of them, and think through the important considerations concerning the logic of inquiry.

Clarity and Relevance of the Study Purpose
Reducing postoperative distress is indeed relevant and useful to nursing. Knowing if a specific training program can achieve it would contribute to nursing knowledge and perhaps even alter and make more effective the nature of "standard" preoperative preparation. Thus, our sample study is both clear and relevant insofar as its purpose and value for nursing are concerned.

Box 7-3   Sample Study Proposal

Title:

Training in Cognitive Coping Skills and the Reduction of Postsurgical Distress

Purpose:

Nursing's major goal after a patient experiences surgery is his or her uncomplicated recovery. Most patients who are admitted to a hospital for surgery experience anxiety and feel helpless. They are surrounded by unfamiliar machinery and subjected to invasive procedures. Yet ample literature supports the conclusion that the events themselves rarely cause patient anxiety but rather the patients' views and information about the events. This study will demonstrate that training in cognitive coping skills can reduce patient anxiety and contribute to a less distressing postsurgical recovery. Implications of this study are that nurses will have empirical support for their role as a health educator, and patients will experience surgery as less traumatic because they feel more independent and in control of their experience. In sum, the specific question for this research is whether cognitive-coping skills training can reduce postsurgical distress in adult patients.

Hypothesis:

The specific hypothesis to be tested in this study is: Patients who are trained in the use of cognitive coping skills before surgery experience less postoperative distress than similar patients who do not receive such training.

Review of Related Literature and Conceptual Framework:

The conceptual framework for this study is drawn from related literature in the fields of nursing and psychology. Meichenbaum, Golfried, Mahoney and colleagues have demonstrated that an individual's internal dialogue and images influence not only feelings related to a situation but also a person's behavior. Langer and associates (1975) trained surgical patients to use cognitive coping skills, including reappraisal and rehearsing positive aspects of a surgical experience, and found that in their sample there was a significant reduction in postsurgical distress. Further clinical evidence of the value of using cognitive coping skills was present in studies by Meichenbaum and Wine (1970). In their research, students after receiving training in coping skills began to label physiological arousal like sweating, increased heart and respiratory rate, and the like as coping rather than debilitating. Other studies have likewise reported reductions in test and speech anxiety following similar training (Wine 1971, Sarason 1973, Norman 1974). Based on the literature cited above, it seems reasonable to assume that surgical patients' internal dialogue and images related to their surgical procedures may influence their postsurgical distress. This study addresses the question of whether a surgical patient's postsurgical distress can be reduced by altering his or her views about the surgical experience through coping-skills training.

Definition of Terms:

Cognitive-coping-skills training: a process by which a nurse teaches patients to change distress-provoking thoughts and styles of thinking in order to produce thoughts that decrease distress.

Box 7-3   (continued)

Postsurgical Distress: constitutes the dependent variable in this study and will be measured operationally using the following indicators:

1. length of stay in the recovery room
2. frequency of pain medication requested
3. time required before eating again by mouth
4. length of hospital stay
5. time required to attain normal routine at home
6. self-report of experience after discharge
7. incidence and severity of postoperative complications

The cognitive-coping-skills training program constitutes the independent variable in this study and will be carried out for all sample members according to the following procedure:

I. Educational Phase:

The purpose of the first phase is to convey the idea that there is no 1 : 1 correlation between a situation and a feeling; rather, it is the individual's style of thinking and images that are the major influencing factors in distress.

This section will incorporate didactic and experiential examples of the idea above. Discussion involving members will be encouraged. Charts and diagrams will be used to aid in understanding the relationship between events and thoughts. Patients will be told that they probably have not been aware of the influence of thoughts on behavior because they were taught to believe that there is a correlation between the two. They will be told that thinking and thinking styles have become routine and automatic, and thus we are not aware of them. Demonstration of this concept of automatic thinking will be carried out.

There will be a homework assignment given to members to bring back the following day. The patients will be asked to visualize the situation of their upcoming surgery and to record their thoughts, images, and feelings concerning the surgery.

II. Rehearsal Phase:

The next day, we will work with the data provided by each member in the following way:

Cognitive Reappraisal
1. Identify with the patients their distressful thoughts (for example, "I am going to die").
2. Teach the patients to identify their assumptions and distinguish them from facts. (Assumptions are neither true nor false but are only probabilities.)
3. Teach the patients to counter their assumptions, using thoughts and images that are incompatible with the original distress-producing thoughts.

A homework assignment will be given to reinforce what the patients have learned.

continued

Box 7-3   (continued)

III. Calming Self-Talk:

Patients will be taught how a stress situation occurs and how to prepare themselves. Examples will be given.

Stress comes about in stages:

Stages	*Examples of Calming Self-Talk*
1. what we say to ourselves when preparing for surgery	1. "I can develop a plan to deal with this situation."
2. the actual situation (the surgery)	2. "One step at a time. I can handle this situation."
3. coping with being overwhelmed	3. "When fear comes, just pause."
4. reinforcing self-statements	4. "I can be pleased with my progress."

IV. Cognitive Control Through Selective Attention:

Patients will be shown that selection of a particular focus (regular breathing, repeating a statement) is incompatible with negative thoughts that produce distress.

Data Collection Procedures and Methodology:

Settings for this study will be four private and public hospitals in a West Coast urban area. Patients of either sex who are in the age range 30–55, have had no previous surgery, have no clinically documented illness, are scheduled for a cholecystectomy without common duct exploration, are willing to give informed consent, and have their physician's referral will be admitted to the study *sample* until a total *n* of 100 patients is achieved. Patients will be assigned alternately to Group A or Group B. Group A will receive cognitive-coping-skill training, and Group B, the control group, will receive no special preoperative preparation other than standard care.

The training will be done by the same nurse with special skills in this method and take 1 hour for each of four days before admission to the hospital for surgery. Patient data will be obtained from the following data sources:

1. the recovery room chart
2. the ward patient chart
3. telephone interviews to obtain self-reports
4. one follow-up home visit conducted one month after discharge

Limitations in the form of uncontrolled *extraneous variables* that are acknowledged consist of the following:

1. Patients at the younger end of the age range may recover more quickly than patients at the older end.
2. Self-report data may be influenced by sample members' attempting to please the interviewer.
3. No comparable preoperative intervention for the control group leaves unanswered the questions of whether any differences are due to the training per se or just any form of special attention.

Box 7-3   (continued)

Data Analysis

The following mock tables reflect the data analysis plan. Scores will be constructed for frequencies of behaviors, summarized in Table I, and frequency of negative and positive comments reported in postoperative phone and home-visit interviews, reflected in Table II. Statistical-analysis procedures will include descriptive data summaries that characterize the study sample and specific techniques appropriate for comparing frequencies for significant differences. Expectations are that the hypothesis will be supported and that both statistically and clinically significant differences will be found between Group A and Group B on the dependent variable of postoperative distress.

Table I: Frequency of Postoperative Distress Behaviors

Distress Behavior	Total Frequency Group A	Total Frequency Group B
1. Length of stay in recovery room (hours)		
2. Number of pain-medication requests		
3. Time required to begin eating by mouth (hours)		
4. Length of hospital stay (hours)		
5. Time required to attain normal routines at home (hours)		
6. Numbers of postoperative complications		

Table II: Self-Report on Postoperative Distress

Number of Negative Comments		Number of Positive Comments	
Group A	Group B	Group A	Group B
Total	Total	Total	Total

SOURCE: Adapted from a research proposal B.E.U. Stroud Rhonert Park, Calif.: Sonoma State University, 1977.

Researchability of the Study Problem   The investigator has met many of the standards for a researchable study problem. The problem can be answered by collecting or measuring empirical data. The investigator has explicitly asked the question: "Can training in cognitive coping skills reduce postsurgical distress in adult patients?" Coping-skills training has been identified as the independent variable and been given an operational definition. Postsurgical distress has been identified as the dependent variable and provided with an operational definition. A specific hypothesis to be tested in the study has been stated: that the training will reduce postsurgical distress. And the study question is accurate and consistent with the title, purpose, and literature review.

The investigator includes some of the study's limitations. But—and this is a rather big *but*— *justification* for accepting the study with those limitations is not included. The influence of age could be controlled for, either through sampling techniques that matched comparative groups by age or through using statistical means to account for any differences in findings that could be attributed to age differences rather than to the independent variable. Similarly, strategies to minimize the Hawthorne effect—the likelihood that any significant differences between Groups A and B are due to the fact that Group A got some kind of "special attention" for four extra hours plus homework activities and group support—could have been incorporated into the study design. Four hours of other individual or group interaction could have been provided to the control group (for example, a general discussion group with the nurse in which the coping skills were *not* taught). Finally, the possibility of biased self-report data could have been decreased by using a mailed, objective self-report form rather than a face-to-face or even telephone conversation with the nurse (particularly if the nurse doing the follow-up interviews was the same one who did the training program).

Adequacy and Relevance of the Literature Review   Again the investigator has met a number of the standards for an acceptable literature review. The references are pertinent to the subject under investigation, are integrated and logically organized, and provide a rationale for the present study. We can also note the following deficiencies, however:

1. The references are dated (not current).
2. We are left unsure about how this particular study will extend prior work.
3. One of the dates is omitted from the references.
4. The literature review does not provide us with the investigator's rationale for measuring the dependent variable of postsurgical distress in the manner chosen.
5. We really don't get much insight into the researcher's awareness of the range of opinion and extent of research findings in the problem area. For example, we don't know if this is a well-studied area or whether the references incorporated represent the totality of the work previously done on this topic.

Agreement of Purpose, Design, and Methods   Although the study has been designed to try to answer the research question, we must notice that a number of omissions make it difficult to conclude that efforts to increase its validity and reliability will be successful. For example, the investigator does not ever actually discuss the choice of a study design and therefore does not comment on its strengths and weaknesses. Because sample members are not randomly selected or assigned, we can surmise that this is a quasi-experimental design with a comparative group. But we are not assured that the two groups are actually comparable once they have been constructed, because analysis of demographic data is not included in the analysis plan. We have commented earlier on the ways in which the procedures fail to control for some of the extraneous variables that could affect the study findings. We also have no results of pilot studies or power analyses on which to base any decisions about the reliability and validity of data-collection operations and adequacy of sample size. For example, is it correct to assume that the number of requests for pain medication is necessarily an indicator of postoperative distress? Might cultural or personal preferences about taking medication be a factor here? The investigator also does not provide us with copies of the data-collection and data-recording tools, making it hard to assess exactly how self-report data, in particular, will be obtained and making it impossible to actually replicate the study. Not knowing what tools or instruments will be used makes it impossible for us to know the sources of them, their tested validity and reliability, or how they were developed—if they were. Finally, although conditions were apparently to be the same for all members of Group A, who experienced the experimental treatment, conditions for Group B were not comparable to those for Group A, and we have no reason to believe that the rater or interviewer was blind when collecting the postoperative data on the dependent variable.

Suitability of the Sampling Procedure   The investigator does tell us the size of the intended sample, the fact that it will be collected from four different hospital settings, and the criteria used to enter eligible sample members into the study. What we find missing is the rationale for these choices. Why not a random sample and assignment to groups? On what basis was the sample size of 100 made? Addition of more of the sampling logic and reporting on the characteristics of the two groups in the study's final report both represent areas for improvement.

Correctness of Analytic Procedures   The logic of analysis of data in the study is underdeveloped and incomplete. Why focus exclusively on absolute frequencies? Are they all of equal weight or importance? What, specifically, will be performed statistically to answer the study question and test the hypothesis for significant differences between the two groups. The analysis section is perhaps the weakest single aspect of the study proposal. We are unable to answer any of the questions appropriate for conducting a critique of a study's analytic procedures, even though sample tables are incorporated. For instance, we don't know the name of the statistical tests to be applied, the probability associated with significant values, how any extra qualitative data might be analyzed or if it will be, whether the intended statistical tests are appropriate to the level of measurement and study question, and what the researcher intends to do about clinically significant findings that may not be "statistically" significant.

Clarity of Findings   Because this is a study proposal rather than a study report, there are, of course, no research findings. Instead, review the questions under this criterion and apply them to a report of findings in a current nursing research journal. And remember that it is neither just nor reasonable to criticize a piece of work such as the simulated proposal we have just dissected for failing to be or do something that the author never intended for it. Our sample proposal could, however, be improved by a less abrupt conclusion that would serve as an abstract or summary of the entire study (see Chapter 8).

Critiquing Research—Some Final Tips

The preceding criteria, questions, principles, and illustrations are all intended to serve as guidelines in critiquing research proposals or reports of study findings. It is never justifiable to apply them without giving sufficient rationale for your opinion that they are appropriate and your conclusions in relation to them. Try to keep in mind the audience for whom the research was intended, and think about the work as a whole even as you scrutinize it for details like the ones suggested in the questions associated with each of the seven criteria. Remember to avoid nitpicking about trivial details and thereby sacrificing the good in favor of the perfect. How you evaluate a piece of research may influence the decisions of others to replicate it or base their practice on it. Try to consult experts and other resource persons on technical aspects that you may feel uncertain about in order to ensure the accuracy and precision of your interpretation. Be considerate in your language. *Science* magazine

advises its reviewers: "If you find you have to devote the last paragraphs of your critique to correcting a false impression [about the quality of the research], reconsider your criticisms of it." This doesn't mean that you should withhold criticism, but the merits of the work (or the lack of them) should emerge as the overriding theme of your critique. Be concise, readable, rational, sensitive, accurate, and impartial. Offer explanation and examples. And practice.

Summary of Key Ideas and Terms

- In order to adequately fulfill the role of research consumer, expected of all nurses regardless of their educational preparation, you must acquire skills of critiquing research.

- Conducting a good critique of a study proposal or report of findings requires not just a list of pertinent questions to ask but criteria or standards against which to evaluate answers to the questions and a comprehension of the rationale for asking and answering them in the first place.

- A *research critique* is a critical estimate of a piece of research that has been carefully and systematically studied by a critic who has used specific criteria to appraise its general features.

- A *research review* identifies and summarizes the major features or characteristics of a study.

- The critic's challenges are to determine what a researcher has tried to do, to evaluate the strategies used in light of the realistic constraints of the study, and to present both criteria and evidence for making judgments about the quality of the research.

- A competent critique ought to represent a contribution to knowledge and scholarly exchange and be helpful to the author of the research.

- A helpful critic uses strategies to differentiate his or her criticism from destructive criticism and trivial nit-picking.

✔ Seven conventional criteria can be used as a basis for conducting a critique of a research proposal or report of study findings. These are: (1) clarity and relevance of the study purpose, (2) researchability of the study problem, (3) adequacy and relevance of the literature review, (4) agreement of purpose, design, and methods, (5) suitability of the sampling procedure and sample size, (6) correctness of the analytic procedure, and (7) clarity of findings.

✔ Well-presented tables ought to conform to a set of characteristic hallmarks.

✔ Avoiding a "cookbook" approach to critiquing research requires that the reader attempt to comprehend scientific issues that underpin the theoretical and logical basis of inquiry.

✔ A high-quality critique can be influential in that others may make decisions to replicate studies or base practice decisions on it. It should strive to be concise, readable, rational, sensitive, accurate, and impartial as well as offering explanations for judgments made.

References

American Nurses' Association: *Preparation of Nurses for Participation in Research*. Kansas City, Mo.: American Nurses' Association, 1976.

Blalock HM Jr: *Causal Inferences in Nonexperimental Research*. Chapel Hill: University of North Carolina Press, 1964.

Field WE: Clinical nursing research: A proposal of standards. *Nurs Leadership* December 1983; 6:117–120.

Fleming JW, Hayter J: Reading research reports critically. *Nurs Outlook* March 1974; 22:172–175.

Flemming J: Teaching nursing research content. *Nurse Educator* 1980; 5:24–26.

Horsley J, Crane J: *Using Research to Improve Nursing Practice: A Guide*. New York: Grune & Stratton, 1982.

Kaplan A: *The Conduct of Inquiry*. San Francisco, Chandler, 1964.

Kramer M et al: The teaching of nursing research. Parts 2, 3. *Nurse Educator* 1981; 6:30–37.

Krampitz SD, Pavlovich N (editors): *Readings for Nursing Research*. St. Louis: Mosby, 1981.

Leininger MM: The research critique: Nature, function and art. Pages 20–32 in: *Communication Nursing Research: The Research Critique*. Boulder, Colo: WICHE, 1968.

Mallick MJ: A constant comparative method for teaching research critiquing to baccalaureate nursing students. *Image* Fall 1983; 15:120–122.

Sjoberg G, Nett R: *A Methodology for Social Research*. New York: Harper & Row, 1968.

Wilson HS: Teaching research in nursing: Issues and strategies. *West J Nurs Res* 1982; 4:365–377.

Further Readings

Chater S: The research critique: The coronary patient. *Nurs Res* Summer 1966; 15:246–251.

Huck SW et al: *Reading Statistics and Research*. New York: Harper & Row, 1974.

Norbeck JS: The research critique: A theoretical approach to skill development and consolidation. *West J Nurs Res* 1979; 1:296–306.

The research critique. Editorial. *Nurs Res* Summer 1966; 15:195.

Schwab JJ: *The Teaching of Science*. Cambridge, Mass.: Harvard University Press, 1966.

Stetler CB, Marram G: Evaluating research findings for applicability in practice. *Nurs Outlook* 1976; 24:559–563.

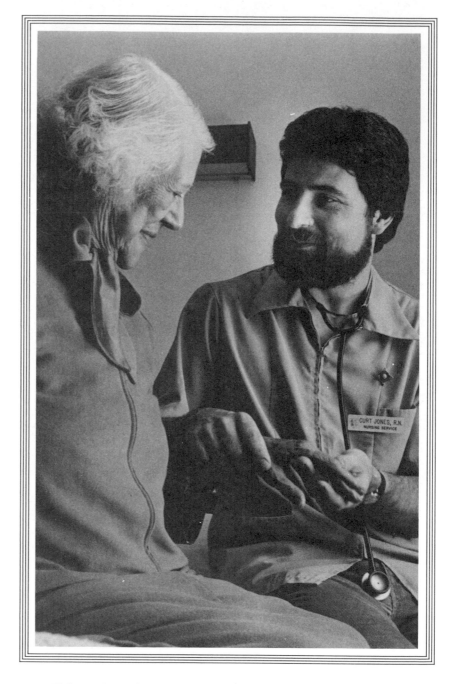

"Science does of course involve a process of proof.
But it also involves a spirit of discovery."

H. S. Wilson (1982)

3

Conducting Research in Nursing

Chapter 8

Writing a Research Proposal

The Practical Imagination at Work

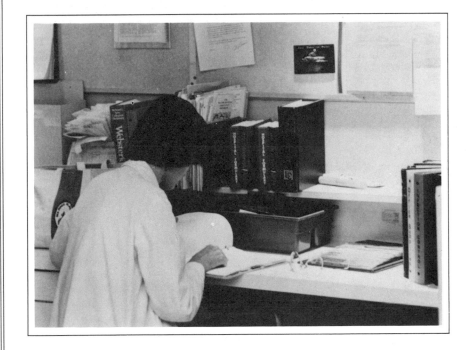

A well-written research proposal convinces members of the scientific community that the research is significant and that the methodological procedures and logic of inquiry are adequate to conduct it.

Chapter Outline

Chapter Objectives

After reading this chapter, the student should be able to:

- Analyze circumstances that might influence what format a research proposal should take
- List the basic components of a research proposal that ought to be included, whatever the format may be
- Interpret the implications of (1) considering one's audience and writing for strangers, (2) making the proposal attractive, and (3) achieving a balance of detail and flexibility in planning the proposal
- Formulate a specific research proposal that reflects an effective synthesis of the six steps of proposal writing: (1) problem statement; (2) theoretical framework and literature review; (3) design, methods, and procedures; (4) timetable or work plan; (5) personnel, budget, facilities, and resources; and (6) abstract, title, and cover letter
- Evaluate one's own (or a colleague's) formal study proposal against conventional criteria for scientific merit
- Explain six strategies that are likely to increase one's chances of finding public or private funding for a proposed research project
- Describe the function of the peer review panel as it is used by the Division of Nursing of the U.S. Department of Health and Human Services in reviewing research grant proposals
- Appreciate the value of proposal-writing skills to the advancement of nursing education, nursing administration, and nursing clinical practice, as well as nursing science in the next decade

In This Chapter . . .

In the opinion of many authorities, the core of a research project is the soundness and coherence of its logic. You communicate this logic more or less effectively through your written research proposal. Here you have the chance to relate your study question to a scientific tradition or the problems of a professional discipline, describe and justify the methodology that you've selected, and reasonably project the importance of your possible conclusions. Like all other communication, proposal writing is part science and part art. In the words of Krathwohl (1977):

Classes in painting can instruct an artist in the principles of shading, contrast and perspective, but it is the artist's creativity with these that is critical to success (p. 1).

This chapter presents the basic characteristics of a research proposal in a general way so as to be applicable to a wide range of study designs and methods. A section on "grantsmanship" and finding money offers both checklists for increasing your chances for success and information on why some proposals fail. Although no one set of standards or rules can hope to capture the variety of methods available for approaching the task of proposal writing, this chapter is intended to increase the likelihood that your research ideas are not rejected by research course faculty members, thesis or dissertation committees, or by funding agencies because they were poorly presented.

The reasons for writing a formal written research proposal vary. A proposal might be required by a thesis or dissertation committee or even for a nursing course as evidence that you not only are able to formulate researchable problems that have merit for nursing but also have the ability to plan systematically to address them. Certainly most funding agencies, private or public, require submission of a research proposal. If you are hoping to get a hospital, clinic, or other institution or group to allow you access and entry to collect data, it is usually a good idea to present the official gatekeepers with a study proposal (see Chapter 13). Institutional review boards (see Chapter 3) require an abbreviated proposal or prospectus before approving studies that involve human beings as research subjects, even when research is conducted as part of an educational experience. And finally, investigators themselves often find that it is useful to synthesize and articulate the ideas and plans that have been evolving as they consider the specific topics of problem formulation, design, sampling, data collection, and analysis. A well-written proposal should convince members of the scientific community that your research is significant and reflects mastery of background knowledge, methodological procedures, and the logic of inquiry necessary to conduct it. This chapter sketches out the range of possibilities for successful proposal writing and attempts to offer you a sense of freedom and responsibility in justifying the choices you have made.

Format of a Study Proposal

The exact format for research proposals and the extent of detail expected in them varies with the target review committee or funding agency. Some granting agencies provide their own guidelines, instructions, and proposal formats in an

application packet. Such a packet, if available, is essential so that you can present your proposed study in a way that can be compared by reviewers with other competing studies. Box 8-1 presents an illustration of instructions you would

---

Box 8-1   *Summary of Suggestions for Preparation of Research Proposals*

Preliminary Informal Proposals

Prospective applicants normally find it desirable to submit a proposal in preliminary form as the basis for discussion before a formal request is prepared. This is usually in the form of a letter of a few pages which describes what the prospective applicant proposes to do, the rationale behind the proposed project, the personnel who would be involved, the expected outcome, and the nature and amount of support needed from the supporting agency, as well as support actually or potentially available from other sources.

It is suggested that the proposals be stapled on the left-hand upper corner and include a cover sheet. A brief abstract or summary of the more important objectives and procedures contained in the formal proposal may be inserted following the summary sheet. Certain additional guidelines are generally furnished after program staff members have had an opportunity to review an informal and preliminary inquiry.

General Outline for Preparation of Proposals

1. *Cover page*: The cover page generally contains identifying information.
2. *Abstract*: The abstract generally occupies a single page, identifies a proposal, and summarizes the contents concisely and simply. The abstract must be written in language understandable by an informed layperson and give a clear, succinct summary of the proposed project. At the top of the abstract page the following items should appear on separate lines: title of project, principal investigator, contracting agency, amount of federal funds requested, and proposed beginning and ending dates. The summary portion of the abstract has three parts:

   a. a statement of the purposes, objectives, or nature of the project

   b. an indication of its expected contribution to nursing

   c. a compendium of the procedures or a description of what is to be done
3. *Narrative*: The narrative of the proposal communicates the project director's plan and its probable effectiveness. It should be clear, concise, forthright, and complete. Within the body section, there are ordinarily four parts, which should be adapted as appropriate for the particular kind of proposed activity to be undertaken.

---

find in such a packet. A human subjects committee (or institutional review board) is interested in a brief prospectus that will enable the members to assess the risk–benefit ratio of your proposed study and whether you've included adequate provisions for obtaining informed consent from prospective research subjects. A thesis or dissertation committee will probably be interested in the intricate details of your background knowledge, design, and methodology to ascertain that your study would be feasible and has sufficient scientific merit. Most research faculty members subscribe to the belief that the clearer and

more precise the original study proposal is, the smoother the actual conduct of the research project itself will be, because you will in effect be carrying out a previously designed plan that has received thorough review and critique by a mentor.

Perhaps the major exception to this position exists among field researchers, who inductively generate a conceptual analysis from qualitative, observational, and interview data (see Chapter 14). Such investigators make a conscious attempt to avoid premature closure on what exactly is important to study until they immerse

Box 8-1   (continued)

a. *Problem and objectives*—The first part tells *why* the proposed activity should be undertaken. It includes a statement of the problem or purposes, review of literature and related research, concise statement of objectives, or any other information necessary to establish a sound rationale.

b. *Description of activities (procedures)*—This part tells *what* is to be done, *when* and *how*. It is the basis for determining the degree to which the proposed activity can be expected to accomplish the objectives or satisfy the needs set forth in the first part of the proposal narrative. It delineates procedures, outlines program arrangements, describes materials to be produced, or otherwise explains how the activity leads to results and how evaluation will be accomplished. Allowances for alternatives, if any, should be noted. A time schedule for completion of the project is usually provided near the end of the proposal. The amount and kind of detailed information will vary according to the type of activity.

c. *Relevance of the findings*—This part tells what new knowledge or contribution toward nursing can be expected and what steps should follow to build on the outcomes. This part tells how the results of the activity may be disseminated or implemented.

d. *Personnel and facilities*—Personnel and facilities are a major determinant of capability. Personnel with major responsibilities are listed by name, position, title, experience, responsibilities within the project, percentage of time committed to the activity, and the extent to which this commitment has been assured. Consultants who have agreed to serve should be similarly identified (otherwise, the application should state the type of consultative assistance required). Facilities should be described, and the extent to which their use has been assured should be indicated.

4. *Budget*: The budget section of the proposal should make reasonable estimates, with enough detail to show careful analysis of expected costs and understanding of fiscal responsibilities in connection with conducting the proposed activity.

5. *Appended items*: Appended items should include:

a. report of other projects

b. agreement with cooperating agencies

c. data-gathering instruments

d. prior approval

e. clearance

f. other items

SOURCE: Sonoma State University, Office of Educational Development, 1971.

themselves in the natural conditions of "the field" (see Chapter 13). Furthermore, the field researcher assumes an attitude of pragmatism about data-collection and analysis strategies rather than adhering strictly to a prefabricated plan, or blueprint. In short, the predominant attitude among this group of researchers is: if it works to advance the analysis (and it's ethical), try it!

For most other studies, however, the research proposal is regarded as a comprehensive summary of what you intend to do, how it will be done, and why it is important. Whenever an in-

vestigator departs from the originally proposed plan, he or she is usually expected to report such deviations and explain why they occurred. Some institutions and agencies view the written research proposal as an actual *commitment on the part of the researcher to conduct the study in a specific way*, and the study itself must pretty much proceed as originally outlined. In this regard, a detailed, extremely precise proposal may be more constricting than helpful. Whether general or specific, the format for research proposals incorporates the sections listed in Box 8-2.

Box 8-2   Components of a Research Proposal

1. a title
2. an abstract (or summary)
3. a statement of the study problem and purpose
4. the theoretical background and or selective review of related research
5. hypotheses to be tested or research questions to be answered
6. the study setting
7. the sampling procedure and characteristics
8. the data-collection strategies or instruments
9. the plans for storing, retrieving, and analyzing data
10. ethical considerations, such as provisions for informed consent and protection of human rights
11. a timetable or work plan for the conduct of the study
12. a budget and statement of resources available or needed
13. a description of the qualifications of the investigator
14. references

The rest of this text offers you much information about making the decisions necessary to carry out a research project. Later in this chapter we will take up each component of writing a research proposal that explains these decisions in detail. But first we will look at some general hints for increasing the chances that your proposal will show off its true potential to those who read it.

General Hints on Preparing a Proposal

Consider Your Audience, and Write for Strangers

Although *you* have no doubt devoted what might seem like an astounding amount of time to thinking through both your research topic and the approach you intend to take to it, remember that the readers and reviewers of your proposal may not be as well informed in your area of interest as you are. *Explain everything clearly and logically.* Avoid using jargon or abbreviations that may be commonplace in your nursing speciality area but "Greek" to a funding agency review committee. Flaws in structure and internal consistency will be easily identified by readers who are unfamiliar with your subject. De-velop a chain of logic throughout your proposal that hangs together and has no weak links. For instance, objectives of the research must logically flow from the problem statement, and each hypothesis or objective must have a corresponding data-collection and data-analysis procedure that addresses it. Choices of descriptive or inferential statistical methods must be consistent with the purpose of your study and the level of inquiry you are proposing. Check your proposal to be certain that objectives are not dropped along the way or that certain data-collection plans are not advanced without a corresponding plan for analyzing them. Good writing, like good speaking, uses visual aids. Make use of headings and subheadings, underlining, diagrams, flow charts, tables, and other strategies that signal to the reader what the critical parts of your proposal are without requiring him or her to plow through endless pages of undifferentiated prose. On this point, however, keep Krathwohl's (1977, p. 21) admonition in mind: "The writer must also be careful to avoid the opposite extreme, jazzing the copy with . . . more gesture than sense. . . . Remember that research is essentially a scholarly activity."

Package Your Proposal So That It Is Attractive

In addition to not being well informed about your research interest, your reviewers and readers may also be less enthusiastic about the value or importance of your study than you are. It's up to you to convey not only what your project hopes to find out but also why doing it is important to the world, to nursing, or to the funding agency. As Polit and Hungler (1983) point out, "There's no need to brag or promise what cannot be accomplished but . . . it is not inappropriate to do a little selling" (p. 607).

Conveying a sense of enthusiasm for your project does not require Madison Avenue techniques. But making your proposal physically attractive is an effective strategy for increasing its appeal. Although fancy binding and printed covers may not only be overly expensive to produce and mail but also cumbersome to circulate among readers, you should definitely pay attention to the following:

- Type the proposal or have it typed (using letter-quality or double-strike type if it's done on a word processor and printer).
- Proofread it, and proofread it again.
- Put it aside, and then reread it with some critical distance.
- Make revisions where necessary.
- Be sure to correct errors in spelling, grammar, and referencing. (The care you give to such

details in your proposal often conveys something about your attention to the details of your research.)
- Number the pages.
- Make the required number of copies to be sent off, and keep at least two copies in different places for yourself.
- Check your proposal for consistent use of the future tense. (After all, you are proposing to do something in the future.)
- Follow the most recent guidelines and instructions for proposal submission that you can obtain from the agency or committee. (It's often an excellent idea to establish a relationship with a representative of the agency early in the proposal development phase to avoid going astray.)

Finally, your proposed research will be more attractive to a funding source or organization if you have taken the time to match the study it proposes with the organization's goals or fields of interest. Consulting agency publications, previously funded studies, or staff members themselves is invaluable in acquiring this kind of information. Intramural funding for nursing research to improve patient care may receive a favorable view by the board of a private community hospital, but basic research directed exclusively to theory testing may not be within its institutional mission.

Balance Detail and Flexibility

A proposal should reflect a balance between sufficient detail, so that reviewers are convinced that the study is worthwhile and the investigator has the ability to conduct it, and sufficient flexibility. Writing such a plan is a craft that must be finely honed. The issue of length comes up here, and two general guidelines coexist: (1) When in doubt about including or excluding some piece of relevant information bearing on your proposed project, *it's better to include rather than exclude it.* (2) Page limitations are set for a purpose and should be respected. The solution to these seemingly incompatible guidelines is to *use appendices to provide auxiliary information* and not try to crowd details into the main body of the proposal. Appendices can give reviewers the benefit of the findings of a pilot study (see Chapter 1). They can also locate the proposed study within the context of a broader program of research. And they can incorporate the qualifications of the investigator. All these additional pieces of information may assist a reviewer in making a decision about your proposal but without unduly burdening someone who may because of limited time be reading a mass of proposals according to the "skip and skim" approach. According to Krathwohl (1977), the typical sequence that many reviewers use goes something like this:

Read and digest the summary or abstract. Skim enough of the first part of the problem statement to get a feel for it. Skim the literature review to figure out the unique features of this study. Skim the objectives and turn to the work plan and look over the flow chart, PERT diagram or timetable to get a detailed grasp of the study design. Check the qualifications of the investigator to see if the necessary competence seems present. Check the budget to be sure it's not out of line with the work proposed or not padded with equipment or travel that is unrelated to the research (or any other comparatively large budget items) (p. 22).

Some of the suggestions covered in the preceeding three general hints are clearly directed to the experienced professional nurse who is seeking funding for his or her ongoing research. But they are also applicable to undergraduate and graduate students who must learn to develop research proposals either for specific course work or before initiating master's theses or doctoral dissertations. Proposal writing is a relevant skill if the investigative roles of all nurses are to be fostered. In the following section we will tackle a realistic, step-by-step approach to writing one. "In a time of fiscal austerity, nurses involved in education, research or health care innovation can either tighten their belts or sharpen their proposal writing skills and apply for funding" (Sexton 1982, p. 31). The written proposal is frequently the only source of information on which fateful decisions are made.

Steps in Writing a Research Proposal

Step 1: The Problem Statement

The statement of the research problem usually begins a proposal. It must not only convince reviewers that the proposed study is important but also reduce the scope of the problem to manageable terms by specifying a study focus. If any specialized or esoteric concepts or terms are used in the problem statement, they must be defined early and prominently so that reviewers don't base their reading on any misconceptions. The art of identifying and articulating a researchable problem was covered in Chapter 5; many experts believe that this step is, in fact, the art of research, because it requires creativity, perceptiveness, and imagination. Although the study problem must not be too broad or grandiose, the potential generalizability of the findings related to studying the problem must also be explicitly stated. Funding decisions are often strongly influenced by the clarity with which an investigator conveys how a particular piece of research will contribute to theory or overall knowledge of general or specific phenomena.

Thus, *both the general statement of the purpose of the research and the specific study question should be succinctly expressed and even underlined very early in the proposal.* Consider how each of the nurse researchers in the following modified and adapted examples presented their study problems in early proposal drafts.

For the most part, the problem statements in the example below:

- are stated with precision
- justify the problem as meriting study

- admit of possible solution
- are intelligible to a reader who is generally sophisticated but may be relatively uninformed in the specific area of investigation
- suggest the significance of conducting the study

It's not a bad idea to conclude the problem-statement section of a proposal with a sentence that begins: "Therefore, the specific problem for this investigation is . . ."

Remember that the intention of this first section of your proposal is to make the problem

Example: Statements of Nursing Problems

Example 1   The concept of the hospice in the United States has evolved in the last decade. The research literature related to this kind of care is sparse. No one has systematically determined what hospice care givers actually do. Furthermore, no research has been conducted to ascertain from terminally ill persons and their families what it is that hospice care givers do that constitutes effective care. Therefore, the problem of this descriptive study is *to identify the effective and ineffective behaviors of hospice care givers in providing care to terminally ill persons and their families in a home setting* (Hehn, D., 1983).

Example 2   It is estimated that 3 million people suffer from a mental disorder annually. Of these, 1.7 million suffer prolonged, severe disability. These constitute the chronically mentally ill population, and the current overall estimate of how many of them have been deinstitutionalized into the community is as high as 800,000. Research on self-care in the basic aspects of living day to day for this population reveals a gap as to the influences of others on self-care practices. The proposed study investigates the influence of characteristics of social network on the performance of self-care by chronically mentally ill adults in the community (Sheets, S., 1983).

Example 3   Knowledge of one's state of health is a prerequisite for practicing self-care. A lack of knowledge has

consequences that may seriously affect biological integrity and quality of cancer patients' lives when they are receiving radiation therapy. To date, no comprehensive anticipatory approach has been tried to help patients prevent or manage the side effects of radiation therapy before their development. *The problem for the proposed experimental study is to test the effectiveness of presenting side effect management techniques information before the occurrence of experienced side effects on care behaviors* (Dodd, M. J., 1982).

Example 4   The overall purpose of this descriptive study is to develop a valid and reliable instrument to describe and measure the phenomenon of fatigue in cancer patients (Piper, B. F., 1982).

Example 5   The problem for this study is to expand the body of knowledge about the experience of pain in adolescents. The long-range goal is to provide health professionals with information to enable them to deal more effectively with adolescents who are anticipating or experiencing pain. *The specific study question is, "Do adolescents hospitalized for acute or chronic illness describe the pain experience the same as nonhospitalized adolescents?"* (Savedra, M., 1982).

SOURCE: Adapted from unpublished research proposals, University of California at San Francisco, 1982.

area of your study clear to a reader. Many proposal writers accomplish this by first presenting the larger context in which the problem is found and then narrowing down the big picture to the specific study that is being proposed. They demonstrate the relationship between the two and highlight why their study is important. The problem-statement section is often labeled "Introduction" and consists of three subheadings:

- Statement of the Study Problem (including specific hypotheses or study questions and definitions of terms)
- Specific Objectives of the Research (a carefully selected, brief list)
- Significance of the Study (along with any limitations you can reasonably identify)

Although it is possible to reduce this section to a few seemingly simple parts, the art of creating a good statement of the problem in a research proposal is usually the product of vigorous intellectual effort and utmost clarity.

Step 2: Theoretical Rationale and Review of Related Literature

Both nursing research that is designed to solve practical clinical problems and studies that are conducted to test or yield knowledge for knowledge's sake must be placed in the context of what scientific work has gone before. Even Sir Isaac Newton paid tribute to his predecessors by commenting that he had been able to see some things that others had not because he had stood on the shoulders of giants. A review of relevant literature is included in a study proposal to accomplish several purposes:

1. It presents the theoretical basis, rational framework, or organizing scheme of which the proposed study is a part.
2. It offers not a mere bibliography but an analytic and critical appraisal of the important and recent substantive and methodological

developments in your area of interest and indicates how your proposed study will refine, revise, extend, or transcend what is now known.

3. It informs and lends support to your assumptions, operational definitions, and even methodological procedures by demonstrating to your reader that the proposed study has profited from scholarly and scientific work that has preceded it.

Critics of this section of study proposals report that the single most obvious flaw is that authors tend to cite theory and prior research that have only the most tenuous connection with the study being proposed. As a result, this section has a disjointed quality, because it looks like a mere catalog or listing of marginally related work lacking in a thoughtful, well-developed integration. Avoid statements that imply either that nothing has been done in your research area or that so much has been done that it is impossible for you to summarize. Statements of this sort are usually taken as indications that the investigator proposing the study does not really have a command of relevant literature and knowledge in his or her field. Tables 8-1 and 8-2 accompanied and summarized one research student's literature review.

Step 3: Design, Methods, and Procedure

By this point in your proposal you have presented the problem(s) you intend to study, the objectives your research will accomplish, the importance and exact meaning of both of these, and the theoretical and empirical background of the present study. Now you must tell your readers or reviewers how you are going to bring about your results, that is, what activities you will conduct to accomplish your study objectives or test your study hypotheses (see Chapter 9).

Label the Design Begin by labeling the general approach, or design, of your study (histori-

Table 8-1   Needs of the Chronically Mentally Ill Identified in the Literature

Source	Material	Personal	Psychological
Bassuk & Gerson (1978)	Money	Safety	Vocational rehabilitation
	Decent housing	Guidance in coping with mechanics of daily living	Sheltered employment or job referrals
	Transportation		Activities and interaction with others
		Adequate follow-up treatment	
		Recreation	
Paul & Lentz (1977)		Resocialization and assistance with ADL	Vocational/role performance or "salable" skills
		Reduction of bizarre behavior	Sheltered employment or job referrals
			Supportive "roommate" in the community
Stein & Test (1978)	Money	Freedom from a pathological, dependent relationship	Supportive other and motivation to persevere and to remain involved with life
	Food		Coping skills
	Housing		Assertive support system
	Transportation		

SOURCE: Used with permission of Sandra L. Sheets, RN, *The Influence of Social Networks on the Performance of Self Care by the Chronically Mentally Ill Adult in the Community*. Dissertation proposal, University of California at San Francisco, 1984.

cal, survey, experimental, quasi-experimental, field study, case study, and so on). In effect, this general label allows you to quickly communicate your proposed procedure for inquiry and gives you an opportunity to anticipate questions about why you have selected the design that you have (see Chapter 6). In short, you should not only identify your plan but also substantiate the reasons for choosing it.

Specify Data-Collection Approaches Following this labeling and accounting, you should state the exact steps you intend to take to answer every question or test every hypothesis proposed in your study. One organizational technique used by proposal writers is to divide a sheet of paper into columns. Label the first column "Objective #1" or "Hypothesis #1," the second column "Method for #1," and the third "Evaluation or Analysis for #1." This strategy helps you to be certain that you indeed have a plan for

dealing with all aspects of the problem that you have introduced and that you have set up a data-collection and analysis mechanism or procedure to address each of them.

Describe the Study Setting Your methods or procedures section should also describe your research setting, if setting is a relevant consideration.

Example: The Study Setting

The proposed study will be conducted at a 450-bed community hospital located in the greater Pittsburgh area. It has the only accredited cancer care program in the immediate area, and the investigator is currently the oncology clinical nurse specialist employed by this hospital. Furthermore, she is familiar with referring physicians.

Table 8-2   Social Network Dimensions Differentiating Mentally Ill from Normals

Dimension	Source
Size	Hammer (1978)
	Pattison (1975)
	Tolsdorf (1976)
	Sokolovsky et al. (1978)
Connectedness or density	Pattison (1975)
	Tolsdorf (1976)
	Sokolovsky et al. (1978)
Symmetry or reciprocity	Pattison (1975)
	Tolsdorf (1976)
	Sokolovsky et al. (1978)
Content or multiplexity	Tolsdorf (1976)
	Sokolovsky et al. (1978)
Frequency and/or amount of contact	Strauss & Carpenter (1972)
	Brown et al. (1972)
	Henderson et al. (1976)
	Vaughn & Leff (1976, 1981)
Network primarily kinship	Pattison (1975)
	Tolsdorf (1976)
	Turner (1979)
Orientation	Tolsdorf (1976)
Satisfaction	Hirsch (1979, 1980)
	[Note: With normals]

SOURCE: Used with permission of Sandra L. Sheets, RN, *The Influence of Social Networks on the Performance of Self Care by the Chronically Mentally Ill Adult in the Community*. Dissertation proposal, University of California at San Francisco, 1984.

Discuss Your Study Sampling   You should discuss the nature and size of the sample and the rationale behind these decisions. The sampling procedure should be identified and explained in adequate detail *so that your study can be replicated and so that the extent of generalizability of your findings can be determined* (see Chapter 9). If your sample members must meet specific crite-

ria, these should be listed. For example, one pediatric nurse engaged in a descriptive study of adolescent cancer patients' experience of fatigue proposed the following sampling criteria:

Cancer patients ($n = 40$) will consist of adolescent leukemia patients admitted to any of three city hospital inpatient units or seen in these institutions' outpatient clinics. Furthermore, they must be able to read, write, and speak English as a primary language, be able to complete data-collection instruments, and be willing to maintain daily diary recordings. Finally, they must have confirmation of their cancer diagnosis. Exclusion criteria include patients who are (1) under psychiatric care; (2) taking antidepressants, sedatives, or thyroid medications; and (3) diagnosed as having diabetes, anemia, or thyroid disease.

Discuss Confounding Variables   Confounding variables that might plague your study need to be addressed in your procedures section (see Chapters 4 and 6). You may eliminate some of them by using random sample selection and random assignment to comparative groups. Some may be addressed by your sample size or exclusion criteria. Others may be controlled for with certain statistical operations (see Chapter 15). But still others may be beyond any of these attempts to reduce their influence and must be identified as limitations of your study or constraints on the generalizability of your findings. Most authorities agree that it is preferable for you to acknowledge problems, errors in design, or limitations rather than attempting to ignore or disguise them. It is important to indicate that whatever compromises you have made with regard to the control of extraneous variables were given careful thought, that you are definitely aware of which variables need to be controlled in order to preserve the integrity of your study, that you have chosen not to control some, and why you believed it was not possible to do so. Krathwohl summarizes these points well (1977, p. 31):

This is a place to demonstrate mastery of the problem. Probably nobody knows better than the researcher the multiple sources of contamination which might affect the study. Convincingly indicate the nature and basis of the particular compromise(s) being proposed and the reasons for accepting them. . . . Avoid expediency as a reason.

Most reviewers of research proposals are experienced scientists and scholars themselves, although they may not be experts on your specific study problem. They will recognize weaknesses and flaws in a study design such as lack of control or comparative groups, a Hawthorne effect, a regression effect, pretest effects, and a biased sample. (See Chapter 6 for a complete discussion of validity and reliability threats to study designs.) Your design discussion ought to show how you have attempted to make your study as precise as is practical to do.

Present Data-Collection Tools or Instruments You must also enumerate and discuss the data-collection instruments you propose to use. If you expect to use published and previously tested tools for data collection, you need to tell your reader why you selected them and how they are appropriate to measure the variables that are important to your study question. The discussion of this relationship often appears in connection with the operational definition of each of your study variables. The measures that you elect to employ must not only be consistent with the variable's operational definition but also have empirical evidence attesting to their validity, reliability, and objectivity (see Chapters 11, 12, and 13). Assistance in evaluating certain instruments can be found in annual test reviews and compendia such as Oscar Buros's *Mental Measurement Yearbooks*, (1938–present) and others included in Chapter 11 of this text. If no instruments exist or are available to investigate the variables of interest to you, it is probably better to propose a methodological study to develop tools rather than to argue that instrument plans will be forthcoming. If "homemade" or "self-developed" instruments are to be used, be sure to justify them in terms of their fit with the operational definition of your study variables. Discuss the procedures you plan to use to de-

velop them, and then establish their reliability and validity.

Present Your Analytic Procedures Finally, the methods or procedures section should present a method of analysis that is consistent with your study questions and levels of measurement. The assumptions of the statistics should fit the data that will be obtained. Most authorities seem to agree that it is not always possible to anticipate every analysis procedure that will be used. It is to your advantage, however, to expose your readers and reviewers to evidence that you have thought through each step that you will need to take to test every hypothesis or respond to every question in your study problem. Many advisers will encourage you to generate mock tables that will organize your data before you collect any, so that others know what you have in mind when it comes to analysis (see Chapter 15). For many proposal writers, this is a very appropriate point at which to consult a computer programmer or statistician who can make suggestions for your analysis plan or even your data-collection procedures (see Chapter 16). Table 8-3 represents yet another type of table that is frequently used in research proposals to clearly demonstrate the structural organization of a study.

A careful plan and procedures section of your proposal need not prohibit discovery of serendipitous findings or inhibit your creativity. Instead, it must support your contention that you know how to answer the research question and possess the attributes of a serious scholar, at least with regard to using an approach that is consistent with systematic inquiry.

Step 4: Timetable or Work Plan

A work plan or timetable accomplishes two main aims:

1. It clarifies for the reader a grasp of the overall flow of research-related activities. (This point is particularly important when the research project is a very complex one.)

Table 8-3   Visual Illustration of Study Plan

Q/H	Instruments	Who Is the Sample	n	Collection				Data Analysis			
				How	When	Where	By Whom	How	When	Where	By Whom
1											
2											
3											

SOURCE: Prepared by James C. Stone and approved by the Academic Review Committee, Department of Education, University of California, Berkeley, January 30, 1979.

2. It constitutes evidence that you have carefully and realistically considered exactly what you intend to do to carry out the proposed study.

The timetable or work plan can be presented by using a number of different formats, but in all cases, it must provide a clear, sequential statement of the operations that will be carried out in your study and must be consistent with the descriptive sections of your written proposal. Whether a table, graph, flow chart, PERT diagram or path analysis is used, the following information should be included:

1. the tasks or project activities
2. an estimate of the amount of time required for each, and scheduled dates
3. personnel requirements for each activity

Accurately estimating the time and resources that will be needed to accomplish project tasks is difficult and often must depend on careful tracking during prior experiences. It is easy to underestimate, for example, the time that can be required to recruit and process project staff, the delays that can be associated with releasing funds to an organization, and the impact that peak times for other work (the beginning and end of the semester or fiscal year) can have on the progress of one's own work. Obviously, when unanticipated events delay the research progress, accommodations such as shifting of funds to hire temporary staff and work plan rearrangements become necessary. The simplest way to portray a work plan or timetable in a research proposal is simply to list research activities and associated dates or blocks of time. One oncology nurse represented her time schedule for the data-collection part of her research on fatigue in cancer patients in a table similar to Table 8-4.

Researchers employ a number of different formats for diagramming the schedule of work in a research project. One of the most familiar ones is the *program evaluation review technique*, or *PERT*. Many authorities believe that such diagrams or similarly constructed flow charts are more informative than simple timetables, because they are a better way of indicating the interrelationships among work that is going on simultaneously or that overlaps. In the generic PERT diagram that appears in Figure 8-1 each arrow stands for a task, and circles indicate the beginning and end of each activity. Numbers in the circles refer to the list of activities. Events that the researcher considers particularly important can be designated by a square or rectangle, and events where two or more lines of work meet can be marked with a triangle. The time line along the bottom shows the months during which the work is scheduled to take place. Clearly, it will be easier to present your work plan or timetable with such a highly detailed

Table 8-4   Time Schedule for Data Collection

	Pilot Study	Descriptive Study		
Time Period:	3/15/84–5/15/84	6/1/84–3/31/85		
Subjects:	n = 18 (9 students; 9 lung cancer patients	n = 60 (20 graduate students; 20 leukemia patients; 20 lung cancer patients)		
Data Collection:		Time 1 (Entry)	Time 2 (3 mos)	Time 3 (5 mos)
	Demographic data Medical history Fatigue diary (daily for 4 wks)	Demographic data Medical history Fatigue diary (daily for 4 wks)	Medical history Fatigue diary (daily for 2 wks)	Medical history Fatigue diary (daily for 2 wks)

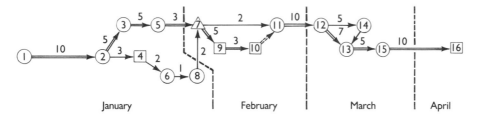

January   February   March   April

PERT Activity List

Begin and End Events	Activity	Estimated Working Days	Symbol Code
1-2	Hire staff	10	◯ Begin or end event
2-3	Write questionnaire	5	▢ Milestone event
2-4	Develop sampling plan	3	△ Interface event
4-6	Procure mailing lists	7	→ Workdays for activity denoted by arrow
3-5	Pre-test questionnaire	5	
5-7	Revise questions and prepare for mailing	3	⇒ Critical path
6-8	Selection of the sample	1	---- Constraint on arrowed
8-7	Prepare mailing envelopes	2	activity by completion
7-9	Prepare interim reports	5	of or product form pre-
9-10	Clear questionnaire with sponsor and submit interim report	5	ceding activity
7-11	Send questionnaire	3	
11-12	Wait returns	10	
12-13	Analyze intials returns	7	
12-14	Interview sample of non-respondents	5	
13-15	Integrate interview data in analysis	5	
15-16	Prepare final report	10	

Figure 8-1 Sample survey analyzed as a PERT diagram, time-scaled by months. (Adapted from D. R. Krathwohl, *How to Prepare a Research Proposal*, 2nd ed., Syracuse, N.Y.: Syracuse University Bookstore, 1977, p. 39. Reprinted with permission.)

approach if you can anticipate all the steps that will be involved. Exploratory studies and field studies make this degree of specificity almost impossible, and a rougher rendition of the work plan or timetable would be expected.

Step 5: Sections on Personnel, Budget, Facilities, and Resources

Personnel   This section of your proposal tells reviewers about the people who will be needed to conduct your study. It is, of course, crucial that the principal investigator, project director, or codirectors be identified and that their qualifications be convincingly presented. Educational preparation, both formal and informal, professional experience, prior research positions in the field, and previous publications related to the proposed study all strengthen one's case. Although it may be expedient to opt for including a "canned" biographic sketch that is already available in your files, reviewers are more likely to be impressed by a presentation of project person-

nel, their "job descriptions," and background information *that has been carefully selected to highlight particular competencies relevant to this study*. A form for each participant's biographical sketch is often included in an application packet (see Figure 8-2). If you are proposing a large, complex study that will involve a lot of people, an organizational chart illustrating their relationship to one another is a good idea. Be alert to the fact that it is considered improper to list as consultants to your project people you have not first contacted. In fact, many agencies expect you to append letters of support or agreement from any consultants you intend to use. Researchers sometimes include the names of members of an advisory committee to attempt to add credibility to their proposal. Again, written consent to serve in such a capacity should be obtained in advance. Box 8-3 illustrates an excerpt from the personnel section of a nursing education proposal submitted to a national health agency for funding.

Budget   Krathwohl, Sexton, Polit and Hungler and other authors agree that the budget sec-

Figure 8-2 Biographical sketch form.

Give the following information for key professional personnel listed on page 2, beginning with the Principal Investigator/Program Director. Photocopy this page for each person.			
NAME		TITLE	BIRTHDATE *(Mo., Day, Yr.)*
EDUCATION *(Begin with baccalaureate or other initial professional education and include postdoctoral training)*			
INSTITUTION AND LOCATION	DEGREE *(circle highest degree)*	YEAR CONFERRED	FIELD OF STUDY

RESEARCH AND/OR PROFESSIONAL EXPERIENCE: Concluding with present position, list in chronological order previous employment, experience, and honors. Include present membership on any Federal Government Public Advisory Committee. List, in chronological order, the titles and complete references to all publications during the past three years and to representative earlier publications pertinent to this application. **DO NOT EXCEED TWO PAGES.**

Box 8-3   Nursing Education Proposal (Personnel Section)

NAME	TITLE OF POSITION	%/HRS.	SALARY	FRINGE BENEFITS	TOTAL
Mary W. Smith	Program Director		-0-	-0-	
Holly S. Wilson	Project Coordinator				
	Spring & Fall, 1977	25%	$ 4,839	$ 658	
	Summer 1977	50%	3,227	310	
Harold C. Jones	Research Associate	50%	8,298	1,129	
Jane Barnes	Research Associate	100%	16,596	2,257	
(Vacant)	Student Assistants (10)	200 hr each	5,000	480	
(Vacant)	Department Secretary	100%	9,024	1,227	
(See continuation page for itemized list)					
		(SUBTOTALS)	$46,984	$6,6061	
	ENTER TOTAL SALARY AMOUNTS PLUS FRINGE BENEFITS				$53,045

tion of a proposal "states your project in monetary or financial terms." The total dollar amount is usually determined by the nature of the study you are proposing, the guidelines and policies of the funding agency, or both. The goal in preparing a budget is to make it realistic. If it is padded to include funds for desirable but not necessarily essential costs, such as extra travel or additional equipment, you risk being eliminated in competition with other proposals. If you have underbudgeted, you may not have sufficient resources to carry out your proposed plan of activities. The application kits provided by federal funding agencies include budget forms (see Figure 8-3) and detailed instructions for completing them. Foundations and private organizations may offer only general limits. Most grant applications, however, allow you to request funds in two categories: direct costs (the money that you spend to carry out the project tasks) and indirect costs (based on an established formula that your in-

stitution requires in exchange for serving as the institutional or administrative site for the grant). Indirect costs cover such things as providing heat and light to the building. They can be as low as 8% and as high as 40% of the direct-cost base number. A written budget narrative should accompany the actual list of costs, in order to explain the reasons for requesting certain items and to link up the budget details with the project activities.

It is always a good idea to consult with your institutional grants and contracts officers early in the process of preparing a research proposal budget. They not only review it for its agreement with institutional policies and salary schedules but can also give you the benefit of past experience with successful and unsuccessful requests. Although it may be time consuming, it is better to actually telephone airlines, printers, the post office, secretarial services, computer resources, and the like to obtain at least general estimates of

Figure 8-3 Project cost estimates (federal support only).

PROJECT DIRECTOR _____ INSTITUTION OR AGENCY _____

PROPOSED DURATION: (mos) _____ STARTING DATE: _____ ENDING DATE: _____

A.	DIRECT COSTS	
	Personnel Salaries**	51***
	Employee Benefits (charged as direct)	52
	Travel	53
	Supplies and Materials	54
	Communications	55
	Services	
	Duplicating and Reproduction	56
	Statistical	57
	Testing	58
	Other	59
	Final Report Production	60
	Equipment	61
	Training Program Costs	
	a. Trainee Support Costs	62
	b. Institutional Allowance	63
	Other Direct	64
	Subtotal, Direct Costs	65
B.	INDIRECT COSTS	66
C.	TOTAL COSTS (Federal Support)	67

*   For projects longer than 18 months in duration, use one sheet for each 12 months of activity and a summary sheet for totals.

**   Consultants: Show rate and number of days under Personnel, transportation and per diem under Travel.

*** Numbers are for computer usage

what various tasks and activities are going to cost rather than merely guessing. Even after all this initial effort, many budgets are renegotiated after a decision to support a project has been made and before funds are released.

Facilities and Other Resources You should indicate the special facilities that are available to you in carrying out your proposed study. One customarily mentions the libraries (and their holdings), computer resources, special equipment or laboratories, office space, and secretarial support services. In many cases, institutions that have been successful in winning grants have this information already compiled and available to researchers who are preparing proposals. Although using such "canned" material can save time, be sure to edit it so that it is relevant to the research at hand. Astute reviewers will be more impressed with your proposal if you do.

If your study requires you to collect data in organizations or institutions other than your own setting, evidence of their willingness to cooperate with you, in the form of letters of agreement or contracts, should be attached. Many funding sources view an institution's willingness to allow you to use their facilities as added support for your proposal.

Step 6: Abstract, Title, and Cover Letter

Most proposals begin with a short (approximately 300-word) abstract, or summary. Even though it usually appears at the beginning of the document, most researchers write it last. The purpose of an abstract is to convey the essence of your proposed study to the reviewers. It not only introduces your study's importance to reviewers but may also be used as the basis for subsequent press releases or publications and may be used as the basis for entering your project into a computerized record-keeping system. It goes without saying, then, that your abstract should be composed carefully, accurately, and clearly. An abstract should include the most important points that you wish to stress about your proposed research and should provide the maximum amount of pertinent information as concisely as possible. A well-written abstract not only presents the central idea of the study but also convinces the reader or reviewer that it is both interesting and important. It should whet the appetite and prepare the reader for the body of the proposal. (See Appendix B for an example.) The title serves similar purposes but in an even more abbreviated way. Try to avoid jargon and clichés in study titles. Instead, use key terms that will orient a reader to the nature of your study and *make sense*.

Finally, your cover or transmittal letter should indicate the agency, office, or grant competition for which your proposal is intended and may make reference to any contacts you may have had with agency staff during its preparation. Send the required number of copies by certified mail or an express service to assure that your proposal meets the required deadline date.

Agencies' Criteria for Evaluating Proposals

All agencies, be they public or private, evaluate proposals that they receive according to sets of criteria. Knowing about such criteria helps you anticipate what will be scrutinized when your proposal is evaluated. Although some funding sources are more detailed in their criteria than others, common themes typically characterize proposal review checklists and you should become familiar with them (see Box 8-4).

Box 8-4   Evaluation Checklists

I. National Institutes of Health (Checklist of deficiencies)

    A. *The Problem*
- The problem is not of sufficient importance or is unlikely to produce any new or useful information.
- The proposed research is based on a hypothesis that rests on insufficient evidence, is doubtful, or is unsound.
- The problem is more complex than the investigator appears to realize.
- The problem has only local significance, is one of production or control, or otherwise fails to fall sufficiently clearly within the general field of interest to the prospective sponsor.
- The problem is scientifically premature and warrants, at most, only pilot study.
- The research as proposed is overly involved, with too many elements under simultaneous investigation.
- The description of the nature of the research and of its significance leaves the proposal nebulous and diffuse without clear research aim.

    B. *The Approach*
- The proposed tests, methods, or scientific procedures are unsuited to the stated objective.
- The description of the approach is too nebulous, diffuse, and lacking in clarity to permit adequate evaluation.
- The overall design of the study has not been carefully thought out.
- The statistical aspects of the approach have not been given sufficient consideration.
- The approach lacks scientific imagination.
- Controls are either inadequately conceived or inadequately described.
- The material the investigator proposes to use is unsuited to the objectives of the study or is difficult to obtain.
- The number of observations is unsuitable.
- The equipment contemplated is outmoded or otherwise unsuitable.

II. U.S. Office of Education (List of shortcomings)

    A. *Problem*
- Limited significance
- Local significance only
- Incomprehensible; not spelled out
- Not appropriate to this granting agency
- Overly ambitious objectives

    B. *Procedures*
- Insufficient detail; vague
- Evaluation procedures inadequate
- Selection of subjects unclear, undefined and/or unrealistic
- Research design inadequate
- Variables uncontrolled
- Discrepancy between objectives and procedures
- No theoretical construct or rationale
- Research design overly complex; too many research components

Box 8-4   *(continued)*

- Statistical procedures unspecified
- Pilot study necessary
- Time schedule inappropriate

C. *Personnel and Facilities*
- Inadequate training and/or experience
- Time commitment inadequate or unspecified
- Consultants needed
- Personnel not specified
- Duties not specified
- Personnel specified but insufficient information provided

D. *Economic Efficiency*
- Budget too high for expected result
- Request for operational or support money

III. National Science Foundation

A review of the evaluation instructions provided to outside reviewers of National Science Foundation research proposals reveals concern about the same general areas noted above for the U.S. Office of Education and the National Institutes of Health. The instructional letter for one program area asks the review to comment on such points as the scientific merit of the research that is proposed and the qualifications of the applicant. It also requests a response to the following questions:
- Is the research well planned?
- Is the research important?
- Is the applicant aware of recent developments in the field?
- Is the applicant adequately trained to undertake the project?
- Is the support requested appropriate for the project?

The definitions of rating terms used by another NSF program may provide further insight into the criteria employed:

Excellent	— The problem is very important and well defined in the proposal. The investigators are highly competent and fully capable of doing the job. Strongly deserves support.
Very Good	— The problem is important and adequately defined in the proposal. The investigators are competent and the research will contribute to their growth. Deserves support.
Good	— The problem may be important, but the research is not well defined. The approach is routine, but might contribute to graduate education or developing the potential of the principal investigator. The proposal is marginal in its present form.
Fair	— The problem is probably unimportant or not well enough defined in the proposal to allow evaluation. The approach is questionable. The proposal is not deserving of support in its present form.
Poor	— The problem is unimportant, subprofessional, or has been solved by others.

SOURCE: Sonoma State University Office of Educational Development, 1974.

Finding Grants

Although this chapter has been developed as a resource for any nurse who must plan and formally prepare a research proposal, much of what has been presented is directed toward the challenges associated with obtaining money to support your studies. In some cases, of course, finding funding for your proposed research will not be a major problem. You may find yourself enrolled in a graduate or undergraduate course on the topic of, for example, constructing or testing data-collection instruments appropriate for nursing studies. As part of the course requirements you will become involved in selectively piloting the instrument with a small sample of subjects. In this case, any costs that may be associated with administering the instrument and coding or analyzing data acquired through its use may be subsumed under the operational budget for the course. In other instances, costs will be sufficiently low as to be covered by students themselves simply as a school-related expense. Collaborative programs of research, in which student research represents a "spinoff" from a program of faculty research and thereby benefits from the funding bases of the overriding project, may minimize the necessity for students and novice investigators to make their own applications for funding.

In an era of fiscal austerity, however, and in the face of clear needs for studies that genuinely contribute to the knowledge base of nursing rather than merely demonstrating methodological mastery, skill in the art of "grantsmanship" is becoming more and more valuable. It is helpful not only to nurse scientists but also to nurse educators, who must plan and systematically evaluate teaching programs; nurse executives, who must often rely on supplemental funds to implement an innovative demonstration project; and nurse clinicians, who seek scientific grounds for their clinical decisions. Sexton (1982) identifies the following seven steps in preparing a proposal for submission to a funding source.

Step 1: Establish Priorities

You must first identify projects that you need money for and studies that you wish you had money for. This step requires that you think about what you want to do, what kind of expenses and resources will be involved, and whether grant funds are in fact going to be necessary.

Step 2: Identify the Money Available

As most of us know, public money granted through the federal government's Department of Health and Human Services has been the largest source of funds for projects related to health. Each federal department or division supports projects that are related to its specific mission, and priorities within a department's mission may change from one year to the next. A Nursing Research Grants Program announcement describing the types of grant eligible for support and other key information is reproduced in Box 8-5.

Most academic institutions have research funds that are available on a competitive basis for seed money to conduct pilot projects or methodological studies—for example, increasing the likelihood that the investigator will be ultimately more competitive and successful when he or she applies for external funds.

Although public funding has predominated in nursing's past, more and more contemporary nurse researchers are approaching private foundations, of which there are over 25,000, or corporations that award grants to health-related projects. Many of the national voluntary health organizations, such as the American Cancer Society, have supported nursing research. Each February the American Nurses' Foundation announces the availability of its competitive extramural grants program, which supports nursing research directed by registered nurses. The foundation specifically encourages proposals in the areas of clinical nursing and nursing administration. Many of the most distinguished doctoral dissertations conducted by nurses have been supported in whole or part by the ANF.* Since its inception in 1955 it has awarded 172 grants for a total of approximately $950,000 for work in cancer research, pain management, and care of the elderly and dying, to name only a few. The deadline for submitting proposals to the ANF is July 1, and awards are announced by October 1 of each year. The maximum grant amount has been $2,500.

Step 3: Learn About Funding Organizations

The *Federal Register* (published Monday–Friday) informs the public of the missions, regulations, and grant-funds priorities of federal programs. The *Foundation Directory* contains program and funding information for at least 3,000 private funding agencies. Your reference librarian or grants officers can guide you to other resources that detail foundation funding, including lists and indices of prior recipients and the topics of their projects.

Sexton (1982, p. 33) and others acknowledge that "less information is available about corporate philanthropy than about foundations." But she does list four useful sources of information on corporations:

- *Bank of America Corporation's Bibliography of Corporate Social Philanthropy*
- *Standard and Poor's Register of Corporations, Directors, and Executives*
- *The Handbook of Corporate Social Philanthropy*
- *The Trade Association Directory*

*The ANF is a nonprofit corporation affiliated with the American Nurses' Association and located at 2420 Pershing Road, Kansas City, Missouri.

Physicians have been extraordinarily successful in acquiring funding for their research programs from drug companies. In fact, some critics believe that the quest for the commercial dollar threatens to tarnish the ethics of certain clinical research. But nurses of the future will be turning more in the direction of corporations for money. Because of their relationship to nurses or their public position on fostering health, companies may prove to be substantial investors in supporting nursing studies.

Step 4: Compare Available Funds with Your Needs

Obtain the key information from these sources and compare the facts you acquire with your own potential projects and financial needs. Sexton (1982) alerts us that the following categories of information about any potential funding source will probably be valuable.

- geographic distribution of awards
- types of project funded
- types of institution funded
- number of grants awarded
- amount of average award and range

Step 5: Consult with Officers in Your Institution

Consultation with representatives of the research development office can ensure that your proposal is consistent with institutional policies about indirect cost rates, copyrights, and protection of human subjects and that the proposal is acceptable to the institution in relation to matters such as the availability of space and use of equipment.

Step 6: Get to Know the Funders

Develop contacts with representatives of the funding agency before completing and submit-

---

Box 8-5   *Grants Announcement of U.S. Department of Health and Human Services*

Purpose:

To enlarge the body of scientific knowledge that underlies nursing practice, nursing education, and nursing services administration; and to strengthen these areas through the utilization of such knowledge.

Types of Grants:

Nursing Research Project Grants support discrete, specified, circumscribed projects in an area representing the investigator's interest and competencies.

Nursing Research Program Grants support clusters of at least three studies focused upon a single theme.

New Investigator Nursing Research Awards (NINRA) support small studies of high quality carried out by new investigators.

Utilization of Research in Nursing Awards (URNA) support projects to bridge the gap between the generation of knowledge through research and the utilization of such knowledge in nursing practice, nursing education, or nursing services administration.

Nursing Research Emphasis Grants for Doctoral Programs in Nursing (NRE/DPN) stimulate nursing research in areas that emphasize special health needs of the nation, and advance the research efforts and resources of faculty in schools of nursing offering doctoral programs.

Guidelines:

Upon request, specific guidelines are available for all programs except Nursing Research Project Grants.

Eligibility:

Any individual, corporation, public or private institution or agency, or other legal entity.

   Principal investigators of NINRA projects must be first-time principal investigators for a Public Health Service-supported research project. Applicants should consult with Division of Nursing staff concerning the choice of application best suited to their needs.

   NRE/DPN projects are specifically designed for schools of nursing that offer doctoral programs.

Period of Support:

1–5 years

   NINRA Awards are limited to periods up to 3 years.

   NRE/DPN projects are also limited to 3 years, but additional support may be awarded to applicants for renewal of funded projects for periods not to exceed 5 years of total support.

Application Procedure:

1. Research grant application kits (PHS 398, Rev. 5/82) are available through the research offices of most institutions.

Box 8-5   (continued)

2. Early in the process of developing an application, prospective applicants should contact the Nursing Research Support Section, Division of Nursing, to discuss plans. Section staff provide technical advice, and sometimes review drafts of proposals in advance of submission. Prospective applicants are advised to consider review of their proposals by local scientists or other experts.

3. Before submitting an application, all applicants should provide the Nursing Research Support Section with the following information: title of the proposal, name of the principal investigator, applicant institution, and expected data of submission.

4. Applications are submitted to a clearinghouse, the Division of Research Grants, National Institutes of Health, rather than to the Nursing Research Support Section. Address labels are included in application kits. Applications are assigned to the Division of Nursing on the basis of nursing relevance.

Application Receipt Deadline Dates:

Program and URNA Applications	Project, NINRA, and NRE/DPN Applications	Renewal and Supplemental Applications	Review Completed	Earliest Possible Funding
February 1	March 1	February 1	September/October	December
June 1	July 1	June 1	January/February	April
October 1	November 1	October 1	May	July

Applications are accepted at any time. They should be submitted to the Division of Research Grants, National Institutes of Health, Room 240, Westwood Building, 5333 Westbard Avenue, Bethesda, MD 20205.

Review Process:

Applications assigned to the Division of Nursing are subject to peer review for scientific merit by an interdisciplinary group of scientists. Recommendations of this group are forwarded to the National Advisory Council on Nurse Training for final recommendations.

Further Information:

Nursing Research Support Section
Nursing Research and Analysis Branch
Division of Nursing, BHPr, HRSA
Parklawn Building, Room 5C-09
5600 Fishers Lane
Rockville, MD 20857
Telephone: (301) 443-6315

Box 8-6   *Guide for Reviewer's Comments on Research Grant Applications*

Please use this guide to prepare written comments on the application(s) which you have been asked to review. The comments will be used for two important purposes: (1) to inform the Ad Hoc Nursing Research Review Group when it meets, and (2) to assist the Division of Nursing staff to prepare an accurate summary of the Review Group's comments for the National Advisory Council on Nurse Training. The Summary Statement also serves as feedback to the principal investigator. Only the primary reviewer must write a description; secondary and tertiary reviewers should write comments on all other categories. Collateral reviewers should address issues related to their particular area of expertise.

I. Description (Primary reviewer only)

Clearly and concisely describe the proposed objectives and procedures, including the theoretical framework, aims, and methodology. Report facts provided by the applicant *only*, and reserve your own evaluative statements for inclusion in the critique. If an application is related to a previous application, please indicate that it is a supplemental, competing continuation, revised, or deferred application (as appropriate), and describe progress and/or changes, as indicated.

II. Critique

A. *Scientific Merit*

Provide a comprehensive evaluation of the proposal, including the significance and originality of the proposed study in relation to its scientific field, the validity of the hypotheses or research questions, the logic of the aims, and the feasibility and adequacy of the procedures for the proposed research. Assess whether the research is likely to produce new data and concepts, and whether alternate routes to the solution of the problem have been provided.

Your comments should include answers to the following questions:

1. Are the aims logical and appropriately conceptualized?
2. What is the significance of the project in relation to the "state of the art" and the needs for research in this area?
3. Are variables adequately defined theoretically and operationally? Are extraneous variables a problem?
4. Is the suggested method appropriate, adequate, feasible?
5. Does the method correspond logically with the specific aims of the project?
6. Are sampling procedures appropriate and feasible, and is the sample size adequate?
7. Are data-collection methods sound?
8. Has the investigator adequately addressed the psychometric properties of any instruments to be used in the project?
9. Are plans for data analysis appropriate to the aims and methods?

Provide specific examples to document your evaluation. For competing continuation and supplemental applications, evaluate progress to date. Be sure to address both strengths and weaknesses, so that the report accurately reflects all critical aspects of the proposal. Do not repeat descriptive comments in this section.

Box 8-6   (continued)

B. *Protection of Human Subjects; Animal Welfare; Hazardous Materials and Procedures*

    1. *Protection of human subjects.* Explain concerns about possible physical, psychological, or social injury individuals might experience while participating as subjects in this project and any concerns about the protection of the rights and welfare of such individuals.

    2. *Animal welfare.* If animals are to be used in the project, discuss whether they will be given proper care and humane treatment so that they will not suffer unnecessary discomfort, pain, or injury.

    3. *Hazardous materials and procedures.* Describe any potentially hazardous materials and procedures, and comment on whether the proposed protection provided by the investigator will be adequate.

C. *Investigators*

    1. *Principal investigator.* Analyze the competence of the principal investigator to conduct the proposed research, including academic qualifications; research experience; publications—especially in refereed journals; clinical expertise; and any special attributes.

    2. *Other project personnel, including consultants.* Analyze the competence of key staff and consultants to perform the roles described for them in the application. Evaluate whether the total research team is adequately qualified to conduct the proposed study, including academic qualifications; research experience; publications—especially in refereed journals; clinical expertise; and any special attributes.

D. *Resources and Environment*
Discuss the adequacy of the resources and environment for accomplishing the proposed project. Comment on the availability of appropriate human subjects and essential laboratory, clinical, animal, computer, or other resources. If applicable, include comment on the extent of departmental and interdepartmental cooperation.

E. *Budget*
Determine whether all items of the budget are realistic and justified. Discuss any overlap with active or pending support. Be specific about each item, if you suggest modification in amount or duration of support. For supplemental applications, comment on the requested budget in relation to the parent grant.

III. Overall Recommendation

Approval, disapproval, or deferral for additional information (by mail or site visit). Recommendation for increase or decrease in budget and/or time. Please provide key reasons for your recommendation(s).

IV. Additional Information

    A. *Conflict of Interest*
To avoid a conflict of interest, real or apparent, a reviewer is prohibited from reviewing applications submitted by his or her own organization. Reviewers should avoid any actions that might give

continued

Box 8-6   (continued)

---

the appearance that a conflict of interest exists. For example, a consultant should not participate in the review of any application from or involving a recent student, a recent teacher, or a close personal friend. Also, reviewers should not participate in the review of an application from a scientist with whom the reviewer has had long-standing differences which could reasonably be viewed as affecting objectivity. All questions addressed to reviewers by applicants should be referred to the Nursing Research Support Section staff.

B. *Additional Information or Collateral Review Needed*
If you feel that additional information is needed from the principal investigator prior to review, or if you feel that another opinion is indicated, please call the Nursing Research Support Section staff immediately. Suggest names of individuals who might provide such a review.

Nursing Research Support Section
Nursing Research and Analysis Branch
Division of Nursing, BHPr, HRSA, DHHS
Parklawn Building, Room 5C-09
5600 Fishers Lane
Rockville, MD 20857
Telephone (301) 443-6315

---

ting your proposal. Many executive staff personnel are able to offer a great deal of specific advice, such as to which department or division a particular proposal should best be directed and how to prepare an acceptable budget. In some cases, your contact person at the funding agency may be willing to read a draft of your proposal before its final submission. Learn what you can about the review process and the criteria according to which your research application will be reviewed. An illustration of such criteria appears in Box 8-6.

Step 7: Follow the Rules

Write and rewrite the final grant application, conforming as closely as possible with the format, agency assurances, administrative approv-

als, number of copies, and deadline dates. Remember that the purpose of this final step is to persuade the funding agency that your study is worthwhile and merits being funded. Berthold's 1973 study of what influenced approval or disapproval of nursing research grant proposals in two national granting agencies revealed that

approval or disapproval . . . is independent of investigator background variables [but] not of the judged adequacy of the investigative team to pursue and complete the specific project for which funding is requested. . . . In general funding is related to the judged adequacy of the proposal as submitted for peer group evaluation. Increased sophistication in asking relevant questions and in designing means for answering research questions in nursing should therefore yield a higher proportion of acceptable proposals (p. 298).

Your Proposal's Review

This chapter offers you a comprehensive guide to the challenging task of writing a formal study proposal, be it for funding or another purpose. Sexton (1982) summarizes what happens if, in fact, you do submit your proposal to a government funding agency. It will be reviewed by the staff members who serve as intermediaries between grant applicants and review committees. If additional information or clarification is needed, they will request it, although they can no longer provide you with consultation. Once they have established that your proposed research is relevant to the goals and priorities of the respective department or division they represent, two advisory panels will review your proposal. First, a *peer review panel* critiques its scientific merit and recommends (1) approval, (2) approval with conditions, (3) approval with communication, (4) disapproval, or (5) deferral for additional information. The reviewers then assign a *priority rating* to each approved application, yielding a funding priority score. Finally, the National Advisory Council of the agency reviews your application's face sheet, the recommendations of the peer review panel, the priority score, and the significance of the project. You are notified of the review's final outcome within a few weeks of the National Advisory Council meeting. If (alas) your study is not approved, you can arrange with the staff representative to have the anonymous comments of the reviewers sent to you. If your proposal is approved, you may enter into some negotiations about the budget and then finally receive an official *Notice of Grant Award* that spells out terms and conditions. Because most projects are funded on a year-to-year basis, it will not be long before you feel as if you must start the grant application process all over again. Fortunately, success breeds success, and surmounting the obstacles won't be quite as difficult the next time around, particularly if you learn from past experience.

Summary of Key Ideas and Terms

☞ In an era when fiscal retrenchment coexists with nursing's goal of building a scientific basis for practice, writing research proposals that can relate a particular project to a scientific tradition, describe and justify the methodological procedures, and present the importance of possible conclusions is becoming acknowledged as an essential skill for all nurses.

☞ Because the exact format and guidelines for preparing a proposal may vary with the target review committee, it is essential to obtain an application packet or a set of guidelines from the agency, institution, or committee and conform to them as closely as possible when preparing your proposal.

✔ Some institutions and agencies view the written research proposal as a commitment on the part of the investigator to conduct the study in the way it was outlined and approved or else report and explain any deviations or changes.

✔ Regardless of the specific format for a research proposal, the following components will be included in some way: a title; an abstract or summary; a statement of the study problem and purpose; the theoretical background and review of related research; the hypotheses to be tested or questions to be answered; the study setting; the sampling procedures and sample characteristics; the data-collection strategies or instruments; the plans for storing, retrieving, and analyzing the data; ethical considerations of the study; a timetable or work plan; a budget statement that includes resources available and needed; a description of the qualifications of the investigator; and references.

✔ General hints for effective proposals: (1) Consider your audience and explain everything clearly and logically. (2) Package your proposal to generate interest in it, so that it is physically appealing and matches the mission or goals of the funding agency. (3) Balance detail and flexibility, and maximize the thoughtful use of appendices to your proposal.

✔ The steps in writing a research proposal involve preparing the problem statement; the theoretical rationale and review of related literature; the explanation of design, method, and procedures; the timetable or work plan; sections on personnel, budget, facilities, and resources; and the abstract, title, and cover letter.

✔ The problem statement a research proposal should include:

- A statement of the specific study problem, including hypotheses, study questions, and definitions of terms

- the specific purposes or objectives of the research

- the significance of or need for the study

✔ The theoretical rationale and review of related literature serves three purposes: (1) It presents the organizing scheme or theoretical framework of which the proposed study is a part. (2) It indicates your grasp of the important and recent developments in your area of interest and how your study will refine, revise, extend, or transform what is known. (3) It lends support to your assumptions, operational definitions, and methodological choices.

✔ A complete explanation of design, methods, and procedures should consist of seven parts:

- Label the general design.
- Specify data-collection and analysis approaches for each study question or hypothesis.
- Describe the study setting.
- Discuss the sampling procedure and sample characteristics.
- Discuss confounding variables.
- Present data-collection tools or instruments.
- Present analysis procedures.

↙ A timetable or work plan should, either in a table or more detailed flow chart or PERT diagram, communicate the tasks or activities to be undertaken, an estimate of the amount of time required for each, and scheduled dates and the personnel requirements for each activity.

↙ The personnel section of a proposal should highlight the competencies specifically required to conduct the proposed study. The budget section includes direct and indirect costs and should be prepared in close consultation with your institution's financial officers so as to make it accurate, realistic, and congruent with institutional policies. Accompanying letters of agreement should reflect facilities and resources available for your project, and a statement of rationale should accompany requests that resources be provided by the funding agency.

↙ The abstract, or summary, should be written last. It should convey the essence of the proposed study in 300 words or less and convince readers that the study is interesting and worthwhile.

↙ Avoid jargon and clichés in study titles, and include a cover letter when submitting a proposal to a review group.

↙ Most review committees have similar criteria for evaluating the scientific merit of research proposals, and these should be considered carefully.

↙ Success in finding funding for your research from public or private sources will be more likely if you:

- Begin by identifying research projects that require grant funding.
- Next identify the money available, using announcements, organizational publications, and your reference librarian.

- Identify relevant resources for learning about the missions, regulations, and grant priorities of various funding sources.

- Obtain key information from these sources, and match the facts you acquire with your potential research projects.

- Consult with staff members in your own institution's research development office.

- Develop contacts with representatives from your target funding agency before even beginning to write your proposal.

- Write and rewrite the final proposal, conforming as much as possible to the funding agency's format, guidelines, deadlines, and so on.

✔ The *peer review system* employed by scientific panels in reviewing grant applications requires that nurses increase their sophistication in developing concise, well-documented proposals for nursing research.

✔ One way of learning to improve your proposals is to request the anonymous critical comments from your reviewers after a proposal is disapproved or assigned a low priority rating for funding.

References

Berthold JS: Nursing research grant proposals: What influenced their approval or disapproval in two national granting agencies? *Nurs Res* July/August 1973; 20:292–295.

Buros OK: *Mental Measurement Yearbooks*. Highland Park, NJ, 1938–present.

Krathwohl DR: *How to Prepare a Research Proposal*, 2nd ed. Syracuse, N.Y.: Syracuse University Bookstore, 1977.

Polit D, Hungler B: *Nursing Research: Principles and Methods*, 2nd ed. Philadelphia: Lippincott, 1983.

Sexton DL: Developing skills in grant writing. *Nurs Outlook* 1982; 30:31–38.

Sheets SL: The relationship of social networks to the performance of self-care by the chronically mentally ill adult in the community. Dissertation proposal, University of California at San Francisco, 1984.

Stone JC: *Visual Illustration of a Study Plan*. Department of Education, University of California at Berkeley, 1979.

Further Readings

Allen EM: Why are research grant applications disapproved? *Science* November 1960; 132:1532–1534.

Bloch D et al: The Nursing Research Grants Program of the Division of Nursing, United States Public Health Service. *J Nurs Adm* March 1978; 7:40–45.

Campos RG: Securing information on funding sources for nursing research. *J Nurs Adm* 1976; 6:16–18.

DeBakey L: The persuasive proposal. *Journal of Technical Writing and Communication*. 1976; 6: 5–25.

Dixon J: Developing the evaluation component of a grant application. *Nurs Outlook* February 1982; 122–127.

Eaves GN: Who reads your project-grant applications in the National Institutes of Health? *Federal Proceedings* January/February 1972; 31:2–9.

Finin L (editor): *Sponsored Fund Administration: A Bibliography*. Albany, N.Y.: Research Foundation of SUNY, 1976.

Fuller EO: The pink sheet syndrome. *Nurs Res* 1982; 31:185–186.

Geitgey DA, Metz EA: A brief guide to designing research proposals. *Nurs Res* 1969; 18:339–344.

Kaiser LR: Grantsmanship in continuing education. January 1973; 12:12–20.

Margolin JB: *About Foundations: How to Find the Facts You Need to Get a Grant.* New York: Foundation Center, 1975.

Notter LE: Improving our skills in developing research protocols. (Editorial.) *Nurs Res* 1973; 22:291.

Phillips TP: What is the difference between a research grant and a research contract? *Nurs Res* September/October 1975; 24:388–389.

Plotkin HM: Preparing a proposal, step by step. *J Systems Mgmt* 1972; 23:36–38.

White VP: *Grants: How to Find Out about Them and What to Do Next.* New York: Plenum Press, 1975.

Chapter 9

Getting Started on Your Study

by Sally Hutchinson RN, PhD

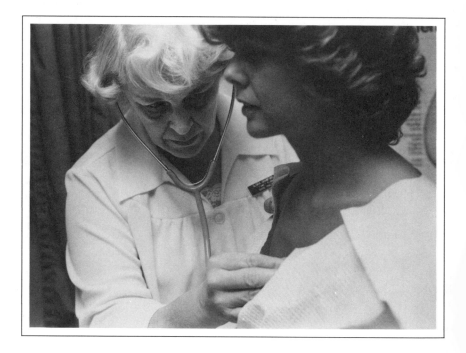

Once you recognize the seed of a worthwhile research idea, you are faced with the challenge of refining it into a researchable question and devising a design to answer it.

Chapter Outline

Chapter Objectives

After reading this chapter, the student should be able to:

- Formulate a research question
- Differentiate between levels of inquiry (Levels 1, 2, 3)
- Specify the steps in a literature review
- Specify the scope of a literature review
- Specify the rationale for a literature review
- Formulate a statement of purpose
- Formulate hypotheses, if appropriate
- Recognize criteria for and types of hypothesis
- Identify variables
- Formulate operational definitions
- Choose an appropriate design for the study purpose
- Classify sampling methods according to probability and nonprobability methods
- Discuss the relevant issues related to sample size
- Discuss sampling with special population groups
- Discuss the relationship of sampling to external validity

In This Chapter . . .

Florence Nightingale, known as the first nurse statistician, can also be credited with advocating that nursing research focus on nursing practice. In 1975, Notter, former editor of *Nursing Research*, echoed Nightingale, and in 1979, Hodgeman predicted such a move in the practice setting, with the actual research to be done by practicing nurses. If nursing is to be based on scientific knowledge, practicing nurses are vital in identifying relevant, researchable problems and participating in the research process. It is toward this end that this chapter moves.

As a practicing nurse or a nursing student in a diploma, A.D., B.S.N., or graduate program you may find yourself in a number of situations that force or encourage you to get started doing research. Suppose a physician or a faculty member is involved in research and asks you to collaborate; or you are working on your B.S.N. degree and as part of your senior practicum you are required to do a research project; or you are a student in a master's program and choose to do the thesis option that earns you an M.S.N. degree; or the director of nursing of the hospital where you work is making resources available for nurses involved in clinical practice to do scientific studies. Furthermore, you recognize that promotions and merit increases for nurses in the future are going to reflect this new emphasis on research productivity. Finally, research can be exciting, intellectually stimulating, and rewarding.

Although you may not be initially aware of it, you have many research ideas. Each nurse has observed some aspect of patient behavior or patient treatment that is perplexing or annoying. These observations can lead you to formulate a general research question, which after a literature review can be refined into a research purpose (see Chapter 5). The research purpose is the objective for your study.

After choosing a research design that is appropriate for your purpose, you select a sample. It is soon time to collect data. By now you are more than halfway through the research process and are on your way toward making a much-needed contribution to nursing knowledge.

Each step of the research process requires that you make decisions. This chapter was written to help you make them. It deals with the questions "How do I formulate a research question?" "What literature do I review, and what do I do with it after I review it?" "How do I state my research purpose?" "How big should my sample be?" "Do I need hypotheses?" "What type of research design is appropriate for my study?" This chapter covers the research process from choosing a question to sampling. Other chapters in this book will discuss the rest of the research process, from data collection to data analysis and discussion. Reading and reflecting on this chapter and on the illustrations from nursing studies that it contains will help you get started as a nurse researcher.

The Research Question

Planting the Seed

Imagine that you are a cardiac rehabilitation nurse and notice that many cardiac bypass patients do not comply with the suggested regimen of diet, exercises, and no smoking. You wonder what sort of nursing intervention would increase their compliance, giving them the opportunity to reap the benefits of their surgery and to live a more comfortable life.

Or assume that you are new to the medical unit of a small community hospital. You notice that hospital procedure requires the application of ice to the injection sites of patients who are receiving heparin, for 15 minutes before the injection and 15 minutes after the injection. You are told by coworkers that the ice is used to decrease bruising from the heparin. You recently worked in a hospital in the nearest large city, and ice was also applied to the heparin site there. You wonder if the ice really does what it is supposed to do.

Or perhaps you work in the labor and delivery units of an urban hospital. You notice that the fathers who go through Lamaze training classes are participating in the labor and delivery process. Men who do not go through the training are excluded from the delivery room. You wonder if the two groups of fathers differ in their feelings about their partner's birth experience or their new baby.

Or imagine that you read in a nursing journal that young male schizophrenics who have female counselors are more likely to keep follow-up appointments and call for help than those who have male counselors. You wonder if this is an accurate picture of the mental health clinic in which you work.

The above situations contain examples of research problems in the early phase of development. The seed of an idea appears, and you must cultivate and nurture it until it becomes a full-grown research project. As you learned in Chapter 5, research problems can come from your experiences, observations, and reading of articles, books, or study reports. Nursing theory or theories from other disciplines, if they are relevant to nursing practice, are excellent sources of research problems and are discussed in Chapter 10.

Determining Your Level of Inquiry

Once you recognize the seed of a worthwhile idea, you are faced with the task of refining the idea into a researchable question and designing the procedures for answering it. Brink and Wood (1983) view research questions as existing on three levels.

Level I Inquiry Level 1 questions are used when little knowledge is available about a topic. (You can determine this through your literature review.) Level 1 questions begin with "What" (see Box 9-1). These questions are used in *exploratory and descriptive research.*

Nurses often become concerned when their literature review (something we'll discuss later in the chapter) reveals very little available information on their research question. The references are often only indirectly related to their specific interest. In nursing a dearth of information is a common occurrence, because nursing is a new and evolving science, and nurses have been actively engaged in research for a mere 20 to 30 years.

Writing a Level 1 question is the perfect solution to the problem of minimal information. If very little information exists, you can design a study to explore and describe your subject, and your findings can be the basis for subsequent

---

Box 9-1	*Level 1 Research Questions*	
Stem	**Topic**	
1. What . . .	are the experiences of fathers who are in the delivery room with their wives?	
2. What . . .	are nurses' attitudes toward obese patients?	
3. What . . .	do insulin-dependent diabetic patients want to know about their disease?	

Table 9-1   Variables and Populations for Three Level 1 Research Questions

Question	Variable	Population
Question 1:	Experiences	Fathers in the delivery rooms
Question 2:	Attitudes	Nurses
Question 3:	Knowledge	Insulin-dependent diabetic patients

higher-level studies. In this way scientists build knowledge and develop theory. Each level of inquiry contributes to the process of maturation as a science.

After you formulate your specific research question, Brink and Wood (1983) suggest, you should check it to be sure that it has (1) one variable or topic and (2) a reference to the population in which the variable or topic will be found (p. 14). The variables and populations in the three questions in Box 9-1 are summarized in Table 9-1.

Level 2 Inquiry   Level 2 questions look for the *relationship between variables*, and they begin by asking, "What is the relationship?" Your literature review will be useful in helping to determine if the research question should be a Level 2 question. If the variables you are interested in are discussed in the literature, you must then come up with a theoretical rationale for the suggested relationship implied in the question. If

you ask, "What is the relationship between the public's political beliefs (liberalism versus conservatism) and their image of nurses?" the literature review that you have conducted should support the idea that the variable *public's political beliefs* is related to the variable *public's image of nurses*. The literature will not specify the precise nature of the relationship between the variables, but it will give you enough information so that you can make a conceptual leap in assuming that the relationship might logically exist. For example, the literature may report that people who have conservative political views tend to prefer that women remain in traditional roles. Those with liberal political views are better able to see women in a variety of roles. A researcher can assume, then, that conservative people may view nurses (97% women) in the traditional role of dependent handmaiden to the physician. In contrast, those with liberal views may more readily see the nurse as being more autonomous, creative, and professional. Other examples of Level 2 research questions are summarized in Box 9-2.

Level 2 questions make reference to two variables. (Remember, Level 1 questions have only one variable and identify the population in which the variable is of interest.)

A *variable* is any factor that varies, so be sure that any variables you choose to examine do, in fact, vary (see Chapter 4). In the variables listed in Table 9-2—patient education, patient compliance, in-service education, and turnover rate—every factor can vary. There may be a patient education program or the absence of such a program—thus, the variability. Patients may or

Box 9-2   Level 2 Research Questions

Stem	Topic
1. What is the relationship . . .	of patient education to patient compliance in a cardiac rehabilitation program?
2. What is the relationship . . .	of continuing in-service education in their specialty to the turnover rate of cardiac care unit (CCU) nurses?

Table 9-2   Variables and Populations for Two Level 2 Questions

Question	Variables	Population
Question 1:	(a) Patient education (b) Patient compliance	Cardiac rehab patients
Question 2:	(a) In-service education (b) Turnover rate	CCU nurses

may not comply, or they may comply in part. There may be continuing specific in-service education, no education, or just general education. The turnover rate can be stated as a percentage of nurses leaving over a certain period of time.

If you asked, "What is the relationship of the discussion method of in-service education to the nurse turnover rate?" you would soon recognize that the factor of "discussion method of in-service education" does not vary as stated. Consequently, you would need to change the "variable" to the more general category of "method of in-service education," which would allow you to examine the discussion method versus the lecture method versus videotape, demonstrating the variability of methods.

Level 3 Inquiry   Level 3 inquiry assumes a relationship, either causal or influential, between two variables and asks "Why?" Your literature review will reveal theory (or other findings) that predict the nature of the relationship. For ex-

ample: "Why does a behavior modification program decrease the acting out of adolescent patients on a psychiatric unit?" Learning theory (classical conditioning) is used to predict how rewards (for not "acting out," for "good" behavior) act as a stimulus to elicit the desired response of more "good" behavior (Wilson & Kneisl 1983, pp. 553–554). Two other examples of Level 3 questions appear in Box 9-3.

Level 3 questions require (1) two variables, one that is predicted to be causal and one that is the effect, or outcome, variable; (2) a population; and (3) a predicted direction (see Table 9-3).

Depending on your literature review, questions may be written at different levels. For example, you may initially write a Level 2 question: "What is the relationship of patient education to patient compliance in a cardiac rehabilitation program?" As you search the literature, you find theory to support the notion that a patient education model using lecture and discussion is more effective in changing behavior than one using videotapes. Therefore, the original question could be rewritten to a Level 3 question: "Why does a lecture and discussion form of education increase patient compliance in a cardiac rehabilitation program?" *If there is theory to predict the nature of the relationship between the variables, then use a Level 3 question.*

One mark of a good research study is that the research question is written at the appropriate level. As you refine your research question, be sure you meet the criteria for the level at which you are writing it. Aim for clarity and conciseness.

Box 9-3   *Level 3 Questions*

Stem	Topic
1. Why . . .	do self-care behaviors increase the feelings of well-being in patients with chronic illness?
2. Why . . .	does attending Alcoholics Anonymous meetings decrease the drinking behavior of alcoholics?

Table 9-3   Variables for Two Level 3 Questions

Question	Variables		Population	Direction
	Causal	Effect		
Question 1	Self-care behaviors	Feelings of well-being	Patients with chronic illness	Increase
Question 2	Attending AA meetings	Drinking behavior	Alcoholics	Decrease

Review of the Literature

After you have written your question, the next step is to return to the literature and conduct a systematic search to find out more precisely what is known about your topic. As we have seen, the level of your question may change after you do an extensive review of the literature. One nurse wrote a Level 1 exploratory question, "What are the experiences of young women with cancer?" His literature review revealed hundreds of articles dealing with psychological and physiological effects of cancer, but none of them focused on young women. The nurse could have written a Level 2 question and examined any number of variables to test for a relationship, and he could have found a theory (perhaps crisis theory) and tested the relationship of selected variables. But because his interest was in *young* women, he elected to formulate a Level 1 question. This example demonstrates that questions can often be written at different levels of inquiry, but as you become more clear about what you specifically want to know about your topic, the question level will also become more apparent.

Steps in Conducting a Literature Review

Do a Computer Search   To begin your literature review, use a computerized search (see Chapter 16). First, select a few key words from your question, and discuss with a reference librarian the appropriate terms to put into the computer. The review should include all variables (key terms) relevant to your study. For example, if you are interested in the question "Why do self-care behaviors increase the feelings of well-being in patients with chronic illness?" you will look up Orem's theory of self-care (1980), articles on self-care behaviors in patients with chronic illness, and articles on patients' feelings of well-being. Reference librarians are incredibly helpful in selecting key words that elicit relevant printouts of references.

Second, check the appropriate indices—medical, nursing, sociology abstracts, and the like (see Chapter 2 for more detail)—depending on the nature of your question. If you can get one or two good articles, the bibliography at the end is often very useful in suggesting other articles. Because there are only a few nursing research journals (see Chapter 2), you can quickly check the last few years and determine what types of research question have been asked in your problem area.

As mentioned earlier, you may find few directly relevant research articles. However, don't be too easily discouraged. Do an exhaustive search, using the suggested multiple sources, that covers at least the last five years. This way you will really know what the state of knowledge on your topic is. The aim of the search is to enable you to place your question in the context of existing knowledge.

Take Notes   As you read, take notes on cards. Five-by-eight cards are particularly useful, because they can hold a good deal of information. Although note taking may seem like a lot of work at the time, it is very necessary and will prevent you from the fate of one nurse, who did a review of the literature, reading approximately 100 articles. Because she felt none were particularly relevant to her study of fathers' perceptions of their pregnant wives, she took no notes. At the end of weeks of work she had nothing recorded. After reexamining the research purpose and rethinking the level of the study, she recognized that her readings were indirectly related to the topic and thus supported the need for a Level 1 exploratory study. Consequently, she had to start all over again.

Even if an article is only peripherally related to your study, jot it down. Because you may be doing a Level 1 study where little is known, you ought to review studies that are indirectly related to clarify the gap your study is designed to fill.

On your note cards write the bibliography and a few major headings (see Figure 9-1).

Scope of a Literature Review

Your review should include six major types of literature:

1. Relevant nursing research.
2. Theoretical literature. This part of the literature review will be addressed in Chapter 10.

AUTHORS: May, Kathryn

TITLE: Three Phases of Father Involvement in Pregnancy

SOURCE: *Nursing Research*, 1980, 31:337–342.

RESEARCH QUESTION OR HYPOTHESIS:

What are men's experiences of first-time expectant fatherhood?

METHOD: Field study: intensive interviews with 20 expectant couples, short field interviews with 30 additional fathers, participant observation in prenatal classes and clinics, and content analysis of popular literature. The aim was to generate substantive theory.

FINDINGS: Three phases of father involvement include an announcement phase, a moratorium and a focusing phase. The fathers' speed of progression through the phases may affect adjustment to fatherhood.

Figure 9-1   Note reference card.

3. General and specialty nursing literature. If research studies are minimal and you see yourself heading for a Level 1 study, search the general nursing literature—*American Journal of Nursing, Heart and Lung, Maternal Child Nursing*, and the like—and other nonresearch-oriented specialty journals. Reading these journals will give you a feeling for what your colleagues are doing with your topic. In the study on the experiences of young women with cancer, the researcher found no scientific articles relating to experiences but several anecdotal articles in the general nursing literature describing a nurse's experience as a patient with breast cancer.

    With Level 2 and 3 studies, general nursing literature may be interesting, but you need to find research that can support (Level 2) or predict (Level 3) the relationship between two variables.

4. Methodological literature. If you notice that all the studies on your subject use a certain method of analysis, you may want to say something about the method. For example: "All previous studies of patients' psychological responses to myocardial infarctions (MIs) have used specific psychological instruments to determine degrees of anxiety." You may want to read something on instruments dealing with anxiety to give you new ideas or sources for criticisms of the instruments (see Chapter 11). If all the studies deal with psychological instruments, perhaps you want to build a case for using an instrument that measures social or cultural responses. Or maybe you don't want to use an instrument at all but instead to explore (Level 1) the patients' experiences with a myocardial infarction (MI) with in-depth semistructured interviews.

5. Research literature from other disciplines. Most nursing research can benefit from research done in other related disciplines—sociology, psychology, anthropology, political science, physiology, or economics, depending on the nature of your question. Do not limit yourself to nursing research, because multidisciplinary literature can offer useful information about theory and methods. Nursing can be viewed as an applied science, so literature in social and natural science may be relevant. Society's pressing problems today are both political and economic, so literature from these disciplines may offer a broad yet relevant perspective on certain nursing research questions. If you are unsure of yourself in these areas, find an expert—an economist, an anthropologist, a psychologist, a physiologist—and ask for help (see the heading Using Other Resources later in this section).

6. Popular literature. Popular literature includes books like *First You Cry, Anatomy of an Illness, In the Company of Others*, and *Heartsounds*. These are written by patients or family members and in journalistic fashion describe a hospitalization or illness through the eyes of the involved participants or subjects. Often newspaper (professional and popular) and magazine articles deal with health issues. Such reports are not appropriate for a Level 2 or 3 study but may inform for a Level 1 study. The American Medical Association newsletter and the Associated Press reported on a California case in which two physicians were tried for murder for discontinuing life support systems on a patient. Articles such as these would be relevant for a Level 1 study focused on intensive care unit nurses' experiences in caring for nonviable patients. These studies add context and history and emphasize the rich descriptive nature of the problems. They also help in identifying particularly relevant variables, such as the legal aspects, ethical aspects, and physicians' perceptions versus nurses' perceptions of discontinuing life support, for example. The value of reviewing popular literature is not supported by the nurse researchers who conduct Level 2 and 3

studies, but a new trend among selected researchers in several disciplines views such literature as a useful source of information.

For your literature review you will be reading many articles that will not be used in the written literature review. Only those articles that are used for the written review are listed in your references.

How to Review

As you review the six types of relevant literature, you are reading not merely for content but analyzing and comparing.

A literature review requires not just the ingestion of large amounts of information but a criticism of each piece. You critique the research articles for their credibility and soundness (see Chapter 7). If a study has a sample size of five, yet makes generalizations to a larger population, you should be skeptical of it. You may want to critique the research articles on separate index cards, recording any problems. When you compose the literature review, mention the serious flaws that may affect your rationale for doing your particular study. For example, if a study used five subjects in an effort to understand the problems these subjects had feeding their cerebral palsied children, a researcher might want to replicate the study using a larger sample. Or if a researcher used an inappropriate method of data analysis or did not sample the appropriate population, a replication study would be acceptable.

If the popular books written by patients focus mainly on the changing body image after mastectomy, you will want to note this narrow thematic focus in your literature review. And if an instrument for measuring ethical judgment is being used to measure nursing students' levels of decision making but has only been used before on male prisoners, you will want to mention this.

As with most steps of the research process, no rigid rules exist for all studies. At each stage the researcher makes many decisions, presumably based on logical consideration of the factors discussed above. As you critically analyze the books and articles, you will be making decisions about what information is vital and relevant to include in your literature review.

Comparative reading relates all of your readings to one another and to your research question. As your sources increase, you may want to categorize your reference cards based on a scheme that makes sense to you and fits your study question or decision. Perhaps your research literature will be categorized according to those studies with experimental designs and those that are observational. Popular literature could be categorized according to biographical and autobiographical reports. Use any scheme that helps you in comparing your references so as to obtain an overview.

Why Review?

You may wonder why reviewing other literature is important. Why can't you just formulate your question and conduct your study and report the findings? Remember that the purpose of science is to build theory and that research is the tool of science (Chapter 1). Although many studies do not directly contribute to theory—for reasons that will become clear in the next chapter—they need to have contextual links. That is, a study in isolation cannot be clearly evaluated for significance and meaning, whereas a study that links up with previous research or theory provides a sense of context and a sense of history. We can analyze and understand the extent of existing knowledge and can determine where we should go in the future. The relevant books and articles that you read are the references that form the foundation and rationale for your own research.

Rationale for Your Research

Earlier in the chapter I mentioned that your observations and experiences often give rise to a research question. If you derived your question from experience or observations and not exclusively from a literature review, you need to describe the experience to the reader as an integral part of the background literature review. This personal account is usually placed at the beginning or end of the review in a research proposal or report. It can be placed anywhere in the literature review, however, as long as it is integrated in a logical fashion. For example, in her study May says,

In spite of increased interest in expectant fatherhood and father involvement, we know very little about men's experiences of pregnancy prior to the last trimester or how they come to be with their partners in birth classes or the delivery room (1982).

Such an account can lead into the literature related to your topic or can end the literature review by adding a humanistic, experiential element to the existing scientific reports.

Using Other Resources

As you begin the phase of getting research started, you should take advantage of all the resources available, not just the literature. Sometimes this means tracking them down and waiting long periods. If you are doing physiological research and you don't know a physiologist, find one or two or three. Talk with them, share your problems and dilemmas, and ask for suggestions. Ask them for the names of people who may be interested or helpful.

"Networking" in person, by phone, or by mail has many positive payoffs. Don't be intimidated by an author of a research article or by a national leader who does research in your specialty. Rather, view these people as resources, and use them as consultants or as sources of information. Most people who do research are excited about their work and actually enjoy sharing their expertise with others. Talking with one key person can sometimes be more useful than reading 50 articles, so in the interest of

efficiency view people as vital resources in addition to the literature.

Networking occasionally results in several people doing collaborative research. The investigators may represent different disciplines or may be nurses sharing a similar interest. Being part of a joint effort can be exhilarating and can produce a study with more breadth and depth than a project with a single researcher. Collaborative research, sometimes called programatic research, also enables investigators to pool and share resources such as statistical, computer, and editorial assistance.

A New Way of Seeing

Coming up with a research question and doing a literature review are challenging tasks that require much thinking and many rewrites. The process is not always totally efficient. You may read a lot of articles that ultimately are not relevant; you may have several ideas that appeal to you but are not feasible, researchable, or significant; and your final question may evolve to be far different from the original one.

Nurses are often task-oriented, and because of this tendency they may need to learn a new way of seeing and thinking to do research. Recognizing this need from the start should make the task somewhat easier. Try to avoid viewing the research enterprise as linear (step by step) and always efficient. Instead, think of getting started as a time for intellectual exploration; a time for musing and changing your mind; a time for checking things out before making a decision and commitment. All of these considerations take time, but the early phase will solidify a definitive research question that is:

- substantiated by literature and rationale
- feasible (the possibility or practicality of conducting the study)
- significant
- researchable (the problem is a *research* problem and does not request a yes or no answer or values or opinions)

Box 9-4	*Study Levels and Their Statements of Purpose*
Level 1	In a study that asks the question "What are the eating habits of bulimics?" the purpose can be expressed in the statement: *The purpose of this research is to explore and describe the eating habits of bulimics.*
Level 2	In a study that asks the question "What is the relationship between smoking and prematurity in primiparous mothers?" the purpose is written as: *The purpose of the study is to answer the question "Is there a significant relationship between smoking and prematurity in primiparous mothers?"*
Level 3	In a study that asks the question "Why does the teaching of self-care strategies increase the feeling of well-being in chronically ill patients?" the purpose is written as: *The purpose of this study is to test this hypothesis: Chronically ill patients who are taught self-care techniques will have higher scores on feelings of well-being than those who do not receive the teaching.*

Statement of Purpose

The statement of purpose answers the question "Why do the study?" Researchers hold different views about stating a purpose for the research. Some believe that a question or hypothesis is sufficient and that including a statement of purpose is redundant. Others believe that both a statement of purpose and a research question or hypothesis are necessary. Brink and Wood (1983) suggest that the purpose be written as a *statement* for a Level 1 study, as a *question* for a Level 2 study, and as a *hypothesis* (or hypotheses) for a Level 3 study. Box 9-4 illustrates this approach.

Planning your research begins with formulating a research question, moves through a review of the related literature and your rationale, and culminates with a concise statement of purpose.

Writing Hypotheses

A *hypothesis* is the statement of a predicted relationship between two or more variables (see Glossary). In the Level 3 example in Box 9-4, the variables are teaching versus nonteaching and feelings of well-being. The hypothesis suggests that there is a relationship between teaching self-care techniques and patients' feelings of well-being. The hypothesis predicts that those receiving the teaching will have higher scores on a measure of feelings of well-being.

Criteria for a Hypothesis

As you write your hypothesis, think about the following criteria, suggested by Polit and Hungler (1983), that are required if a statement is to be considered a hypothesis:

Testable: In order for a hypothesis to be testable there must be a predicted relationship between variables. For example: "Nursing schools with flexible curricula will retain and graduate more students." Here, there is only one variable (retention and graduation of students), making the hypothesis untestable because there is nothing to compare. If the hypothesis were rewritten as "Nursing schools with flexible curricula will retain and graduate more students than nursing schools without flexible curricula," the hypothesis is testable. You can measure the retention and graduation rates of schools with both curricula—flexible and inflexible (the other variable)—and compare them.

A hypothesis can only be tested if the variables can be observed or measured. Operational definitions have the goal of making the variables observable or measurable. For example, you may wonder what a "flexible curriculum" is. A flexible curriculum can be operationally defined as a curriculum that allows the students to (1) take a test to demonstrate knowledge of lower level courses, (2) challenge upper level courses, and (3) meet at a variety of times and places for classes. An inflexible curriculum refers to programs without these three criteria. Because of this clear definition the variables *flexible curriculum* and *inflexible curriculum* can be measured.

Justifiable: A hypothesis must be justifiable, meaning that you have derived your hypothesis from theory. For example, if you read that behavior modification is more effective in encouraging weight loss in obese people than lectures on nutrition and dieting, you can write a hypothesis to that effect. For example, obese people who participate in behavior modification training lose more weight than obese people attending lectures on nutrition and dieting. This hypothesis clearly is derived from a behavioristic theoretical framework.

However, suppose you have an idea that meditation might help people lose weight, and you write a hypothesis that proposes to look at the relationship between meditation and weight loss in two groups (one with meditation classes and one without). This hypothesis does not meet the criteria of being justifiable, because it was not deduced from a theoretical framework. Rather,

the idea was merely a whimsical thought or personal hunch. It is a good practice to list all possible hypotheses and to follow your hunches to the hypothesis stage, but they must always be justified by some theoretical support. If they are not, a research question is more appropriate.

Components of a Hypothesis

Hypotheses must be written clearly and concisely. Each word should add meaning to the hypotheses and have a purpose. Brink and Wood (1983) identify the three components that are essential to a well-written hypothesis: (1) the experimental group; (2) the expected result, and (3) the comparison group (p. 72). Table 9-4 shows the different parts of hypotheses in studies published in *Nursing Research*.

Types of Hypothesis

Hypotheses can be:

- simple
- complex
- directional
- nondirectional
- research hypotheses
- statistical hypotheses

A *simple* hypothesis predicts the relationship between one independent variable (IV) and one dependent variable (DV), whereas a *complex* hypothesis predicts the relationship between two (or more) independent variables and two (or more) dependent variables. Note the examples in Table 9-5.

As the words imply, a simple hypothesis is easier to test, measure, and analyze than a complex hypothesis. Because nursing research deals with human beings, who are complex, however, a lot of nursing research uses complex hypotheses. The most important considerations for you as a researcher to think about are: (1) What type

Table 9-4   Required Parts of Hypotheses [1]

Hypothesis	Experimental Group	Expected Result	Comparison Group
1. Patients who receive reconditioning have less bladder dysfunction after indwelling catheter removal than patients who receive no conditioning (Williamson 1982)	Patients who receive reconditioning	Will have less bladder dysfunction after indwelling catheter removal	The patients who do not receive reconditioning
2. Patients who are educated before an operation about the possibility of unusual sensory or cognitive experiences will not have such experiences after the operation or will feel comfortable or in control of the experience if they occur (Owens & Hutelmeyer 1982)	Patients who are educated preoperatively	Will not have or will feel comfortable with unusual sensory or cognitive experiences	The group is not mentioned in the hypothesis, but it would be patients who are not educated.
3. Patients having mastectomies for breast cancer will experience more depression than patients undergoing hysterectomy for gynecological cancer or patients undergoing breast biopsy (Krouse & Krouse 1982)	Patients having mastectomies	Will experience more depression	Patients undergoing hysterectomy for cancer and patients undergoing breast biopsy
4. The health-belief scores of adult women who practice breast self-examination will be higher (will reflect greater perceived susceptibility and greater perceived benefits) than the health-belief scores of adult women who do not practice BSE (Hallal 1982)	Adult women who practice breast self-examination	Will have higher health-belief scores	Those adult women who do not practice BSE
5. There is a difference in sleep–wake patterns following minor head injury compared with preinjury sleep–wake patterns (Parsons & Ver Beek 1982)	Patients with minor head injuries	Will have different (the nature of the difference is not predicted) sleep–awake patterns	Those patients who have not sustained a head injury

[1] According to the usual criteria for experimental groups, the patients in examples 3, 4, and 5 are not truly an "experimental" group because they are not randomly assigned to a treatment. Rather, they already have a mastectomy, or practice BSE, or have a minor head injury. However, for purposes of this chart in explaining the required parts of a hypothesis they can be considered the experimental group.

Table 9-5 Simple and Complex Hypotheses and Their Variables

Simple Hypotheses	Independent Variables	Dependent Variables
1. The health belief scores of adult women who practice breast self-examination will be higher (will reflect greater perceived susceptibility and greater perceived benefits) than the health-belief scores of adult women who do not practice BSE (Hallal 1982)	Practice of breast self-examination	Health-belief scores
2. Oxygen inhalation by nasal cannula of up to 6 liters per minute does not affect oral temperature measurements taken with an electronic thermometer (Lim-Levy 1982)	Oxygen inhalation by nasal cannula	Oral temperature measurement
3. Sexually active adolescents are more likely to accept contraceptive counseling at the time of a negative pregnancy test than at the time of a routine medical visit (Marcy et al 1983)	Timing of counseling	Acceptance of contraceptive counseling
Complex Hypotheses		
1. Higher levels of experienced personal control over one's life will be associated with more perceived purpose to one's life, higher self-esteem, and lower self-reported anxiety in late-stage cancer patients (Lewis 1982)	Levels of experienced personal control	Perceived purpose to one's life Self-esteem Self-reported anxiety
2. The longer the history of trauma with no effect by voluntary actions, the lower the level of experienced control over one's health, the higher the self-reported anxiety, the lower the experienced purpose in life, and the lower the individuals' self-esteem in late-stage cancer patients (Lewis 1982)	The length of time of the history of trauma	Level of experienced control over one's health Self-reported anxiety Experienced purpose in life Self-esteem
3. Three months after onset of employment (at a public psychiatric in-patient facility), personal and training variables will be more predictive of tenure status than ward-related and organizational variables (Depp et al 1983)	Personal variables Training variables Ward-related variables Organizational variables	Tenure status

of hypothesis is best for your study? and (2) Is the study you are planning feasible? That is, if a complex hypothesis is appropriate for your study but you cannot collect the data to test it, then by all means write a simple hypothesis.

A *directional* hypothesis specifies the direction of the relationship between variables, whereas a *nondirectional* hypothesis only predicts that there is a relationship. Note the difference:

- *Directional Hypothesis*: Patients who receive reconditioning have less bladder dysfunction after indwelling catheter removal than patients who receive no conditioning (Williamson 1982).

- *Nondirectional Hypothesis*: There is a difference in sleep–wake patterns following minor head injury compared with preinjury sleep–wake patterns (Parsons & Ver Beek 1982).

Because theory always suggests the direction of the relationship, hypotheses should be directional. But you will read many examples of nondirectional hypotheses. Such hypotheses were not derived from theory but generally came from hunches or a literature review. In such situations a research question should be written.

As with much of research, there is controversy over the use of directional and nondirectional hypotheses. Some researchers believe that if you can't write a directional hypothesis, then you should not design your study to test hypotheses but should instead ask a Level 1 or 2 question—"What is . . ." or "What is the relationship between . . ." Other authorities believe that you can use directional or nondirectional hypotheses depending on your level of knowledge about a topic. They suggest that if there is not enough knowledge to predict the relationship, you should use a nondirectional hypothesis. For your research I suggest writing directional hypotheses, because they are clearer and more logi-

cal and because hypotheses should be derived from theory that is sufficiently evolved to deduce them.

A *research hypothesis* states the anticipated relationship between variables; all the examples to this point have been research hypotheses. A *null*, or *statistical*, *hypothesis* is a hypothesis written in the form that predicts *no relationship* between the independent and dependent variables: "There is no relationship between modes of intervention and weight loss in obese people" is an example of a null hypothesis. Principles used in statistical inference require that all research hypotheses be tested in the null form. The probability used to do statistical tests works under the assumption that there are no differences between variables, thus the use of the null (see Chapter 15). For clarity in research studies, however, hypotheses should be stated in the research form, which clearly indicates the thinking of the investigator.

Defining Variables

Now that you have completed the literature review and defined your research purpose as a statement or a question or hypothesis, you are ready to define your study's variables operationally so that you can move on to collecting data. It is impossible to collect data until you have made your variables clear and until you have decided how to study them.

A variable is, as the name suggests, any factor that varies. See Table 9-6 for examples of hypotheses and their variables. For example, age, weight, height, temperature, P_{CO_2} values, stress, political beliefs, and attitudes are all variables, because all vary to some degree. Gender varies from male to female and is an example of a *dichotomous* variable, that is, a variable with only two categories. Age, weight, height, and P_{CO_2} have a range of variability and are examples of *continuous* variables (see Glossary).

Nurse researchers are interested in studying variables, particularly how they vary in relation to one another. For example, how does alcoholism vary with different types of treatment methods? How does surgical patients' anxiety vary with different types of anesthesia? An independent variable can stand alone, whereas a *dependent variable* depends on another variable (see Chapter 4). In some studies, independent variables are thought to influence dependent variables in a cause-and-effect fashion; for example, exposure to the sun over time may cause skin cancer. Independent variables are those that the researcher manipulates. For example, you, through the sampling process, can study people with much sun exposure and people with little sun exposure, thus manipulating the independent variable. Or, the researcher can introduce a cardiac rehabilitation education program (inde-

Table 9-6   Hypotheses and Their Variables

Hypothesis	Variables	Type of Variation
1. Patients who receive reconditioning have less bladder dysfunction after indwelling catheter removal than patients who receive no conditioning (Williamson 1982)	Reconditioning	The patients receive reconditioning or don't receive reconditioning
	Bladder dysfunction	The bladder is dysfunctional or is not.
2. Patients who are educated before an operation about the possibility of unusual sensory or cognitive experiences will not have such experiences after the operation or will feel comfortable or in control of the experience if they occur (Owens & Hutelmeyer 1982)	Preoperative education	Patients receive preoperative education or don't.
	Postoperative experiences	Unusual sensory experiences are present or not.
	Feelings about the postoperative experience	The patient can feel comfortable or in control of the unusual sensory experience or not.
3. Patients having a mastectomy for breast cancer will experience more depression than patients undergoing hysterectomy for gynecological cancer or patients undergoing breast biopsy (Krouse & Krouse 1982)	Type of surgery	Surgery can be mastectomy, hysterectomy, or biopsy.
	Amount of depression	Depression can range from none to severe.
4. The health-belief scores of adult women who practice breast self-examination will be higher (will reflect greater perceived susceptibility and greater perceived benefits) than the health-belief scores of adult women who do not practice BSE (Hallal 1982)	Health belief scores	The scores may range from high to low.
	The practice of BSE	Women may or may not practice BSE.
5. There is a difference in sleep–wake patterns following minor head injury compared with preinjury sleep–wake patterns (Parsons & Ver Beek 1982)	Sleep–wake patterns	The sleep–wake patterns may vary in terms of times and duration.
	Head injury	The patients may be preinjury or postinjury.

pendent variable) and study patients' understanding (dependent variable) of their illness (see Chapter 6).

If you are testing hypotheses (Level 3), you will have an independent and a dependent variable. Since Level 1 studies are exploratory, the relevant variables are not all known at the outset. All variables are assumed to be independent until there is enough of a knowledge base to predict the nature of the variables. In Level 2 studies, in which the researcher asks if there is a significant relationship between variables—for example, "Is there a significant relationship between women's age and sleep patterns?"—there is the underlying assumption or hunch that women's age (independent variable) does affect sleep patterns (dependent variable). But until the research is completed, one cannot justifiably predict a cause-and-effect pattern.

Once your research statement, question, or hypothesis is written clearly, with the appropriate delineation of variables, you need to write *operational definitions* for them. Operationally defining your variables requires that you clearly specify them and say how you are measuring them.

If your variable is age, how will you collect data on the subjects' age? Ask them? Have them write it on a questionnaire? Here, for example, is an operational definition of age: "The age of the subject will be asked during the interview session and will be recorded in number of years and months." An operational definition of sleep pattern is: "Sleeping electroencephalograms will be recorded over one eight-hour period, and the pattern will be assessed according to the Bannon Sleep Pattern Instrument." In both examples you can see clearly what variable is being studied and how it will be measured. The operational definition permits you to go from the abstract idea of variables to a concrete definition of how to measure the specific variables. (See Box 9-5 for examples from published nursing research.)

Variables can be concrete (gender, age, height) or more abstract (stress, depression, political beliefs, spiritual beliefs). Abstract variables can be measured using many different instruments (see Chapters 11, 12, and 13). Stress and depression can be measured psychologically or physiologically; depression can be studied by projective techniques, self-report, or observation. Political beliefs and spiritual beliefs can be assessed by in-depth interviews or questionnaires. Because of all the possibilities, too numerous to list here, you must carefully specify your own approach to measuring your study's variables.

Choosing a Design

In Chapter 6 you learned that a design was a blueprint, or plan, for conducting your research, and you learned about the different types of design. The question that faces all researchers is "What is the best design for my study?" A good design follows logically from the study's purpose. Let's look at a purpose that is to explore and define unstudied variables, such as experiences of ICU nurses caring for nonviable patients. If the purpose is to explore and define variables, the study can also be called a factor-naming study. Certain designs lend themselves to studies that are intended to search for factors and to explore and define a given problem.

Historical and Case Study Designs

A historical design, as we saw in Chapter 6, aims to synthesize facts, thereby extending knowledge. The exploration and description of changes that occurred in public health nursing in the United States between 1900 and 1930 is an example of a historical research purpose (Buhler-Wilkerson 1983).

The descriptive case study design, using in-depth analysis, examines a new problem with an exploratory approach. A case study design would have been appropriate to study the "bubble boy" (who had the rare immunological disease called severe combined immunodeficiency), because he was the first child to spend his entire existence, except for his last 15 days, in sterile plastic chambers (Begley & Shapiro 1984). An exploration and description of his relationships with staff or family members would have made a significant contribution to knowledge. Case study designs are not used much in nursing, perhaps because they require much analytic rigor and much time. However, Meir and Pugh (1983) advocate the case study as a viable approach to clinical research.

Case study designs that use experimental approaches (discussed in more detail in Chapter 6) are useful if you want to use an intervention with one patient and measure a selected dependent variable before, during, and after the intervention. Some nurse researchers are beginning to see the value of this type of case study design, especially in selected situations (Barnard 1983, Holm 1983).

Box 9-5   *Operationalizing Variables—Examples From Nursing Research*

Purpose/Question/Hypotheses

The purpose of this study was to identify procedural components to be used in analog studies of preparatory techniques for childbirth. The questions asked were (1) "which of four laboratory pain stimuli (modified submaximum effort tourniquet technique, Forgione–Barber pain stimulator, cold water stimulus, faradic shock) is most similar to the pain associated with the transition phase of labor?" and (2) "what is the patterning and duration of contractions and intercontraction intervals in this phase?"

Operational Definitions

1. Cold pressor: The CPS involves placing the subject's hand in a bath of ice water at 1° to 2°C (Barber & Hahn).
2. Modified submaximum effort tourniquet technique: The MSETT consists of the application to the upper arm of a standard adult-size blood pressure cuff inflated to 250 mm Hg (Johnson & Rice).
3. Faradic shock: The FS consists of a .6 MA electric shock delivered through a concentric electrode to the nonpalmar surface of the hand (Tursky).
4. Forgione–Barber pain stimulator: The FBPS consists of having subjects place their index finger in a device wherein a Plexiglas wedge is lowered to apply a constant weight (approximately 267 g) to the first joint (Forgione & Barber).

SOURCE: E. Geden et al, "Identifying Procedural Components for Analogue Research of Labor Pain," *Nursing Research*, 1983, 32:80–83.

Purpose/Question/Hypotheses

I. Frequency of pauses will be inversely related to the amount of stress during the conflict-stimulated interaction of a marital dyad.
II. Frequency of laughter will be inversely related to the amount of stress during the conflict-stimulated interactions of a marital dyad.
III. Frequency of interruptions will be inversely related to the amount of stress during the conflict-stimulated interaction of a marital dyad.
IV. Frequency of questions will be inversely related to the amount of stress during the conflict-stimulated interaction of a marital dyad.

Operational Definitions

A *pause* was defined as a hesitation that broke up the continuity of vocal sequences within or between sentences. Pauses ranged between .8 and 5.0 seconds (Goldman-Eisler) and were measured by a stopwatch manufactured by SGA Scientific, Inc.

Laughter was defined as an explosive sound or a continuous gentle sound resembling suppressed mirth and generally understood to constitute a laugh in this culture.

An *interruption* was defined as the listener breaking in with a remark while the spouse was speaking. A silence between any two statements had to be less than .8 seconds (a pause) to constitute an interruption.

A *question* was defined as an interrogative sentence or clause.

Psychological stress was defined as the response to emotionally based, mentally aversive stimulation

Box 9-5   (continued)

produced by the conflictual interaction of a marital dyad resolving disagreements generated by the IMC. Psychological stress was measured by voice analysis using the PSE® and was scored according to a coding manual developed by the Center for the Study of Human Relations at New York University.

Conflict-stimulated interaction was the audio-taped discussion of a marital dyad resolving conflictual marital situations generated by the IMC.

SOURCE: P. M. Hurley, "Communication Variables and Voice Analysis of Marital Conflict Stress," *Nursing Research*, 1983, 32:164–169.

Purpose/Question/Hypotheses

The purpose of this study was to examine the effect of passive range of motion, active range of motion, and isometric exercises of the legs on energy expenditure.

Operational Definitions

Passive and active exercise programs involved the same maneuvers; the only difference was that passive exercises were performed on the subject by the investigator, and active exercises were initiated by the subject. The active and passive exercises involved five components: flexion of the lower leg by bringing the knee toward the chest, raising the entire leg straight into the air, abduction of the leg, internal and external rotation of the leg, and dorsiflexion plus plantar flexion of the foot.

The isometric exercise program involved the tensing and relaxing of each buttock, the pressing of each leg into the bed, an attempt to raise each leg against restraint, the maximum extension of each foot, and the maximum flexion of each foot.

Energy expenditure is measured by:

1. *Oxygen consumption*—measured by a Waters MRM-1® oxygen consumption computer.
2. *Respiratory rate*—measured by notation of upward deflections on a pneumograph.
3. *Heart rate*—determined by notation of R waves occurring on an electrocardiograph.
4. *Blood pressure*—measured by a 7P8 preamplifier Grass Model 7 Polygraph®.

SOURCE: D. Hathaway and E. A. Geden, "Energy Expenditure During Leg Exercise Programs," *Nursing Research*, 1983, 32:147–149.

Survey Designs

Survey designs can have the purpose of describing characteristics, opinions, attitudes, or behaviors as they currently exist in a population (Chapter 6). If you want to explore and describe the attitudes of nurses with associate degrees, bachelor's degrees, and master's degrees toward "no codes," you can do a comparative survey. You are comparing samples from three groups (A.D., B.S.N., and M.S.N. nurses) in relation to specific variables (attitudes toward no-codes). If you study patients' opinions about being treated by nurse practitioners, you can use a descriptive survey design that will portray types of feelings or attitudes about the designated group (nurse practitioners).

A cross-sectional survey design can answer a question, such as "What are the experiences of parents who have two children with a fatal disease (muscular dystrophy, cystic fibrosis) when each child dies?" Remember that the cross-sectional survey design requires subjects who are at different points of an experience. So parents who have lost their first child are surveyed, as are parents who have lost their second. A longitudinal survey would interview these same parents over time, assessing their experiences at predetermined stages.

If the purpose of your research is to answer the question "What is the relationship between X variable and Y variable?" you are doing a factor-relating, or association, study. A correlational survey design is appropriate if you want to discover the magnitude of and direction of the relationship between variables. For example, if you have theoretical reasons to believe that socioeconomic status may be related to how the public views nurses, you can do a survey that has the purpose of assessing that relationship. Or if you wonder how the new, untested method of indirect calorimetry correlates with the accepted Harris Benedict Equation (these are two methods for measuring nutritional needs of patients with chronic obstructive pulmonary disease), you can look for the magnitude of the relationship with a correlational survey design. If the new method has a high correlation with the traditional method, then perhaps either method could be used, depending on cost, the ease of using each, and other relevant factors.

With correlation research, where you are looking for relationships between variables and trying to find whether one or more variables can predict another variable, representativeness is very important (see section on "Sampling" in this chapter). If you wonder whether undergraduate grade-point average or the Graduate Record Examination can predict success in graduate school, you will need to ensure a representative sample, or your study will be unable to accurately predict success.

Evaluation surveys are used to make judgments, to evaluate a program, policy, or method. Such surveys have research questions that ask about the relationship between a program and another variable or variables—for example, "What is the relationship between parent education and child abuse?" An evaluation survey is one way of eliciting the desired information.

Any design that has the purpose of answering a question about the relationship between or among variables is used only after the area of interest has been explored and defined. Factor-relating studies (Level 2) are conducted before there is enough information to design a Level 3 hypothesis-testing study.

Experimental Designs

Level 3 or causal hypothesis-testing studies require a design that maximizes control of variance. Consequently, experimental designs are the best choice, because they demand random selection of the sample, random assignment to groups, and control and manipulation of the independent variable.

If you have a hypothesis that derives from the literature, with operationally defined variables, and if you can randomly assign subjects to control and experimental groups and impose a treatment or intervention, controlling intervening variables, then you should use an experimental design. As we saw in Chapter 2, Lim-Levy (1982) studied the effect of oxygen inhalation on oral temperature. She randomly assigned 100 healthy adults to a control and to three experimental groups that received 2, 4, and 6 liters per minute of oxygen for 30 minutes. She measured oral temperatures before and 30 minutes after the oxygen treatment. Data analysis revealed that the treatment had no significant effect, and this recognition should cause practicing nurses to reevaluate the common practice of taking rectal or axillary temperatures of certain patients receiving oxygen.

Because random assignment and controlling variables in nursing research are so difficult, experimental designs are rare. You should sensitize yourself to your everyday nursing practice, however, and be alert for research questions that may lend themselves to experimental design. Toney's (1982) study on paternal bonding, in which some fathers (experimental group) held the newborn for 10 minutes the first hour after delivery and some fathers (control group) held the newborn 8 to 12 hours after delivery, is another good example of experimental research.

Quasi-Experimental Designs

Quasi-experimental designs are useful if the researcher cannot randomly assign subjects to control and experimental groups. The varieties of quasi-experimental designs are described in Chapter 6. Scott's 1983 study entitled "Anxiety, Critical Thinking and Information Processing During and After Breast Biopsy" is an example of a time-series quasi-experimental design. Scott studied 85 women volunteers who had experienced breast biopsy. She measured state anxiety, critical thinking ability, and judged duration (the difference between subjective judgment of and actual passage of time), and their relationship to coping relatedness and change over time. The women were tested after hospital admission, before diagnostic results were known, and 6 to 8 weeks later; the women whose results were benign were retested when the crisis was expected to be resolved.

Scott used the "before" measures (DV) as a baseline to compare with the "after" measures (after hearing the results were benign = IV). She found that critical thinking was reduced at the time of hospitalization when compared with 6 to 8 weeks after discharge; the anxiety levels of patients before they learned of diagnostic results were extremely high; 6 to 8 weeks after the diagnosis of "benign," state anxiety levels were significantly reduced; patients with high anxiety levels had difficulty in reasoning abilities and decision making; judged duration, a measure of information processing capacity, was not significantly changed between the hospital and postdischarge periods (p. 30). Scott related each variable to the patient's total coping process and suggested that awareness of patients' abilities to cope allows for nursing interventions that increase coping effectiveness.

To combat the disadvantages of the quasi-experimental design (see Chapter 6), Scott could add, as she suggests, a nonequivalent comparison group such as male patients who are diagnosed as having genitourinary carcinoma.

Quasi-experimental designs are the next best thing to experimental designs. Think about experiences that patients face during diagnosis and treatment and imagine how you could design a quasi-experimental study that measures patients on some variables before and after a treatment or compared with another group undergoing a similar experience.

Ex Post Facto Designs

Ex post facto designs are common in nursing research, because they study an event or experience after the fact, thus making many patients perfect subjects because they have had to undergo a certain experience (brain surgery, bone marrow transplant, spinal tap) that warrants close scientific examination. Gierszewski (1983) studied the relationship between weight loss, locus of control, and social support in the female employees of a life insurance company who had participated in a nutrition and weight-control program.

As you look around your work environment and notice patients who have experienced something—a specific nursing intervention, a diagnostic procedure, a crisis of any type—think about how theory could be used to suggest a hypothesis for study. Gierszewski became aware of the women experiencing a nutrition and weight-control program. She then thought about weight control and its theoretical relationship to locus of control and social support, which led to her hypotheses. Patients who sign out against medical advice (AMA) may be a relevant group to study in terms of locus of control. Parents who are child abusers are another group who need to be studied in an attempt to understand related variables, such as self-concept and locus of control.

When you cannot manipulate an independent variable and randomly assign subjects to control and experimental groups, an ex post facto study is appropriate and worthwhile. Just remember that because of the design you are not studying cause and effect but rather correlations among variables. Thus, your conclusions and interpretation need to be clear on this fact.

Methodological Designs

Methodological designs are vital to nursing research. Such studies develop or validate research instruments that are specifically designed to answer nursing questions. Given and his associates' 1983 study entitled "Development of Scales to Measure Beliefs of Diabetic Patients" leads the reader through the process of identifying health-belief concepts and attempts to construct scales for measuring these concepts.

Methodological research is long-term and is often the source of a dissertation. The investigator then follows up testing and validating the instrument in the period after the dissertation. In fact, the development of a valid and reliable instrument to measure some aspect of nursing inquiry could be a life's work and would represent a valuable contribution to nursing theory and practice.

If you decide to develop an instrument, your literature review will include the same types of literature as other studies but will focus on methodological literature—the "how tos" of instrument construction and measurement. Additional examples of methodological studies are given in Chapter 6.

You have now had a glimpse of the design possibilities that may be appropriate for your research purpose. Issues of reliability and validity are vital to any design, and Chapter 6 offers an in-depth discussion of study designs and concerns of reliability and validity. The related issue of bias in sampling is discussed in the next section. Your design will be a good one if it allows you to pursue your research purpose with accuracy and with control of variables (internal and external validity).

Sampling

Assume that you have just been selected to be a taster for the nutrition department of your small community hospital. Your job is to taste 30 low-calorie desserts and rate them according to specific criteria. Eating the entire 30 desserts is probably impossible and unnecessary. Rather, you will take a small bite, a sample, of each, which you assume to be representative of the entire dessert.

In your research you also will be sampling. Sampling is a vital part of the research process, and the strategies for choosing your sample will influence your results and your interpretation of them. Now that you have formulated your purpose and chosen a design, you need to decide who or what you will study. Your research purpose should lead you to *relevant* subjects. If you plan to study disgruntled patients or patients who are unhappy with their nursing care, be sure to select patients who are, in fact, disgruntled.

A *sample*, a subset of the population, is a group (of people, records, organizations) drawn from the *population*. The population is the total group that meets your criteria, and it is often referred to as the *universe* or the *target population*. If you plan to study quadriplegic patients with decubitus ulcers, all such patients are your target population. Because finding and contacting all of these people is impossible, you will choose a sample of quadriplegics with decubitus ulcers. Your sample will come from the *accessible population*, the population that is feasible. Perhaps you have access to two large rehabilitation hospitals, to five general hospitals, or to a home health service, all of which care for quadriplegic patients with ulcers. Any patients you can use as subjects compose your accessible population.

All researchers use sampling, because it is a feasible and logical way of making statements about a larger group based on a smaller group. Investigators can make inferences from the sample to the population if the sample-selection process is a systematic one. The method of selecting a sample is thus crucial to the research design. You must be concerned with how you can get the most *representative* sample possible. You wonder if a certain treatment method decreases the incidence of decubitus ulcers in quadriplegic patients, compared with another treatment method. To be able to say that one method is better than the other, you must be sure that your sample represents the characteristics of the population.

The next obvious question is "How do you make your sample representative?" Probability and nonprobability sampling are the two major approaches to sampling (see Table 9-7). *Probability sampling* is the more rigorous. It requires that every element in the population have an equal chance, that is, a *random* chance, of being selected for inclusion in the sample. *Nonprobability sampling*, in contrast, provides no way of estimating the probability that each element will be included in the sample. With the nonprobability approach the results will be representative of your sample only and cannot be generalized to the accessible population.

Types of Probability Sampling

Simple random sampling The best-known probability sampling approach is simple random sampling. Each individual in the *sampling frame* (all subjects in the population) has an equal chance of being chosen. If you plan to study patients with acquired immune deficiency syn-

Table 9-7   Types of Sampling

Probability Sampling	Nonprobability Sampling
Simple Random Sampling	Accidental or Convenience Sampling
Systematic Sampling	Snowball Sampling
Stratified Random Sampling	Purposive or Judgement Sampling
Cluster Sampling	Expert Sampling
	Quota Sampling

drome, for example, you will need a list of all of these patients who make up the population. To select the sample:

- Assign a number to each member of the population, and go to a table of random numbers (see Table 9-8).
- Close your eyes and with a pencil point to a number on the table.
- Move in a systematic way—up, down, or diagonally—choosing your sample by picking those subjects whose numbers correspond to the table of random numbers.
- Ignore numbers that do not appear on your frame (for example, 100 if your frame only goes to 99).
- Once a number is selected and becomes part of the sample, ignore it if it appears again in the table of random numbers.
- Stop when your sample size is obtained. (Sample size is discussed later in the chapter.)

Other methods of random selection may be used as long as they ensure that each subject has an equal chance of selection. Such methods include putting well-mixed names in a hat or shuffling name cards thoroughly and then selecting the required number from a deck.

Systematic Sampling   Systematic sampling involves drawing every N^{th} element from a population. If you wanted to do a survey of nurses who subscribe to the *American Journal of Nursing*, you could select a systematic sample of 1000. You start, as with the random sample, by closing your eyes and pointing to a number and then choosing every N^{th} number that follows. For example, if you start at number 11, you may decide to pick every tenth number (this is arbitrary). You then pick number 21, 31, 41, 51, and so on until all subjects are obtained. Systematic sampling results in a representative sample if the sampling frame doesn't have any built-in bias. For example, bias would result if the Journal's circulation lists were arranged in such a way that nurse subscribers were listed by state or year of beginning subscription. Instead of getting a sample representative of subscribers, you might be getting a sample that included only nurses in the Northeast or only nurses who had subscribed for 10 years or more. If you decide to do

Table 9-8   Listing of Random Numbers

09 18 82 00 97	32 82 53 95 27	04 22 08 63 04	83 38 98 73 74	64 27 85 80 44
90 04 58 54 97	51 98 15 06 54	94 93 88 19 97	91 87 07 61 50	68 47 66 46 59
73 18 95 02 07	47 67 72 62 69	62 29 06 44 64	27 12 46 70 18	41 36 18 27 60
75 76 87 64 90	20 97 18 17 49	90 42 91 22 72	95 37 50 58 71	93 82 34 31 78
54 01 64 40 56	66 28 13 10 03	00 68 22 73 98	20 71 45 32 95	07 70 61 78 13
08 35 86 99 10	78 54 24 27 85	13 66 15 88 73	04 61 89 75 53	31 22 30 84 20
28 30 60 32 64	81 33 31 05 91	40 51 00 78 93	32 60 46 04 75	94 11 90 18 40
53 84 08 62 33	81 59 41 36 28	51 21 59 02 90	28 46 66 87 95	77 76 22 07 91
91 75 75 37 41	61 61 36 22 69	50 26 39 02 12	55 78 17 65 14	83 48 34 70 55
89 41 59 26 94	00 39 75 83 91	12 60 71 76 46	48 94 97 23 06	94 54 13 74 08
77 51 30 38 20	86 83 42 99 01	68 41 48 27 74	51 90 81 39 80	72 89 35 55 07
19 50 23 71 74	69 97 92 02 88	55 21 02 97 73	74 28 77 52 51	65 34 46 74 15
21 81 85 93 13	93 27 88 17 57	05 68 67 31 56	07 08 28 50 46	31 85 33 84 52
51 47 46 64 99	68 10 72 36 21	94 04 99 13 45	42 83 60 91 91	08 00 74 54 49
99 55 96 83 31	62 53 52 41 70	69 77 71 28 30	74 81 97 81 42	43 86 07 28 34

systematic sampling, be sure to study the list carefully for potential systematic bias.

Stratified Random Sampling A *stratum* is a subpopulation and *strata* are two or more homogeneous subpopulations. Examples of strata of interest to nursing include patients who have certain diseases, patients who live in specified areas, or patients who require certain treatments. Major political polls use stratified random sampling, assessing different strata of the population. To use this method:

1. Select a population, and determine the relevant strata.
2. Sample a number of people in each stratum. The number in a sample should be the same as the proportion of the group in the total population. For example, if your population is patients with collagen diseases and your strata are patients with lupus, (3% of the population), patients with arthritis (95% of the population), and patients with scleroderma (2% of the population), you will use the same proportions in your sample—3% lupus patients, 95% arthritis patients, and 2% scleroderma patients.
3. After you decide on the strata and proportions, choose the subjects within each of the categories according to random sampling methods. Remember, randomly does not mean haphazardly.

When you decide to do a stratified random sample, think carefully about your population and the concept of relevancy. If you know your population composition and its relation to a specific characteristic, *and* if the factors are relevant based on logic and the literature review, stratify your sample. If you do not know your population composition or if the factors are not relevant (for example, the hair color of new mothers who elect rooming in on obstetric units), then do not stratify your sample.

Cluster Sampling *Cluster sampling* requires that the population be divided into groups, or clusters. If you are studying associate degree

nursing students, you may not have the time, money, or ability to get all the individuals' names, but:

1. You have a list of the associate degree schools in the area.
2. You randomly derive your sample from this list of clusters (schools).
3. You sample all students in each chosen cluster, or you sample only randomly selected students from each cluster.

You are randomly sampling both schools and subjects. Depending on your research problem you move in stages from the most complex to the most simple unit, which is why cluster sampling is also called multistage sampling.

Most large-scale surveys use cluster sampling, because simple or stratified random sampling involves too few subjects from too few places, resulting in much wasted time, money, and energy.

A Critique of Probability Sampling Probability sampling is based on probability theory, which focuses on the possibility of events' occurring by chance (Kerlinger 1973, Winer 1962). Probability sampling is less likely to result in a biased sample that is not representative of the population, because it insists that each element in the population has an equal chance of being selected. The ability to obtain representative samples makes probability sampling superior to nonprobability sampling. Ensuring a representative sample avoids bias, making it possible to generalize research results to the accessible population.

Sampling error can be estimated with probability sampling. Sampling error refers to the differences between sample values and population values. Some amount of sampling error is inevitable in any research study, but probability sampling does allow estimates of the degree of expected error. (For more about this see Cohen 1977 and Chapter 15.)

Probability sampling with small populations (for example, patients with liver transplants) may be efficient and effective. If the group is homogeneous, however, then sophisticated sampling is not necessary. In nursing, because we deal with human beings and thus many variables, it is unlikely that our population is ever homogeneous. Most people are different psychologically, culturally, or socioeconomically, bringing homogeneity into question.

In life, it is said, death and taxes are the only certainties. In sampling there is no certainty that a probability sample ensures everyone's participation. If a group is underrepresented or refuses to participate for whatever reasons, a biased sample may result.

Types of Nonprobability Sampling

Nonprobability sampling is nonrandom sampling of subjects. Therefore, there is less chance of obtaining a representative sample. Most nursing research involves nonprobability sampling.

Accidental, or convenience, sampling Accidental, or convenience, sampling allows the use of any available group of research subjects. For example, to study children in well-baby clinics, you might pick a public clinic because of its geographical proximity and because you can readily get access. These children are relevant subjects, and they are available. Because of a lack of randomization in sampling, however, they may not be typical of well babies but may be atypical in some unidentified ways. The investigator has no control over the sampling process—the sample, the sampling representativeness, or the possible biases.

Snowball sampling is a kind of accidental sampling. It involves subjects' suggesting other subjects to the researcher, so that the sampling process gains momentum, like a snowball rolling down a hill. A nurse was studying women prisoners with an in-depth interview technique. Because only certain women were willing to be involved, the researcher asked each prisoner after the interview to suggest one or two other prisoners who might be interested in participating.

This was a convenient and effective way of soliciting subjects. Of course, sampling bias is likely to be present, because women who agree to participate may be different from those who don't.

Snowball sampling is used if subjects are difficult to identify because they are hidden in the population (transsexuals, faith healers, women who have had abortions), but they may be part of an informal network. Brink and Wood (1983) use the term *network sampling* and say it is useful in finding "socially devalued urban populations such as addicts, alcoholics, child abusers, and criminals," because these people are usually hidden from outsiders (p. 143).

Purposive, or Judgment, Sampling In *purposive* sampling the researcher selects a particular group or groups based on certain criteria. In this subjective sampling method the researcher uses his or her judgment to decide who is representative of the population. Because objectivity is lacking, this method is not recommended except in certain circumstances. For example, if you wanted to test an instrument to measure stress in patients who have just been admitted to the hospital, you could use a purposive sample of patients from surgical units, CCU units, labor and delivery units, medical units, and outpatient units. A pretest with such heterogeneous groups might offer interesting information. Or if you wanted to validate an instrument measuring self-concept or locus of control, you might give it to normal adults, normal teenagers, depressed adults, and depressed teenagers. You would expect group differences to be evidenced in the test scores. If there were no group differences, you would question the validity of the instrument.

Expert sampling is a type of purposive sampling that involves choosing experts in a given area because of their access to the information of relevance to your study. The Delphi technique uses expert sampling. Several rounds of questionnaires focusing on a specific topic are sent to experts, with the aim of eliciting their opinions. After data analysis the questions are reformulated and sent out again. The aim is for fairly rapid group consensus. For example, a study at the University of Florida preceded planning for a master's degree in nursing administration. When curriculum planning began, the program director questioned hospital administrators and nursing administrators, using the Delphi technique.

A conscious bias that cannot be measured exists in purposive sampling. Therefore, you should only use it if there are no other sampling alternatives, and you must be very wary in interpreting the data.

Quota Sampling   Quota sampling is different from stratified sampling in two ways. Quota sampling is not random and may or may not sample proportions representative of the population. (Remember, in stratified sampling the proportions are representative.) In quota sampling the researcher makes a decision, based on judgment, about the best type of sample for the study. For example, if you are studying nurses' attitudes toward nurses who have problems with chemical abuse, you may want to get a representative quota of male and female nurses from different age groups and with different educational preparation.

The researcher decides what the strata are depending on the variables that might affect the dependent variable being investigated. The gender and age of nurses probably affects their attitudes toward nurses with chemical abuse problems (dependent variable). Their educational preparation might also be a meaningful stratum. Since 3% of nurses are male and 97% are female, similar percentages can be drawn for the study. Since W% of nurses are between the ages of 20 and 30, X% between 30 and 40, Y% between 40 and 50, and Z% over 50, the sample can reflect these same proportions.

If you study chemically dependent nurses' responses to different treatment programs, you may want to study equal numbers of male and female nurses, and an equal number of nurses from different age groups. In this case, the sample is not representative of or drawn proportionately from the population.

Using quota sampling you can sample *matched pairs*. This means you select your sample on predetermined important characteristics. For example, if you wonder how preoperative education affects cardiac bypass patients' behavior post-operatively compared to angioplasty patients, you might match the patients according to risk factors—age, weight, exercise, smoking.

Quota sampling is used when an investigator cannot select a random sample but aims for more control than is possible with accidental, or convenience, sampling. Subjects are selected if they fit the criteria for each stratum as set by the researcher. The aim is to reduce bias or sampling error.

A Critique of Nonprobability Sampling   In most nursing studies we settle for nonprobability sampling, because the population is too unknown to obtain a random sample or because the expense in time and money of a random sample is too great. Also, informed consent is vital in research, and this requirement decreases the possibility of a random sample. Instead, our subjects are willing, informed participants who have the freedom to withdraw from a study at any time.

Because nursing research studies regularly use nonprobability samples, we need to be knowledgeable about the strengths and limitations of each type and attempt to make the sample as representative as possible. Caution in generalizing findings beyond what is warranted in studies with nonprobability samples is important.

Sample Size

Of vital importance in every researcher's mind is "How many subjects do I need?" As is true of much of the research process, there are no hard and fast rules for sample size. Rather, you must consider the research purpose, the design, and the size of the population. Depending on circumstances, a large or small number of subjects may be appropriate. Actually, however, with the exception of case studies the larger the sample, the more valid and accurate the study, because a larger sample is more likely to be representative of the population. The following general guidelines may be helpful in determining sample size (n):

- If the population is homogeneous, you can use a smaller sample than if it is heterogeneous. On the one hand, a study examining the experiences of breast-feeding mothers will involve much variability, because mothers of all ages, of all socioeconomic groups, and of all ethnic groups breast-feed. A study of the health habits of eighth-grade girls in a private school on the other hand, will have less variability. The girls are approximately the same age and come from the same socioeconomic group, so a smaller sample will be more likely to yield "typical" subjects. The review of the literature and your nursing experience will help you estimate the population variability.

- If you use a research design that requires numerous treatment groups (experimental design), then you must determine the number of subjects needed for the smaller groups (called cells) and not just for the larger group heading. For example, if you study the use by chronically ill geriatric patients of Orem's self-care model, do not base decisions about sample size exclusively on the larger group of geriatric patients needed. Perhaps your design requires you to compare patients in a private hospital with patients in a Veterans Administration hospital or cardiac patients with cancer patients and kidney patients. Because of all the subgroups you will need more subjects than if you merely looked at a single group of chronically ill patients. You should decide the cell size for each subsample or treatment group and then add these together to get your total n. If the cell size is too small (often 10 or fewer), the treatment mean, a frequency calculation, is more likely to be skewed by one atypical number. A cell size of 20 or more generally

yields more accurate results and allows more options when it comes to statistical analyses.

- Survey designs frequently use many more subjects than observational or experimental designs, because telephoning or mailing questionnaires to a large number of people is feasible, whereas observing large numbers of people may not be. One must also plan ahead for the possibility of less than a 100% return rate and of subject attrition over time. However, in experimental research it is not feasible to do experiments with many human subjects. In nursing, because of all the variables we must control, getting a cell size of ten is often very difficult and, at times, impossible. Case studies and case histories require even fewer subjects, usually between one and ten.

- A thorough review of the literature will give you ideas about what size sample is typical for certain types of research questions and designs used in nursing research (see Table 9-9). However, be aware that in many studies the sample size is too small and, therefore, should be viewed with a critical eye.

- The statistical analyses you choose to use may have certain requirements regarding sample size. Be sure you know at the proposal stage of your research what statistical analyses you will use. If you leave this choice until later, your sample size may be too small, prohibiting you from conducting the planned statistical analysis.

- *Power analysis* is vitally important when you are making decisions about sample size. Power refers to the probability that an inferential statistical test (see Chapter 15) will reject the null hypothesis when it is false and allow you to declare that the research hypothesis is supported when, indeed, it should be.

Determining sample size is one way of increasing power; this is in part because a larger sample size decreases variance and increases the degrees of freedom for the test (see Chapter 15). Also, decreasing variance through increasing homogeneity of subjects or by increasing your controls aims to ensure an in-

Table 9-9   Sample Sizes Used in Selected Nursing Studies

Abstract	Design	Sample Size
1. Three groups of women were compared to determine their perceptions and their degree of participation in decision making, the type of anesthesia for delivery, and the presence of their husbands at the births. Forty women had vaginal deliveries, 39 had emergency cesareans, and 43 had planned cesareans. All the women were interviewed and completed self-administered questionnaires 2 to 4 days after delivery. The three groups had significantly different perceptions of the birth experience, with the emergency cesarean birth group having the most negative perception. Among women having cesareans, more positive perceptions were associated with regional anesthesia, presence of their husbands at delivery, and greater participation in decision making. Women in the cesarean groups were less likely to breast-feed, and those having planned cesareans were least likely to attend childbirth classes. Many of the women were unaware of the options available to them that could influence the birth experiences.	Ex post facto	122

SOURCE: M. Cranley et al, "Women's Perceptions of Vaginal and Cesarean Deliveries," *Nursing Research*, 1983, 32:10–15.

Abstract	Design	Sample Size
2. Thirty-seven married first-time fathers attending uncomplicated deliveries of normal infants were randomly assigned to two groups, holding or not holding at delivery. At 12 to 36 hours after birth, bonding-behavior frequencies were recorded during 10 minutes of father–infant interaction. Two observers measured the behaviors: verbal interaction, smiling, eye contact, fingertip and whole-hand touching. Analysis of the data by multivariate analysis of variance (MANOVA) and univariate analysis of variance (ANOVA) revealed no difference between the groups ($p = .05$). More bonding behaviors were noted with increased levels of education, male infants, breast-fed infants, and outlet-forcep or cesarean-section deliveries. Early contact did not appear to enhance bonding, although several other factors seemed to be related, indicating a need for further study on paternal bonding.	Experimental	37

SOURCE: L. Toney, "The Effects of Holding the Newborn at Delivery on Paternal Bonding," *Nursing Research*, 1983, 32:16–19.

Abstract	Design	Sample Size
3. The attitudes of women toward (1) a woman in menopause, (2) comparable male and nonmenopausal female stimulus figures, and (3) themselves were compared using a vignette approach. Vignettes depicting a middle-aged female and a middle-aged male were presented to 152 women between the ages of 18 and 55. The women were asked to rate the vignette subjects on a semantic differential. Approximately half of the women received a vignette of a woman who was identified as being menopausal, and half received the identical vignette without the menopausal condition. Participants then completed a semantic differential rating of themselves and the Tennessee Self Concept Scale (TSCS). There was no difference in the semantic differential ratings of the menopausal and the nonmenopausal vignette characters, nor in the male and the female characters. Although the participants ranked themselves higher than both the female and male characters, there was no difference in the ratings of the vignettes or the self by women with lower versus higher self-esteem.	Descriptive survey	152

SOURCE: A. Muhlenkamp et al, "Attitudes Toward Women in Menopause: A Vignette Approach," *Nursing Research*, 1983, 32:20–23.

continued

Table 9-9   *continued*

Abstract	Design	Sample Size
4. State anxiety, critical thinking ability, and judged duration were tested for coping relatedness and change over time in 85 women, aged 18 to 60, who were experiencing breast biopsy. Participants were tested after hospital admission but before diagnostic results were known. Six to eight weeks later, women whose results were benign were tested again—when an acute crisis is considered concluded. Findings revealed extremely high state anxiety levels prior to biopsy and compromised reasoning ability at a critical time when demands on cognitive functioning were high.	Quasi-experimental	85

SOURCE: D. Scott, "Anxiety, Critical Thinking and Information Processing During and After Breast Biopsy," *Nursing Research*, 1983, 32:24–28.

5. The study investigated the relationship between weight loss, locus of control, and social support. It was hypothesized that internals would be more successful in weight reduction than externals/powerful others or externals/chance; that participants with higher social-support scores would be more successful in weight reduction than participants with lower social-support scores; and that social support would contribute more to success in weight reduction in externals/powerful others than in internals or externals/chance. Subjects were 46 female employees of a large life insurance company who had participated in a nutrition and weight-control program. They were studied 6 months later to assess weight change, locus of control (specifically, using a multidimensional health locus of control scale and a modified weight locus of control scale), and social support (using an investigator-developed scale). Study findings did not support the hypotheses. Rather, a significant negative relationship was found between social support and weight reduction in the case of internals. Possible explanations for the findings were discussed, along with recommendations for practice and further research. For example, it was suggested that it may be most desirable for those attempting weight loss to be sufficiently internal that they believe they are capable of bringing their weight under control, yet sufficiently external that they are amenable to the advice of health professionals.	Ex post facto	46

SOURCE: S. Gierszewski, "The Relationship of Weight Loss, Locus of Control, and Social Support," *Nursing Research*, 1983, 32:43–47.

6. A 63-item questionnaire utilizing the modified Paternal–Fetal Attachment Scale (PFA) (Cranley), the Marital Relationship Scale (Wapner), and the Physical History Scale (Wapner) was tested on 100 expectant fathers who had wives in their third trimester of pregnancy. Scores on the PFA were positively correlated with the strength of the marital relationship as perceived by the expectant father during pregnancy. A positive but weak association was shown between paternal–fetal attachment and the incidence of physical symptoms resembling pregnancy in the expectant father. Further testing of the PFA and related variables is indicated.	Correlational survey	100

SOURCE: R. H. Weaver, "An Exploration of Paternal–Fetal Attachment Behavior," *Nursing Research*, 1983, 32:68–72.

7. The purpose of this study was to identify procedural components to be used in analogue studies of preparatory techniques for childbirth. The questions asked were (1) which of four laboratory pain stimuli (modified submaximum effort tourniquet technique, Forgione–Barber pain stimulator, cold water stimulus,	Correlational survey	40

continued

Table 9-9   *continued*

Abstract	Design	Sample Size
faradic shock) is most similar to the pain associated with the transition phase of labor? and (2) what is the patterning and duration of contractions and inter-contraction intervals in this phase? Forty primiparous women rated their contractions (within 48 hours following delivery) and rated the four laboratory stimuli (6 to 8 weeks postpartum) using the McGill Pain Questionnaire. Significant correlational relationships were found between each laboratory stimulus and contraction ratings. Uterine monitor records were scored to obtain contraction and intercontraction data: X number and duration of contractions, X duration of intercontraction intervals. The general patterning of these variables was relatively stable. In a subsequent laboratory trial using the above parameters, the Forgione–Barber pain stimulator was found to be the stimulus of choice. SOURCE: E. Geden et al, "Identifying Procedural Components for Analogue Research of Labor Pain," *Nursing Research*, 1983, 32:80–83.		
8. (Hypothetical) The purpose of this study is to determine if a 2g sodium diet results in a significant decrease in blood pressure in a newly diagnosed hypertensive patient. SOURCE: K. Holm, "Single Subject Research," *Nursing Research*, 1983, 32:253–255.	Experimental	I

crease of power. A third method to increase power is that of increasing the effect size. Increasing the effect size merely means that you, in any way possible, increase the intensity or frequency of your treatment in an experimental design. For example, if you were applying ice after heparin injections to decrease bruising, you might leave it on longer than the original five minutes to be sure of its effect. Perhaps ice will prevent bruising if it is left on for 15 minutes instead of five minutes. These three methods (1) increasing sample size, (2) decreasing variance, and (3) increasing effect size all serve to increase power.

Cohen (1977) writes authoritatively and extensively about power analysis, but a statistical consultant can be helpful in determining your required sample size with a power analysis. The computational procedures for conducting power analyses are, however, beyond the scope of either this chapter or Chapter 15 on statistics. Tables exist in many statistics books to estimate the probability of a Type 2 (beta) error (i.e., incorrectly labeling a difference as due to chance when it's actually a real difference) for commonly used statistical procedures. Such tables can be used to estimate the needed sample size before research begins. If you know in advance that the sample size is necessarily small—say 20 patients—and you need a larger sample to avoid Type 2 errors, you may choose to redesign or even abandon the project rather than doing research that, from a statistical point of view, is not worth doing.

The major focus in sampling should be on design. You should do everything possible to assure representativeness of the sample to the population; however, a large sample size cannot correct a poor design (Polit & Hungler 1983, p. 427).

Sampling From Special Population Groups

Special population groups present practical and ethical problems to researchers. Access to certain patient groups may be difficult or require extra effort by the researcher. According to Sexton (1983, pp. 378–380), some problems confronting researchers who study the chronically ill (COPD patients) include:

- identification of subjects and their reluctance to participate in studies—a problem of sufficient sample size
- implementation of certain designs (a panel study, longitudinal, experimental, or correlational) due to the exacerbations, remissions, and mortality of the illness—a problem of limited study designs
- consideration of the feasibility of the energy and the abilities required of the patient for each type of data collection—a problem of data collection

Nurses should not be reluctant to pursue research with chronically ill patients but must focus energy on working toward the best and most feasible approach, taking into account the typical problems these patients present.

Children, the mentally ill, the mentally retarded, and the elderly are also people who require special consideration by the nurse researcher. Although "informed consent" (see Chapter 3) aims to protect patient's rights, it sometimes is less than effective. Most informed consent procedures have three conditions:

- The individual subject must volunteer to participate.
- The individual must be mentally competent.
- The individual must be informed of the risks, benefits, discomforts and compensation.

Mitchell (1984) discusses the questions of when children are capable of informed consent, the difference between assent and informed consent, and parental permission versus consent. Nurses historically have been advocates of children and are now (because of new 1983 regulations from the Department of Health and Human Services) legally accountable for protecting children's rights.

Watson (1982) writes on informed consent of special subjects, including captive groups (i.e., prisoners), the acutely ill and dying patients, and the mentally ill and legally incompetent, including children. She raises the question of "What is voluntary consent and who can give it?" (p. 43) Can a subject who is impaired or vulnerable physically or psychologically really give informed consent? Hayter (1979, p. 125) says:

General agreement seems to exist on two points:

1. Persons who are unable to give their own informed consent should not be research subjects if other subjects can be used.

2. The less able a person is to protect himself, the more vigilant the investigator must be in protecting him.

Mann and Whall's (1984) research on informed consent and the deinstitutionalized patient suggests that extra time and additional written explanations about research are useful to this special group. Reminding patients of their right to avoid participation or stop participation at any time also may serve toward the goal of insuring informed consent.

On the other hand Robb (1983) cautions us to beware the "informed consent," and expresses her fear that in our willingness to comply with legal and ethical restrictions we may be "protecting" the elderly to death by avoiding using them as research subjects. She urges "creative solutions" to "the burdens of written consent." Informed consent issues are clearly related to practical considerations of obtaining an adequate sample.

Sampling and External Validity

Your research purpose and design affect how important representativeness, yielding external validity, is. Different types of research question require, to a greater or lesser degree, representative samples. If you are doing descriptive research, which aims to describe behaviors or attitudes of a group, representativeness is very important, because you are aiming for descriptive accuracy (external validity). If your sample is biased or not representative, your description will be inaccurate and invalid.

In methodological studies you will need to be concerned with all types of reliability and internal validity—content-, construct-, and/or criterion-based validity (see Chapter 11). In case studies or case histories, you may be more concerned with illustrating or generating theory, and the issue of representativeness is not critical. In contrast, representativeness and external validity in experimental studies are of great significance. Because obtaining representative samples in experimental nursing studies is often impossible, however, replication studies are useful in establishing external validity.

Sampling is a complex but essential stage in the research process. Some authors have devoted entire books to the various sampling procedures. For more information, review the References and Further Readings listed at the end of the chapter.

As you get started on a research project, constantly evaluate where you are and where you are going. Think of the consistency and the logic of the entire process. (Note the summary of steps in Box 9-6.) Your initial question leads to a relevant literature review, which results in a purpose. Within the purpose, whether you focus on a statement, a question, or a hypothesis, your vari-

---

Box 9-6   Steps in Getting Started

1. Write a research question based on your experience, observations, or literature.

2. Review the literature—nursing research literature, general nursing literature, research from other disciplines, methodological literature, popular literature, theoretical literature.

3. Network—interview resource people.

4. Refine your specific study question.

5. Write your purpose—as a statement, question or hypothesis—depending on the level of inquiry of your question.

6. For Level 2 and 3 studies, operationally define your variables.

7. Choose an appropriate research design.

8. Select a sample.

---

ables are clear and operationalized so they can be measured. Based on the purpose, you choose an appropriate design, which almost suggests a sample. After you ascertain the feasibility of obtaining subjects and carrying out your study, and you get approval from the Institutional Review Board (IRB), you are ready to collect and analyze data. Once you have reached this point conceptually, you are ready to put all your planning into action.

Summary of Key Ideas and Terms

- A *research question* can be derived from observations, experiences, or the literature.

- Classifying research questions into one of three levels of inquiry helps in the choice of a research purpose and design that are appropriate for your question.

- An extensive literature review provides contextual relevance for the research question, suggesting the correct level of inquiry.

✔ *Level 1 inquiry* is used for exploratory, descriptive studies in which there is little available literature on the research question.

✔ *Level 2 inquiry* looks for the relationship between variables. The literature suggests the relationship between variables but does not specify the nature of the relationship.

✔ *Level 3 inquiry* assumes a significant relationship between variables. A literature review reveals theory that predicts the nature of the relationship.

✔ A thorough literature review includes nursing research literature, theoretical literature, general and specialty nursing literature, methodological literature, research literature from other disciplines, and popular literature and covers the last five years.

✔ Writing a research question and doing a literature review are challenging and time-consuming tasks. Allowing time for intellectual exploration is useful. Such exploration involves networking with appropriate experts and thinking about the feasibility, significance, and researchability of the problem.

✔ The statement of the research purpose derives from the level of inquiry. The purpose of a Level 1 question is written as: "The purpose of this research is to explore and describe . . ." The purpose of a Level 2 question is written as: "The purpose of the study is to answer the question . . ." The purpose of a Level 3 study is written as: "The purpose of this study is to test the hypothesis . . ."

✔ A *theoretical framework* that predicts the nature of the relationship between variables is necessary for a Level 3 hypothesis-testing study.

✔ For a hypothesis to be testable, the variables must be able to be observed and measured. The *dependent variable* must be observed under at least two different conditions; variables, to be measured, require operational definitions.

✔ A hypothesis requires three components (Brink & Wood 1983): an *experimental group*, *the experimental result*, and a *comparison group*.

✔ Hypotheses can be simple or complex, directional or nondirectional, and stated as research or statistical hypotheses.

✔ In Level 1 studies (*exploratory*) all variables are assumed to be independent until research is done that indicates the nature of the variables. In Level 2 and 3 studies, independent and dependent variables need to be clearly identified.

✔ After the identification of the variables, operational definitions are written that specify how the variables will be measured.

✔ A good research design follows logically from the study's purpose. Historical and case study designs are appropriate for Level 1 studies. Survey designs, depending on the type, are used in Level 1 or 2 studies. Experimental and quasi-experimental designs and ex post facto designs are used with Level 3 studies. Methodological study designs are used to develop and validate an instrument.

✔ The *research purpose* should lead an investigator to appropriate subjects for the sample. The sampling process, whereby a researcher studies a subset of the population, is a feasible and logical way of making statements about a larger group based on a smaller group. To make such inferences, a sample should be as representative of the total population as possible.

✔ *Probability sampling*, the most rigorous sampling approach, requires that every element in the population have an equal (random) chance of being included in the study. With *nonprobability sampling* the results are representative of the sample only and cannot be generalized to a larger population.

✔ Most nursing studies use nonprobability sampling, because the population is too unknown to obtain a random sample or the expense of time and money of a random sample is too great.

✔ *Sample size* is very important and is dependent upon the research purpose, the design, and the size of the population. Generally, the larger the sample, the more valid and accurate the study.

References

Barnard K: The case study method: A research tool. *Am J Maternal Child Nurs* 1983; 8:327.

Begley S, Shapiro D: The death of the 'bubble boy.' *Newsweek* March 5, 1984:71.

Brink P, Wood M: *Basic Steps in Planning Nursing Research, from Question to Proposal.* Belmont, Calif.: Wadsworth, 1983.

Buhler-Wilkerson K: False dawn: The rise and decline of public health nursing in America, 1900–1930. Pages 89–106 in: *Nursing History, New Perspectives, New Possibilities.* Lagemann E (editor). New York: Teachers College, Columbia University, 1983.

Cohen J: *Statistical Power Analysis for the Behavioral Sciences.* New York: Academic Press, 1977.

Cranley M et al: Women's perceptions of vaginal and cesarean deliveries. *Nurs Res* 1983; 32:10–15.

Depp F et al: Predicting tenure decisions of psychiatric nursing assistants: Individual and work related factors. *Res Nurs Health* 1983; 2:53–59.

Geden E et al: Identifying procedural components for analogue research of labor pain. *Nurs Res* 1983; 32:80–83.

Gierszewski S: The relationship of weight loss, locus

of control and social support. *Nurs Res* 1983; 32:43–47.

Given C et al: Development of scales to measure beliefs of diabetic patients. *Res Nurs Health* 1983; 6:127–141.

Hallal J: The relationship of health beliefs, health locus of control, and self-concept to the practice of breast self-examination in adult women. *Nurs Res* 1982; 31:137–142.

Hathaway D, Geden, E: Energy expenditure during leg exercise programs. *Nurs Res* 1983; 32:147–150.

Hayter J: Issues related to human subjects in *Issues in Nursing Research*. Downs F, Fleming J (editors). New York: Appleton-Century-Crofts, 1979.

Hodgeman E: Closing the gap between research and practice; changing the answers to the "who," the "where," and the "how" of nursing research. *Int J Nurs Studies* 1979; 16:105–110.

Holm K: Single subject research. *Nurs Res* 1983; 32:253–255.

Hurley PM: Communication variables and voice analysis of marital conflict stress. *Nurs Res* 1983; 32:164–169.

Kerlinger F: *Foundations of Behavioral Research*. New York: Holt, Rinehart & Winston, 1973.

Krouse H, Krouse J: Cancer crises: The critical elements of adjustment. *Nurs Res* 1982; 31:96–101.

Lewis FM: Personal control and quality of life in late-stage cancer patients. *Nurs Res* 1982; 2:113–118.

Lim-Levy F: The effect of oxygen inhalation on oral temperatures. *Nurs Res* 1982; 31:150–152.

Mann L, Whall A: Informed consent and the de-institutionalized patient. *J Psychosoc Nurs* 1984; 22:22–27.

Marcy S et al: Contraceptive use by adolescent females in relation to knowledge, and to time and method of contraceptive counseling. *Res Nurs Health* 1983; 6:175–182.

May K: Three phases of father involvement in pregnancy. *Nurs Res* 1982; 31:337–342.

Meier P, Pugh E: *The Case Study: A Viable Approach to Clinical Research*, Unpublished paper, 1983.

Mitchell K, Protecting children's rights during research. *Ped Nurs* January/February 1984; 9–10.

Muhlenkamp A et al: Attitudes toward women in menopause: A vignette approach. *Nurs Res* 1983; 32:20–23.

Notter L: The case for nursing research. *Nurs Outlook* 1975; 23:760–763.

Orem D: *Nursing: Concepts of Practice*. New York: McGraw-Hill, 1980.

Owens J, Hutelmyer C: The effect of preoperative intervention on delirium in cardiac surgical patients. *Nurs Res* 1982; 31:60–62.

Parsons C, Ver Beek D: Sleep–awake patterns following cerebral concussion. *Nurs Res* 1982; 31:260–264.

Polit D, Hungler B: *Nursing Research*. Philadelphia: Lippincott, 1983.

Robb S: Beware the "informed consent." (Editorial.) *Nurs Res* 1983; 32:132.

Scott D: Anxiety, critical thinking and information processing during and after breast biopsy. *Nurs Res* 1983; 32:24–28.

Sexton D: Some methodological issues in chronic illness research, *Nurs Res* 1983; 32:378–380.

Toney L: The effects of holding the newborn at delivery on paternal bonding. *Nurs Res* 1983; 32:16–19.

Watson A: Informed consent of special subjects. *Nurs Res* 1982; 31:43–47.

Weaver RH: An exploration of paternal–fetal attachment behavior. *Nurs Res* 1983; 32:68–72.

Williamson M: Reducing post-catheterization bladder dysfunction by reconditioning. *Nurs Res* 1982; 31:28–30.

Wilson H, Kneisl C: *Psychiatric Nursing*, 2nd ed. Menlo Park, Calif.: Addison-Wesley, 1983.

Winer BJ: *Statistical Principles in Experimental Design*. New York: McGraw-Hill, 1962.

Further Readings

Arkin H, Colton R: *Tables for Statisticians*. New York: Barnes & Nobles, 1950.

Campbell DT, Stanley JC: *Experimental and Quasi-experimental Design for Research*. Chicago: Rand McNally, 1963.

Drew C: *Introduction to Designing and Conducting Research*. St. Louis: CV Mosby, 1980.

Ledman S: *Applied Sampling*. New York: Academic Press, 1976.

Marks R: *Designing a Research Project: The Basis of Biomedical Research Methodology*. Belmont, Calif.: Lifetime Learning Publications, 1982.

Smith M, Naftel E: Meta-analysis: A perspective for research synthesis. *Image* 1984; 16:9–13.

Chapter 10

Relating Your Study to a Theoretical Context

by Sally Hutchinson RN, PhD

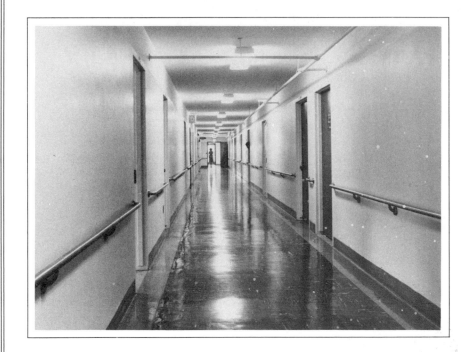

One of the goals of research is to extend the scope of nursing knowledge. To accomplish this successfully, a study is placed in a theoretical context or designed to develop a theoretical context.

Chapter Outline

Chapter Objectives

After reading this chapter, the student should be able to:

- Explain the terms *theory, concept, conceptual framework, construct, proposition,* and *model*
- Differentiate between conceptual and theoretical frameworks on at least four points
- Interpret Kaplan's empirical-theoretical framework and its relevance for nursing theory development
- Explain the purpose of a conceptual map
- Discuss various types of theory
- Describe four purposes of theory in a discipline
- Analyze the relationship of theory and research
- Describe the meaning of paradigmatic, preparadigmatic, and paradigm-transcending research; and discuss where nursing as a science fits into this typology
- Discuss the four questions raised in recent literature concerning nursing theories
- Define *metatheory*
- Analyze and evaluate nursing theories by applying the basic questions in meta-theory
- Discuss the difference between internal and external criticism of a theory
- List and interpret the ten criteria for theory evaluation
- List the four concepts that customarily serve as a focus for a nursing theory
- Understand the intellectual contributions of 11 historically important nurse theorists
- Discuss the use of conceptual models in nursing practice and nursing research
- List some relevant questions to ask about theoretical models for nursing

In This Chapter . . .

The words *theory, concept, construct, theoretical framework*, and *nursing model* have become common in contemporary nursing literature. This chapter aims to make these terms, which frequently evoke anxiety, confusion, and dismay, understandable, palatable, and relevant to the nursing student and practicing nurse who is interested in research.

Theories play a big role in our conceptions of events and people in our everyday life. If you work in a hospital or health care agency you are probably familiar with systems theory. Understanding why a private psychiatric hospital did not survive, for example, was made possible in part through a systems analysis. This process involved analyzing the subsystems of organizational structure, technology, economics, and symbolic systems (Hutchinson 1984). Perhaps you are attempting to analyze why a nurse colleague appears to have a fear of success. Psychoanalytic theory offers a possible explanation, as does feminist theory, if your colleague is a female. Shopping at the grocery store and being forced to pay higher prices for certain items may stimulate reflections on the economic theory of supply and demand. If you have ever cared for

young children, the developmental theories of Piaget (1958) or Erickson (1963) can be helpful in understanding their behaviors at various ages. In a patient care situation the theory of gravity helps us understand why patients with dependent edema due to venous insufficiency are placed in various positions.

Theories from other disciplines, such as those mentioned above, often provide the framework for nursing research. One goal of research is to extend the scope of our knowledge. To do this successfully, a research study must be placed within a theoretical context or be designed to develop one. When a study is placed within a theoretical context, the theory guides the research process from the research question, through the design, to a discussion of the results. This chapter discusses the use of theories from other disciplines and also emerging nursing theories in the research process. You may wonder how a nursing theory differs from any other theory. How do you know a good theory from a poor one? Where do theories come from? And what is a theory anyway? These questions constitute the focus of this chapter, and examples drawn from nursing research serve as illustrations.

Vocabulary of Theory

As you read about theories and their relationship to nursing research, you will immediately become aware of the frequent use of some new and esoteric language. An understanding of this vocabulary is essential for you to be able to appreciate and apply the ideas in your reading and in your practice and research.

Theory

What is a theory? The word *theory* comes from the Greek *theoria*, which means vision. Most people expect theories to be fact, but they really are perspectives on truth or reality. Theories are viewpoints or ways of perceiving. Kerlinger

(1973) gives us a more formal definition of *theory*: "A theory is a set of interrelated constructs (concepts), definitions, and propositions that present a systematic view of phenomena by specifying relations among variables, with the purpose of explaining and predicting the phenomena" (p. 9). Henkel points out that "theories refer to a hypothetical universe—hypothetical in the sense that it encompasses all past, present, and future cases to which the theory applies, wherever they may occur" (1976, p. 84). Examples of theories you have probably heard about and perhaps even used in your practice are psychoanalytic theory, the theory of relativity, the theory of evolution, the theory of gravity, learning theory, systems theory, and the theory of homeostasis.

Concept

Fawcett (1978a) describes *concepts* as the building blocks of theories. Concepts may be concrete (patient, blood loss, temperature elevation) or abstract (wellness, grief, stress) and, therefore, must be clearly defined so researchers understand their real meaning and can attempt to measure them. Concepts should be defined in terms of their relationship to other concepts, and this is called a *constitutive* definition. A concept's *operational* definition links that concept to the real world so it can be observed, controlled, and measured (Fawcett, p. 50) through the research process.

Conceptual Framework or Model   A *conceptual framework*, or *conceptual model*, which you will read about in the literature on nursing theory and in many research studies, refers to concepts that structure or offer a framework of propositions for conducting research. Nurse scientists disagree about whether nursing has true theories or just conceptual frameworks at its present stage of scientific development. Distinctions between the two are summarized in Table 10-1.

Fawcett points out that whereas there is a difference between conceptual and theoretical models, *theoretical model* and *theory* are frequently used interchangeably. In fact, a *theoretical model* "refers to a group of interrelated theories which provide rationale for the hypotheses, policies and curricula of a science, whereas a theory encompasses fewer phenomena" (1978b, p. 19). Later on in this chapter we will look at some criteria for the evaluation and analysis of theories.

Construct   When you read about concepts and theories, you may also read about *constructs*. Constructs are a group of concepts that are directly or indirectly observable (Jacox 1974, p. 6). They are derived from a combination of academic and clinical knowledge and contribute theoretical meaning and scope to a theory (Glaser & Strauss 1967, p. 70). Familiar examples of constructs are *society*, *socioeconomic status*, and *self-concept*. *Theoretical terms*, which are terms specific to a given theory, are not observable. Examples of theoretical terms are *superego* and *Oedipal complex*, from psychoanalytic theory (Jacox 1974, p. 6). *Creating meaning*, from a theory about how nurses survive the horror of some of their work (Hutchinson 1984), and *limiting intrusion*, from a theory about the social processes in a nontraditional treatment setting for psychiatric patients (Wilson 1982), are examples of theoretical terms discovered by nurses in their qualitative research.

Proposition

Theories require *propositions*, and propositions describe the relationship of two or more concepts. As you can see from the definitions, theory development begins with the identification and description of concepts and constructs and proceeds to formulate propositions that describe the nature of the relationships between these concepts. Nursing studies on empathy (Forsyth 1980), privacy (Rawnsley 1980), restlessness

Table 10-1   Differences Between Conceptual and Theoretical Models

Conceptual Models	Theoretical Models
1. They are pretheoretic bases from which substantive theories may be derived	1. They propose frameworks derived from theories
2. They are highly abstract	2. They are less abstract than conceptual models
3. Concepts are related and multidimensional	3. Concepts are narrowly bounded, specific, and explicitly interrelated
4. They provide a perspective for a science	4. They postulate relationships. They are descriptive, explanatory, or predictive (Reilly 1975). In applied science they are prescriptive
5. They are derived from unsystematic empirical observations and intuition	5. They are constructed from available theories and findings of empirical research (Reilly 1975)
6. They are developed through the process of induction	6. They are developed through the processes of induction and deduction
7. They must be evaluated on logical grounds and cannot be empirically tested	7. They permit empirical tests (Torgerson 1958)

SOURCE: Adapted from J. Fawcett, "The 'What' of Theory Development," in *Theory Development: What? Why? How?*, New York: National League for Nursing, 1978, pp. 18–19.

(Norris 1975), and humor (Hutchinson 1976) offer a beginning look at these concepts and their relevance to nursing. Conceptual analysis has as its goal the examination of parts, the operations of, and the interrelated whole of a thing (Chinn & Jacobs 1975). Constitutive and operational definitions are derived from this knowledge. Before nursing can claim to have its own unique theories, it first must have concepts, constructs, and propositions. Figure 10-1 demonstrates that theory building starts with a few concepts, which may be conceptualized into constructs. Concepts and constructs are used to generate propositions, which form the basis for the theory. Clearly nursing research, which has the purpose of conceptual analysis, is very much needed to generate a body of scientific knowledge.

Theories, concepts, constructs, and propositions aim to describe pieces of reality. Most scientists believe that there is a reality "out there" and that it is worthwhile to obtain knowledge about it (see Chapter 1). Theories and their com-

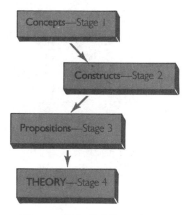

Figure 10-1 Building a theory.

ponent parts refer to, explain, describe, and predict reality in more or less concrete or abstract ways. Kaplan (1964) describes an empirical–theoretical continuum that allows us to view the relationship between what is observed empirically and what is described theoretically (see Figure 10-2).

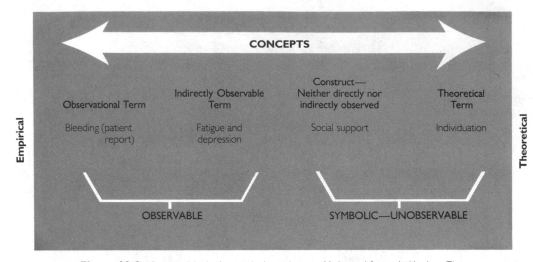

Figure 10-2 An empirical–theoretical continuum. (Adapted from A. Kaplan, *The Conduct of Inquiry*, San Francisco: Chandler, 1964, pp. 57–60. Reprinted with permission.)

Concepts may vary from the empirical, that is, observable (*blood loss*) to the theoretical, that is, abstract (*grief*); constructs tend to be more symbolic (*social loss*); and theoretical terms are generally derived from specific theories (*ego, id, superego, individuation, reinforcement*). Recognition of this continuum from the empirical to theoretical should help when you read theories and attempt to understand how they are linked up with observable reality; or, if you are generating a theory in your own research (see Chapter 14), you need to be aware of where your terms are located on the continuum as you aim for a fit between the empirical and theoretical worlds.

Model

Model is another term you will be confronted with in your education and practice. There are curricular models, administrative models, teaching models, and practice models. Bush (1979) writes, "A model represents some aspect of reality, concrete or abstract, by means of a likeness which may be structural, pictorial, diagrammatic or mathematical" (p. 16). A model, unlike a theory, does not focus on the relationships among phenomena but rather on their structure or function. A model is essentially an analogy, a symbolic representation of an idea. You will probably remember the model of the heart or the eye that you used in anatomy class. The structure of the organs was accurate and complete, but the model did not tell you about how or why the parts were interrelated.

Perhaps in your psychiatric nursing experience you have read Hildegard Peplau's *Interpersonal Relations in Nursing* (1952) and learned how to interact with patients based on her model. Fitzpatrick and her associates (1982), in their book *Nursing Models and Their Psychiatric Mental Health Applications*, examine a number of therapy models (individual, family, crisis) and discuss their relationship to selected nursing models (Rogers, King, Orem, Roy). All of these models essentially offer a system for understanding and analyzing phenomena.

Nurses borrow models from other fields, as they do with theories, if these can explain nursing phenomena. For example, one nursing student analyzed nurse–physician relationships by using a model of exchange from economic theory. Rhythm models, from many disciplines, are useful in examining healthy and unhealthy human functioning such as menstrual and sleep cycles and, as such, have implications for nursing (Floyd 1982). Because these borrowed models often don't fit nursing phenomena exactly, nurse scientists work on adapting them to nursing's perspective, using what works and altering or discarding what doesn't.

Models and Theories   You may now wonder about the relationship between models and theories. Bush (1979) writes elaborately on the subject. She identifies three types of relationship between models and theories:

1. Models may be constructed for theories. For example, Figure 10-3 demonstrates an example of the Orem self-care model. This visual, symbolic model essentially simplifies Orem's theory, making it visible in the same way a model of the eye demonstrates its structure.
2. Models may serve to stimulate theoretical explanations. For example, a biochemical model of how certain cancer cells are believed to behave offers scientists a perspective that encourages theoretical thinking. A proposed nursing model can function in the same way.
3. Mathematical models exist at a higher level of abstraction, are based on theory, yet are functional in suggesting theories in any discipline. A typical mathematical model (Estes 1963) is shown below:

$$gn = \left(1 - \frac{1}{N}\right)(1 - C)n$$

These models transcend the subject matter by proposing a more or less universal structure. Nursing does not yet have these models.

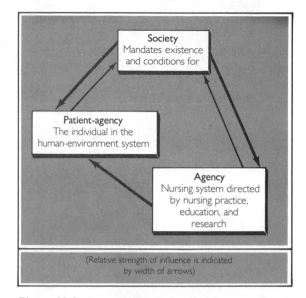

Figure 10-3 A model of Orem's self-care theory. (Based on J. Fitzpatrick et al., *Nursing Models and Their Psychiatric Mental Health Applications*, Bowie, Md.: Robert J. Brady Co., 1982, p. 59. Reprinted with permission.)

Models and Research   The process of research, according to Bush (1979), can be conceptualized by a model. Chinn and Jacobs (1978) offer a model of the scope of the research process for nursing. They view the research process as having four steps:

1. evaluation and analysis of concepts
2. formulation and testing of relational statements
3. theory construction
4. practical application of theory

You can relate this model in part to the levels of research questions discussed in Chapter 9. The first step in developing theory is to explore and describe the relevant variables or concepts in nursing practice. The second step is to test which variables are related to each other and to what degree. Once the variables and the nature of the relationships have been identified, propositions

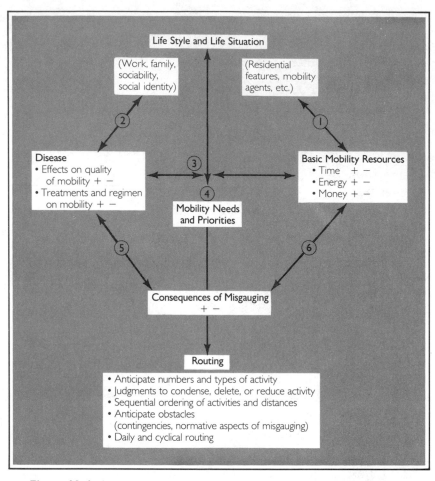

Figure 10-4 A conceptual map: How elderly, indigent patients with emphysema get around. (Adapted from S. Fageraugh, "Getting Around with Emphysema," *American Journal of Nursing*, January 1973, pp. 94–99. Reprinted with permission.)

can be written, and the interrelated system of propositions forms the structure of a theory. Once a theory is proposed, it must be tested and, if necessary, modified until it is useful for nursing. Chinn and Jacobs's model demonstrates the unity that the research–theory relationship should have. You can see by looking at their model how different types and levels of research are all necessary to contribute to nursing knowledge. This supports the idea of pluralism of nursing research.

When you are doing research, you can conceptualize your thoughts by building a model (dia-grammatically, physically, mathematically, or symbolically, depending on what you are studying). Such models simplify and clarify theory (Step 1 above) or stimulate theoretical explanations (Step 2 above).

Artinian's (1982) article "Conceptual Mapping" deals with the value of such maps (which are theoretical models) for understanding the relationship among variables in a study. In experimental and correlational studies, mapping or model making helps in conceptualization of the research problem. If you are doing a qualitative research study with the aim of theory generation (see Chapter 14), mapping helps you see your theory, and this visualization of the interrelationships of the variables is surprisingly helpful in encouraging further conceptualization. Figure 10-4 is an example of a conceptual map. This map illustrates how elderly indigents with emphysema get around.

Conceptual maps can be useful to you at all stages of the research process, from your proposal to the final writing of your report of findings. The conceptualization required for map making results in a logical and organized model, accurately depicting your research.

Types of Theory

The process of theory building occurs in the mind of the researcher, who has more or less interaction with the empirical world. The degree of involvement with the "real" world has an influence on the type of theory that is proposed. Theories can be divided into three types, all of which are described by sociologists. They are *grand* theories, *middle-range* theories, and *abstracted empiricism* (see Figure 10-5).

Grand Theories

Grand theories (Mills 1959) attempt to explain almost everything about a subject. They are composed of numerous global concepts that often are poorly defined and have ambiguous and unclear relationships. Constructs and propositions are nonexistent or are equally vague and appear to have little basis in the practical world. Models of such theories are either impossible or are incomprehensible. Because these theories are not grounded in empirical data, they are usually not useful as guides for nursing practice. Mills accuses them of proposing "irrelevant . . . monolithic concepts" (p. 45).

Nurse theorists who write theories *of* nursing that attempt to look at the relationship between the four accepted variables *humanity*, *society*, *health*, and *nursing* (Yura & Torres 1975) have been accused of wasting time and effort. Such grand theories are often derived from thinking in isolation from reality and from intuitive leaps that ultimately tell us more about the theorists than the world they are attempting to describe. Concepts in grand theories can be used to give a researcher a way to think about data. Blalock (1970) calls these *"sensitizing concepts."* For ex-

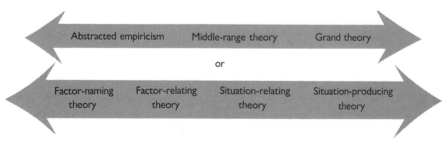

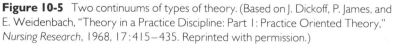

Figure 10-5 Two continuums of types of theory. (Based on J. Dickoff, P. James, and E. Weidenbach, "Theory in a Practice Discipline: Part 1: Practice Oriented Theory," *Nursing Research*, 1968, 17:415–435. Reprinted with permission.)

ample, in an exploratory study of a neonatal intensive care unit (NICU) (Hutchinson 1984), the sensitizing concept of *culture* from anthropology was used. The concept *culture* gave the researcher a beginning way to view a new, overstimulating, and confusing environment. Sensitizing concepts help in the initial organization of data.

Middle-Range Theories

Merton (1968), a sociologist, describes *middle-range theories* as those that look at a piece of reality and identify a few key variables. Propositions are clear, and hypotheses can be derived to test the theory. Substantive theories (theories about a substantive or empirical area—for example, the social processes in the emergency room, the functions of self-help groups, the patient/staff interactive patterns in a psychiatric hospital) are middle-range theories. In order to develop middle-range theories, the researcher is very close to the empirical world, often using the methods of field research—participant observation and interviewing (see Chapter 13). The scope of the problem is limited, which encourages an in-depth exploration and analysis of a selected topic. Examples of middle-range theories include Glaser and Strauss' classic studies *Awareness of Dying* (1965) and *Time for Dying* (1968), Wilson's study on *Deinstitutionalized Residential Care of the Mentally Disordered: The Soteria House Approach* (1982), and Hutchinson's study entitled *Survival Practices of Rescue Workers: Hidden Dimensions of Watchful Readiness* (1983). Middle-range theories, more so than grand theories, fit the empirical world from which they are derived and, as such, permit suggestions for nursing practice.

Middle-range theories are often developed by inductive methods (see Chapter 14) such as grounded theory or ethnographic methods and require that the researcher be theoretically sensitive to the data. The researcher conceptualizes empirical data. Honigman (1976) makes it clear that data are

. . . not reflections of facts or relationships, existing independently of the observer. In the process of knowing, external facts are sensorily perceived and immediately transferred into conceptualized experience, the observer being an active factor in the creation of knowledge, not a passive recipient or register [p. 245].

Abstracted Empiricism

Abstracted empiricism (Mills 1959) is on the far left of the continuum, revealing its concrete and nearsighted focus on only empirical phenomena. Abstracted empiricism implies that the empiricism or facts are in isolation from any theory. For example, nurses go about their practice without theory to guide them, functioning instead on the basis of facts or beliefs. In some hospitals nurses use ice before giving heparin injections because they believe ice should decrease bruising because it causes vasoconstriction. In other hospitals nurses don't use ice, either because they have never thought to use it or perhaps because they believe that vasoconstriction prevents the absorbtion of heparin, thereby encouraging bruising. These nurses are basing their care on authority or tradition rather than on theoretical protocols, which ideally guide practice. Jacox (1974) points out that the underlying assumption of the abstracted empiricist approach to theory development is that the accumulation of many pieces of data will ultimately and clearly suggest relationships among the data. She writes: "This is analogous to a collection of bricklayers, each making a brick in isolation from other bricklayers, and with no blueprint to follow. They throw these bricks together into a large pile, confident that, somehow, a house will emerge" (p. 11).

It is to prevent isolated fact collecting that some research faculty members at colleges of nursing are insisting that research be directly linked to either nursing theory or theory from other disciplines. If the state of knowledge or a particular study question make this impossible, then it behooves a researcher (student, faculty member, or practicing nurse) to do Level 1 studies (see Chapter 9) that aim at descriptions of subjects relevant to nursing. Only in this way can nurses formulate the theoretical base necessary to direct practice decisions. Other nurse scientists advocate the idea of groups of nurses working on research problems from different perspectives, and with different methods, so as to expand the knowledge base; or a nursing career can be built around a narrow focus, which over time yields depth. Anderson's work from 1975 to 1983 with sucking and newborns is an example of this in-depth approach. Specialty groups (cardiac care nurses, psychiatric nurses) in some areas can collaborate and specify specialty-linked research priorities that, when linked with theory, combat abstracted empiricism.

Dickoff, James, and Weidenbach, two philosophers and a nurse scientist, present another typology for theories. Their typology is similar to that of Diers (1979), described in Chapter 6 (see Figure 10-6).

1. *Factor-isolating theories* (also called factor-naming theories). These theories involve the identification and classification of concepts or variables relevant to nursing. Naming, according to Dickoff and his colleagues (1968a), "is the verbal counterpart of creating or inventing conceptual unities" (p. 421). The authors emphasize the importance of this early theory development by pointing out that all disciplines must have terms that are usable and known to the participants. Without such words there is no common language or knowledge base.

2. *Factor-relating theories* (situation-depicting theories). Once factors are identified and named, they must be related. Situations involving several variables are described or depicted, which increases general understanding.

3. *Situation-relating theories* (predictive theories). Predictive theory developmentally must follow descriptive theory and allow the nurse to predict that if *A* happens, *B* will happen. The two situations of *A* and *B* are causally related. Promoting or inhibiting theories attempt to conceptualize the relationships between *A* and *B* so as to be able to suggest what factors promote *A*'s production of *B*, what factors inhibit *A*'s production of *B*, what the related variables of *A* producing *B* are, and what the conditions that influence *A* producing *B* are. Promoting and inhibiting theories are prerequisites for the prescriptive theories.

4. *Situation-producing theories.* Prescriptive theory accepts as given the importance of *A* in producing *B* and predicts how to get *A* to produce *B* faster or how to facilitate *A*. If using the symbols *A* and *B* is confusing, substitute a nursing intervention (preoperative patient education) for *A* and a patient response (having less anxiety) for *B*, and re-read the preceding third and fourth levels of theories. Dickoff and his associates (1968a, p. 422) emphasize three points about prescriptive theories:

- The prescription is a command.
- This directive commands action toward a specified end.
- The command is directed to some specified agent.

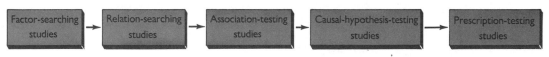

Figure 10-6 Diers's continuum of nursing studies. (Based on D. Diers, *Research in Nursing Practice*, Philadelphia: Lippincott, 1979. Reprinted with permission.)

The Purpose of Theories

Why does nursing need theories? Ellis (1968) suggests four purposes that theories serve:

1. Theories allow us to distinguish fact from pseudofact. *Facts* are derived from multiple congruent and similar observations of the same phenomena over time. Theories help us determine what is "true" and what isn't true.

2. Because nursing is holistic, it needs to integrate facts from many fields—biology, physiology, psychology, sociology—and make them useful for nursing. Theories will help in this process of synthesis.

3. Theoretical knowledge gives direction to practice, and theory should be tested in practice. If theories are ineffective, they must be modified or discarded and new theories conceptualized.

4. Theory is useful as a framework for storing knowledge available in the literature. In this case the isolated facts in the literature can be put together in a cohesive fashion when they are related to a theory. The theory serves as a guide for retrieval and use of information.

Kaplan (1964), in his classic book *The Conduct of Inquiry*, makes another very important point:

Theories are not just means to other ends, and certainly not just to ends outside the scientific enterprise, but they may also serve as ends in themselves—to provide understanding, which may be prized for its own sake [p. 310].

Fawcett (1978a) makes a strong point for the need to relate research to theory when she says that to do research or to develop theory in isolation from each other is to take an "excursion into the trivial" (p. 49). She views research and theory as a *double helix*, as two intertwining parts that are inextricably linked to each other (see Figure 10-7):

Theory is one helix, spiralling from the conception of an idea through modifications and extensions to eventual confirmation or refutation. Research is the second helix, spiralling from identification of research questions through data collection and analysis to interpretation of findings and recommendations for further study. The core of the double helix is the pairing of theory development with the research process. In the core, theory directs research and research findings shape the development of theory [p. 50].

Nursing has been criticized for:

- not having a theoretical base for its practice
- producing many pieces of isolated research that do not have an integrating theoretical framework and that, when completed, are not placed in any theoretical context
- not encouraging students to begin to develop

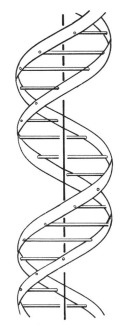

Figure 10-7   The double helix structure of DNA.

theories at the descriptive level but, rather, encouraging premature experimental research

The major point of all this criticism is that Fawcett's double helix of theory and research is not yet fully realized in nursing science. Let's look at a historical perspective of nursing research in an attempt to more fully understand these problems.

In Search of Paradigms

Using Thomas Kuhn's (1970) typologies, nursing can be said to be in a preparadigmatic state. This means that nursing, because it is a developing science, simply does not have sufficient consensus about its dominant *paradigms* (models or theories) to guide research. Paradigms, which do exist in the natural sciences and, to some degree, in the social sciences, supply a foundation for much research. Paradigms specify the types of research question to be asked and the appropriate methods for answering them. Paradigms include methods and laws, and they offer a perspective that guides research and forms the basis for a discipline's tradition. For example, anthropologists are known for using the concepts *culture, symbolic systems, kinship,* and *community* as frameworks for research. They are also known for "doing ethnographies"—descriptive studies, generally of other cultures—using the method of fieldwork with participant observation and interview (see Chapter 13). Past and present paradigms in the natural sciences include thermodynamics, particle physics, and relativity. Two nurse researchers, Donaldson and Crowley (1978), make the point that paradigms provide both the *substantive* structure (content) and *syntactical* structure (methods) of a discipline.

Researchers who work within the more established disciplines of the natural or physical sciences and social sciences learn the acceptable theoretical frameworks and methods during their education. They are inevitably taught by mentors who frequently have students participating in their research in an apprenticeship model. Students do not question the existing paradigms; to do so is heretical and is to desert the discipline. Students and scholars in the field aim to contribute to the existing body of knowledge by testing the acceptable theories. As Meleis, Wilson, and Chater (1980) write, they "solve meaningful puzzles" (p. 119).

Unlike those in the more mature disciplines, nurses have no acceptable paradigms to take for granted. Nursing is in an emerging state and, as such, is described as preparadigmatic. When the other disciplines such as psychology and sociology were developing, they, too, were attempting to establish some foundations and theories to guide their research and to establish a scientific tradition. During a discipline's emergence, researchers typically grasp unsystematically at any piece of knowledge or any method that appears even remotely useful. All facts seem equally relevant, because there are no criteria to aid in discriminating the useful from the nonuseful. Hardy (1978b) points out that this preparadigmatic phase is often frustrating and confusing to all members of the discipline, giving rise to heated arguments about the value of particular theories and research methods. Another problem that nursing has experienced as a result of being in the preparadigmatic phase of its evolution is premature rigor, the tendency toward tunnel vision that focuses on minute and sometimes trivial rules of research methods. With premature rigor we limit our options and do not foster the spirit of inquiry that is so vital to an emerging discipline. On the positive side, most nursing leaders accept research pluralism, which means the testing of a variety of theories from other disciplines and the use of multiple methods. Such pluralism permits the refinement and testing of multiple paradigms that are contenders for paradigms specific to nursing. Research pluralism is highly appropriate for this early phase in nursing's scientific and intellectual history.

Paradigm-transcending research, which Kuhn proposes as the basis for scientific revolutions, has the goal of discovering new theories and methods. And these new theories, or paradigms, will subsequently guide further inquiry. Meleis, Wilson, and Chater (1980) offer the discovery of the oxygen theory of combustion as an example of paradigm-transcending research. In this discovery the paradigm of pneumatic chemistry was significantly altered. Examples of paradigm-transcending research in nursing include studies by Hutchinson (1983), Stern (1982), and Wilson (1982). Nursing needs more paradigm-transcending studies that aim to develop theories that explain and predict empirical phenomena relevant to the discipline. The counterpart to the development of theories is the testing of existing theories (remember the double helix). Nursing is progressing in the testing of hypotheses derived from existing nursing theories that will expand the scope of nursing knowledge. For example, see Gill and Atwood's (1981) study that uses Martha Rogers's theory.

Whither Nursing Theories?

Let's now examine some issues surrounding the development of nursing theories. We have established that the discipline of nursing needs theories, but of what type, and for what purpose? Questions raised in the recent literature include:

1. Is nursing research basic or applied (Crawford, Dufault, & Rudy 1979; Donaldson & Crowley 1978)?

2. Is nursing theory borrowed or unique (Donaldson & Crowley 1978)?

3. Should we have grand theories of nursing or practice theories (Beckstrand 1978, 1980; Collins & Fielder 1981; Crawford, Dufault, & Rudy 1979; Wald & Leonard 1964)?

4. What paths to knowledge and development exist (Crawford, Dufault, & Rudy 1979)?

These issues were the dominant focus of three nursing theory conferences in the 1960s. Nurse theorists presented papers that examined the questions in detail. Although many diverse opinions and beliefs were evident, there appeared to be unity around several points.

Basic or Applied Research?   Debating whether nursing knowledge is "basic" or "applied" raises the question of whether nursing research should aim to discover new knowledge (thus expanding the knowledge base for the sake of acquiring more knowledge) or to develop knowledge that can be used expressly to guide nursing practice. An example of research in nursing that contributes to our knowledge may be a physiological study about how respiratory exchange works with cardiopulmonary disease patients. Early on, this research may not have a clear application for practice, but ultimately its utility would be recognized once scientists understood the process. Such understanding surely would suggest appropriate nursing intervention measures.

This example illustrates a point that many nurse scientists make: It is foolish and wasteful to spend time discussing the philosophical questions about whether nursing research is basic or applied. Rather, nursing needs all kinds of research, basic and applied, and inevitably most basic research in nursing results in practical suggestions that will affect patient care (see Chapter 2).

Borrowed or Unique Theory?   A second question asks if nursing theory is borrowed or unique. There is agreement among nurse scientists that *nursing theory is both borrowed and unique*. That is, nurses use knowledge from many disciplines (psychology, sociology, physics, physiology, education); however, this knowledge only becomes integrated into nursing theory if nurses adapt it and alter it to fit the unique needs and perspectives of nursing. Nursing theories are those that are systematically derived from studies of nursing practice and that reveal a unique nursing perspective.

Grand Theories or Practice Theories? The nursing literature is replete with articles addressing the third question of whether we should seek one or several grand theories *of* nursing, or theories *for* practice. As you learned earlier, grand theories of nursing concern the profession in general—what it is, what the responsibilities are, and how work is viewed. A grand theory is "a generalized theory capable of supporting an overall concept of a process of nursing . . ." (Putnam 1965, p. 430.) In contrast, practice, or prescriptive, theories offer nurses *direct guides for action*. Theories *for* rather than *of* nursing aim to improve practice so as to "help individuals cope with health problems when their own strength, will or knowledge is insufficient" (Ellis 1968, p. 218).

Efforts to develop grand theories for nursing are not likely to succeed and are not as necessary as working toward middle-range, empirically based theories that can guide practice. Grand theories are less useful, because their large scale inevitably makes them vague and diffuse and, consequently, difficult to test. Beckstrand (1980) argues forcefully against a focus on grand theories of nursing: "Identifying the concepts relevant to nursing as an activity will not help nursing develop comprehensive scientific knowledge of its clients' problems and how to deal with them" (p. 76). Ultimately, perhaps, a grand theory could be developed if numerous practice theories could be synthesized and conceptualized clearly enough to suggest some overriding or transcendent concepts and constructs that are unique to nursing.

One practice theory is obviously not enough to cover the complexity of all nursing; therefore, emphasis should be placed on generating multiple practice theories appropriate to specific problems and areas in nursing—for example, theories of pain alleviation or care of the dying (Jacox 1974). If some unity could ever be derived from a conglomeration of practice theories, then perhaps a general practice theory could be synthesized. At this time, the likelihood of achieving such a goal is remote. Furthermore, some nurse scientists question the worth of such a huge undertaking.

Beckstrand (1978, 1980), a solo voice, argues in a series of articles against practice theories at all. Instead, she believes that knowledge of science, ethics, metatheory, and philosophy is sufficient for nursing.

What Paths to Knowledge? The fourth question concerns the appropriate paths for knowledge development for nursing science. Again, pluralism in methodology seems to be praised. Nurses need to generate theory inductively, test theory deductively, and also embrace the use of philosophical, phenomenological, and historical methods of research. The method chosen should not become an end in itself, but rather must be appropriate for answering the question. (See Chapter 6, on study designs.) Platt (1964) cautions us:

Beware of the man who is method-oriented rather than problem-oriented. The method-oriented man is shackled; the problem-oriented man is at least reaching freely toward what is most important [p. 353].

A major goal for nursing is to decide what questions are relevant to and significant for nursing. Donaldson and Crowley (1978) warn us that we can no longer assume that we all have a tacit understanding of "the nursing perspective" and "the essence of nursing." Rather, we must be able to articulate our unique perspective so it makes clear our knowledge and our philosophy. According to Hardy (1978b), we are aiming for a metaparadigm, "the broadest consensus within a discipline . . . which provides the general parameters of the field and gives scientists a broad orientation from which to work" (p. 38).

Evaluation and Analysis of Theories

Metatheory is a type of philosophical theory, a philosophy of science, that studies the logical and methodological foundations of a particular discipline (Carnap 1966, p. 188). Wilson and Kneisl (1983) point out that problems of metatheory "raise general issues [and] provide criteria of choice or standards" (p. 78) that allow us to make informed decisions about the value of proposed nursing theories. Metatheory gives us a structure, in the form of questions, to analyze and evaluate nursing theories. The customary questions are:

1. Is it a theory? What is our shared definition of a theory?

2. Is it a nursing theory? That is, what, if any, theoretical orientations compose and inform nursing's unique body of knowledge?

3. Is it any good? What are the standards we use to evaluate a theory or a fragment of a theory (Wilson & Kneisl 1983, p. 78)?

Is It a Theory?

In this chapter you have already been exposed to multiple definitions and conceptualizations of theory, from naming theory to practice theory, from grand theory to abstracted empiricism, from basic to applied, borrowed to unique, a theory *for* nursing and *of* nursing. In spite of all the varied definitions most scientists would agree that the purpose of a theory is to describe, explain, and predict truths about the subject of study.

Concepts that serve as the focus for nursing theories are the *person*, *society* or *environment*, *health*, and *nursing* (Yura & Torres 1975, Fawcett 1978b).

Recall Kerlinger's (1973) definition of a theory: "A theory is a set of interrelated constructs (concepts), definitions, and propositions that present a systematic view of phenomena by specifying relations among variables, with the purpose of explaining and predicting the phenomena" (p. 9). A nursing theory, therefore, would demonstrate the relationships among nursing, humanity, society, and health.

For a theory to be considered a theory, the following components must be present:

1. concepts that describe the empirical world

2. definitions of concepts (constitutive and operational)

3. constructs or propositions

4. links among the concepts and constructs that explain and predict phenomena

Developing a theory is complex, laborious, and time-consuming work requiring superior conceptual abilities. Only the mature sciences can boast that they have theories to guide them in research. In nursing this work has just begun.

Is It a Theory Unique to Nursing?

Contemporary debate focuses on the feasibility and desirability of developing theories unique to nursing. On one side are those scientists who believe that one's interests should dictate the pursuit of knowledge. Therefore, regardless of one's discipline, any scientist is free to explore and study any phenomenon, ultimately making a contribution to knowledge in general that may be useful to nursing or to the other sciences. Another group, also opposed to working toward developing nursing theories, believes that theories do not and will not have special relevance for nursing. Rather, theories from other disciplines (physiology, psychology, anthropology, and economics) can be modified and applied to nursing problems.

In the opposite camp are those who advocate

working toward unique nursing theories. They are fearful that scientists outside of nursing will not have the depth of interest and effort required to generate nursing knowledge. And unique nursing knowledge is mandatory to guide our practice. Borrowing from other disciplines will not contribute comprehensive in-depth knowledge necessary for scientific practice.

Wilson and Kneisl (1983) quote Immanuel Kant:

To yield to every whim of curiosity and to allow our passions for inquiry to be restrained by nothing but the limits of our ability, shows an eagerness of mind not unbecoming to scholarship. But, it is wisdom that has the merit of selecting from among the innumerable problems which present themselves, those whose solution is important to mankind [p. 79].

This philosophy suggests that nurse scholars focus in on problems that are unique to nursing in an effort to develop nursing theories (see Chapter 5).

Criteria for Judging a Theory

Stevens * presents one set of standards for theory evaluation. She advocates internal and external criticism. "Internal criticism deals with how theory components fit with each other. Internal criticism asks (given the premise that a theory assumes), does the theory logically follow? Do its pieces relate in a logical pattern" (p. 50)? The following four criteria are used to judge internal construction:

1. *Clarity* means that a theory is presented in such a way that the definitions of concepts and propositions and their relationships are easily understood. Glaser and Strauss (1967) emphasize the crucial nature of this criterion and call it a theory's "grab" for the practi-

---

* From B. Stevens, *Nursing Theory: Analysis, Application, Evaluation.* Boston: Little, Brown, 1979.

tioner or actor in the social world under investigation.

2. *Consistency* requires that the theory be consistent in the meaning of terms, interpretations, principles, and methods of reasoning (Stevens 1979, p. 52). A term used in one part of the theory must mean the same thing when used later on in the theory; and if a phenomenon is interpreted one way, it should be interpreted with the same meaning throughout the theory.

3. *Logical development* demands that the reasoning process be logical and lead logically to conclusions. The premises for the "argument" must be true and logically yield the conclusions. For example, "All patients are sick," "All mentally ill people are sick," and therefore "All patients are mentally ill" is an *illogical* sequence. Here, the premise may be wrong (patients may not be sick, depending on the definition), and the conclusions are surely wrong, based on illogical thinking.

4. The *level of theory development* must be assessed in order to understand the theory in a context of knowledge. You will assess whether it is a conceptual analysis, or a descriptive theory, or a situation-relating or more advanced situation-producing theory.

The next six criteria refer to *external criticism*; that is, how does a particular theory relate to the world of people, health, environment, and nursing (the four key variables in most nursing theories)?

1. *Adequacy* refers to the ability of the theory to satisfactorily deal with the nurse scientist's perspective of nursing. There must be adequacy of principles, interpretations, and methods. Do you accept the basic principles that are the foundation of the theory? Does the theorist's perception or interpretation of nursing make sense and accurately mirror the real world? Does the method of the theory permit research, and if so, what

types of research are appropriate (deductive, philosophical)?

2. *Utility* requires that a theory be useful in education, research, or practice. Glaser and Strauss (1967) talk of "fit," which means essentially the same thing as utility. The concepts and propositions must "fit" the work world of the nurse and must be operationalized so they can be applied and tested.

3. *Significance* refers to the requirement that a theory address issues basic and relevant to nursing and aim toward increasing nursing knowledge. The theory's significance should be obvious and should lead to further discovery of knowledge through research.

4. *Discrimination* requires that the theory clearly define its boundaries so that its relatedness to nursing is obvious. The theory must discriminate between what nursing is and what it isn't.

5. *Scope* is an indication of whether the theory has a narrow or broad focus. Earlier in this chapter you read about different levels of theory (from "abstracted empiricism" to "grand" and from "factor isolation" to "situation-producing"), so you are aware that there is some disagreement over how broad in scope a theory should ideally be. However, most nurse scientists recognize the current need for limited scope theories to actually guide practice decisions.

6. *Complexity and parsimony* are two sides of a coin. Parsimony is a property of a theory, meaning that it explains as much as possible with the fewest possible variables. This is sometimes called the power of a theory. A powerful theory is one that makes few assumptions and that clearly separates the critical variables from the diffuse background. Some scientists believe that in aiming for parsimony, one may miss the essence. Rather, one should strive for complexity because it examines the relationship between many

variables. In fact, the nature of the subject matter should dictate to what degree a theory is complex or parsimonious (Stevens 1979).

Theoretical models can be classified as developmental, interaction, or systems. Thibodeau elaborates, saying "developmental models use life-span physiological, cognitive, and psychosocial theories to define the four assertive components (people, environment, health, nursing) of the nursing paradigm. Systems models use general systems theory as the basis for defining the four components. Interaction models have symbolic interaction and role theories as their base" (1983, p. 43). An eclectic model combines several types, offering a diversified perspective. As you read theories, evaluate and analyze the theoretical perspective and determine if they are consistent throughout.

Other nurse scientists (Duffey & Muhlenkamp 1974, Ellis 1968, Hardy 1978a, Johnson 1974) have proposed some similar and different criteria for theory evaluation. Any or all of these criteria offer a useful structure for you to evaluate any theoretical model for nursing. Two final points are important regarding the evaluation of theoretical models:

1. Recognize that both internal and external criticism are necessary to thoroughly understand a nursing model.

2. Criticize a model only after you fully understand it, because *unbiased* criticism is the only fair and helpful criticism (see Chapter 7). To criticize a model because you intuitively don't like it or because your values are different from those inherent in it is not appropriate. Rather, view it for what it is, and use theoretical rather than emotional criteria for your evaluation. Chapter 7 offers some useful points about the art of criticism in a research study that are equally applicable to nursing theory evaluation.

Theoretical Models in Nursing—Some Examples

This section of the chapter offers you a brief encounter with 11 nursing theorists. This overview can acquaint you with the major perspective of each model and give you a feeling for the historical development of nursing theory. Perhaps one or more models will catch your interest, and you can read in more depth by going directly to the writings of the particular theorist or an authoritative source on nursing theory such as Meleis (1984) or Stevens (1984).

Florence Nightingale

Nightingale can be considered to be the first nursing theorist if we accept evidence that she offered a theoretical orientation to nursing without calling it one. Her focus was on the physical environment (as opposed to the psychosocial environment), which was appropriate for the difficult conditions of the Crimean War. Her table of contents in *Notes on Nursing: What It Is and What It Is Not* (1946) clearly illustrates her environmental approach: Ventilation and Warming, Health of Houses, Petty Management, Noise, Variety, Taking Food, What Food? Bed and Bedding, Light, Cleanliness of Rooms and Walls, Personal Cleanliness, Chattering Hopes and Advices, and Observation of the Sick (p. 5). Nightingale believed that if nurses altered the environment in a positive fashion, the reparative process could begin.

Lydia Hall

Hall's theory presents the three "aspects of nursing": the person (or the core of nursing), the disease (or the cure of nursing), and the body (the care of nursing) (see Figure 10-8). Her philosophy developed from her work at the Loeb Center of Montefieore Hospital in the Bronx.

Patients had recovered from their acute illnesses and were recuperating in this long-term, patient-centered treatment center. Depending on the patient's problems, each of the three aspects of nursing might be emphasized or deemphasized, demonstrating the changing nature of their relationships.

Virginia Henderson

Henderson wrote her famous *definition* of nursing in 1955:

Nursing is primarily assisting the individual (sick or well) in the performance of those activities contributing to health or its recovery (or a peaceful death) that he would perform unaided if he had the necessary strength, will, or knowledge. It is likewise the unique contribution of nursing to help the individual to be independent of such assistance as soon as possible [p. 4].

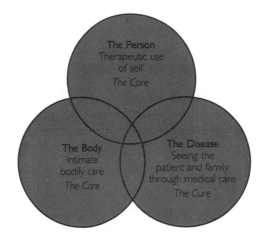

Figure 10-8 Hall's three aspects of nursing. (From Nursing Theories Conference Group, *Nursing Theories: The Base for Professional Nursing Practice*, © 1980, p. 44. Reprinted by permission of Prentice-Hall, Inc., Englewood Cliffs, N.J.)

Box 10-1   Henderson's Components of Basic Nursing Care

1. Breathe normally.
2. Eat and drink adequately.
3. Eliminate body wastes.
4. Move, and maintain desirable postures.
5. Sleep and rest.
6. Select suitable clothing—dress and undress.
7. Maintain body temperature within normal range by adjusting clothing and modifying the environment.
8. Keep the body clean and well groomed, and protect the integument.
9. Avoid dangers in the environment, and avoid injuring others.
10. Communicate with others in expressing emotions, needs, fears, or opinions.
11. Worship according to one's faith.
12. Work in such a way that there is a sense of accomplishment.
13. Play or participate in various forms of recreation.
14. Learn, discover, or satisfy the curiosity that leads to normal development and health and use of the available health facilities.

SOURCE: V. Henderson, *The Nature of Nursing*, New York: Macmillan, 1966, pp. 16–17.

Following up her philosophical definition with concrete examples, Henderson listed 14 components of basic nursing care (see Box 10-1). These components focus on "helping the patient with the [listed] activities or providing conditions under which he can perform them unaided" (1966, pp. 16–17). You can see by her list that Henderson recognized physiological, psychological, and spiritual needs.

Hildegard Peplau

Peplau, a psychiatric nurse, presented her theoretical model in *Interpersonal Relations in Nursing* (1952). According to Peplau, nursing is a "significant therapeutic interpersonal process. . . . Nursing is an educative instrument, a maturing force, that aims to promote forward movement of personality in the direction of creative, constructive, productive, personal, and community living" (1952, p. 16) (see Figure 10-9).

Peplau's theory focused on the four phases of the nurse–patient relationship (see Figure 10-10).

1. Orientation—the nurse and patient meet in response to the patient's "felt need" (p. 18).
2. Identification—the patient responds to the nurse if he or she offers needed help (p. 30).
3. Exploitation—the patient uses the nurse as a resource person (p. 37).
4. Resolution—when the patient's needs are met, he or she relinquishes ties to the nurse (p. 40).

Wilson and Kneisl (1983) say that Peplau's phases of the relationship represent precursors to the phases of the nursing process (assessment, planning, intervention, evaluation).

Fay Abdellah

Abdellah classifies nursing problems into 21 categories (see Box 10-2). She views the nurse as a problem solver whose goal is to identify and then remedy these biopsychosocial problems. Abdellah's list is comparable both to Henderson's 14 nursing care components and to Maslow's hierarchy of needs (Falco 1980).

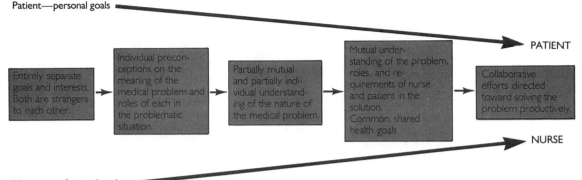

Figure 10-9 A continuum of the changing nurse–patient relationship. (From H. Peplau, *Interpersonal Relations in Nursing*, New York: Putnam's, 1952, p. 10. Reprinted with permission.)

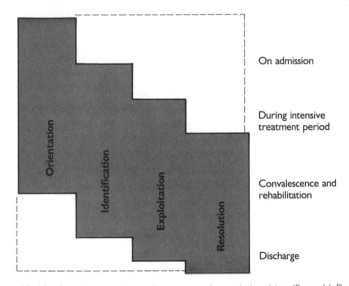

Figure 10-10 Overlapping phases in nurse–patient relationships. (From H. Peplau, *Interpersonal Relations in Nursing*, New York: Putnam's, 1952, p. 21. Reprinted with permission.)

Dorothea Orem

Orem's theory of self-care appeared in the nursing literature in 1959. Her theory centers on the individual: "Self-care is the practice of activities that individuals personally initiate and perform on their own behalf to maintain life, health, and well-being. . . . It is an adult's personal, continuous contribution to his own health and well-being" (1971, p. 13). Orem proposes six categories of universal self-care requisites (see Box 10-3). If an individual cannot meet self-care needs because of illness, injury, or disease, the nurse enters and offers "health deviation

---

Box 10-2   Abdellah's List of Nursing Problems

1. to maintain good hygiene and physical comfort
2. to promote optimal activity: exercise, rest, and sleep
3. to promote safety through the prevention of accidents, injury, or other trauma and through the prevention of the spread of infection
4. to maintain good body mechanics and prevent and correct deformities
5. to facilitate the maintenance of a supply of oxygen to all body cells
6. to facilitate the maintenance of nutrition of all body cells
7. to facilitate the maintenance of elimination
8. to facilitate the maintenance of fluid and electrolyte balance
9. to recognize the physiological responses of the body to disease conditions—pathological, physiological, and compensatory
10. to facilitate the maintenance of regulatory mechanisms and functions
11. to facilitate the maintenance of sensory function
12. to identify and accept positive and negative expressions, feelings, and reactions
13. to identify and accept the interrelatedness of emotions and organic illness
14. to facilitate the maintenance of effective verbal and nonverbal communication
15. to promote the development of productive interpersonal relationships
16. to facilitate progress toward achievement of personal spiritual goals
17. to create and/or maintain a therapeutic environment
18. to facilitate awareness of self as an individual with varying physical, emotional, and developmental needs
19. to accept the optimum possible goals in the light of limitations, physical and emotional
20. to use community resources as an aid in resolving problems arising from illness
21. to understand the role of social problems as influencing factors in the cause of illness

SOURCE: F. Abdellah et al., *Patient Centered Approaches to Nursing,* New York: Macmillan, 1960, p. 16.

Box 10-3   Orem's Universal Self-Care Requisites

1. air, water, and food
2. excrement
3. activity and rest
4. solitude and social interaction
5. hazards to life and well-being
6. being normal

SOURCE: From D. E. Orem, *Nursing: Concepts of Practice,* New York: McGraw-Hill, 1971, pp. 21–28.

self-care." The nurse assesses the patient's level of functioning and ability to care for himself or herself and then gives "wholly compensatory," "partially compensatory," or "supportive–educative" care. Orem calls these three types of assistance "nursing systems," and each one describes the patient's and nurse's role. Orem's theory has great interest in contemporary nursing with its renewed focus on self-care.

Martha Rogers

Rogers published her book *An Introduction to the Theoretical Basis of Nursing* in 1970, draw-

---

Box 10-4   Rogers's Principles of Homeodynamics

1. Principle of resonancy

   the continuous change from lower to higher frequency wave patterns in human and environmental fields

2. Principle of helicy

   the continuous innovative, probabalistic increasing diversity of human and environmental field patterns characterized by nonrepeating rhythmicities

3. Principle of integrality[a]

   the continuous mutual human field and environmental field process

[a] Formerly called the principle of complementarity. From The Second National Post-Master's Conference, April 5–6, 1984.

SOURCE: M. Rogers, Department of Nursing. New York University. Handout, 1984.

---

ing on knowledge from anthropology, sociology, religion, philosophy, mythology, and general systems theory. Her theory has changed somewhat and become clarified over the years. *At the present time, she views the "unitary" person as the basis of nursing's uniqueness.* The science of nursing is "the study of the nature and direction of unitary human development and the derivation of descriptive, explanatory, and predictive principles that are basic to nursing practice." The practice of nursing is "the use of the body of knowledge in service to people." The purpose of nursing is "to help individuals and groups achieve maximum well-being within the potential of each" (Rogers 1982).

Rogers views science as humanistic, not mechanistic. People and the environment are two energy fields that are always open, have pattern and organization, and change continuously and creatively (Rogers 1984). Rogers identifies three principles of homeodynamics that postulate the nature and direction of change. (See Box 10-4.)

Myra Levine

Levine proposes four conservation principles that aim to alter patients' adaptation processes in positive ways. Levine writes: "Conservation means 'keeping together' (L. *conservatio*), but it should not imply minimal activity. In nursing, to keep together means to maintain a proper balance between active nursing intervention coupled with patient participation on the one hand, and the safe limits of the patients' ability on the other" (1971, p. 46). The nurse first identifies the patient's specific pattern of adaptation and then uses the following principles to plan nursing intervention:

1. the principle of the conservation of patient energy. Nursing intervention is based on conserving the individual patient's physiological and psychological resources.

2. the principle of the conservation of structural integrity. Nursing intervention is based on conserving the individual patient's body form and function.

3. the principle of conservation of personal integrity. Nursing intervention is based on conserving the individual patient's self-identity and self-respect.

4. the principle of conservation of social integrity. Nursing intervention is based on conserving the individual patient's ethnic, religious, and subcultural affiliations (1967, pp. 46–59).

Levine views her principles as offering new directions for holistic approaches to patient care.

Sister Callista Roy

Roy's adaptation theory (1976) views us as bio-psychosocial beings who have to continually adapt to a variety of stimuli, which she calls "focal," "contextual," and "residual" (p. 12). The focal stimulus has to do with a degree of change (e.g., a temperature variation); contextual stimuli include other stimuli present (e.g., humidity); and residual stimuli involve beliefs and attitudes that affect a given situation (p. 13). Roy identifies four adaptive modes that help people cope with the changing environment—basic physiological needs, self-concept, role function, and interdependence (p. 18). These four adaptive modes are essentially methods of coping that appear between a need and a behavior. For example, if the environmental temperature changes, a person may be hot or cold, and these feelings elicit an adaptive mode. The person feels the need and acts to address the need. Roy views basic needs as underlying the adaptive modes. The nursing process is used to promote the patients' adaptation in each mode. In her book, Roy (1976) gives examples of nursing interventions for specific adaptation problems.

Imogene King

King (1978) proposes a general systems theory about the human level of functioning. *People, environment, nursing,* and *health* are her four basic concepts. She postulates three dynamic interacting systems (see Figure 10-11): Each individual is a *personal system.* These individuals interact among one another to form *interpersonal systems,* such as dyads, triads, and groups. The interpersonal systems then form *social systems,* which are comprehensive levels of functions of human beings (1978, p. 12). A person's "personal system" is dependent largely on one's perception of self. These perceptions directly influence behavior. The nurse–patient nursing process is implemented in the interpersonal system. The social systems—family, religious, edu-

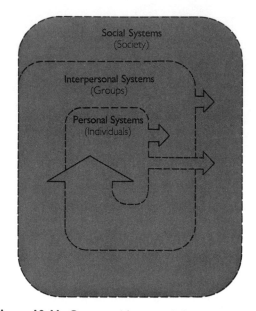

Figure 10-11 Conceptual framework for nursing. (From I. King, *Toward a Theory for Nursing,* New York: John Wiley, 1981. Reprinted with permission.)

cational, and health care systems (King 1981)—provide a context in which nurses work. To help patients achieve goals, nurses must interact effectively with social systems. King views her theory as "organizing complexity and variety in nursing . . . [and] in looking for relationships within this complexity and variety" (p. 15).

Betty Neuman

Neuman (1982) proposes a health-care systems model, which views the person as a complete system with parts and subparts that interrelate. Neuman sees human beings as subject to stressors, which she identifies as intrapersonal, interpersonal, and extrapersonal, and as having flexible lines of resistance that help defend against these stressors (see Figure 10-12). Nursing assessment focuses on gaining information about the relationship among physiologic, psychologic, sociocultural, and developmental variables; nursing intervention can be primary,

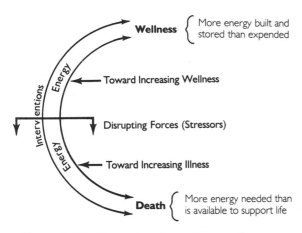

Wellness { More energy built and stored than expended

Toward Increasing Wellness

Disrupting Forces (Stressors)

Toward Increasing Illness

Death { More energy needed than is available to support life

Figure 10-12 Neuman's wellness–illness continuum based on a systems model. (From B. Neuman, *The Neuman Systems Model*, Norwalk, Conn.: Appleton-Century-Crofts, 1982, p. 11. Reprinted with permission.)

secondary, or tertiary. The nursing process, including nursing diagnosis, nursing goals, and nursing outcomes, is expected to facilitate the use of the model (1982, p. 119).

The 11 theoretical models just discussed offer a perspective on where nursing science originated and how far it has progressed. Although the theorists presented can be considered

dominant, other nurse scientists—for example, Dickoff and James (1968), Johnson (1980), Orlando (1961), Weidenbach (1969)—have contributed to the development of nursing theory.

Upon close analysis and evaluation, you will be able to recognize similarities and differences in philosophy and focus. As nursing evolves as a science, its paradigms will become clear and will serve as a guide for research, education, and practice. It is only when this happens that we will be able to consider nursing a scientific discipline.

To further emphasize in a more concrete fashion the implications of nursing theories, I refer you to Roy's *Introduction to Nursing: An Adaptation Model* (1976). Suppose that in your practice you care for a patient with a mastectomy, an anxious elderly male, or a teenager with endocrine problems. Roy's adaptation model offers a framework with which to view these diverse problems and many others. The book presents theoretical knowledge for understanding patients' psychological and physiological needs, factors to consider in the assessment of the problem, and specific suggested nursing interventions. As nurses learn about such theories and begin to put them into practice, their usefulness will become clear.

Conceptual Frameworks to Guide Nursing Practice

Nursing theories and theories adapted from other disciplines guide practice decisions. Wilson and Kneisl (1983) discuss four conceptual frameworks used in psychiatric nursing: medical–biological, psychoanalytic, behavioristic, and social–interpersonal. Table 10-2 demonstrates clearly how each of these models affects patient care. A necessary question for psychiatric nurses to ask when they are applying for a new job is always, "What is your treatment philosophy, your conceptual model?" The question is vital because if you are hired in a setting that uses a medical or custodial model, as the chart shows,

you will not be viewed as a therapeutic agent but rather will spend time delivering medications and monitoring patients after electroconvulsive therapy treatments.

Neuman's book *The Neuman Systems Model* (1982) devotes an entire section to application of the conceptual model to nursing practice. Plans for nursing intervention with patients' specific problems are derived from the model. Gudmundsen (1982) says:

One models nursing as one models all else: by proposing symbolic systems that can be identified with spe-

Table 10-2 A Comparative Analysis of Major Features of Four Conceptual Frameworks

Conceptual Framework	Assessment Base	Problem Statement	Goal	Dominant Intervention
Medical–biological	Individual client symptoms	Disease	Symptom control Cure	Somatotherapies
Psychoanalytic	Intrapsychic Unconscious	Conflict	Insight	Psychoanalysis
Behavioristic	Behavior	Learning deficit	Behavior change	Behavior modification or conditioning
Social–interpersonal	Interactions of individual and social context	Dysfunction	Enhanced awareness and quality of interactions	Group and milieu therapies

SOURCE: H. Wilson and C. Kneisl. *Psychiatric Nursing.* 2nd ed. Menlo Park, Calif.: Addison-Wesley, 1983, p. 37.

cific nursing phenomena in specific situations by means of observation and experimentation. . . . The criteria for judging all models are the same, however, deriving from their general role in the developing of nursing science: scope, adequacy to their chosen data base, extendability, predictive power, communicability, simplicity [p. 265].

Numerous clinical studies are presented, which serve to test the model and practice. Breckenridge (1982) adapted the model for renal patients. She found the model's focus on prevention and on the total person useful, because renal patients present with multiple problems. The Neuman framework permits assessment of the patient and evaluation of resources available to help the patient cope with stressors. Intervention then focuses on decreasing stress from a variety of areas. Primary, secondary, and tertiary preventive measures are included (see Figure 10-13). For example, the normal line of defenses is the patient's existing level of wellness. In renal patients, primary prevention focuses on teaching how to prevent an infection (due to immunosuppressive drug therapy) and, thus, strengthens the patient's defenses. Secondary prevention is used when the normal lines of defense are interfered with, as with renal failure. At this time,

hemodialysis or transplantation may be required. When the stressor is serious, the body's lines of resistance, which are internal (increase of leukocytes), rally to fight the infection. Behavior modification that also can strengthen resistance to infection is an example of tertiary prevention. Behavior modification aids in increasing patient compliance to a rigorous regimen, including diet, medications, and the avoidance of contact sports (1982, pp. 268–270). Figure 10-14 demonstrates the three levels of intervention—primary, secondary, and tertiary—and the three levels of stressors—interpersonal, intrapersonal, and extrapersonal. All preventions aim to increase the patient's lines of defense. The following example illuminates the use of terms in a case history.

Neuman views prevention as circular. That is, tertiary prevention includes primary and secondary prevention. For example, the transplant is secondary prevention, and tertiary prevention aims to help the patient reach an optimal level of wellness. The Neuman assessment–intervention tool measures the patient's adjustment: If the patient and the nurse recognize the threat of infection, then tertiary measures include, along with behavior modification, the primary measures of education to prevent infection. After the

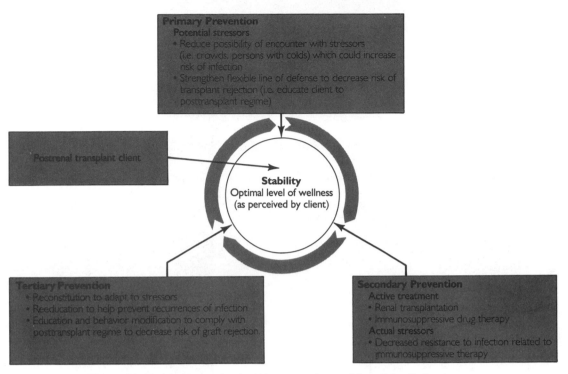

Figure 10-13 Health care for the kidney transplant recipient. From D. Breckenridge, "Adaptation of the Neuman Systems Model for the Renal Client," in B. Neuman, *The Neuman Systems Model*, Norwalk, Conn.: Appleton-Century-Crofts, 1982, p. 271. Reprinted with permission.)

Example: Preventions Used to Increase Patient's Line of Defense

Mr. J has had chronic renal failure for eight years which he perceives as a life-term illness.

Intrapersonal physiologic stressor

He has received maintenance hemodialysis for six years at a community life-support center.

Secondary prevention-treatment intervention

Mr. J. receives daily shunt care by his wife or health-care providers to decrease the risk of infection.

Tertiary prevention-reconstitution intervention

He may be faced with early retirement, due to a recent worsening of his condition.

Extrapersonal physiologic and developmental stressor

Because of his illness, family and friends cater excessively to him, making him feel different.

Intrapersonal sociocultural stressor

SOURCE: D. Breckenridge, "Adaptation of the Neuman Systems Model of the Renal Client," in *The Neuman Systems Model* by B. Neuman, Norwalk, Conn.: Appleton-Century-Crofts, 1982, p. 268.

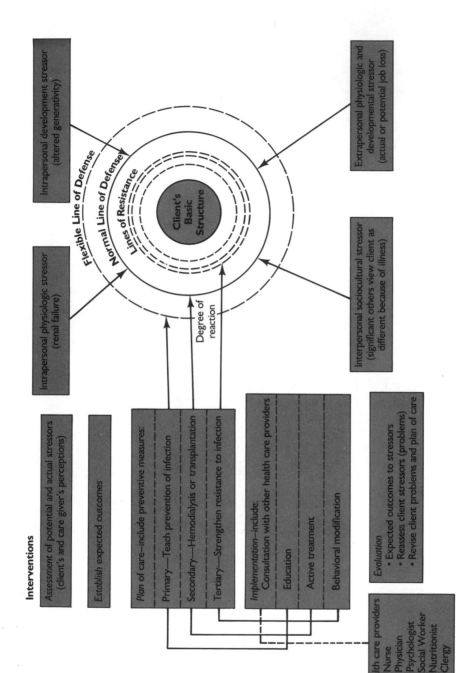

Figure 10-14 Clinical practice framework for the renal client. (From D. Breckenridge, Adaptation of the Neuman Systems Model for the Renal Client," in B. Neuman, *The Neuman Systems Model*, Norwalk, Conn.: Appleton-Century-Crofts, 1982, p. 269. Reprinted with permission.)

client is functioning well (tertiary prevention), the focus is then on primary intervention to prevent an infection, to help the client at the optimal level of wellness.

Many other examples of using conceptual models in practice can be found in Neuman (1982).

Conceptual Models in Nursing Research

As we progress in our theory development, more and more research will derive from conceptual models. As with nursing practice, the conceptual model structures the entire research process. Nursing models or models from other disciplines can be used. See Box 10-5 for examples of contemporary research studies and their conceptual frameworks. Dickoff and his colleagues (1968b) make the following point about "borrowing" models from other disciplines: "Practically speaking, what is needed is for a nurse researcher to develop both her self-surveillance and her self-esteem so as to be able to take advantage of the help and securities of established disciplines without thereby sacrificing her nursing impetus or nursing identity" (p. 553).

Models From Other Disciplines

As early as 1968, Myrtle Irene Brown wrote on the use of the concept of socialization (from sociology) in geriatric nursing research. She calls her early classifications "primitive" yet emphasizes that her work aimed "to describe the socializing behavior of nurses with the aged and to identify related variables" (p. 216). This is an appropriate first step in research and theory development, at least according to Dickoff and his associates' idea of levels.

Other nurse scientists have made efforts to adapt existing theories to nursing. For example, Ann Whall (1980) has examined existing theories of family functioning and shown their relationship to nursing theories. She discusses the

similarities between Peplau's (1952) approach and the psychoanalytic approach in family functioning, between King's (1978) theory and the communicationist approach, and between Rogers's (1970) theory and the family systems approach. Whall's work demonstrates her assertion that existing theory must "be examined and, if relevant, be formulated or adapted in terms of nursing theory" (p. 67). After such reformulations, propositions can yield hypotheses that can be tested, thus forming the basis for nursing research.

Questioning Nursing Models

In a similar quest for useful models for nursing research, Cronenwett and Brickman (1983) discussed four models of helping and coping in childbirth. After describing each model and its assumptions and the pros and cons, they concluded the article by raising some relevant questions for nursing research (pp. 87–88). Some or all of these questions could be adapted and asked about many other models for nursing:

1. Are some helping models generally better than others?

2. Are different models best for different clients?

3. Are client–provider teams using the same (congruent) models most effectively?

4. Is it better to apply one model to a client consistently or to change as the client's needs, situations, and skills change?

Box 10-5   *Contemporary Research Studies and Their Conceptual Frameworks*

Title:	Duration of Pain Condition and Physical Pathology as Determinants of Nurses' Assessments of Patients in Pain
Author:	Taylor, Ann Gill, Skelton, James A., & Butcher, Jan
Source:	*Nursing Research* (1984), *33*(1), 4–8

Abstract:

This article is based on an experiment that examined features distinguishing chronic from acute pain syndromes, and their influence on nurses' estimates of patient suffering, pain relief actions, and attitudes toward patients. Two hundred sixty-eight nurses received one-paragraph descriptions of patients complaining of severe pain. Descriptions varied on the dimensions of duration (acute vs. chronic), signs of physical pathology (positive vs. negative), signs of depression (positive vs. negative), and diagnostic category (low back vs. headache vs. joint pain). Subjects estimated the intensity of the hypothetical patient's suffering, indicated priorities for specific pain relief actions, and rated the patient on a series of trait dimensions. Subjects attributed less intense pain when the patient had no signs of pathology and when duration was long-termed and chronic. They also assigned lower priorities to medication-related nursing actions when signs of pathology were negative. Finally, more negative personality and behavioral traits were attributed to the patient when signs of pathology were negative. The results reflect a dichotomous, organic versus psychogenic model of pain on the part of health care staff. Since the data indicate the chronic pain sufferer is negatively stereo-typed by staff, a need exists to develop and disseminate more integrative models of the pain experience.

Conceptual Framework: The authors draw on literature about classic pain theory and the biomedical model of pain. They point out that, according to many researchers, "classic pain theory discounts the role of emotional and psychological factors in the pain experience" (p. 7). They advocate more knowledge of chronic pain (possibly a suggestion for the development of a theoretical model).

Title:	Effects of Modeling and Information on Reactions to Pain: A Childbirth-Preparation Analogue
Author:	Manderino, Mary A., & Bzdek, Virginia M.
Source:	*Nursing Research* (1984), *33*(1), 9–14

Abstract:

A labor-preparation analogue study was conducted to examine the efficacy of videotaped information and modeling as pain-reducing techniques for women during labor and delivery. Sixty nulliparous college female undergraduates were randomly assigned to four treatment conditions: (a) videotaped modeling; (b) videotaped information; (c) videotaped information and modeling combined; and (d) control (irrelevant) videotape. Assessments of the effectiveness of these treatments were made during a one-hour session involving twenty 80-second exposures to the Forgione-Barber pain stimulator. The timing and sequencing of the pain

Box 10-5 (continued)

stimulus was patterned to resemble labor contractions. Dependent variables included self-reported pain, heart rate, systolic and diastolic blood pressure, frontalis electromyogram, and respiratory rate. The group that received information and modeling combined reported significantly lower pain ratings than each of the other three groups. Analyses conducted on the physiological dependent variables failed to demonstrate significant treatment effects. The implications of these findings are discussed from the perspective of developing more effective methods of preparing women for the experience of childbirth.

Conceptual Framework: *Bandura's Social Learning Theory* (1969), which demonstrates that learning can occur vicariously (p. 9).

Title: Therapeutic and Physical Touch: Physiological Response to Stressfui Stimuli

Author: Randolph, Gretchen Lay

Source: *Nursing Research* (1984), *33*(1), 33–36

Abstract: Sixty female college students were exposed to a stressful stimulus and treated by therapeutic or physical touch. Groups were compared on levels of physiological response through electromyographic, skin conductance, and peripheral skin temperature measures. The hypotheses predicted that the therapeutic touch group would remain more relaxed than the physical touch group. None of the hypotheses were confirmed using a one-way analysis of covariance.

Conceptual Framework: Therapeutic touch

Title: Therapeutic Touch: Is There a Scientific Basis for the Practice?

Author: Clark, Philip E., & Clark, Mary Jo

Source: *Nursing Research* (1984), *33*(1), 37–41

Abstract: The research-related literature on the topic of therapeutic touch is critically reviewed. The purpose of the review is to explore the current scientific basis for the teaching and practice of therapeutic touch as a treatment modality. An examination of published research literature indicates that empirical support for the practice of therapeutic touch is, at best, weak. The results of well-designed, double-blind studies have been transient, of no significance, or are in need of independent replication. Current practice of therapeutic touch is empirically little more than practice of placebo. Considerations for further nursing research are also presented.

Conceptual Framework: As the abstract explains, this article reviews research-related literature on the conceptual framework of therapeutic touch. The authors point out that unless the framework is supported by empirical research, "nurse practitioners of therapeutic touch will be relegated to the practice of 'placebo mumbo jumbo'" (p. 40).

5. Are some models better for providers?

6. Do organizational structures determine the choice of helping model?

7. Does professional role socialization determine the choice of helping model?

8. Has there been a historic evolution of the dominant helping models applied to childbearing families? (pp. 87–88)

The search for theories and models for helping and coping in many areas of nursing is a most useful endeavor. Cronenwett and Brickman's beginning look at models generates many varied ideas and approaches for further study.

In 1981 Gill and Atwood published a study in which they used Martha Rogers's conceptual model to derive hypotheses for testing. Essentially, they attempted to explain the relationship between epidermal growth factor and epidermal wound healing. In 1983 Kim responded to Gill and Atwood's article by raising three questions:

1. Is the logic used to derive the research hypotheses adequate, appropriate, and rigorous?

2. Is the research methodology used in the study appropriate for testing Rogers's model?

3. If problems exist with respect to the above two questions, how might they be resolved? (p. 89)

Kim concluded that problems exist in Gill and Atwood's original conceptualization of wound healing, and if this conceptualization is erroneous, all else that follows is inevitably inappropriate. Kim's article points out the necessity for dialogue among nurse scientists on how to derive hypotheses from abstract models, such as Rogers's, that are "adequate, appropriate, and rigorous" (p. 89). Nursing research needs to use nursing conceptual models as theoretical frameworks, but similar to borrowing and adapting theories from other disciplines, we must continue to discuss and evaluate all theories to ensure that they are being interpreted correctly and offer a useful framework for nursing research.

This chapter has aimed to emphasize the interdependence of nursing theory, research, and practice. Dickoff and his associates (1968) offer a meaningful model and summary statement: "Theory is born in practice, is refined in research, and must and can return to practice if research is to be other than a draining-off of energy from the main business of nursing and theory more than idle speculation" (p. 415).

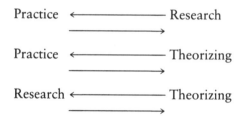

Developing a body of knowledge about nursing and for nursing practice is critical if we are to move from a discipline based on tradition and authority to a discipline based on science. Placing nursing studies within the context of our evolving theoretical base is essential to that goal.

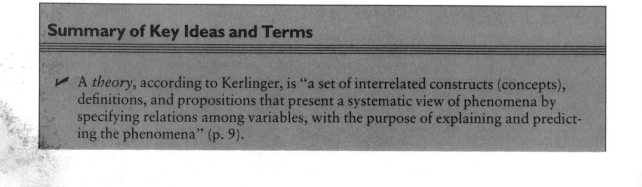

Summary of Key Ideas and Terms

✔ A *theory*, according to Kerlinger, is "a set of interrelated constructs (concepts), definitions, and propositions that present a systematic view of phenomena by specifying relations among variables, with the purpose of explaining and predicting the phenomena" (p. 9).

✔ *Concepts* are the building blocks of theories, and may be concrete (patient) or abstract (wellness).

✔ A *conceptual framework* or model refers to concepts that essentially structure or offer a framework of propositions for conducting research.

✔ A *construct* is a group of concepts that are derived from a combination of academic and clinical knowledge and contribute meaning and scope to a theory (Jacox 1974, Glaser & Strauss 1967).

✔ *Propositions* describe the relationship of two or more concepts.

✔ The empirical–theoretical continuum demonstrates the relationship between what is observed empirically and what is described theoretically.

✔ A *model* depicts structural or functional relationships "by means of a likeness which may be structural, pictorial, diagrammatic or mathematical" (Bush 1979).

✔ *Conceptual mapping* is a theoretical model for understanding the relationship among variables in a study.

✔ Types of theories include grand, middle range, and abstracted empiricism. *Grand theories* are global and vague and attempt to explain almost everything about a subject. *Middle range theories* focus on an empirical area and have clear propositions from which hypotheses can be derived and have implications for practice. *Abstracted empiricism* focuses only on empirical phenomena, i.e., facts which are in isolation from any theory.

✔ Looking at levels of theory is another way to categorize theories. *Factor-isolating theories* (factor-naming theories) involve the identification and classification of concepts or variables. *Factor-relating theories* (situation-depicting theories) relate factors to each other. *Situation-relating theories* (predictive and promoting or inhibiting theories) allow predictions that if *A* happens, *B* happens, and can suggest what factors influence the causal relationship and in what way. *Situation-producing* theory is prescriptive theory.

✔ According to Ellis, theories serve four purposes: (1) theory allows us to distinguish fact from pseudofact; (2) they help synthesize facts from many fields; (3) theoretical knowledge gives direction to practice; (4) theory acts as a framework for storing knowledge available in the literature.

✔ Prior to the 1980s, most nursing research was conducted without a theoretical framework. Rather, frameworks from other disciplines were used or the researcher used no theoretical framework, but rather chose specific research instruments to collect data on some variable.

✔ *Paradigms* specify the type of research questions to be asked and the appropriate methods for answering them.

✔ Nursing is preparadigmatic (before paradigms) because it is an emerging science. Consequently, nurse scientists are attempting to develop useful paradigms to guide nursing practice and research.

✔ Paradigm-transcending research is research that has the goal of developing new theories and methods. Nursing needs more of these studies that explain and predict empirical phenomena relevant to our discipline.

✔ Nursing theory is both borrowed from many disciplines and unique in that some theories are derived systematically and directly from nursing practice.

✔ Nurses need to encourage pluralism in research methods and in theory testing and theory generation.

✔ A theory may be evaluated on four criteria that refer to the internal construction of a theory: (1) clarity; (2) consistency; (3) logical development; and (4) level of theory development (Stevens 1979).

✔ A theory may be evaluated on six criteria that refer to the external criticism of a theory: (1) adequacy; (2) validity; (3) significance; (4) discrimination; (5) scope; and (6) complexity/parsimony (Stevens 1979).

✔ Theoretical models can be classified as developmental, systems, or interaction. Developmental models use life span theories to define the four components of the nursing paradigm—people, environment, health, and nursing. Systems models use general systems theory, and interaction models have symbolic interaction and role theories as their theoretical bases (Thibodeau 1983, p. 43).

✔ Conceptual frameworks from nursing and from other disciplines can be used to guide nursing practice and nursing research.

✔ Nursing theory is dependent on nursing practice; practice is dependent on theory; and research is dependent on practice.

References

Abdellah F et al: *Patient Centered Approaches to Nursing.* New York: Macmillan, 1960.

Anderson G: Infant colic: A possible solution. *Am J Maternal Child Nurs* 1983; 8:185.

Anderson G: A preliminary report: Severe respiratory distress in two newborn lambs with recovery following nonnutritive sucking, *J Nurse Midwifery* 1975; 20:20–28.

Artinian B: Conceptual mapping: Development of the strategy. *West J Nurs Res* 1982; 4:379–393.

Beckstrand J: The notion of a practice theory and the relationship of scientific and ethical knowledge to practice. *Res Nurs Health* 1978; 1:131–136.

Beckstrand J: A critique of several conceptions of practice theory in nursing. *Res Nurs Health,* 1980; 3:69–79.

Blalock H: *An Introduction to Social Research.* Englewood Cliffs, N.J.: Prentice-Hall 1970.

Breckenridge D: Adaptation of the Neuman systems model for the renal client. In Neuman B: *The Neuman Systems Model,* Norwalk, Conn.: Appleton-Century-Crofts, 1982.

Brown M: Social theory in geriatric nursing research. *Nurs Res* 1968; 17:213–217.

Bush H: Models for nursing. *Advances In Nursing Science* 1979; 1:13–21.

Carnap R: *Philosophical Foundations of Physics.* Gardner M (editor). New York: Basic Books, 1966.

Chinn P, Jacobs M: Theory development in nursing. Tape series. Denton: Nursing Sciences Tape Library, Texas Woman's University, 1975.

Chinn P, Jacobs M: A mode for theory development in nursing. *Advances in Nursing Science* 1978; 1:1–11.

Clark P, Clark M: Therapeutic touch: Is there a scientific basis for the practice? *Nurs Res* 1984; 33:37–41.

Collins R, Fielder J: Beckstrand's concept of practice and theory: A critique. *Res Nurs Health* 1981; 4:317–321.

Crawford G et al: Evolving issues in theory development. *Nurs Outlook* May 1979; 27:346–351.

Cronenwett L, Brickman P: Models of helping and coping in childbirth. *Nurs Res* 1983; 32:84–88.

Dickoff J, James P: A theory of theories: A position paper. *Nurs Res* May/June 1968; 17:197–203.

Dickoff J, James P: Theory development in nursing. Pages 45–92 in: *Nursing Research.* Verhonick PJ (editor). Boston: Little, Brown, 1975.

Dickoff J et al: Theory in a practice discipline: Part 1 Practice oriented theory. *Nurs Res* 1968; 17:415–435. (a)

Dickoff J et al: Theory in a practice discipline: Part II Practice oriented research. *Nurs Res* 1968; 17:545–554. (b)

Diers D: *Research in Nursing Practice.* Philadelphia: Lippincott, 1979.

Donaldson S, Crowley D: The discipline of nursing. *Nurs Outlook* February 1978; 26:118–120.

Duffey M, Muhlenkamp A: A framework for theory analysis. *Nurs Outlook* 1974; 22:571.

Ellis R: Characteristics of significant theories. *Nurs Res* May/June 1968; 17:217–222.

Erikson E: *Childhood and Society.* New York: Norton, 1963.

Estes WK: Growth and function of mathematical models for learning. In: Marx M (editor), *Theories in Contemporary Psychology.* New York: Macmillan, 1963.

Fageraugh S: Getting around with emphysema. *Am J Nurs* 1973; 73:94–99.

Falco S: Faye Abdellah. In *Nursing Theories.* Nursing Theories Conference Group (editor). Englewood Cliffs, N.J.: Prentice-Hall, 1980.

Fawcett J: The relationship between theory and research: A double helix. *Advances Nurs Sci* 1978; 1:49–62. (a)

Fawcett J: The "What" of theory development. Pages 17–33 in: *Theory Developments: What? Why? How?* New York: National League for Nursing, 1978.(b)

Fitzpatrick et al: *Nursing Models and Their Psychiatric Mental Health Applications.* Bowie, Md.: Robert J Brady, 1982.

Floyd J: Rhythm theory: Relationship to nursing conceptual models. In Fitzpatrick J et al: *Nursing Models and Their Psychiatric Mental Health Applications.* Bowie, Md.: Robert J Brady, 1982.

Forsyth G: Analysis of the concept of empathy: Illustrations of one approach. *Advances Nurs Sci* 1980; 2:33–42.

Gill P, Atwood J: Reciprocity and helicy used to relate mEGF and wound healing. *Nurs Res* 1981; 30:68–72.

Glaser B, Strauss A: *Awareness of Dying.* Chicago: Aldine, 1965.

Glaser B, Strauss A: *Discovery of Grounded Theory.* Chicago: Aldine, 1967.

Glaser B, Strauss A: *Time for Dying.* Chicago: Aldine, 1968.

Gudmundsen AM: Conceptualization of the Neuman model for nursing practice by nursing students. Pages 265–266 in Neuman B: *The Neuman Systems Model*. Norwalk, Conn.: Appleton-Century-Crofts, 1982.

Hardy M: Evaluating nursing theory. In: *Theory Development: What? Why? How?* New York: National League for Nursing, 1978.(a)

Hardy M: Perspectives in nursing theory. *Advances Nurs Sci* 1978; 1 : 37–48.(b)

Henderson V: *The Nature of Nursing*. New York: Macmillan, 1966.

Henkel R: *Tests of Significance*. Beverly Hills: Sage, 1976.

Honigman J: The personal approach in cultural anthropological research. *Curr Anthro* 1976; 17 : 243–261.

Hutchinson S: Humor: A link to life. In: *Current Issues and Trends in Psychiatric Nursing*. Kneisl C, Wilson H (editors). St. Louis: CV Mosby, 1976.

Hutchinson S: *Survival Practices of Rescue Workers: Hidden Dimensions of Watchful Readiness*. Lanham, Md.: University Press of America, 1983.

Hutchinson S: Creating meaning out of horror. *Nurs Outlook* 1984; 32 : 86–90.

Hutchinson S: The hospital of broken dreams: A systematic investigation of a moribund psychiatric hospital. *Issues in Mental Health Nursing*, November 1984.

Jacox A: Theory construction in nursing: An overview. *Nurs Res* 1974; 23 : 4–13.

Johnson D: Development of theory: A requisite for nursing as a primary health profession. *Nurs Res* September/October 1974; 23 : 372–377.

Johnson D: The behavioral system model for nursing. In: Riehl J, Roy Sister C (editors), *Conceptual Models for Nursing Practice*. New York: Appleton-Century-Crofts, 1980.

Kaplan A: *The Conduct of Inquiry*. San Francisco: Chandler, 1964.

Kerlinger N: *Foundations of Behavioral Research*. New York: Holt, Rinehart & Winston, 1973.

Kim H: Use of Rogers' conceptual system in research: Comments. *Nurs Res* 1983; 32 : 89–91.

King I: The "why" of theory development. *Theory Development: What? Why? How?* New York: National League for Nursing, 1978.

King I: *Toward a Theory for Nursing*. New York: John Wiley, 1981.

Kuhn T: *The Structure of Scientific Revolutions*. Chicago: University of Chicago Press, 1970.

Levine M: The four conservation principles of nursing. *Nurs Forum* 1967; 6 : 45–59.

Levine M: Holistic nursing. *Nursing Clinics of North America*, 1971; 6 : 253–264.

Manderino M, Bzdek V: Effects of modeling and information on reactions to pain: A childbirth-preparation analogue. *Nurs Res* 1984; 33 : 9–14.

Meleis A et al: Toward scholarliness in doctoral dissertations: An analytical model. *Res Nurs Health* 1980; 3 : 115–124.

Meleis A: *Theoretical Nursing: Development and Progress*. Philadelphia: Lippincott, 1984.

Merton R: *Social Theory and Social Structure*. New York: Free Press, 1968.

Mills CW: *The Social Imagination*. New York: Oxford University Press, 1959.

Neuman B: *The Neuman Systems Model*. Norwalk, Conn.: Appleton-Century-Crofts, 1982.

Nightingale F: *Notes on Nursing: What It Is and What It Is Not*. Philadelphia: Lippincott, 1946.

Norris C: Restlessness: A nursing phenomenon in search of meaning. *Nurs Outlook* February 1975; 23 : 103–107.

Orem D: *Nursing: Concepts of Practice*. New York: McGraw-Hill, 1971.

Orlando IJ: *The Dynamic Nurse–Patient Relationship*. New York: Putnam, 1961.

Peplau H: *Interpersonal Relations in Nursing*. New York: Putnam, 1952.

Piaget J: *The Growth of Logical Thinking from Childhood to Adolescence*. New York: Basic Books, 1958.

Platt JR: Strong inference. *Science* 1964; 146 : 347–353.

Putnam P: Conceptual approach to nursing theory. *Nurs Sci* December 1965; 430–442.

Randolph G: Therapeutic and physical touch: Physiological responses to stressful stimuli. *Nurs Res* 1984; 33 : 31–36.

Rawnsley M: The concept of privacy. *Advances in Nursing Science* 1980; 2 : 25–31.

Reilly D: Why a conceptual framework? *Nurs Outlook* September 1975; 23 : 556–567.

Rogers M: *An Introduction to the Theoretical Basis of Nursing*. Philadelphia: FA Davis, 1970.

Rogers M: *Nurse Educators' Conference*. New York, December 1982.

Rogers M: *The Second Post-Masters' Nursing Conference.* Savannah, Ga., April 1984.

Roy Sister C: *Introduction to Nursing: An Adaptation Model.* Englewood Cliffs, N.J.: Prentice-Hall, 1976.

Stern P: Affiliating in stepfather families: Teachable strategies leading to stepfather–child friendship. *Western Journal of Nursing Research* 1982; 4: 74–83.

Stevens B: *Nursing Theory: Analysis, Application, Evaluation.* Boston: Little, Brown, 1979.

Taylor A, Skelton J, Butcher J: Duration of pain condition and physical pathology as determinants of nurses' assessments of patients in pain. *Nurs Res* 1984; 33: 4–8.

The Nursing Theories Conference Group: *Nursing Theories: The Base for Professional Nursing Practice.* Englewood Cliffs, N.J.: Prentice-Hall, 1980.

Thibodeau J: *Nursing: Analysis and Evaluation.* Monterey, Calif.: Wadsworth Health Sciences Division, 1983.

Torgerson S: *Theory and Methods of Scaling.* New York: Wiley, 1958.

Whall A: Congruence between existing theories of family functioning and nursing theories. *Advances Nurs Sci* 1980; 3: 59–67.

Wald F, Leonard R: Towards development of nursing practice theory. *Nurs Res* Fall 1964; 13: 309–313.

Weidenbach E: *Meeting the Realities in Clinical Teaching.* New York: Springer, 1969.

Wilson H: Limiting intrusion-social control of outsiders in a healing community. *Nurs Res* 1977; 26: 103–111.

Wilson H: *Deinstitutionalized Residential Care of the Mentally Disordered: The Soteria House Approach.* New York: Grune and Stratton, 1982.

Wilson H, Kneisl C: *Psychiatric Nursing,* 2nd ed. Menlo Park, Calif.: Addison-Wesley, 1983.

Yura H, Torres G: *Today's Conceptual Frameworks Within Baccalaureate Nursing Programs.* NLN publication #15-1558. New York: National League for Nursing, 1975, pp. 17–25.

Further Readings

Chenitz WC: Entry into a nursing home as status passage: A theory to guide nursing practice. *Geriatric Nurs* March–April 1983: 92–97.

Fawcett J: *Analysis and Evaluation of Conceptual Models of Nursing.* Philadelphia: FA Davis, 1984.

Galligan A: Using Roy's concepts of adaptation to care for young children. *Am J Maternal Child Nurs,* January–February 1979: 24–28.

Henderson V: *Basic Principles of Nursing Care.* Geneva, Switzerland: International Council of Nurses, 1972.

Mercer R: A theoretical framework for studying factors that impact on the maternal role. *Nurs Res* 1981; 30: 73–77.

Millor GK: A theoretical framework for nursing research in child abuse and neglect. *Nurs Res* 1981; 30: 78–83.

Neuman M: *Theory Development in Nursing.* Philadelphia: FA Davis, 1979.

Roy Sister C, Roberts S: *Theory Construction in Nursing: An Adaptation Model.* Englewood Cliffs, New Jersey: Prentice-Hall, 1981.

Stevens B: *Nursing Theory: Analysis, Application, Evaluation,* 2nd ed. Boston: Little, Brown, 1984.

Welton B: Operationalization of Martha Rogers' theory throughout the nursing process. *Internat J Nurs Studies* 1979; 16: 7–20.

Chapter 11

Collecting Data With Psychosocial Instruments

by Jane S. Norbeck RN, DNSc

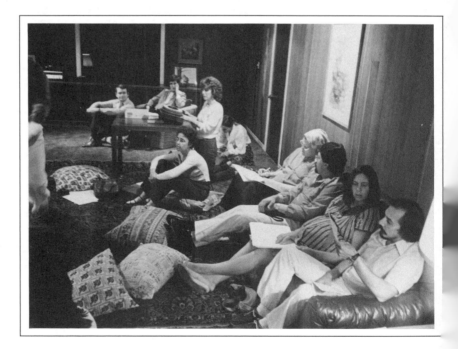

In nursing research, locus of control and social support are among the varied and extensive concepts being measured by using psychosocial instruments.

Chapter Outline

Chapter Objectives

After reading this chapter, the student should be able to:

- Discuss at least five psychological or social phenomena that can be measured by psychosocial instruments
- Classify psychosocial instruments as subjective or objective and as direct or proxy
- Develop a sample item to illustrate each of the following types of measurement: rating scale, semantic differential, sorting technique, paired comparison, patient log, ability test, test of knowledge, and projective test
- Discuss the concepts of reliability and validity and distinguish among the various types that can be established
- Evaluate a psychosocial instrument in relation to the four ideal qualities of measurement instruments, including various types of reliability and validity
- Demonstrate the ability to locate an existing instrument to measure a selected psychosocial variable by using appropriate compendia
- Discuss major reasons for conducting pilot testing of psychosocial instruments
- Evaluate an information-gathering questionnaire in relation to the four areas of decisions for evaluating questions
- Compare and contrast the advantages and disadvantages of self-administered and face-to-face methods of data collection with psychosocial instruments
- Demonstrate the ability to develop a hand-scoring or computer-scoring protocol that reduces the likelihood for error

In This Chapter . . .

We have all filled out a variety of psychosocial instruments, ranging from highly structured intelligence tests to open-ended questionnaires about a course we have completed. Perhaps you were required to participate in research in undergraduate psychology courses in which you completed large batteries of instruments. From these experiences you know that some instruments make sense and seem appropriate to the purpose; others may seem mystifying, irrelevant, or poorly developed. Some instruments are easy and even fun to complete; others may be confusing, repetitious, tedious, or annoying. These reactions are important for you to consider, because they may affect the extent or quality of your own research subjects' responses. In addition to these qualities of acceptability are the measurement properties of reliability and validity, which instruments must have to satisfy scientific standards.

This chapter, then, deals with the data-collection phase of research and examines the problems and challenges of measuring psychosocial concepts. A wide range of topics or constructs can be measured by psychosocial instruments, but many of these represent phenomena that cannot be measured directly, as can many physiological variables (see Chapter 12). Instead, instruments are developed to measure attitudes, perceptions, or self-ratings that are intended to represent the psychosocial variable.

Several thousand psychosocial instruments have been developed over the years in the fields of anthropology, nursing, psychology, and sociology. Yet every year hundreds of new instruments are developed in these fields, many times duplicating, but not necessarily improving on, previous instruments. In fact, Chun, Cobb, and French (1975) noted that 63% of the instruments in their compendium of published instruments had been used only once, and only 3% had been used ten or more times. Moreover, comparisons of the development and testing of these instruments revealed that the more frequently used measures were not qualitatively any better than the less popular ones.

Because the process of developing and testing an instrument is extensive and time consuming, your awareness of existing instruments—or sources for locating instruments—will be important in planning your research. Aside from a brief discussion about developing a questionnaire to collect specific information, this chapter considers the decisions you will make in selecting and evaluating psychosocial instruments and the actual process of administration and scoring data. Examples from specific instruments illustrate common issues that arise in planning and conducting nursing research.

Ways of Measuring With Psychosocial Instruments

The range of phenomena included in psychological and social investigation is vast, and "new" concepts are continually being created along with the development of nursing theories and theories of human behavior (see Chapter 10). Thus, it probably isn't possible to compile an

exhaustive list of topics in this field. Table 11-1 outlines major concepts or phenomena that are being measured with psychosocial instruments. In nursing many existing concepts are further refined to increase their specific relevance to nursing problems. For example, a measure of children's coping with new situations might be modified to measure children's coping with hospitalization, and the variable *locus of control* has been adapted to measure health locus of control (Wallston, Wallston, & DeVellis 1978).

To demonstrate the importance of psychosocial instruments in nursing research, I analyzed the data-gathering techniques used in all the studies published in 1983 in *Nursing Research* (Volume 32) and *Research in Nursing and Health* (Volume 6). Table 11-2 shows that of the 72 data-based articles, 78% used psychosocial instruments, compared with 12% using physiological measures and 10% using qualita-

Table 11-1   Phenomena Measured by Psychosocial Instruments

Concept or Phenomenon	Examples
Abilities	intelligence
Attitudes	political, religious
Communication	nonverbal
Coping	style
Development	infant, adolescent
Emotional states	anxiety, depression
Family functioning	cohesion, interaction
Individual functioning	activities of daily living, adjustment
Interests	vocational
Knowledge	sex information
Mental functioning	cognitive stage
Needs	affiliation, achievement
Occupational functioning	job stress
Personality	traits
Role	conflict
Self-concept	ideal versus actual self
Sociometric standing	social class, popularity
Social behavior	social network, social skills
Social environment	ward atmosphere
Stress	recent life events
Values	moral, interpersonal
Well-being	life satisfaction

Table 11-2   Analysis of Data-Gathering Methods in Published Nursing Research

Data-Gathering Method	Number of Studies	Percentage
Psychosocial instruments	56	77.7
Psychosocial qualitative methods	7	9.7
Physiological measures	9	12.5

SOURCE: All studies published in 1983 by *Nursing Research* (Vol 32) and *Research in Nursing and Health* (Vol 6). Total number of articles: 81; Number of data-based articles: 72.

tive methods, such as content analysis and field methods (see Chapter 13). Other conclusions drawn from analysis of these published articles will be discussed later in the chapter.

Objective and Subjective Measurement

Many of the concepts in Table 11-1, such as well-being or coping, can be measured either objectively or subjectively. If you wanted an *objective measure* of patients' understanding of the teaching they had received about their diagnosis and treatment, you might administer a written or oral test with items about the material covered in the teaching. You would obtain a *subjective measure* if you asked them questions face to face or in a questionnaire about their perception of the adequacy of their knowledge of their diagnosis and treatment. Because of the nature of many psychosocial phenomena, observational methods of behavior would be required to obtain objective measures. Instead, self-report measures are often used to obtain subjective appraisals of these psychosocial variables. Subjective appraisals are consistent with many theoretical approaches in nursing and the social sciences. For example, the stress and coping theory of Lazarus (1966) emphasizes the individual's *appraisal* of the situation rather than an outside view of how stressful a given event or demand may be. In this view, there can be no objective determination of the stressfulness of particular events, because similar events or demands are actually different for different individuals (see Chapter 1).

Certain of the psychosocial variables listed in Table 11-1 can be measured directly. For example, you can obtain a *direct measure* of a person's age, income, years of education, or number of children. The vast majority of psychosocial variables cannot be measured directly, however, and a *proxy measure*—a measure or count of something that stands for an object or quality—is developed to represent the construct. Thus, for example, the number of items describing anxious behaviors or feeling states that a person checks as applicable at a given time is taken as a proxy measure for the person's actual anxiety level. Extensive testing of such instruments should be done to validate that the items do indeed measure the intended construct. In the case of anxiety measures, the psychometric testing to establish validity has included correlations between the questionnaire score and physiological measures of anxiety, comparisons of scores between psychiatric patients and nonpatients, and anxiety-arousing experiments in which pre- and posttesting scores are used to demonstrate that the score on the anxiety questionnaire does indeed increase after the anxiety-arousing experience. Different types of validity and ways to establish them will be discussed later in the chapter.

Looking again at the analysis of published studies in nursing, Table 11-3 shows that most of the measurement of psychosocial variables was done with proxy measures. Of the 125 psychosocial instruments used, only 7% were direct measures of actual behavior. Examples of direct measurement included analysis of vocal behavior—for example, pauses, laughter, and interruptions—reported by Hurley (1983); analysis of verbal communication patterns by Kishi (1983); and measurement of falling asleep behaviors of hospitalized children (White, Wear, & Stephenson 1983).

The remaining 116 instruments (93%) used proxy measures for a wide variety of variables, such as anxiety, interpersonal needs, job satisfaction, locus of control, perceptions of well-being, quality of life, and many other variables. Of these, 89% were measured by rating scales and the rest by a variety of methods that will be discussed in the next section.

Types of Measure Frequently Used

Many forms of question are used in psychosocial instruments. Some are similar in format to those commonly used in educational testing: true–false, multiple-choice, short-answer, and open-

Table 11-3   Type of Data-Gathering Method Used in 56 Psychosocial Nursing Studies[a]

Data-Gathering Method	Number of Instruments	Percentage
Direct measurement	9	7.2
Proxy measurement	116	92.8
Types of proxy instrument:		
Rating scales	103	88.8
Tests of knowledge, ability, or performance	9	7.8
Sorting[b]	(3)	
Behavioral log	2	1.7
Semantic differential	1	.9
Ranking	1	.9
	116	100.1

[a]Based on the analysis of all published research in two nursing research journals for 1983 (see Table 11-2 for details).

[b]Sorting techniques in these studies were used as preliminary methods and not in the resulting instruments administered to study subjects.

ended essay questions. These four types of question are useful for obtaining factual information and for testing a person's ability or knowledge. The questions in Box 11-1, developed for a demographic data checksheet, are examples.

In addition, several types of scale have been developed for psychosocial testing, particularly to assess attitudes, interests, and values. Commonly used scales are based on rank-ordering a list of stimuli, sorting stimuli into categories, making comparisons between pairs of objects or stimuli (paired comparisons), and rating techniques. Of these, rating techniques are most frequently used in psychosocial instruments, and they were used in the vast majority of the nursing studies described in Table 11.3. Each of these scales will be described, along with examples of their use in nursing research.

Commonly Used Rating Scales   Several formats are used in creating scales for rating a set of items, but each involves selecting a step in a scale that can be assigned a numerical value. Figure 11-1 illustrates variations of graphic and numeri-

cal scales. Rating scales also vary in the number of steps provided for responses. Only two steps are used for bipolar adjectives (for example, *effective* or *ineffective*), whereas 10 steps might be required for a rating scale based on percentages—for example, "for each item, estimate the percentage of time you spent in each activity." Whether an odd or even number of steps is preferable depends upon dual considerations: is the middle (neutral or uncertain) step important to measure, or would this step encourage noncommittal responses and thereby reduce the discriminating power of the data? An even number of steps is usually preferable for scales that range across opposite dimensions (for example, from *agree* to *disagree*), thus forcing the respondent to select either *slightly agree* or *slightly disagree*.

Instruments based on scaling techniques usually have several items to be rated for each construct. (As you will recall from Chapters 4 and 10, a *construct* is a concept used in a theory to account for relationships in observable events.) The ratings for each item are added to obtain a score for the construct. This method of measure-

---

Box 11-1   Sample Questions From Demographic Data Checksheet

A. Multiple-Choice Questions

1. Sex

   _____ 1. male

   _____ 2. female

2. Marital status

   _____ 1. single,
   never
   married

   _____ 2. married

   _____ 3. divorced
   or
   separated

   _____ 4. widowed

B. Short-Answer Questions

3. What is your

   age? _____

4. How many years of
   education have you
   completed beyond high

   school? _____

C. True–False Question

5. Are you currently
   employed?

   _____ 1. yes

   _____ 2. no

D. Open-Ended Essay Question

6. Describe the most
   stressful aspect of your
   current or most recent
   employed position.

   _____

   _____

   _____

---

ment is referred to as a *Likert scale* after the person who developed it for use in measuring attitudes.

An example of a rating scale that is used frequently in nursing research is the State–Trait Anxiety Inventory (STAI), an instrument with 20 items to measure state anxiety (transitory responses) and 20 items to measure trait anxiety (stable individual differences in anxiety-proneness) (Spielberger 1983). Each item describes a particular aspect of anxious behavior or feelings. This type of scale is also called a summative instrument, because the ratings for each item are added to obtain the score. Because some of the items may have been worded negatively to avoid creating a *response set*—that is, a tendency to respond to items in a consistent manner based on an irrelevant criterion, such as responding *true* to all items in a true–false test or agreeing with all the statements that appear to be more "socially desirable" than others—the scores for the negative items are reversed in scoring so that the scores for all of the items have the same meaning (high anxiety). After making this correction, the ratings from all 20 items are added to obtain the anxiety score. Because anxiety is an abstract concept with many defining features, it is important to have several items, including both anxious behaviors and conscious feelings, to increase the likelihood of measuring all of the variations that might occur among individual subjects.

Other Types of Scale or Measure   Another type of rating scale technique is the *semantic differential*, which is typically used to measure attitudes. The concept or object to be rated is written at the top of a page, followed by a list of bipolar adjectives (*responsible* and *irresponsible*, *bad* and *good*). The respondent rates the concept or object along a seven-point scale for each adjective pair. If more than one concept or object is subjected to the same list of adjective pairs, comparisons of attitudes can be made based on the ratings. For example, Muhlenkamp, Waller, and Bourne (1983) compared the

1. Graphic Scales Without Numbers

Completely agree _/_ _/_ _/_ _/_ _/_ _____ Completely disagree

| Not at all effective | Slightly effective | Moderately effective | Very effective | Extremely effective |

2. Graphic Scale With Numbers

Completely agree _/_ _/_ _/_ _/_ _/_ Completely disagree
1   2   3   4   5   6

3. Numerical Scales

1. Completely agree	a. extremely well
2. Mostly agree	b. very well
3. Slightly agree	c. fairly well
4. Slightly disagree	d. hardly at all
5. Mostly disagree	e. not at all
6. Completely disagree	(numbers implied)

4. Numerical Scale Expressed in Percentages

0   10   20   30   40   50   60   70   80   90

Figure 11-1 Types of rating scale.

attitudes of women toward menopausal women, nonmenopausal women, and males by comparing the ratings on 15 pairs of adjectives for each of these stimulus objects.

Sorting techniques involve giving respondents a stack of cards with one item per card and asking them to sort them into piles based on some specified dimension (for example, difficulty level or attractiveness). Respondents may be free to develop as many piles as they wish, with as many or few cards in each pile as they choose, or these decisions may be predetermined by the researcher. The *Q-sort* is an example of a constrained sorting technique, in which respon-

dents are limited to a certain number of items at the extreme ends of the continuum of the piles but can place more items in the middle ranges. This method yields a normal distribution of responses, and the items that the respondent most strongly agrees or disagrees with are identified. Jacobson (1983) describes a modified Q-sort in which Neonatal Intensive Care Unit (NICU) nurses sorted 52 incidents describing stressful experiences in neonatal intensive care nursing into categories of most to least stressful. The results of the sorting were used to identify the high and low stress incidents for subsequent study of coping strategies.

Similar to sorting techniques, *ranking techniques* involve considering a set of stimuli in relationship to other items in the set. Respondents are asked to rank-order the objects or stimuli on the basis of some property. Because only one item is assigned for each rank, however, a smaller number of stimuli can be accommodated than with sorting techniques. An example of a ranking task is to ask students to rank from one to ten the most important features of a course that should be retained if the course were to be revised. The list of ten stimuli to be ranked might include specific readings, films, lecture topics, or simulated experiences.

An example of a modified ranking procedure used in a study of factors related to the selection of an obstetrician is reported by Brien, Haverfield, and Shanteau (1983). Expectant parents were given a list of 24 items and asked to rank the 4 most important items with a value of 1, the 4 second most important with a value of 2, and so on. Although this was a paper-and-pencil test, it actually was more like a sorting technique than a ranking technique, because the items were ranked into groups of four rather than having each item higher or lower than every other item.

The method of *paired comparisons* involves asking people to choose between two objects or stimuli in each of a series of items. All possible pairs of the items are presented, to allow for comparisons of the relative values of each item in relation to each other item. This technique is often used in studying a person's values or interests.

A method that has emerged in recent reports of nursing research is the use of *patient logs* to record data on a daily (or more frequent) basis. These logs may vary from open-ended to highly structured checklists—for example, of symptoms, food choices, or moods. Woods (1981) outlined several potential uses as well as problems in the use of patient logs. She indicated that more research is needed to determine which types of variable are best suited to this approach.

A recent use of patient logs was reported by Hayter (1983). Two types of structured record were kept by patients to study sleep behaviors of older persons: a record of usual sleep-related activities during a 24-hour period—time for arising, naps, total time in bed, and so on—and a chart of sleep–awake state for each 30-minute period of the 24 hours.

Intelligence tests, achievement tests, skill tests, and many other types of *ability test* are used to study certain psychosocial variables. Some of these tests are developed for use in educational, vocational, or counseling settings. These tests are often highly developed measures that have normative data available for various population subgroups. In a nursing study of the effects of the 12-hour shift, the signs of fatigue were studied by using a reasoning test and a vital signs performance test (Mills, Arnold, & Wood 1983).

Tests of knowledge are probably most familiar to you because of your long history of taking examinations. When used in nursing research, tests of knowledge usually involve either the nursing knowledge required of practitioners or the knowledge of health behaviors required by patients. In a study of adolescent contraceptive use (Marcy, Brown, & Danielson 1983), knowledge of sex and contraception was determined by the Sex Knowledge Test, which had been developed to evaluate sex education programs in high schools.

Projective tests have had limited use in nursing research. They were developed for use in psychiatric diagnosis or psychological evaluation. These tests are based on the premise that unconscious material is not readily accessible to most people but that this material is often "projected" onto ambiguous stimuli. Thus, the skilled clinician can interpret the symbolic meaning in patients' responses to these stimuli and learn about their emotional needs, conflicts, and personality. Because extensive training is required to learn how to interpret the data from these tests, their use in research is limited.

Ideal Qualities of a Measurement Instrument

After the study problem and design have been clearly developed (Chapter 9), a series of decisions about how to measure the identified variables must be made. In exploratory studies the variables pertinent to the study question may not yet be known, and the researcher is likely to use open-ended methods for collecting data (Chapter 13). In studies that build on previous findings or that are designed to test theoretical propositions, however, specific variables are defined in the research question and hypotheses. Decisions about the measurement of psychosocial variables should take into account four general considerations:

1. the congruence of the measurement instrument or approach with the variable to be measured
2. the psychometric properties of the instrument
3. the feasibility of using a particular instrument within the research plan
4. the acceptability of the measurement instrument or approach to the study respondents

Each of these considerations is taken up below.

Congruence With Variable to Be Measured

Many psychosocial instruments are developed within the context of a theoretical framework for interpreting the meaning of the construct to be measured. Thus, an instrument to measure clinically significant indicators of depression in psychiatric practice might not be a valid measure of depressive mood states in nonpsychiatric populations. For example, many scales of depression include the "vegetative" symptoms of depression, including appetite and sleep distur-bances. Because these symptoms are frequently associated with normal pregnancy, such items would spuriously increase the depression scores for pregnant women. An instrument that tested only depressive mood would be preferable for this clinical group.

Another problem in assessing the congruence of the construct with the variable identified in the study problem stems from the lack of agreement on the definitions or components of many psychosocial constructs. Depending on theoretical definitions, self-concept can be seen as distinct from or similar to self-esteem. Many instruments to measure self-concept or self-esteem exist, but they differ in what aspects of the larger construct they actually measure.

The State–Trait Anxiety Inventory described above is a good example of the refinement of measurement to keep pace with conceptual development in the field. Before the development of the STAI, anxiety measures combined transitory anxiety states and the more enduring anxiety-proneness trait in single measures of anxiety. Many research studies now specify one or the other form of anxiety from the STAI as the operationalized version of the concept of anxiety based on the theoretical model that was used to guide variable selection for the research.

Psychometric Properties of the Instrument

Beyond the theoretical considerations described above, any instrument used in research should have at least minimal levels of reliability and validity established. Box 11-2 outlines the usual types of reliability and validity that are tested in the development of an instrument. *Reliability* of measurement refers to the consistency, accuracy, and precision of the measures taken. *Validity* refers to relevance: does the instrument really

Box 11-2   *Types of Reliability and Validity Testing*

I. *Reliability Estimates*
    A. Test–retest reliability
    B. Parallel forms; alternate forms
    C. Internal consistency: split halves
II. *Validity Estimates*
    A. Content validity
        1. Face validity
        2. Logical, or sampling, validity
    B. Criterion-related validity
        1. Predictive-validity coefficient
        2. Concurrent-validity coefficient
    C. Construct validity
        1. Group differences
        2. Changes
        3. Correlations
        4. Processes
        5. Multitrait–multimethod
        6. Factorial validity

SOURCE: Adapted from *Introduction to Measurement Theory*, by M. J. Allen and W. M. Yen. © Copyright 1979 by Wadsworth, Inc. Reprinted by permission of Brooks/Cole Publishing Company, Monterey, Calif.

measure what it claims to measure? Because so much of the measurement of psychosocial variables involves proxy measures, considerations of reliability and validity are very important in nursing research. In fact, even well-designed research is unlikely to be published in scientific journals if the psychometric properties of the measurement strategies cannot be demonstrated.

Reliability   What constitutes minimal levels of psychometric testing of an instrument? Considering reliability, we want assurance that, as with a ruler, we will obtain the same reading each time the measurement is used (unless a "real" change in the value has occurred). This type of reliability is usually established by administering the instrument on two or more occasions to the same respondents with a time interval long enough to avoid carryover effects and short enough to avoid actual changes in the construct that is being measured. This is called *test–retest reliability*.

If more than one version of an instrument is developed, *parallel-forms*, or *alternate-forms*, *reliability* is determined by comparing scores from the various versions for equivalence. Additionally, we want assurance that the items within the instrument are all working in relatively the same way—that is, are consistent with one another. This type of reliability, *internal consistency reliability*, is usually tested by comparing parts of the instrument with one another. In the *split-half reliability* testing method, half of the test is compared with the other half. Or each item may be compared with the entire set of items through statistical procedures such as coefficient alpha, which calculates the reliability of the whole test. Depending on the nature of the measurement instrument, certain statistical methods of estimating reliability are more appropriate than others; these considerations are discussed in detail in standard texts on measurement theory (for example, Allen & Yen 1979).

Validity   Minimal levels of validity cannot be specified for all cases, because the appropriate methods will vary for different types of instrument. It can be stated, however, that *content validity*, although necessary, is not a sufficient indication that the instrument actually measures what it is intended to measure, because it is based on subjective judgments. Content validity includes subjective judgments about face validity and logical or sampling validity.

Face validity involves subjective judgments by experts or respondents about the degree to which the test appears to measure the relevant construct. This assessment is sometimes called "armchair" validity, because it does not involve actual use of the instrument to evaluate its performance.

Logical, or *sampling*, *validity* refers to the extent that the items in a test adequately represent the content of the topic or construct covered in the test. It is usually established by having experts in the field evaluate the congruence between the construct and the instrument, including whether all aspects of the topic or construct are covered.

If you wanted to establish the content validity of an instrument to measure job stress in critical-care nursing, you might have experts in job stress *and* critical-care nurses evaluate the face validity of the instrument. To establish logical, or sampling, validity, however, you would determine the categories of job stress in critical-care nursing identified in the literature and have experts evaluate the extent to which your items covered these categories, as well as theoretical aspects of job stress in general.

At least one type of criterion-related validity or construct validity (see below) is also needed beyond content validity to give *minimal* assurance that the instrument may be valid. And in addition to internal consistency reliability, test–retest reliability should be established. Further analysis of the published studies in nursing described in Tables 11-2 and 11-3 was done to explore the extent to which nursing research

meets this standard. Table 11-4 shows that in studies that made use of existing instruments, 68.6% of the instruments met this standard (the sum of levels 3, 4, and 5). In studies that made use of an "investigator-developed" instrument designed for that study, however, only 3% of the instruments met the standard.

Criterion-related validity refers to the extent that the score on the instrument can be related to a criterion (the behavior that the instrument is supposed to predict). As shown in Box 11-2, criterion-related validity may be either *predictive* or *concurrent*, depending on when the criterion variable is measured. If the criterion measure is obtained at the same time as the measurement under study, concurrent validity is assessed. If the criterion measure is obtained at some future time (after the predictor instrument was used), predictive validity is assessed. For both types, the correlation between the instrument and the criterion measure is used as the criterion-related validity coefficient. For example, in a study of the effects of job stress on job satisfaction, concurrent validity would be tested through the correlation between the job-stress

Table 11-4   Types of Reliability and Validity Established for 116 Psychosocial Instruments[a]

Type of Instrument	Percentage at Each Psychometric Level[b]					
	0	1	2	3	4	5
Existing instrument (n = 86)	8.1	16.3	7.0	40.7	15.1	12.8
Instrument developed for study[c] (n = 30)	73.3	16.7	6.7	3.3	0	0

[a]Based on the analysis of published research in two nursing research journals for 1983 (See Tables 11.2 and 11.3).

[b]Ratings of Psychometric Levels are as follows:
  0 = No reliability or validity established.
  1 = Content validity and/or coefficient alpha reported.
  2 = In addition to Level 1, reliability testing includes test–retest reliability.
  3 = In addition to Level 2, one other type of validity beyond content validity has been established.
  4 = In addition to Level 2, two or more additional types of validity beyond content validity have been established.
  5 = In addition to Level 4, extensive psychometric testing, including establishing normative data, has been completed.

[c]Excluding cases in which instrument development and testing was the focus of the article.

measure and a job-satisfaction measure. Predictive validity might be tested through the correlation between the job stress measure and *subsequent* job turnover.

Construct validity refers to the degree to which an instrument measures the theoretical construct or trait that it was designed to measure. It can be assessed in several ways but never definitively established. Predictions of group differences in scores for "known groups" can be tested to validate an aspect of construct validity. For example, a test of developmental stages in the acquisition of certain cognitive structures can be administered to children of different ages. If the children in the younger age groups perform significantly worse than children in older age groups, some evidence of the validity of the developmental aspect of the construct has been established. Several other methods for testing construct validity exist. One is the complex multitrait–multimethod validity testing developed by Campbell and Fiske (1959) to establish *convergent* (highly related to measurement of the same trait by a different method) and *discriminant* (unrelated to the scores from tests measuring different traits) validity. As in the case of reliability testing, standard texts on measurement theory provide detailed descriptions of the various methods for establishing validity (for example, Allen & Yen 1979).

Feasibility Within the Research Plan

Thus far, we have considered theoretical and psychometric qualities of measurement instruments. Practical considerations must also be taken into account, because the instrument is used in a larger context that may influence its appropriateness. The research plan specifies how subjects will be recruited and tested. The various methods of approaching subjects differ in the amount of face-to-face contact, the opportunity for explanation or clarification, the time and setting for completing the materials, and many other facets of the data-gathering process.

Consider the differences between receiving a packet of questionnaires in the mail and sitting down with a researcher who is available to answer questions about the various instruments. On the one hand, instruments with complex instructions may not be filled out appropriately or completely if the respondent cannot obtain help or is subject to frequent interruptions. On the other hand, the anonymity of the mails may increase the likelihood that respondents will provide sensitive information such as income level, sexual orientation, or drug habits.

Another aspect of the research context to consider when selecting a measurement instrument is the overall data-gathering plan. Other variables are often measured at the same time. Not only must the overall time of the testing session be within reasonable limits, to prevent fatigue effects, but how the various instruments might influence one another must be taken into account. For example, if one instrument in the battery measures attitudes toward handicapped children and another measures attitudes toward public expenditures for health and welfare, the responses to the second instrument might be influenced by the feelings evoked by thinking about handicapped children.

All instruments administered at the same time need to be compatible in their method of administration. For example, a Q-sort, which requires the presence of the research assistant, would not be possible in a mailed self-administered method. It is possible, however, to combine methods if more than one contact is planned with the respondents. Thus, a battery of self-administered questionnaires can be mailed to the respondent, followed (or preceded) by a face-to-face interview or testing session.

Acceptability to Respondents

Another practical issue for consideration is how the subjects are likely to respond to the measurement instrument that is selected for use in the study. Obviously, the instrument must be appropriate for the literacy and educational level of the respondents. Constructs that are likely to vary in specific content or expression for different cultural, ethnic, age, or sex groups should be measured with instruments that have been validated for the intended population in the study.

Less obvious, but equally important, is the fit between the implied values or sensitivities of the instrument and what would be considered acceptable to the respondents. For example, an attitude scale that seems to emphasize conservative attitudes might be regarded as irrelevant to college-age respondents who might refuse to answer parts or all of the questionnaire. This problem becomes particularly acute when the format of the questionnaire involves forced choices between pairs of alternatives, neither of which seems acceptable.

Some instruments have built-in devices to evaluate test-taking behavior. For example, consistency of responses is checked by presenting the same question more than once in the instrument and comparing the responses. Other devices attempt to assess the tendency for the respondent to "fake good" or "fake bad," as in psychological tests that assess personality or functioning. Respondents differ in their tolerance for these techniques, and they may refuse to complete the instrument if they find these features too annoying.

Selecting an Instrument

Locating Suitable Instruments

Considering the great diversity of concepts or phenomena that might be measured in nursing and psychosocial research and the wide range of potential population groups that might be studied, is it likely that an instrument already exists to measure the variables the researcher has identified in the study problem and design? From the proliferation of "investigator-developed" instruments described in research articles, one would doubt that relevant instruments existed in the majority of cases. This conclusion is usually not warranted, however. A conservative estimate of the number of psychosocial instruments that have been developed and tested to some extent over the last several decades is between 5000 and 8000. These instruments vary widely in the soundness of their theoretical basis and the extent that reliability and validity have been established. *Nonetheless, a great deal of unnecessary effort is expended in research because of the failure of investigators to search thoroughly for available instruments.*

Instruments developed for many nursing studies—particularly those that never reach publication—are often not subjected to adequate reliability and validity testing. Another problem stemming from the proliferation of new instruments is that comparison of findings from study to study is difficult if similar constructs are measured by many different instruments.

Sources of Information About Existing Instruments Several important resources have been developed to help investigators locate instruments. These compendia differ in the type of information they provide and their method of use. Table 11-5 summarizes the features of key resources. Depending on the type of variable that is to be measured, some resources are more useful than others. For example, if the variable is an attitude, the book by Shaw and Wright (1967), which specifically deals with attitude measures, might be the most useful in locating an instrument.

The resources that provide detailed information about the instruments, sometimes including

Table II-5   Key Compendia for Locating Psychosocial Instruments [a]

Title or Author of Compilation	Number of Entries	Type and Amount of Information
Tests in Print III (Mitchell 1983)	2672	Brief description of test and citations for reviews and applications
Mental Measurements Year-book (Buros 1978; Mitchell in press). Monthly updates online from Bibliographic Retrieval Service.	1184	Critical reviews on new and revised instruments (8th edition has 898 reviews); same as *Tests in Print* for other instruments
Bonjean et al (1967)	2080	Brief descriptions for 47 instruments; citations for the other instruments
Cattell and Warburton (1967)	612	Descriptions of each instrument and its use
Chun, Cobb, and French (1975)	3000	Citations of original sources and applications
Comrey, Backer, and Glaser (1973)	1100	Brief description of instrument, reliability, and validity
Johnson and Bommarito (1971); Johnson (1976)	1200	Description of instrument, reliability, and validity; sample items
Robinson and Shaver (1973)	127	Complete instrument; description of instrument, reliability, and validity; evaluation
Shaw and Wright (1967)	176	Complete instrument; description of instrument, reliability, and validity; evaluation
Straus and Brown (1978)	813	Description of instrument, reliability, and validity; sample items
Sweetland and Keyser (1983)	3000	Description of instrument
Ward and Fetler (1979) Ward, Lindeman, and Bloch (1979)	118 140	Complete instrument; description of instrument, reliability, and validity; evaluation

[a] For details and other sources, see Compendia of Psychosocial Instruments at the end of this chapter.

complete copies, are the easiest to use, because the suitability of the instrument can be evaluated without having to locate other references. At the other extreme, the book by Chun, Cobb, and French (1975) provides only references for instruments, and one must locate the references to obtain information about the instrument and its use. Although this book is more difficult to use, it has so many entries that it may be superior in determining whether any instruments exist to measure a construct.

Two resources are of particular relevance to nurse researchers: *Instruments for Measuring Nursing Practice and Other Health Care Variables* (Ward, Lindeman, & Bloch 1979) and *Instruments for Use in Nursing Education Research* (Ward & Fetler 1979). These books provide both descriptive and evaluative information about the instruments, as well as copies of each instrument. Together they describe over 250 instruments used in nursing research. A sample of the descriptive information provided for each instrument appears in Box 11-3.

Searching for an Instrument When the variable to be measured has been clearly delineated, the researcher should conduct a systematic search to locate an existing instrument by following these steps:

1. If the variable falls into a special category, compendia that feature specialized instruments, such as measures for use with children, should be consulted first.
2. The next resource to consult would generally be the current edition of *Tests in Print* or other compendia that index a wide variety of published instruments.
3. Compendia that index unpublished instruments should be consulted next.
4. Recent instruments might be located by using citation abstracts for works that have not yet been compiled in compendia (for example, *Psychological Abstracts*, *Index to Nursing Literature*).

In addition to whole instruments that measure the variable, your search should include instruments that might measure the variable as a *subscale*, one of several specific measures that contribute to a broader measure. Personality tests, such as the Minnesota Multiphasic Personality Inventory (MMPI), for example, often measure a number of elements in the construct of personality that are labeled as subscales, such as paranoia or depression. Tests that measure needs often have subscales for each of the needs postulated—for example, need for affiliation, need for control, and need for achievement. The subscales are usually imbedded in the instrument in such a way that the entire instrument must be administered in order to be valid. In these cases,

though, only the subscale that measures the variable you want to study needs to be scored.

Evaluating Instruments

When appropriate instruments have been located, they should be evaluated according to the qualities described earlier in this chapter. Some compendia provide evaluative information about the psychometric properties of the instruments. Others range from providing no information to summarizing the available data on reliability and validity for the user to evaluate.

If the instrument was listed in *Tests in Print*, it is likely that detailed reviews have been published in one or more of the editions of *Mental Measurements Yearbook*. These reviews not only summarize available information on reliability and validity but also compare the instrument with others in the field. The manuals that are developed for published instruments provide information about psychometric testing, but this information must be evaluated by the prospective user, because it is usually presented in a favorable light to promote marketing of the instrument.

In addition to evaluating the instrument itself, you must also assess the appropriateness of the instrument for the intended study population and the method of administration. In my work with single parents and pregnant women, for example, instruments designed to measure stress from the accumulation of recent life events tended to be sex-biased and lacked many items of particular relevance for women (Norbeck 1984). This is not surprising in view of the fact that the early instruments in this field were developed for use with naval shipboard personnel.

A common mistake in instrument selection is to assume that an instrument is sound because it is widely used. Certainly, many widely used instruments are excellent, but worth needs to be determined on a case-by-case basis. For example, the Edwards Personal Preference Schedule, which produces subscales for 15 needs, is

Box 11-3 Descriptive Information of Instrument

Key Concepts: Functions; preparedness; proficiency

Title: ADN GRADUATE LEVEL OF FUNCTIONS

Author: PRIMM, Peggy L.

Variables

Degree of preparedness or level of functioning of graduates of AD nursing degree programs as perceived by the directors and faculty of such programs

Description

Nature and Content:

There are two forms of the instrument. The form for faculty members asks respondents to answer the questions according to their perception of what is being taught in their associate degree nursing (ADN) program. The form for program directors asks that they respond with reference to the written goals and objectives of their nursing education programs.

The first 53 items are identical for the two forms—24 four-category rating-scale items address graduate nurses' levels of functioning with responses representing the following hierarchy: (1) task-oriented non-evaluative behavior; (2) an increasing amount of assessment of the task; (3) an evaluation of the need for, outcome of, or effeccctiveness of the nursing task; and (4) feedback or change in planning on the basis of evaluation. The items are grouped into three subscales identified on the instrument reproduced here, i.e., communication, care, and management. Six items deal with the amount of time judged to be required for graduates to become competent for various nursing roles. Eight items ask whether the ADN program graduate is competent to function in various agencies. Fifteen questions ask if the ADN program graduate is competent to function in various hospital units. On the form to be completed by program directors, one question asks the numbers of years of experience needed as a hospital staff nurse before taking a teaching position in an ADN program. Five forced-choice items address types of courses relevant to preparation for a position as an ADN program faculty member. The remaining items address various background characteristics of the respondent.

Administration and Scoring:

Self-administered, requiring 15 to 20 minutes for completion. Information relevant to scoring procedure was not provided.

Development

Rationale:

The instrument was based on program outcomes as perceived by faculty currently teaching in ADN programs and on program objectives as perceived by directors of the same programs. It was designed to measure the similarity of current programs with the original ADN program proposal by Montag (1) and the congruence of expectations held by faculty and directors within and between programs.

Source of Items:

Items addressing levels of functioning were based on statements of nursing functions found in the relevant literature.

Box 11-3 (continued)

Procedure:

Items addressing levels of functioning were pilot tested three times to: (1) obtain agreement that the functions were common and noncontroversial to the role of nursing in a general hospital setting; (2) ensure agreement on the hierarchy of behavioral levels; and (3) improve clarity, appropriateness, and completeness. The 24 resulting scales were grouped into three categories: patient care, management/leadership, and communication. One scale, number 3, did not fit into one of these categories but was retained because of its importance to the study's purposes (2).

Reliability and Validity

Internal consistency reliability estimates of the 24 levels of functioning subscale items were assessed using a convenience sample of 251 faculty and 36 program directors. Reported alpha values were: .76 for the communication subscale; .88 for the care subscale; .74 for the management subscale.

Some degree of content validity is ensured by the procedures used for the development of the instrument and the source of the items.

Use in Nursing Education Research

Primm (2) developed and used the instrument in her doctoral research of ADN program outcomes. Her sample included faculty members and program directors of 41 ADN programs in 5 midwestern states and Dr. Mildred Montag. The purposes of her study were to compare responses across and between programs, to compare faculty and administrator responses with Montag's, and to compare responses with findings in the literature on ADN programs.

Comments

Some researchers may find that the instrument contains content not relevant for their purposes, especially items following the initial 24 levels of functioning items. Some of the rating choices should be made more homogeneous in content and should be edited accordingly. Item analysis can be used to refine items and options within each subsection.

The reliability data are encouraging but need to be assessed by other users in other situations with different respondents.

References

1. Montag, Mildred L. *The education of nursing technicians*. New York: Wiley, 1951.
2. Primm, Peggy L. *Faculty/administrators' perceptions of associate degree nursing graduates functional levels*. Unpublished doctoral dissertation, University of Iowa, 1978.

Contact for Information

Peggy L. Primm, R.N., Ph.D.
Division of Nursing
Marycrest College
Davenport, Iowa 52804

SOURCE: From P. L. Primm, "ADN Graduate Level of Functions." In M. J. Ward and M. E. Fetler, *Instruments for Use in Nursing Education Research*. Boulder, Colo.: Western Interstate Commission for Higher Education, 1979, pp. 1–2.

consistently one of the most widely used instruments listed in the *Mental Measurements Yearbook* series. But the critical reviews over the years clearly state that the validity testing for this instrument is sketchy and inadequate (Heilbrun 1972, McKee 1972).

Instruments With Incomplete Psychometric Data

What if you locate an instrument that appears to measure the variable that you want to study, but the instrument has not been tested sufficiently to establish its reliability and validity? In such a case, you may decide to conduct some testing to validate the instrument. The type and amount of testing required will depend on what was established by the author of the instrument or by other researchers who have subsequently used it. Naturally, before investing time and effort in testing an existing instrument, you should have confidence in its design and content. Nonetheless, it is certainly easier to complete areas of psychometric testing on a partially established instrument than to develop items and test all aspects of reliability and validity for a new instrument.

Pilot Testing

When you locate an instrument that meets the criteria of theoretical congruence, psychometric adequacy, feasibility, and acceptability, you should pilot-test it to validate these judgments. Pilot testing can establish:

1. exactly how long it takes to complete the instrument or battery of instruments
2. whether any instructions are not clear
3. whether subjects find anything objectionable or inappropriate about the instrument

Subjects' responses to the questionnaires should be elicited to learn whether there are any other unanticipated problems with the instrument that has been selected. Potential problems in scoring the data from the instrument can also be detected and corrected at this stage. Fox and Ventura (1983) list 23 issues that can be addressed in a small-scale trial run of the study instrument and outline 15 suggestions to maximize the benefits in conducting this testing. This excellent methodological reference should be consulted when you plan these preliminary steps of your research to avoid carrying unnecessary faults and problems into the actual study.

Developing a Questionnaire

It is beyond the scope of this chapter to describe the complex process of developing an instrument to measure a nursing construct. Standard textbooks on measurement theory and instrument development should be used, in conjunction with statistical consultation, to develop a systematic plan to develop and test any new instrument.

In many research questions, however, there are situations in which information of a more factual or discrete nature is needed. You can develop a questionnaire designed to elicit this specific information. Although this type of information gathering is more straightforward

than measurement of complex psychosocial constructs, the questionnaire should still be pretested with respondents similar to those who will eventually be used in the research.

A useful checklist has been developed by Selltiz, Wrightsman, and Cook (1976) for evaluating questions that have been developed for a questionnaire. This checklist identifies four areas of decisions about the construction of the questionnaire that should be considered:

1. decisions about question content
2. decisions about question wording

3. decisions about the form of the response requested
4. decisions about the sequence of questions in the questionnaire

The questions these authors pose for each of these areas are listed below. The authors also present a detailed discussion about each question, with examples and suggestions.*

A. Decisions about question content
   1. Is this question necessary? Just how will it be useful?
   2. Are several questions needed on the subject of this question?
   3. Do respondents have the information necessary to answer the question?
   4. Docs the question need to be more concrete, specific, and closely related to the respondent's personal experience?
   5. Is the question content sufficiently general and free from spurious concreteness and specificity?
   6. Do the replies express general attitudes and only seem to be as specific as they sound?
   7. Is the question content biased or loaded in one direction, without accompanying questions to balance the emphasis?
   8. Will the respondents give the information that is asked for?

B. Decisions about question wording
   1. Can the question be misunderstood? Does it contain difficult or unclear phraseology?
   2. Does the question adequately express the alternatives with respect to the point?
   3. Is the question misleading because of unstated assumptions or unseen implications?

   4. Is the wording biased? Is it emotionally loaded or slanted toward a particular kind of answer?
   5. Is the question wording likely to be objectionable to the respondent in any way?
   6. Would a more personalized or less personalized wording of the question produce better results?
   7. Can the question be asked better in a more direct or a more indirect form?

C. Decisions about form of response to the question
   1. Can the question best be asked in a form calling for a check answer (or short answer of a word or two, or a number), free answer, or check answer with follow-up answer?
   2. If a check answer is used, which is the best type for this question—dichotomous, multiple-choice ("cafeteria" question), or scale?
   3. If a checklist is used, does it adequately cover all the significant alternatives without overlapping, and in a defensible order? Is it of reasonable length? Is the wording of items impartial and balanced?
   4. Is the form of the response easy, definite, uniform, and adequate for the purpose?

D. Decisions about the place of the question in the sequence
   1. Is the answer to the question likely to be influenced by the contents of preceding questions?
   2. Is the question led up to in a natural way? Is it in correct psychological order?
   3. Does the question come too early or too late from the point of view of arousing interest and receiving sufficient attention, avoiding resistance, and so on?

*From C. Selltiz, L. Wrightsman, and S. Cook: *Research Methods in Social Relations*, 3rd ed. New York: Holt, Rinehart & Winston, 1976, pp. 552–574. Reprinted with permission.

An ideal way to obtain information to answer these questions is administering the questionnaire to respondents and asking them to write any questions or reactions they have about the questions in the margin. This method allows you to discover potential problems with the questionnaire even if the pilot respondents answer the questions appropriately. A marginal note can reveal, for example, that the respondent had to decide between two possible interpretations of the question, even though the response appeared appropriate.

Further evaluation of the adequacy of the questions and the format can be obtained from scoring the answers. In checking the response alternative to indicate the age of a child, a re-

spondent had checked two alternatives: 6–12 months and 1–2 years. In this example, scoring the pilot data revealed that the response alternatives were not free from overlap—a 1-year-old child can fit into both response alternatives.

After scoring the data from the pilot questionnaires, you can check the adequacy of the data obtained by conducting the statistical tests that you have planned for the actual sample. At this stage it may be discovered that a particular variable was not measured in a useful way. The question can be redesigned for the final version of the questionnaire to obtain additional information so that this variable can be scaled.

Administering Psychosocial Instruments

Just as selecting appropriate instruments is crucial in the measurement of psychosocial variables, selecting the most appropriate method of administration will influence the results of your data-collection efforts. Many psychosocial instruments can be self-administered, but there are situations in which it may be more appropriate to allow for more face-to-face contact. Depending on the characteristics of the respondents, the situation, and the design of the study, the same instrument might be administered through a self-administered mailing, through an interview, or through a combination of methods.

When you are planning how to recruit and test subjects, one of the easiest methods that comes to mind is mailing packets of questionnaires to potential subjects. The apparent ease of mailing compared with locating and recruiting subjects one by one is sometimes offset by disadvantages. But there are also situations that are ideal for mailed administration. Areas to consider when selecting the method of administering instruments are:

1. anticipated response rate
2. characteristics of the potential subjects

3. complexity of the instructions or task
4. quality of data required

Anticipated Response Rate

Generally, the response rate is higher when you can recruit subjects for your study through direct contact. This contact allows you to "sell" your study and to answer questions. When study instruments are mailed to potential subjects, the response rate is much lower. Although there are no absolute rules, response rates of 50% for mailed administration of questionnaires are considered adequate, and rates of 70% are considered very good (Babbie 1973). Lower response rates are subject to question regarding *response bias*; that is, the sample might not be representative of the population in some systematic way—perhaps having a higher level of education than the nonrespondents. Thus, the validity of your research would be undermined if you obtained too low a response rate. As is the case with any method of administration, you should compare the characteristics of your sample with the characteristics of the full population—for example, all the patients who use the agency where you recruited your sample—to determine whether your sample is representative or biased in some way.

Another consideration regarding response rate is the projected sample size required to fulfill the design of your study (see Chapter 9). If you have determined that you need at least 100 subjects to conduct the appropriate statistical analyses to test your hypotheses, but the pool of potential subjects is only 200, you may not have a sufficient margin to use a mailed administration. Sometimes, however, the response rate is greater than might have been anticipated. A pilot study can help you estimate what the response rate is likely to be for the actual study.

There are techniques for increasing the response rates for mailed administration. These include an enticing cover letter, the promise to report the study findings, and follow-up mailings to remind or urge the person to participate. Similarly, strategies are used to increase the response rate in face-to-face recruitment. By imagining the point of view of your potential subjects you can anticipate some barriers or inducements that influence a patient's decision about participating. Some respondent barriers are logistical, such as needing child care while participating in the study; others reflect the level of motivation to participate in research.

A variety of motivations exists for participating in research. For well-educated respondents, the promise of feedback of the study findings tends to be motivating. A small monetary reimbursement for the respondent's time and effort may facilitate recruiting patients who are highly stressed or overburdened. Patients who have experienced a particularly difficult illness or treatment frequently say that it is rewarding to think that their participation might help others in similar situations.

Characteristics of the Potential Subjects

The most appropriate method of administration depends in part on the subject's educational level, age, eyesight, hearing ability, language, and past experience (or lack of experience) with psychosocial instruments. Patients who have difficulties with any area of functioning that may be needed to complete the instrument would not be appropriate for self-administration methods. Because clinical populations in nursing often do not meet the "ideal" of being healthy, well-educated, and experienced research subjects, creative efforts are required to reach potential participants who are often excluded—for example, non–English speakers or hard-of-hearing patients—in order to increase the clinical relevance of research.

Complexity of the Instructions or Task

Some methods of data gathering, such as the Q-sort, require direct contact with the subjects because the apparatus includes a large stack of cards to be sorted into piles. Other instruments require direct contact because the instructions are too complex for most individuals to understand without some assistance. Decisions about the complexity of the instructions or the task have to be made in relation to the characteristics of the potential respondents. If the study subjects are all expected to have advanced educational degrees, even instruments with very complex instructions or task requirements can safely be self-administered. Most samples are likely to have a range of individuals, however, and highly complex instruments are not likely to be filled out correctly by all respondents without some direct assistance.

Quality of the Data Required

Different methods of administering psychosocial instruments result in somewhat different responses from subjects. On the one hand, a research interview, as opposed to self-administered questionnaires, permits probing to obtain more detailed data, allows the establishment of rapport to facilitate less superficial responses, and provides for checking the completeness and the accuracy of the data (Isaac & Michael 1981). The quality of the data is usually better—for example, there are fewer "missing data"—when the researcher is available to answer questions and check on the completeness of the responses before the respondent leaves.

On the other hand, self-administered instruments, if well constructed, allow for greater uniformity of responses; provide anonymity, which may encourage frankness and honesty; and may be more feasible and economical to reach a larger number, or more representative sample, of people (Isaac & Michael 1981).

As in the case of evaluating the suitability of individual instruments, the methodological reference by Fox and Ventura (1983) should be consulted to aid you in the preliminary small-scale administration of your study instruments to evaluate the entire procedure of recruiting and testing subjects you have selected.

Scoring Psychosocial Instruments

Scoring instructions are usually provided for instruments, but they can be very complex. Investigators should check their interpretation of the instructions with others and should devise methods to reduce the likelihood of errors in the repetitive task of scoring raw data.

Techniques to Increase Accuracy and Sensitivity

The instructions provided by the developer of the instrument assume that you will use methods to avoid introducing errors into the data. Special care should be taken in identifying the appropriate items for each subscale and in the handling of *reverse-scored items* (items worded in the opposite way to avoid response set bias). If the instrument will be hand-scored, templates should be developed for the various groupings of items (subscales, reverse-scored items) to prevent errors at the item level. *Templates* are cardboard or plastic overlays with holes that allow only certain items to be visible. For an instrument with several subscales, for example, there would be a separate template for each subscale. When a template is placed on the questionnaire, only the items for the one designated subscale are visible. The scores for this subscale are calculated according to the instructions on the template, and

then the next subscale template is placed on the questionnaire.

Computer scoring not only reduces the time to score data but also greatly reduces the chance of errors (see Chapter 16). Program statements for scoring are developed to reverse the scores for the items indicated, to compile subscales from designated items, and to calculate any other weightings or transformations of the scores. Obviously, the instructions to the computer must be checked for accuracy or the entire data set will be scored incorrectly.

The computer can be used to check for certain types of error in hand- or machine-scored data. After calculating the highest and lowest score that could possibly occur for each subscale or variable, you can have the computer search for any scores lower or higher than the specified ranges. Depending on the nature of the instrument, other values can be determined to check for errors in the data. Naturally, errors that fall within the allowable range of scores cannot be detected by this method.

Handling Inconsistencies in Raw Data

In dealing with actual data, there will be inconsistencies due to the respondents' interpretations of instructions, omitting of items, or other irregularities. In the case of the omission of a small number of items from a scale, the scoring instructions might call for substituting the mean score for the missing items or some other standardized method. For example, in a scale of 20 items the mean might be substituted for a small number of missing responses. Such a correction should not be used if too many items have missing responses; a score for such respondents should not be calculated.

Patterns of unanticipated responses may appear in the data. To score these data, the research team should develop *decision rules* to be used consistently whenever a similar response occurs. These decision rules ensure that such unusual responses will be scored in the same way for all respondents. For example, on a social support scale a few respondents listed entire families rather than individuals on some lines of their network list. In order to score all respondents

in a similar way, the investigators (Norbeck, Lindsey, & Carrieri 1981, 1983) established a uniform way to score the few occasions in which entire families appeared as a single entry on the list. This decision rule reduced the likelihood of experimenter bias in unconsciously manipulating scores for individual respondents. Thus, regardless of the size of the network for the respondent who listed an entire family, the scores for entire families were handled in the same way whenever they were encountered. A log should be kept to document such decision rules as they are developed.

Normally, few unusual responses are found in scoring data. In some instances, however, many unusual responses occur. By keeping a log of these responses it is sometimes possible to discover a pattern after many instruments have been scored. In fact, it is sometimes found that a typographical error in some versions of the instrument accounted for the unusual responses.

Final Note

Throughout this chapter, emphasis has been placed on careful selection, conceptual and methodological accuracy, examination of context, and evaluation of judgments. These skills and behaviors are not an end in themselves, however. They are meant to help make methodology a matter of course, so you can have confidence in the mechanical aspects of research while reserving your creative energy to develop thoughtful, relevant research questions in psychosocial nursing.

Summary of Key Ideas and Terms

✔ Unnecessary effort can be expended in research because investigators fail to search for an appropriate existing instrument.

✔ Developing an original instrument to measure a nursing construct is a lengthy and complex process.

✔ *Concurrent validity* is a type of criterion-related validity calculated as the agreement between the instrument and criterion scores obtained at the same time; *predictive validity* is observed at a future time.

✔ A concept, defined in terms of observable events, used in a theory to account for relationships in data is a *construct*.

✔ *Construct validity* is the degree to which an instrument measures the theoretical construct or trait it was designed to measure. Testable predictions to establish construct validity may be based on group differences, changes, correlations, processes, and content- or criterion-related validity relationships.

✔ *Content validity* is the degree to which the items in an instrument measure the domain intended, as determined through two types of rational analysis (face validity and logical or sampling validity).

✔ *Convergent validity* is a type of construct validity that shows the degree to which the scores from a measure resemble the scores from a different measure of the same construct.

✔ A proved, accepted, valid measure of some variable is a *criterion measure*.

✔ *Criterion-related validity* is the extent to which the scores from an instrument can be related to a criterion, measured either at the same time (concurrent validity) or at a future time (predictive validity).

✔ *Decision rules* are preestablished methods for handling unusual data that will be applied consistently in all cases.

✔ A *direct measure* is a measure or count of an object or quality itself; a *proxy measure* stands for an object or quality.

✔ *Discriminant validity* is determined from evidence that a measure of a construct is measuring only that construct, and thus is not highly related to other unrelated constructs.

✔ *Face validity* is a type of content validity that is a subjective judgment of the degree to which a test appears to measure what it purports to measure.

✔ The degree to which the items or groupings of items in an instrument obtain the same results is *internal consistency reliability*.

- An attitude scale in which respondents are presented with statements and asked to indicate how much he or she agrees or disagrees with each statement is called a *Likert-type scale*.

- *Logical* (*sampling*) *validity* is a type of content validity that is a subjective judgment of the extent to which the items adequately cover the content of the domain that the instrument purports to measure.

- *Objective measure* is the actual behavior, knowledge, or some other quality exhibited by a person.

- *Parallel-forms* (*alternate-forms*) *reliability* is the degree to which two or more forms of an instrument are equivalent.

- Measurement devices that provide ambiguous stimuli for the respondent are *projective methods*. Interpretation of the responses is based on the assumption that the respondent will project values, needs, and attitudes into responses.

- *Q-sort* is a sorting technique in which people are given a set of stimuli (e.g., statements, names, pictures) and asked to sort them into piles based on some criterion, such as attractiveness, personal relevance, etc.

- The property of an instrument related to consistency and accuracy in results is its *reliability*.

- *Response set* is a systematic tendency for a person to respond to items in an instrument in a stereotypical way, unrelated to the actual content of the instrument; for example, to give responses that seem the most socially desirable.

- *Scale* is a measuring instrument composed of several items that have a logical or empirical relationship to each other in which the subject is asked to give ratings, rankings, or some other response.

- *Subjective measure* is based on respondents' subjective perceptions about their behavior, knowledge, needs, or other characteristics.

- The degree to which the same results are obtained in two or more administrations of the same instrument, separated by a time interval when no basis exists for expecting a difference in the actual value is called the *test-retest reliability*.

- The property of an instrument related to relevance—it measures what it is supposed to measure—is its *validity*.

References

Allen MJ, Yen WM: *Introduction to Measurement Theory*. Monterey, Calif.: Brooks/Cole, 1979.

Babbie ER: *Survey Research Methods*. Belmont, Calif.: Wadsworth, 1973.

Brien M et al: How Lamaze-prepared expectant parents select obstetricians. *Res Nurs Health* 1983; 6:143–150.

Campbell DT, Fiske DW: Convergent and discriminant validation by the multitrait–multimethod matrix. *Psychol Bull* 1959; 56:81–105.

Chun K-T et al: *Measurement for Psychological Assessment: A Guide to 3000 Original Sources and Their Applications*. Ann Arbor, Mich.: Survey Research Center Institute for Social Research, 1975.

Fox RN, Ventura MR: Small-scale administration of instruments and procedures. *Nurs Res* 1983; 32:122–125.

Hayter J: Sleep behaviors of older persons. *Nurs Res* 1983; 32:242–246.

Heilbrun AB Jr: Review of the Edwards Personal Preference Schedule. Pages 148–149 in: *Seventh Mental Measurements Yearbook*. Highland Park, N.J.: Gryphon Press, 1972.

Hurley PM: Communication variables and voice analysis of marital conflict stress. *Nurs Res* 1983; 32:164–169.

Isaac S, Michael WB: *Handbook in Research and Evaluation*, 2nd ed. San Diego: Edits, 1981.

Jacobson SF: Stresses and coping strategies of neonatal intensive care unit nurses. *Res Nurs Health* 1983; 6:33–40.

Kishi KI: Communication patterns of health teaching and information recall. *Nurs Res* 1983; 32:230–235.

Lazarus RS: *Psychological Stress and the Coping Process*. New York: McGraw-Hill, 1966.

Marcy SA et al: Contraceptive use by adolescent females in relation to knowledge, and to time and method of contraceptive counseling. *Res Nurs Health* 1983; 6:175–182.

McKee MG: Review of the Edwards Personal Preference Schedule. Pages 149–151 in: *Seventh Mental Measurements Yearbook*. Highland Park, N.J.: Gryphon Press, 1972.

Mills ME et al: Core-12: A controlled study of the impact of 12-hour scheduling. *Nurs Res* 1983; 32:356–361.

Muhlenkamp AF et al: Attitudes toward women in menopause: A vignette approach. *Nurs Res* 1983; 32:20–23.

Norbeck JS: Modification of recent life event questionnaires for use with female respondents. *Res Nurs Health* 1984; 7:61–71.

Norbeck JS et al: The development of an instrument to measure social support. *Nurs Res* 1981; 30:264–269.

Norbeck JS et al: Further development of the Norbeck social support questionnaire: Normative data and validity testing. *Nurs Res* 1983; 32:4–9.

Selltiz C et al: *Research Methods in Social Relations*, 3rd. ed. New York: Holt, Rinehart & Winston, 1976.

Spielberger CD: *Manual for the State–Trait Anxiety Inventory*, rev. ed. Palo Alto, Calif.: Consulting Psychologists Press, 1983.

Wallston KA et al: Development of the Multidimensional Health Locus of Control (MHLC) Scales. *Health Education Monographs* 1978; 6:160–170.

White MA et al: A computer-compatible method for observing falling asleep behavior of hospitalized children. *Res Nurs Health* 1983; 6:191–198.

Woods NF: The health diary as an instrument for nursing research: Problems and promise. *West J Nurs Res* 1981; 3:76–92.

Compendia of Psychosocial Instruments

Bonjean CM et al: *Sociological Measurement: An Inventory of Scales and Indices*. San Francisco: Chandler, 1967.

Buros OK (editor): *Personality Tests and Reviews*. Highland Park, N.J.: Gryphon Press, 1970.

Buros OK: *The Eighth Mental Measurements Yearbook*. Highland Park, N.J.: Gryphon Press, 1978.

Cattell RG, Warburton F: *Objective Personality and Motivation Tests*. Urbana: University of Illinois Press, 1967.

Chun K-T et al: *Measurement for Psychological Assessment: A Guide to 3000 Original Sources and Their Applications*. Ann Arbor, Mich.: Survey Research Center Institute for Social Research, 1975.

Comrey AL et al: *A Sourcebook for Mental Health Measures*. Los Angeles: Human Interaction Research Institute, 1973.

Goldman BA, Busch JC (editors): *Directory of Unpublished Experimental Mental Measures.* Vols 2–4 (1971–1976). New York: Human Sciences Press, 1978, 1982, 1984.

Goldman BA, Saunders JL (editors): *Directory of Unpublished Experimental Mental Measures.* Vol 1 (through 1970). New York: Human Sciences Press, 1974.

Johnson OG: *Tests and Measurements in Child Development: Handbook II.* Vols 1 and 2. San Francisco: Jossey-Bass, 1976.

Johnson OG, Bommarito JW: *Tests and Measurements in Child Development: A Handbook.* San Francisco: Jossey-Bass, 1971.

Lake DG et al: *Measuring Human Behavior: Tools for the Assessment of Social Functioning.* New York: Teachers College Press, Columbia University, 1973.

Lyerly SB: *Handbook of Psychiatric Rating Scales,* 2nd ed. New York: Research and Education Association, 1981.

Miller DC: *Handbook of Research Design and Social Measurement,* 4th ed. New York: Longman, 1983.

Mitchell JV Jr (editor): *Tests in Print III: An Index to Tests, Test Reviews, and the Literature on Specific Tests.* Lincoln: University of Nebraska Press, 1983.

Mitchell JV Jr (editor): *The Ninth Mental Measurements Yearbook.* Lincoln: University of Nebraska Press. [In press.]

Reeder LG et al: *Handbook of Scales and Indices of Health Behavior.* Pacific Palisades, Calif.: Goodyear, 1976.

Robinson JP et al: *Measurement of Occupational Attitudes and Occupational Characteristics.* Ann Arbor, Mich.: Survey Research Center Institute for Social Research, 1969.

Robinson JP et al: *Measures of Social Psychological Attitudes,* rev ed. Ann Arbor, Mich.: Survey Research Center Institute for Social Research, 1973.

Shaw ME, Wright JM: *Scales for the Measurement of Attitudes.* New York: McGraw-Hill, 1967.

Straus MA, Brown BW: *Family Measurements Techniques: Abstracts of Published Instruments, 1935–1974,* rev ed. Minneapolis: University of Minnesota Press, 1978.

Sweetland RC, Keyser DJ (editors): *Tests: A Comprehensive Reference for Assessments in Psychology, Education and Business.* Kansas City, Mo.: Test Corporation of America, 1983.

Walker DK: *Socioemotional Measures for Preschool and Kindergarten Children.* San Francisco: Jossey-Bass, 1973.

Ward MJ, Fetler ME: *Instruments for Use in Nursing Education Research.* Boulder, Colo.: Western Interstate Commission for Higher Education, 1979.

Ward MJ et al (editors): *Instruments for Measuring Nursing Practice and Other Health Care Variables.* Vols 1 and 2. DHEW Publication No. HRA 78-53. Washington, D.C.: U.S. Government Printing Office, 1979.

Further Readings

American Psychological Association: *Standards for Educational and Psychological Tests,* rev. ed. Washington, D.C.: American Psychological Association, 1974.

Anastasi A: *Psychological Testing,* 5th ed. New York: Macmillan, 1982.

Blalock HM Jr: *Conceptualization and Measurement in the Social Sciences.* Beverly Hills, Calif.: Sage, 1982.

Bradburn NM, Sudman, S: *Improving Interview Method and Questionnaire Design.* San Francisco: Jossey-Bass, 1979.

Hulin CL et al: *Item Response Theory: Application to Psychological Measurement.* Homewood, Ill.: Dow Jones-Irwin, 1983.

Nunnally JC Jr: *Introduction to Psychological Measurement.* New York: McGraw-Hill, 1970.

Chapter 12

Collecting Data on Biophysiologic Variables

by Ada M. Lindsey RN, PhD
Nancy A. Stotts RN, EdD

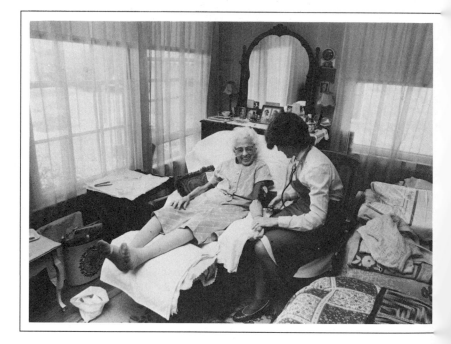

Nursing research that examines biophysiologic variables is in a preliminary stage. The findings that result may have a significant impact on patient outcomes.

Chapter Outline

Chapter Objectives

After reading this chapter, the student should be able to:

- Propose a plan to identify the biophysiologic variables that have been studied and the measurement techniques used
- List available resources for gaining information about biophysiologic instruments that can be used for measurement of variables
- Discuss analytically the guidelines in selecting an instrument to manipulate or measure a biophysiologic variable
- Compare and contrast at least one direct and one indirect measurement for a selected biophysiologic variable
- Compare and contrast the criteria for selection of a paper-and-pencil versus other measures of biophysiologic variables

- Give at least two examples of biophysiologic variables for which measurement will yield interval-level data
- Give two examples of equipment/instruments used in measuring a biophysiologic variable of interest
- Explain how reliability of equipment may be tested
- When given a research study that includes biophysiologic variables, evaluate the instrumentation used for the independent and the dependent variables
- Critique the methods section of research reports relative to inclusion of information about instrumentation used for measuring biophysiologic variables

In This Chapter . . .

Is it common practice to withhold iced beverages from patients with a myocardial infarct? Do you know what effects the drinking of ice water or some other iced noncaffeinated beverage will have on the myocardium of patients with a myocardial infarction? Does the degree of coldness, the volume consumed, the time over which it is consumed, or the position assumed for drinking the fluid make a difference in the effects? How would you determine or measure these effects?

Do you know what effects the provision of sucking opportunities for premature infants during tube feedings will have on their weight or the length of time until they can be bottle fed? Will the sucking opportunities adversely affect these infants? How much energy is required for sucking? How would you determine or measure these variables?

Do you know what effects therapeutic touch or conversation about the patient's condition will have on the intracranial pressure of unconscious head-injured patients? How can you define therapeutic touch? When should you measure intracranial pressure? How many data points are needed? Is a mean pressure over some specified period of time sufficient to capture the nature of change in the dependent variable, intracranial pressure?

These are only a few of the examples and questions that can be addressed in collecting data on biophysiologic variables. This is an exciting and challenging area for nurse researchers, and the findings that result may have a significant impact on patient outcomes.

Nursing research often includes variables which require physiologic *instrumentation* for their measurement. For example, if you wanted to determine the effects of some specific nursing activity, such as turning, on the intracranial pressure of head-injured patients, instrumentation would be necessary to quantify changes in the dependent variable (intracranial pressure) as influenced by the independent variable (turning). If you wanted to examine the effect of use of the bedside commode on oxygen consumption and heart rate in myocardial infarct patients, instrumentation also would be required to quantify those dependent variables.

In this chapter, measurement of biophysiologic variables is presented from the perspective of the research process. Conceptualization of these variables is acknowledged as being particularly critical to the selection of instruments for measurement. Prior research frequently provides the foundation for further study. Thus, critical consideration and evaluation of the conceptualization, operationalization of the variables, instruments used for measurement, and analysis of the findings are areas emphasized in this chapter, specifically in relation to measurement. A means to summarize prior research is proposed to assist you in identifying existing knowledge in the field and to help you to conceptualize the area of your research interest. The wide array of instruments available as well as the strengths and limitations of some of the instruments are explored. Practical issues such as whether the "ideal" instrument is available, whether a noninvasive measure can be used instead of an invasive one, and issues pertinent to cost involved in various measurement techniques are areas addressed in this chapter. Threats to validity and reliability of instruments are repeatedly emphasized. These themes are illustrated with examples of nursing research in

which biophysiologic variables were measured.

Specifically, five major content areas of concern to nursing are used as the scheme for organizing the review of research examples. These five areas are feeding alterations, activity and position, patient education, healing and infection, and environmental stimuli. These specific problem areas were selected as being exemplary of research areas of particular interest to nursing and for which several studies have been reported recently in the nursing literature. The process of measurement of biophysiologic variables, from conceptualization to interpretation of findings, is presented and illustrated with examples from these five conceptual areas.

Preparing for Your Study

Background literature and research reports relevant to the problem area will help you conceptualize the specific research questions you want to study and determine which variables are of greatest importance to your problem area. Once the variables of interest have been identified, from the theoretical, empirical, and clinical perspective of the research problem, you need to develop an operational definition for each of them (see Chapters 4 and 9). These operational definitions provide specific information about how the variables will be measured.

Read Broadly

Seeing how other investigators have defined and measured the same or similar variables will help you select measurement instruments. Initially, as you begin to address your problem area, it is useful to read broadly. Determine what questions others have addressed, identify problems

in the design or measures used previously, and think about what remains unknown.

Use Summary Charts

In our experience with reviewing previous work, it has been particularly helpful to develop summary charts (Lindsey et al 1981; Lindsey 1982, 1983). An example of such a chart is given in Table 12–1. A summary of studies in which the effects of activity on intracranial pressure were examined is another example of this kind of review (Mitchell 1980). On the summary chart, always identify the following information:

- Authors
- Source of their report
- Purpose(s) of the study
- Research questions or hypotheses
- Independent and dependent variables

- Measures and equipment that were used to quantify the variables
- Study sample
- Specific procedures described for the data collection
- Major findings and conclusions

Preparing the information from each related study in this manner will make it easier for you to evaluate studies, to analyze designs and data collection techniques, and, if possible, to compare findings across studies. It is absolutely essential for you to do this kind of a review of prior work in your problem area and to integrate and synthesize the ideas about what is known and what remains unknown.

Make Decisions Based on Information From Prior Studies

From this kind of a review you should be able to determine the focus for subsequent research in your problem area. It is also useful in helping you make decisions about the measurement of the variables you have selected for your study.

Table 12-1   Chart for Summarizing Studies in a Problem Area

Authors Source of report Purpose of study	Research questions or hypotheses	Variables: independent and dependent	Instruments or equipment	Sample and procedure	Major findings and conclusions
1.					
2.					
3.					

Discuss Your Study With Others

Once you have formulated your study, talk about it to other clinicians and researchers. Specifically, discuss the questions you will be attempting to examine and the measurement aspects of your research problem. Others may be able to assist you in refining your work and in providing insight to potential problems. It is much better to trouble-shoot all possible contingencies *before* you begin your data collection. Think, talk, read, rethink, continue to talk, and reread. These activities are most frequently associated with better research outcomes.

Biophysiologic Instruments

An enormous array of biophysiologic phenomena and variables are of interest to nurse researchers. A considerable range of equipment has been used, and it varies widely in level of sophistication. In some situations the equipment is used to create the independent variable, such as equipment for oxygen administration, for suctioning, or for administering tube feedings. In other cases the equipment and instruments are used to measure the dependent variables of interest, such as a thermometer, a scale, a sound-level meter, or an *electroencephalogram* (EEG) or *electrocardiogram* (ECG) tracing. Whether equipment is used for the independent or the dependent variable depends entirely on the research design and the research questions or hypotheses to be examined.

Examples of equipment used include the cardiac monitor, sphygmomanometer, stopwatch, protractor, treadmill, strain gauge, infusion pump, femoral arteriovenous shunt flow meter, thermometer, gastric motility recording device, scale, tape measure, motorized rocking hammock, rocking bed, audio tape player, wrist accelerometer, electric surface stimulator, hand positioning device, transcutaneous oxygen monitor, Holter monitor, Douglas bag, and biofeedback equipment. And the list goes on. A few biophysiologic instruments and the parameters they measure are given in Box 12-1.

Resources That List Instruments

Information about biophysiologic instruments and their characteristics such as usability, valid-

---

Box 12-1   Four Biophysiologic Instruments and What They Measure

Cardiac monitor:	Sphygmomanometer:	Flow meter:
Rate	Systolic blood pressure	Blood pressure
Rhythm	Diastolic blood pressure	Volume
Conduction pattern	Mean blood pressure	Rate
Infusion pump:	Pulse pressure	
Volume		
Pressure		
Rate		

ity, and reliability has not been organized into a single source like those available for psychosocial instruments. Available resources that describe biophysiologic instruments are not as comprehensive as those in other fields, but the following may be of help to you:

- instrument compilation texts
- review articles
- published research reports
- equipment catalogues from manufacturers
- exhibits at major meetings

The second volume of *Instruments for Measuring Nursing Practice and Other Health Care Variables* (Ward & Lindeman 1978) includes a few descriptions of instruments used for measuring biophysiologic variables. Very few of the nursing research texts address measurements of biophysiologic variables in any detail. Content about such instruments is usually so well integrated that it is not readily accessible. Biophysiologic phenomena and variables that were studied by nurse investigators from 1970 to 1980 were identified by Lindsey (1982, 1983, 1984). Reviews are an important source of information; in addition, you should read the original published articles. Reviews provide a compilation of research, and comparisons of specific instruments can be made. Most investigators are willing to share information about the equipment they used. Another source for information about instruments is catalogs from manufacturers of equipment; these may be obtained directly from the company or from sales representatives. Information about equipment can also be obtained by visiting the exhibits at major nursing meetings. Using a combination of these resources will supplement your review of studies and will help you select the most appropriate instrument.

Guidelines for Selecting Biophysiologic Measures

In making decisions about measuring variables, there are several factors to consider. Consideration of these areas will facilitate your selection of the optimal instrument(s).

Availability

Availability of appropriate equipment is a major factor. From your clinical experience you will have some ideas about the equipment that is used in the patient population from which you will be selecting your study sample. If the desired equipment is not used routinely in the settings where you plan to collect data, it may be possible to obtain it from other sources. You may be able to borrow it from another setting or obtain it on loan from the company that manufactures it, or perhaps it will be necessary to purchase it.

Direct or Indirect Measure

Another factor to consider is whether or not it is possible to obtain a direct measure of the variables. Whenever a direct measure is available, it is ideal to use it. For example, if you are interested in the effect of body position on blood pressure, an arterial line (not a cuff sphygmomanometer) is the most direct measure for obtaining a blood pressure.

In some cases you may have to use an indirect measure of the variable. If you were interested in comparing the energy expended in two types of bathing—for example, a bed bath versus a standing shower—you would have to select an indirect measure of energy expenditure, such as oxygen consumption. If you were interested in determining the stress response to some stressor, such as observing resuscitation of other patients in the coronary care unit, you would select several indirect measures to quantify the response. Examples include heart rate, blood pressure, plasma cortisol levels, and urinary excretion of catecholamines.

Single Versus Multiple Measures

This last example illustrates another important notion. For some variables it may be important to use multiple measures to assess the effect of the independent variable on changes in the outcome variable(s) of interest. One measure may not be adequate to demonstrate change; it may not be sufficiently sensitive to show the effects of the independent variable. With a single measure, the changes observed also could be due to other events; multiple measures would help control for this possible problem. The uncontrolled existence of these other factors poses competing hypotheses and reduces the strength of the study findings. For example, caffeine consumption and body position, as well as the introduction of some independent variable stressor such as a treadmill, influence heart rate and blood pressure. The point is that the findings will be less credible unless all the other major factors which influence the dependent variables (e.g., heart rate and blood pressure) are held constant or are accounted for. When you make the final decision about the operational definitions, you have taken into account the potential threats, and the definitions that emerge direct the instrumentation. That is why creating the operational definitions for the variables is such a critical step in the research process. If measurement of the variables is not sufficient to capture the phenomena, it will be impossible for others to believe or to use the findings.

Sensitivity, Validity, and Reliability

The instruments selected to measure the study variables should be the most appropriate ones available. They should be sufficiently sensitive to show changes in the parameter being measured, and they should be valid and reliable. Issues related to the use of the transcutaneous oxygen monitor illustrate this point. The more traditional and accurate approach for measuring change in the blood gases has been via collection of arterial blood samples. Obtaining arterial blood for gas analysis is considered an *invasive procedure*, and multiple samplings may adversely influence an already compromised patient. Transcutaneous oxygen and carbon dioxide monitors have been developed to alleviate this problem; a heated electrode is used as a *noninvasive* sensing device. These monitoring devices are used frequently for the short-term gestation infant because the blood gas values obtained from the monitors and from the actual blood samples are more nearly identical (except at hypoxic levels) than those values obtained when the monitors are used for adults.

Invasive Versus Noninvasive Measures

This example also illustrates several other issues involved in selecting instruments to quantify changes in biophysiologic variables. One issue is that of selecting invasive versus noninvasive techniques. On the one hand, the only true or credible measure for a variable may require an invasive procedure, and in some patient populations the clinical state of the desired study population may preclude the use of such techniques (see Chapter 3). On the other hand, these subjects may already have invasive lines from which it is possible to quantify changes in the variable of interest. For example, if you wanted to determine the effects of the patient's position on reading central venous pressures, it would be possible to do this study in subjects who had a central venous line connected to a monitor with either a polygraph tracing or a digital readout.

Level of Data Obtained

Another consideration in instrument selection is the type of data that can be obtained. Measurement of many biophysiologic variables yields interval-level data, because values for the variables usually lie along some continuum (see Chapter 15). For example, heart rate, respiratory rate, temperature, oxygen consumption, body weight, serum albumin, urinary output, and age yield data points distributed at equal intervals. Such continuous data points allow the use of more powerful statistical analyses. (Refer to Chapter 15 for the benefits of collecting interval-level or ratio-level data.) With some paper-and-pencil measures you are unable to get interval-level data, but in some circumstances these measures must be used, nonetheless, because they best capture the variable of interest.

Cost

The last issue influencing equipment selection is cost. Of course, it is essential to select an instrument that is both affordable and appropriate. You may need to find a source of funds—for example, working with another researcher who has grant or institutional support, submitting an application to a funding source to obtain your own support, or obtaining assistance from the manufacturer whose equipment you will be using in your study (see Chapter 8). As illustrated in subsequent sections of this chapter, it is also pos-

sible to conduct studies that require no additional costs for instrumentation.

Serious consideration should also be given to the cost of the research to the subjects—that is, cost of equipment, cost of time, cost of privacy, and attendant risks—and the potential benefits to be gained. When these costs and the benefits are made explicit, most subjects willingly consent to participate in research that they perceive to have merit (see Chapter 3).

Summary of Guidelines

All these issues must be examined in determining the measurements to be made for all the study variables. Major questions to ask yourself when selecting an instrument are summarized below:

- What instruments are routinely used in your setting to measure the variable of interest?
- Are the instruments you want to use readily available?
- Is direct or indirect measurement most meaningful and practical?
- Will the instrument be sensitive enough to detect changes in the variable?
- Are multiple measures needed to capture the breadth of the variable(s) of interest?
- Do the measures yield interval-level data?
- Are the instruments considered to be valid and reliable?
- If invasive measures are needed, are they a routine part of the care for the patient population of interest?
- What is the cost of the instruments you are planning to use?

The selected instruments must be able to measure the variable(s), be sensitive to changes in the variable(s), be valid and reliable, and be affordable.

Paper-and-Pencil Instruments to Measure Biophysiologic Variables

Some biophysiologic phenomena are more subjective than objective in nature; pain, fatigue, and nausea are three examples. To quantify these phenomena, the investigator must rely on the subject's perception and evaluation of the magnitude or changes in the sensation experienced. In these instances paper-and-pencil instruments are used frequently to measure the sensation. The McGill-Melzack Pain Questionnaire (Melzack 1975), the Fatigue Symptom Checklist (Yoshitake 1971), and the Symptom Distress Scale (McCorkle & Young 1978) are examples of paper-and-pencil instruments for which some validity and reliability have been established. In addition, visual analog scales have been devised for subjects to rate the magnitude of the perceived sensation. These have a straight line with anchoring words placed at either end of the line. At one end the phrase could be "the worst I have ever had," while at the opposite end, "the least I have ever had" could be used. The subjects are given directions to place a mark along the line that best represents what they feel with respect to the dimension being assessed, for example, pain or nausea. An example is shown in Figure 12–1.

Some biophysiologic phenomena are assessed according to written criteria developed to quantify the status (or change in status) of individuals. The criteria were determined in respect to the accepted range of normal values. An example is the Glasgow Coma Scale; it is used to evaluate an individual's responsiveness to specific graded stimuli (Teasdale & Jennett 1974). After the subject's responses to the listed items are evaluated, a composite score is determined by summing the ratings. Three areas in which the responses are rated are eye opening, best verbal response, and best motor response. The scale is short, and the responses are rated according to well-defined criteria such as eyes open spontaneously = 4, eyes open to speech = 3, to pain = 2, and none = 1. This scale is used clinically as well as for research to assess level of consciousness. Another example is the Short Portable Mental Status Questionnaire; it is frequently used to assess the mental status of elderly subjects (Pfeiffer 1975). Ten questions are used, and if fewer than six correct answers are given, the elderly subject is considered to be unreliable in providing accurate information. In essence, this instrument taps cognitive function.

The guiding force for instrument selection, in all cases, must be the conceptualization of the phenomena to be studied. There is no inherent value in using a sophisticated invasive measure, such as serum level of lactic acid, if it does not capture the real effect of the variables being studied. Do not dismiss paper-and-pencil instruments to measure phenomena just because the variable is physiologic. Remember the guideline of appropriateness; the instrument must measure the phenomena of concern sensitively, reliably, and validly.

When walking up one flight of stairs, I feel

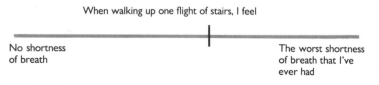

No shortness
of breath

The worst shortness
of breath that I've
ever had

Figure 12–1 Visual analog scale for measuring one dimension of the biophysiologic variable breathlessness. Using a ruler, the distance from the left end of the scale to the vertical cross line is the measurement.

Instrumentation: Independent and Dependent Variables

Some equipment is used to create and specify the independent variable. An example is the *treadmill*; it is a platform covered with a moving walking surface. The speed of the moving surface and the angle of the platform can be altered to produce a known physiologic demand. The treadmill is used frequently in research. It is set at certain speeds and at certain gradients to establish variable levels of activity as the independent variable; thus the effects of various levels of activity can be studied.

Other equipment is used to quantify changes in the dependent variables. For example, the cardiac monitor (ECG tracing) is used to determine changes in cardiac rhythm, rate, and conduction patterns in response to varying activity levels. These same dependent-variable parameters could be used to assess the effects of drinking ice water on the myocardium in infarct patients. The independent variable, drinking ice water, could be varied by temperature (degree of coldness), amount given, and position assumed for ingestion of the water. In these two rather different studies, the same outcome measures could be used to show changes. The determination of what parameters to quantify is based on the operational definitions of the study variables.

Instruments Used to Manipulate the Independent Variable

The considerations for selecting instruments to manipulate the independent variable are really the same as those for choosing instruments to measure the dependent variable. Thus, of concern is the ability of that equipment to manipulate or affect, under the specified experimental conditions, the phenomena of concern. For example, if you wanted to assess the effects of the temperature of dressings (independent variable) on wound healing (dependent variable), you would need to be sure that your equipment provided the specific temperature required for the dressing. Material to provide insulation for the dressing would also be necessary to prevent an influence of environmental temperature on the temperature of the dressing. These conditions have the potential of influencing the dependent variable, wound healing. Conceptual considerations and the operational definitions for the independent variable also provide direction for selection and use of the instruments.

Biophysiologic Phenomena: Measurement of Variables

There are diverse types of measures to quantify biophysiologic variables. The researcher's conceptualization of the variable provides the referent frame for determining the measurement strategy and for selecting the measurement instrument(s). Some measures are more physical in nature, such as body temperature, while others are more biochemical in nature, such as serum albumin. It is possible that a number of measures, diverse in nature, may be used as a composite to quantify changes in some variable(s).

For example, if the outcome variable of interest is nutritional status, a composite of anatomical, physical, and biochemical measures may be used; these include temperature, weight, caloric intake, activity, nitrogen balance, and serum albumin. While it is possible to categorize the measures as being physical, anatomical, or biochemical, it is more useful from a research perspective to select the appropriate measures on the basis of how variables are conceptualized and defined operationally for the specific study.

Instrument selection, as we have seen, is based on conceptualization of the research questions. Biophysiologic phenomena studied previously by nurse investigators have been reviewed by Lindsey (1982, 1983, 1984), Kinney (1984), and Foster, Kloner, and Stengrevics (1984). The number of these phenomena examined in nursing studies is large and quite varied. Within the limits of this chapter, it is possible to address only five of these research areas. For each problem area included, one or more studies will be used to show how nurse researchers have measured some of the variables and to address some of the more salient points about the selection and use of instruments to quantify the study variables. The five phenomena to be included are *feeding alterations, activity and position, patient education, healing and infection, and environmental stimuli.*

Feeding Alterations

The majority of the reported research on feeding alterations has addressed two problem areas: the effects of tube feedings and nausea and vomiting associated with administration of anticancer therapy. Several studies representative of these problem areas are used to illustrate the measurement techniques selected to quantify the variables of interest.

Instrumentation and Measurement Issues

Tube Feeding   This can be an uncomfortable experience for many patients. By altering the variables of tube feeding (such as temperature, rate, and volume) and studying the effects, researchers may be able to determine the optimal conditions that will cause the least discomfort.

Using six paid volunteers, Kagawa-Busby and colleagues (1980) conducted a study to "evaluate the effects of nasogastric tube feedings (NGTF) administered at three different temperatures on gastric motility, total gastrointestinal transit time, diarrhea and adverse subjective symptoms" (p. 277). The independent variable was the temperature of the tube feeding, and the dependent variables quantified were the gastric pressure (used as an indi-

rect measure of gastric motility), stool transit time, intragastric temperature, and subjective symptoms reported by the subjects. The materials and equipment required to conduct this study included nasogastric tubes, liquid diet, an infusion pump, a nonabsorbable stool marker, a thermistor, gastric strain gauge and pressure recording device, and a system for the subjects to indicate their subjective sensations during the tube feedings.

Two similar studies had been reported previously; one using five adult volunteers (Hanson 1973) and one using two rhesus monkeys (Williams & Walike 1975). In each of these reports the instruments used and the procedures are well described.

Heitkemper and colleagues (1977) conducted a study to determine the effects of rate and volume of tube feeding on tolerance of subjects to the feedings. Rate, as one independent variable, was set at 30, 60, and 85 mL/min, and volume, as the second independent variable, was given as 200, 350, and 500 mL. Tolerance was operationalized to include frequency of subjects' subjective responses, frequency and severity of observed adverse effects, and gastrointestinal disturbances (indirectly assessed by measuring pressure changes within the gastrointestinal tract). This study also used six paid volunteers, and materials and equipment similar to those desribed above were used for data collection. The instruments and procedure are desribed in the report.

In these studies the number of subjects included was inadequate, but the studies represent preliminary work. They provide examples of questions about biophysiologic phenomena of interest to nurses.

Nonnutritive Sucking   Feeding alterations of another kind occur in premature infants. The sucking reflex of a premature is poorly coordinated, and the general weakness of these vulnerable infants may preclude them from obtaining sufficient formula via sucking. Usually these infants (34 weeks or less gestation) are given tube feedings, and few to no opportunities for sucking are provided during this period.

Nurse researchers designed a study to test the effects of nonnutritive sucking (using a pacifier nipple) on the clinical course of premature infants (Measel & Anderson 1979). Opportunities for nonnutritive sucking were provided during and for 5 minutes after every tube feeding. Operational definition of the dependent variable, clinical course, included morbidity, time of initiation of bottle feeding, weight, and time of discharge. Fifty-nine premature infants were alternately assigned to the experimental or to the control group. Exclusion criteria and description of the sample are described in the research report.

The equipment needed to create the independent variable, sucking, was made by the investigators. The equipment is not expensive and is readily available. The report includes a description of the construction of the pacifiers as well as the manipulation. Although not used in this study, an electronic suckometer has been devel-oped and can be attached to a research nipple so that sucking can be quantified.

These investigators also developed a feeding evaluation scale that was used at the time of the first bottle feeding. The remainder of the data was collected from the chart or from observation. Unfortunately, from the perspective of the research design, infants in both groups were allowed to have pacifiers at any time, and the frequency and duration of these extra sucking opportunities were not reported. Another limitation to credibility of the findings acknowledged by the investigators is that complications between the two groups were different. It is difficult to control confounding variables in clinical research; however, attempts to control or account for these variables should be made. The researchers did report that the infants in the experimental group gained more weight (2.6 gm/day), that bottle feeding was initiated earlier (3.4 days), and that they were discharged earlier (4 days).

Nausea and Vomiting   Studies in which nausea and vomiting were examined primarily have been conducted with cancer patients. Several different examples illustrating different measurement issues are given.

In one study the relationship between anxiety, hopelessness, pain, specific demographic characteristics, and the degree of nausea and vomiting experienced by 26 cancer patients receiving chemotherapy for the first time was investigated (Zook & Yasko 1983). The subjects were receiving a variety of cytotoxic agents and a variety of antiemetics; the study could have been strengthened if both of these confounding variables had been controlled by sample selection criteria. (This is important, because different chemotherapy agents have a different propensity for causing nausea and vomiting.) Standardized instruments were used to measure some of the specified variables—for example, the Spielberger State–Trait Inventory, the Beck Hopelessness Scale, and the McGill-

Melzack Pain Questionnaire. A nausea and vomiting scale was developed specifically for this study.

When investigators develop instruments for a study, validity and reliability data are usually not established (see Chapters 4, 7, and 11). Lack of these data always creates a question about the findings, because one cannot assume that the scale is, in fact, measuring accurately and reliably what it is purported to measure. This study, however, is a good example of the use of paper-and-pencil instruments to quantify the subject's perception of biophysiologically related sensations.

In another study, Cotanch (1983) tested the use of progressive muscle relaxation (PMR) in reducing nausea and vomiting and psychologic averseness associated with cancer chemotherapy. The nine subjects were all experiencing refractory drug-induced nausea and vomiting. They were being treated aggressively with a variety of experimental cytotoxic agents, and all were receiving antiemetic agents. Again, control of these confounding variables could have strengthened the study. Progressive muscle relaxation was the independent variable. The investigator provided the PMR training individually to each subject, and they were given audiotapes to take home to practice PMR twice a day and while receiving chemotherapy. One question that remains unanswered is the extent to which each subject achieved PMR. This is an important notion, because PMR (the independent variable) was being tested for its influence on the outcome variables (nausea and vomiting) of interest. Baseline values were obtained, and then data were collected at subsequent cycles of chemotherapy administration. However, the study was not initiated at the first cycle of therapy. Data for several variables were collected. They include physiologic arousal (operationally defined as blood pressure, pulse, and respiration), state–trait anxiety (Spielberger's inventory), food and fluid intake for two days after therapy, change in weight, and degree and frequency of nausea and vomiting. The use of antiemetics for 48 hours was recorded.

This is an example of a quasi-experimental study (no randomization and no control group) (see Chapter 6) in which the intervention had a biophysiologic component, and the effects of the PMR were assessed by measuring nausea and vomiting as the dependent variables.

Because anxiety as a state or trait and food and fluid intake may also influence the nausea and vomiting experienced, measurement of these moderating, or intervening, variables was included in the study design. Accounting for or measuring the extent or existence of other variables that may have some potential contribution in influencing the magnitude of the outcome variables is of critical importance in research. If it is known or suspected that food and fluid intake would contribute to nausea and vomiting, the dependent variables of interest, then control of or measurement of food and fluid intake becomes important in explaining the findings obtained. Think about all the major possible explanations that could account for the findings other than the independent variable being tested (such as PMR), and attempt to control for or to measure those other variables. This will increase the credibility of the results obtained (see Chapter 6).

Nutritional Status Nurses have become more interested in determining the nutritional status of various populations. From clinical observations, it is apparent that the patient's nutritional status may influence the health outcome. Those with less than an adequate nutritional status are at risk for a variety of effects such as prolonged hospitalization, increased incidence of infection or other complication, and decreased tolerance to therapy. Patients with cancer or anorexia nervosa or those who are obese or elderly are populations for whom assessment of nutritional status is particularly important. Nutritional status is one of those biophysiologic variables, like the stress response, that requires measurement of multiple parameters. Because there is no one best measure, researchers must use several.

Layton and colleagues (1981) evaluated, over a three-month period, the nutritional status of eight allogeneic bone marrow recipients who were given total parenteral nutrition. The laboratory tests and the other parameters monitored are well described in this research report.

This is an example of a study in which measurement of the biophysiologic parameters requires obtaining blood and urine samples and sending them to a laboratory for analysis.

Laboratory Analysis Each laboratory establishes the normal values for each parameter based on the specific analytical procedures used in making the determination; in some cases, these normal values may vary from laboratory to laboratory. Usually the investigator reports the normal range of values from the laboratory in which the analyses were performed. You need to consider this fact when reading and comparing findings from several research reports and in designing and conducting your own study. In the above cited study the parameters for which laboratory analysis was used include serum albumin and 24-hour urinary creatinine and nitrogen.

In addition to the use of lab values, other measures included in this study to determine the subject's nutritional status were body weight, triceps skinfold thickness, and arm muscle circumference. Using established formulas, nitrogen balance was calculated from intake and output measures of nitrogen, and the creatinine height index was calculated from the 24-hour urinary creatinine excretion. Several pieces of equipment were used: a scale, a plastic tape measure, and calipers designed to measure skinfold thickness.

Reliability Because this study was longitudinal and thus data were collected at several points in time, determining the reliability of the equipment in collecting these values over time is important. For example, the same scale should be used for determination of the weight or prior to weighing the subject an object with a known weight should be used and the scale adjusted accordingly. This is one method for achieving reliability of measurement over time. This same attention to reliability is necessary for the calipers as well. Although one of the manufacturers of calipers reports an accuracy of measurement within a 1-mm error range, a small metal block with specified varying thicknesses can be used to calibrate the calipers to ensure reliability. This is important when measuring parameters at several different times, particularly if you are interested in determining changes over time.

As you are aware, determining the reliability of an instrument is different from determining *interrater reliability* (see Chapter 11). Establishing interrater reliability is also essential if more than one individual will be collecting the data. For instance, if your study requires collection of data using the calipers, all those who will be measuring the skinfold thickness should practice repeatedly on several different individuals with the calipers and record their measurements. Comparison of the values obtained will provide evidence of the similarity or dissimilarity in the measurements made by the raters. If the measurements obtained on the same individuals are statistically different between the raters, there is obviously a problem in ensuring interrater reliability. The point is that both reliability of the instrument in measuring the parameter as well as reliability across raters in obtaining the measurements must be established. Both of these kinds of reliability issues influence data collection. This kind of information should be included in research reports and clearly must be part of the research plan.

Nurse researchers have conducted a number of other studies in which various aspects of feeding alterations were examined. Some of the variables and instruments used are listed in Table 12-2. The studies just cited were selected to illustrate a variety of considerations that are important to the conduct of research in which biophysiologic variables are measured.

Table 12-2   Feeding Alterations: Four Examples With Variables and Instrumentation

Variables		Instrumentation	
Independent	Dependent	Independent	Dependent
1. Temperature, volume, and rate of liquid diet (tube feeding)	Subjective sensations Stool transit time Gastric motility Intraluminal temperature	Method of maintaining temperature and flow rate of tube feeding	Assessment tool for sensations Nonabsorbable stool marker Strain gauge Thermistor
2. Sucking Opportunities	Weight change Time to first bottle feeding Success with first bottle Time to discharge	Nipples Electronic suckometer	Scale Medical record Evaluation instrument for bottle feeding
3.	Nausea Vomiting		Instruments to quantify incidence, frequency, duration, and amount
4.	Nutritional status		Scale Tape measure Skin fold thickness calipers Laboratory analysis of selected serum and urine components Diet intake records

Activity and Position

Studies in the area of activity and position have focused on the effects of increases or decreases in activity and the effects of various positions or of changing position. Examples are the effects of ankle flexion against a footboard, a specific activity regimen as part of a stroke rehabilitation program, or the mobilization of a patient after surgery. Dependent variables in this type of study have included electrocardiographic responses, various vascular pressures, energy expenditure, fatigue, and intracranial pressure. Understanding the approaches used to measure the effects of activity and position will help you formulate your own research or appreciate the studies that have been conducted to determine the effects of daily patient activities and the measurements which have been used to quantify the magnitude of the effects. Examples of the variables which have been studied and the instruments used are given in Table 12-3.

Instrumentation and Measurement Issues

Energy Expenditure   Oxygen consumption is one of the variables frequently used to measure the effects of activity. It is often used to measure energy expenditure.

Table 12-3   Activity and Position: Four Examples With Variables and Instrumentation

Variables		Instrumentation	
Independent	Dependent	Independent	Dependent
1. In-hospital bathing	Oxygen consumption Hemodynamic responses EKG responses	Thermometer	Portable EKG recorder Cuff sphygmomanometer Stethoscope Stopwatch Max Planck respirometer Beckmann automatic gas analyzer
2. Arm extension Hip flexion Turning supine to right Turning right to supine Turning supine to left Turning left to supine Head rotated right Head rotated left	Intracranial pressure		Ventriculostomy drainage with #8 French tube Open bore manometer Ruler
3. Backrest position: Flat and 20°	Cardiac output	Carbon dioxide injector Protractor	Thermodilution catheter Cardiac output computer
4. Backrest position: 0°, 20°, 30°, 45°	Pulmonary artery pressure (systolic, diastolic, mean) Pulmonary capillary wedge pressure	Ruler	Strain gauge Thermodilution catheter Gould brush recorder

Oxygen consumption was used by Johnston, Watt, and Fletcher (1981) to examine the effect of standard in-hospital bathing practices undertaken by immediate post-myocardial infarction patients. Twelve patients with documented transmural infarctions were the convenience sample for the study. The independent variable, standard bathing techniques, included three levels of bathing activity—standing shower, bed bath, and tub shower. The dependent variables were oxygen consumption as well as other responses determined by hemodynamic and electrocardiographic changes observed in response to the bathing treatment. The variable oxygen consumption was operationalized as the volume of oxygen consumed per kilogram of weight per minute (V_{O2}), the total ventilation of expired air at ambient temperature pressure saturated (VE_{ATPS}), metabolic equivalent units (METS), and respiratory quotient (RQ). Oxygen consumption was measured using the *Max Planck respirometer* technique. The method of calibration of the gas meter was described, and a known reference gas was used.

The validity of the technique was established by comparing the *Douglas bag technique* with that of the Max Planck respirometer. Equations were not explicitly stated for the oxygen calculations, but a reference was cited for those calculations. The reported detail of the methodology would permit the study to be replicated. Oxygen consumption is a complex and expensive measure to obtain but quite an accurate approach to quantifying an important variable.

In a study of the effects of various lifting techniques on the energy expenditure of subjects (Geden 1982), the lifting techniques of concern were mechanical lift, rocking axillary, self-lift, shoulder assist, and straight pull. Geden was interested in determining the effects when nurses used each of these specific techniques with normal subjects. The dependent variables were energy expenditure, heart rate, respiratory rate, and blood pressure. Energy expenditure was operationally defined as oxygen consumption; the Waters MRM-1 Oxygen Consumption Computer was used to measure it in this study. The authors noted that this instrument is comparable to Douglas bag gas sampling.

What is important to recognize is that there are many instruments available to measure oxygen consumption. The Douglas bag technique is considered the "gold standard"—that is, the ideal against which all other measures are evaluated. When you are reading or planning a study and the techniques noted by others for measuring a physiologic variable are not familiar to you, it will be necessary to find a reputable source to increase your understanding of the technique. Normally, authors cite references they have used for instrumentation, and this is a good place to begin your search for further information. In addition, the validity of that instrument—that is, how accurately it measures the variable under consideration—is a critical consideration. The reliability of the instrument also is important, because it tells you how reproducible the findings are. Information about both of these aspects of an instrument should be noted in a study report or found in the references cited in the article.

Hathaway and Geden (1983) built on this work when they studied the effect of various types of leg exercises on energy expenditure. They used a convenience sample (see Chapter 9) of 36 healthy adults, half men and half women. The independent variable of various types of leg exercise was divided into three levels—passive range-of-motion exercises, active range-of-motion exercises, and isometric exercises. In this study energy expenditure was measured by oxygen consumption, respiratory rate, heart rate, and blood pressure. The type of instrument used to collect each variable is described as well as its model number; this detail about instrumentation adds credibility to the findings.

Position   The effects of position and activity on other aspects of biophysical functions also have been reported. Intracranial pressure is one of those areas.

Mitchell, Ozuna, and Lipe (1981) examined the effects of turning the body to four positions, with two passive range-of-motion activities, and with head rotation right and left on intracranial pressure. The independent variable was two activities—arm extension, hip flexion—and the four positions—supine to right, right to supine, supine to left, left to supine. Also, the effects of head rotation left and head rotation right were evaluated. The dependent variable of intracranial pressure was operationalized as ventricular fluid pressure (VFP). The authors describe its normal variations and the effects that various maneuvers have on VFP. Lengthy descriptions are provided of the VFP system used, its insertion, associated equipment, and the technique for measuring intracranial pressure. In addition, the authors discuss the assets and limitations of this system in producing valid and reliable data and why these data could be used to accomplish the purpose of the study.

This aspect of the study provides an excellent model for the new researcher to follow in describing his/her instruments and for the critical consumer of research findings to use in evaluating the study (see Chapter 7).

Backrest position has been studied to determine its effect on parameters obtained from a pulmonary artery catheter. For the critical care nurse, such studies add to the scientific basis of nursing practice.

Grose, Woods, and Laurent (1981) reported one of the first studies in which the effect of backrest position on cardiac output measured by the *thermodilution technique* was examined. The two positions evaluated were flat and 20-degree backrest elevation. Instrumentation for both the independent variable and the dependent variable is important in this study. A protractor was used to determine accurately and consistently the angle of the backrest.

Although studies in which physiologic variables are measured are sometimes quite technologically advanced, the operationalization of this independent variable illustrates that the instrumentation selected must be appropriate to the purpose of the study and need not always be expensive or technically complicated.

The procedure for determination of the cardiac output is well described. Measurement of cardiac output with a pulmonary artery catheter requires the injection of a solution and the distal measurement of its temperature to calculate the flow through the heart, that is, the cardiac output. The authors controlled extraneous contamination from other variables when they standardized the pressure, timing, and volume of injectate; they did this by the use of a carbon dioxide injector, which provided a uniform rate and volume of injectate. In addition, cardiac output was measured two times, and the average of these two samples was used for the study (see Chapter 6). Also, when the cardiac output was read off the digital readout, it was checked by two investigators. These various details of the

design were planned by the investigators to increase the internal validity of the measures and were then reported so readers could know what precautions had been taken. The detailed descriptions that Grose, Woods, and Laurent provided would allow others to build on their work.

Backrest position was also addressed by Chulay and Miller (1984). They looked at its effect on pulmonary artery and pulmonary capillary wedge pressure measurements in cardiac surgery patients. They had an interesting way to operationalize the four angles of backrest—0, 20, 30, and 45 degrees. They used basic geometry and defined the distance of elevation of the backrest by the sine of the angle (for example, sine 20 degrees = $11/32$); the backrest was elevated 11 inches vertically, because the backrest portion of the bed that was to be elevated was 32 inches (see Figure 12–2).

Again, in this study information about all of the instrumentation is provided in detail. It includes use of the phlebostatic axis, placement of the transducer, and the types, models, and brands of the various pieces of equipment used. A brush recorder was used to record the *waveform* from which the dependent variables of pulmonary artery pressure and pulmonary capillary wedge pressure were derived. Although the authors indicated that data were read at end-expiration and that data were rounded off to the nearest torr (millimeter of mercury), they could have further strengthened the instrumentation (internal validity) if they had indicated who had interpreted the waveforms and who had validated the readings that the first person obtained.

The effects of a lateral position compared with a supine position on pulmonary artery pressures also have been explored (Kennedy, Bryant, & Crawford 1984). The dependent variable of pulmonary artery pressure was measured using instruments comparable to those in the

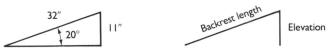

Figure 12–2 Example of use of geometry to determine angle of elevation for backrest.

Chulay and Miller study. These authors, however, had to solve the problem of how to keep the transducer at the level of the left atrium when patients were in the lateral position.

From the consumer's perspective, what this tells you is that although instruments such as the pulmonary artery catheter have a high degree of validity and reliability, consideration must be given to appropriate use so the data generated can be meaningful. You, therefore, must have a clear understanding of the conditions for use of instruments to measure biophysiologic variables in order to gain the valuable quantitative data they are capable of producing.

Activity and position have been examined in a variety of other studies, and data on the physiologic effects of activity and position are being accumulated. Sufficient replication of these studies will help provide a scientific base for nursing care related to activity and position in various patient populations.

Patient Education Outcomes

The value of patient education is frequently measured by multiple dependent variables. These variables often include measures of knowledge gained, psychologic adjustment, and physiologic function. The focus of this section will be the biologic measures used to examine some outcomes of patient education.

Instrumentation and Measurement Issues

The content of a teaching program dictates the measures that can logically be used to measure the effectiveness of education provided. To some extent, the nature of the content also determines the manner in which, as well as the instruments by which, the independent variable is delivered.

For example, when the effects of structured and unstructured preoperative education were compared (King & Tarsitano 1982), part of the content of the structured program focused on coughing and deep breathing. Thus, the authors selected pulmonary function measures to evaluate the effectiveness of the program. The specific pulmonary function tests selected in this case were decided, in part, by the fact that this study was a replication of a study by Lindeman and Van Aernam (1971). Measures of the dependent variable of pulmonary function included vital capacity, maximum midexpiratory flow rate, and forced expiratory volume. In this case another pulmonary function test, expiratory reserve volume, was added because of a recommendation arising from the original study. Length of hospital stay was the second dependent variable.

Length of time in the hospital is frequently used as a general category to evaluate the complete status of biologic variables. It is a gross measure of sickness and is often used because data to calculate the length of hospitalization are easy to collect, inexpensive to obtain, and positively correlated with the cost of hospitalization.

The conceptual framework for the study usually indicates the theoretical considerations that dictate the nature of the instruments to be used. This is an important point to consumers of research, because it means that part of your role in deciding to use data from a study will be based on whether there is logical consistency between the conceptual framework and the instruments selected to measure the selected variables. If the instrument measures, directly or indirectly, the variable under consideration, then you can be more assured that the correct instrument has been selected. When the conceptual framework and the operationalization of the variables, and thus the instruments, are not congruent, or the measurement is a remote approximation of the variable under consideration, then there is the possible threat that the instrument cannot measure what the researcher intended it to measure. King and Tarsitano's study (1982) is an example of a good fit between the conceptual framework and the instrumentation.

In Hill's study (1982) of the effect of providing various methods of preoperative information on the recovery of older people undergoing cataract surgery, the independent variable was type of information. The four types were behavioral information, sensory information, both behavioral and sensory information, and general information. The dependent variables were postoperative orientation, mood states, and performance. Performance was operationalized with physiologic measures such as ambulation, length of postoperative hospitalization, and time of first venture from home after discharge.

It is somewhat difficult to standardize the instrumentation for the independent variable in educational studies where people deliver the content. However, reliability among nurses can be established and needs to be addressed to minimize the confounding variables. Hill (1982) could have strengthened this study if interrater reliability of the nurses, in applying the independent variable (type of information), had been addressed. A strength of this study, however, was the cluster of physiologic measures plus the psychologic measures used in this case to capture the essence of recovery.

The effectiveness of the educational component of a rehabilitation program was examined in Perry's study (1981). Perry operationally defined effectiveness as subjective evaluation by the patient that the day was "good"; the reported number of symptoms experienced; the symptoms treated by the patient; the appropriateness of the treatment for the symptom; and a change in the number of and types of treatment used by patients. Thus, in this study self-report is used to determine the effectiveness of education on physiologic functioning.

Self-report is fraught with the potential for threats to validity because of its subjective nature. It is possible that the use of more objective measures for some of the physiologic data would have strengthened the measurement portion of the study—for example, the addition of measures of changes in pulmonary function values or changes in blood levels of drugs used.

Another set of pulmonary parameters was used by Janson-Bjerklie and Clarke (1982) to determine whether asthmatics could learn to control bronchial diameter by the use of biofeedback. Whole body *plethysmography* was used to obtain measures of thoracic gas volume, total respiratory resistance, and change in airway resistance. This involved putting the patient in a box that looked like a telephone booth, in which respiratory gas volume and composition were controlled. Dependent variable values were obtained by measuring the pressure and flow of the gases.

This measurement provides information about bronchial diameter. As bronchial diameter increases, airway resistance decreases; thus, airway resistance is a direct measure of airway diameter and, as a part of airway diameter, bronchial diameter. Although the research topic seems deceivingly simple, the instrumentation needed to answer the question is complex and expensive. The researchers selected an appropriate instrument to measure the dependent variable to assess the effectiveness of use of biofeedback to control bronchial diameter.

The effects of teaching various types of relaxation to patients have also been explored. A wide range of biophysical responses has been used as the dependent variable.

Wells (1982) examined the effects of a relaxation technique on postoperative muscle tension and pain. Using a two-group, pretest–posttest design (see Chapter 6), the author compared relaxation with routine preoperative instructions. She used a surface *electromyograph* (EMG) and a visual analog scale to measure pain intensity and distress. There was a separate scale for pain intensity and distress. (See Figure 12-1 for an example of a visual analog scale.) Both of these instruments are described.

For the EMG, the accuracy of the measurement is said to have been 1%. This small percentage of error makes the data generated more credible. But it would be helpful to know how the validity of the EMG was tested. In addition, the validity of the analog scale is said to have been investigated in the author's laboratory, but how the author concluded that it would separate

the two components of the pain experience is not stated. As a consumer of research, you must look for the validity and reliability of the tools used for measurement and for specific descriptions of how those conclusions were reached (see Chapter 7).

The effects of relaxation therapy also were addressed by Nath and Rinehart (1979). They investigated the effect of teaching relaxation individually and in groups on the blood pressure of subjects with essential hypertension. Blood pressure was measured with an aneroid sphygmomanometer, with the cuff placed 2.5 cm above the antecubital space; the bag was deflated at 2–3 mmHg per second.

The blood pressure cuff is commonly used in the clinical area and is considered an accurate instrument. It does need to be calibrated periodically, and the authors make no mention of whether calibration was done, whether the same sphygmomanometer was used for all subjects, or whether blood pressure was consistently measured by a single individual on all of the subjects. Statements about these aspects of instrumentation would have strengthened the measurement portion of the study. Knowing what the researcher did to assure the validity of the instruments adds credibility to the findings obtained.

Measurement of the physiologic effects of patient education may be of interest in a study you are reading or designing. Examples of measures that investigators have used to examine the specific effects of patient education are found in Table 12-4. Serious attention must continue to be focused on identifying and using measures that are sensitive to physiologic effects produced by patient education and on clustering those measures to capture the full impact that such education may have.

Table 12-4   Patient Education: Four Examples of Variables and Instrumentation

Variables		Instrumentation	
Independent	Dependent	Independent	Dependent
1. Level of structure of the teaching program	Pulmonary function (vital capacity, maximum mid-expiratory flow rate, forced expiratory volume, expiratory reserve volume) Length of hospital stay		Spirometer
2. Types of information: Sensory Behavioral Sensory and behavioral General	Ambulation Length of postoperative hospitalization First venture from home after discharge		Chart Self-report
3. Bronchial diameter	Total respiratory resistance Functional residual capacity Airway resistance	Computer with analog to digital converter Oscilloscope	Respiratory resistance unit Whole-body plethysmography
4. Educational component of a rehabilitation program	Number of "good" days Changes in number of symptoms Whether symptoms were treated by the patient		Self-report

Infection and Wound Healing

Studies by nurse researchers in the area of healing and infection have focused largely on care of invasive lines or local wounds. The independent variable(s) of concern have included various skin preparation techniques and products, various dressings, and administration of drug therapy. The dependent variables in these studies have focused on infection rate, phlebitis, and healing. Instrumentation is a challenge when these areas are studied, and appreciation of the equipment needed to manipulate the independent variable(s) and assess the dependent variable will allow you to plan more clearly your study design and to critique related studies. Examples of variables and instruments used in the area of healing and infection are given in Table 12-5.

Instrumentation and Measurement Issues

Infection   Antibiotics are frequently prescribed prophylactically and as therapeutic treatment for infection. The nursing responsibility inherent in this medically prescribed regimen lies in the manner in which the antibiotic is administered.

Table 12-5   Wound Healing and Infection: Four Examples With Variables and Instrumentation

Variables		Instrumentation	
Independent	**Dependent**	**Independent**	**Dependent**
1. Methods of administration of antibiotic	Quantity of antibiotic administered	IV sets with and without volume control chamber	Spectrophotometer
2. Frequency of changing intravenous tubing and percutaneous site	Incidence of phlebitis		Subjective evaluation of pain, erythema, elevated temperature
3. Site and type of thermometer	Temperature reading		Electronic and mercury thermometers Calibration plug for electronic thermometer Water bath NBS certified thermometer
4. Epidermal growth factor	Migration of keratinocytes Rate of differentiation of keratinocytes	Dermatome	Biopsy equipment Histologic slides
	Rate of healing	Grading of ulcers	Kundin wound tool

Kerr and her colleagues (1979) examined two commonly used methods of administering antibiotics to see if there was a difference in the quantity of the antibiotic remaining in the tubing between the primary bottle and the volume control chamber when the tubing was clamped and when it was unclamped. The quantity of antibiotic was simulated with the dye methylene blue, which has the same pH as ampicillin and was provided in concentrations approximating those used for ampicillin administration. The color comparisons between the various concentrations of the dye administered by the two different methods was evaluated using a *spectrophotometer*, an instrument that quantifies the density of the color present, with the more concentrated solutions having a greater density. The dilutions and the readings from the spectrophotometer were checked by two investigators. A visual evaluation was also completed.

plicability of the findings to the clinical area. The instrument used to quantify the dependent variable is a well-accepted measure of color density, but the question of how adherent methylene blue is to the inside of the IV equipment in comparison with the antibiotics raises another problem. That is, solutions of varying molecular weight and composition have different adherency properties; and these differences between the two solutions were not addressed. Nevertheless, the researchers demonstrated ingenuity in approaching a clinical problem using the more controlled laboratory environment with its sophisticated instruments to find an answer.

Some problems, however, are examined using the clinical setting. When the study design is well controlled, findings can be generalized for the population that has been examined.

This rather elaborate laboratory study is a fine example of testing a clinical problem in the laboratory, and in this case, there is direct ap-

One such study, undertaken by Nichols, Barstow, and Cooper (1983), sought to determine the relationship between the incidence of phlebitis and the frequency of changing the intravenous tubing and the percutaneous site. The dependent variable in this study was the incidence of phlebitis, with the operational definition for phlebitis being the presence of two of the three classic signs of inflammation: pain, erythema, and elevated temperature.

It is not clear from the narrative in the study whether the elevated temperature was a local or systemic phenomenon. Such details in operational definitions have implications for both the validity and reliability of the measures selected and used. These authors have provided a model for the clustering of symptoms to measure a dependent variable. The strength of their definition of phlebitis lies in its conceptual basis, which is made explicit in the conceptual framework of the study (see Chapter 10). Here is another example in which the test of internal consistency shows a logical link between the theoretical underpinnings of the study and the measurement technique.

An interesting series of studies has been conducted on the validity and reliability of thermometers as a measure of temperature. These studies are included here because one cardinal sign of infection is elevated temperature. These studies as a whole are presented because they illustrate the variability that a single instrument may give under different environmental conditions and when applied using different techniques. The research consumer must constantly read with a cautious eye to see what precautions the investigator has taken to minimize these threats to instrument validity and reliability (see Chapter 6).

Erickson (1980) examined the effect of sublingual site and type of thermometer on oral temperature. The three sublingual sites were the right and left sublingual pockets and the front sublingual area. The two types of ther-

mometers were electronic and mercury in glass. A second purpose of the study was to examine the effect of insertion technique on temperature readings and thermometer response time. This researcher compared the thermometers to be used in the study against a bath of a known temperature to establish their validity. The electronic thermometers were then calibrated, and the amount of error of the mercury-in-glass thermometers was noted.

This researcher used acceptable methods to ensure the validity of her measuring tool. Without this information the data would not be meaningful. The rigor in this approach is important.

Schiffman (1982), who examined the difference between axillary and rectal temperatures in neonates, used the same method to establish the validity of measurement by the thermometers. The researcher and three additional data collectors took the temperatures of the neonates, and the researcher noted that interrater reliability in reading the thermometers was established when the validity of the thermometers was evaluated.

Description of the validity and reliability of instruments was critical to this study. The procedures used to establish validity and reliability make the data believable.

Hasler and Cohen (1982) examined the effects of various means of oxygen administration on oral temperature readings in healthy subjects. They compared subjects' temperatures before oxygen administration with those during oxygen administration. They built on the work of Erickson (1980) in selecting their thermometer placement. No check was made on the validity of measurement by the thermometer, although the investigators did standardize the thermometer used. Because of the failure to check the accuracy of the thermometer, the findings from this study must be questioned.

As a consumer of research, you must consider what role the establishment of validity of measures of physiologic variables has for drawing implications from the study for practice application (see Chapter 2). Appreciating the need to establish the validity of such a simple measure as taking a temperature suggests that in more sophisticated instruments validity procedures must also be undertaken.

Wound Healing Several studies of wound healing are of interest from an instrumentation perspective. Instruments used to manipulate the independent variable(s) as well as to measure the dependent variable(s) must be considered.

Gill and Atwood (1981) reported a study that sought to establish a dose–response curve for epidermal growth factor and wound healing in the pig model. Specifically, they were interested in the effect of epidermal growth factor on migration of keratinocytes over the wound, the mitotic index, and rate of differentiation of keratinocytes. The independent variable was the epidermal growth factor, and the dependent variable was histologic evaluation of keratinocytes.

This study is an example of a nursing research study that blends a basic science framework with a nursing science framework (see Chapters 1 and 10). Gill and Atwood manipulated a factor that influences cell growth—that is, epidermal growth factor, and described this manipulation from the nursing science framework of Rogers, specifically in terms of the principles of reciprocy and helicy. The interpretation of this model has been criticized (Kim 1983), and the authors have replied to this criticism (Atwood & Gill-Rogers 1984). This debate increases our understanding of their perspective of the conceptual framework for the study. The use of a combination of frameworks is an important model for nursing to acknowledge and use. The framework for a study need not arise from one discipline. It must, how-

ever, be logical and internally consistent. Again, it is important that the conceptual perspective drive the choice of the independent variable and the instruments used to measure it.

Biologic instruments are an important part of manipulating the independent variable as well as measuring the dependent variable in this study. Use of an instrument was critical in making wounds on the pig's back. The wounds had to be partial thickness (not all of the layers of the skin are removed), and the depth of them had to be uniform so the effects of the various concentrations of growth factor could be examined. A *dermatome* is a standard approach to creating such wounds, but in this case the instrument employed was not described. For measurement of the dependent variable, tissue biopsies were performed. The specific technique and instrument are not described, nor is the manner in which the cells were prepared for histologic examination. Interpretation of the microscopic evaluation of the cells also was critical to the credibility of the findings of the study. Yet who did the evaluation and whether this was confirmed by an independent rater were not mentioned. The authors did take steps to control for bias in that they randomly selected the wounds to be biopsied. Another strength of the study is the authors' acknowledgement that it was a pilot study.

Two treatments for decubitus ulcers were evaluated in a consortium study directed by Roesler (1983). The independent variable in this study was type of treatment for decubitus ulcers. The specific dressings evaluated were Op-Site, which was used on all stages of decubiti, and Vigilon Primary Wound Dressing, which was used on stage III and IV ulcers. Subjects were included in the study when a Stage I–IV ulcer was present. The stages of ulcers were defined, and these categories were mutually exclusive. Training of nurses in use of the wound care products is described.

How or whether reliability was established among the nurses in staging the ulcer or applying the treatments is not stated. Incorrect staging could result in serious threats to the findings, as could inconsistent application of the wound care agents. Description of the steps used to control for this variation would have strengthened the study. When multiple care givers are involved and multiple research sites used, consideration must be given to the reliability of the instruments and to the people who use them.

The dependent variables for this study were the rate of healing, nursing time required to perform the treatments, and cost effectiveness. Rate of healing was measured with the *Kundin wound tool*, which assesses volume of missing tissue by measuring the depth of the wound and its circumference. Stage I ulcers were defined as reddened skin that is intact, and stage II ulcers as reddened and broken skin that may be excoriated or vesiculated. The Kundin wound tool provides for measurement of circumference but not depth for these two stages of decubiti. The nurses were taught to use the tool, but how reliability between raters was evaluated is not described.

Instrumentation to measure healing in the clinical area has been problematic because the available tools are indirect, disrupt healing, or are not sensitive to subtle daily changes in healing. Some currently used measures of wound healing have the potential of causing disruption of the healing process, for example, tissue biopsy by punch or scraping. This is a threat to subsequent measures in terms of validity and reliability in assessing healing of those disrupted wounds. Repeated sampling may delay healing. A Wound Assessment Instrument to assess healing has been developed (Stotts & Cooper 1984) which allows evaluation of the physical attributes of the wound, such as color of tissue and adherence of exudate. Once reliability of this instrument has been established on a patient population, it may be used in studies to improve measurement of healing without causing disruption of the healing process.

Nursing time in the Roesler study (1983) was operationally defined as the amount of time recorded by nurses to complete the treatment. It was noted in the definition that nursing time did not include the time it took for turning and positioning the patient. The nurses kept a flow sheet for this purpose. Six hospital sites and clients of one Visiting Nurses Association were used for this study, and a self-report method was a practical approach to determining the time it took for the daily care. Cost effectiveness was quantified as the amount of cost of the products for the three treatments and additional supplies needed for that treatment. All the variables are operationally defined, which would make replication of the study possible.

The areas of healing and infection are often under the control of the nurse. Appreciation of the instrumentation needed to manipulate variables and assess their effects will facilitate mounting of studies in this area and improve the interpretation of findings.

Environmental Stimuli

Nurse investigators have been interested in the effects of different environmental stimuli on a variety of dependent biophysiologic variables. In some cases the effects of naturally occurring environmental stimuli have been examined. In other studies the investigators have created diverse environmental stimuli as the independent variables (see Table 12-6 for examples).

Instrumentation and Measurement Issues

Sound   An example of a study using naturally occurring stimuli was reported by Helton and colleagues (1980). They examined the mental effects of sleep deprivation in 62 critically ill subjects. In another study naturally occurring

Table 12-6   Environmental Stimuli: Four Examples With Variables and Instrumentation

Variables		Instrumentation	
Independent	Dependent	Independent	Dependent
1. Kinesthetic stimulation	Growth Development Neurological function	Motorized hammock Rocking bed Movement of limbs	
2. Suctioning	Oxygen tension	Suctioning equipment	Transcutaneous oxygen monitor Blood gas analyzer
3.	Sleep		Observation records Videotape recording EEG, EMG tracings
4. Touch therapeutic or physical		Person trained in techniques of touch	Cardiac monitor Intracranial pressure monitor Thermistor Thermograph Dermograph Electrodes

sounds were measured in two different hospital units, using a sound level meter (Woods & Falk 1974).

In another descriptive study, the relationship between selected sounds in a coronary care unit (CCU) and the heart rate responses of subjects in the CCU was determined (Marshall 1972). An audiotape recorder was used, and the ECG recordings of the subjects yielded the heart rate.

The major problem with the instrumentation for this study was that the tape recorder and ECG system were not synchronized for the simultaneous recording of unit sounds and ECG tracings. This coordination of timing of the data collection is necessary for moment-to-moment analysis in determining the effects of specific environmental sounds on heart rate responses.

Therapeutic Application of Stimuli   Nurse investigators have also manipulated environmental stimuli. Short-gestation infants are used as the subjects in a number of such studies. Examples of the stimuli used include cycling-motion exer-

cise of upper and lower limbs (Porter 1972), auditory stimulation (playing the recording of a heart beat), and kinesthetic stimulation (using a motorized hammock or a rocking water bed) (Barnard 1973, Neal 1977). The outcome measures included growth and development and neurologic function. Several nurse investigators, using *animal models*, studied the effects of thermal applications to the abdomen on local and systemic tissue temperatures (Dyer & Bagnell 1970, Martinson & Anderson 1978). The question these studies raise is the extent to which animal findings can be applicable to humans. Beyond access to animals and training in the techniques of handling, the equipment needed for these two studies was rather simple. It included equipment for quantifying and maintaining the temperature specified for the thermal application. As the outcome, or dependent, variable was local and systemic tissue temperature change, the major piece of equipment needed was a thermometer that was sensitive and reliable. In another study the association between insertion of a rectal thermometer and changes in heart rate and rhythm was examined in 19 acute myocardial infarct patients (Gruber 1974). Again, the equipment needed to conduct this study was readily available.

As shown in these studies, measurement of some biophysiologic variables is not complicated. What is important is that the instruments selected do, in fact, measure directly or are considered to be the best indirect measures of the variables under study, that they are sensitive to the changes expected, and that they are reliable.

Coronary Precautions   Many commonly accepted nursing practices have not been based on empirical data. Specific procedures described in older editions of nursing fundamentals texts and some that have been passed along by tradition need to be subjected to empirical testing (see Chapters 1 and 2). For example, a number of nursing practices, referred to as coronary precautions, are believed to control environmental stimuli that might adversely affect the individual with a myocardial infarct—for example , prohibiting ice-water ingestion (Kirchhoff 1981). The effects of some of these environmental stimuli are being examined by nurse investigators. These studies need to be replicated to determine if the findings are consistent. If the reported findings are confirmed, they will form the basis for change in nursing practice, and some of these coronary precautions will be retired as myths. The two major notions are that the effects of commonly used clinical nursing therapies need to be studied and that more than one study is needed to justify changes in practice. Similar studies, using similar patient populations, in which similar questions are addressed and in which similar measurements are used, need to be conducted to demonstrate confirmation or refutation of findings across these multiple studies. Findings from only one study, regardless of the quality of the study, are insufficient to use as a basis for change in practice.

Kirchhoff (1982) conducted a national survey using 240 hospitals with critical care units to determine the restrictions imposed on myocardial infarct patients. She reported that "despite findings that cast doubt on the practices of restricting ice water and rectal temperature measurement, coronary precautions are commonly practiced" (p. 196). Two recent research reports illustrate the study of one of the coronary precautions, oral temperature.

To determine the effect of oxygen inhalation by a nasal cannula on oral temperatures, 100 healthy adults were randomly assigned to four groups—a control group and three groups to which oxygen was administered for 30 minutes at 2, 4, or 6 liters per minute (Lim-Levy 1982). The oral temperature of each subject was measured before oxygen was administered and after 30 minutes of exposure while oxygen was still being given. No significant effects of oxygen administration on oral temperature were found.

From these findings the investigator suggested that there was a need to review the practice of using less acceptable sites (axillary or rectal) for obtaining the temperature in patients receiving oxygen. However, several critical questions must be addressed before these findings can be used to change practice. One question is whether findings from a healthy adult population would be similar to those obtained in a clinically ill population. Another question is whether changes would be found if the subjects received oxygen over a period of time greater than 30 minutes, which is the case in a clinical population.

An adequate description of the instruments used is included in the research report. A single electronic solid-state thermometer capable of registering 94 to 108° F $\pm$ .2° was used for measuring the dependent variable, the oral temperature of each subject. When the subject's maximum temperature was reached, a red light and an audible tone signaled the investigator.

The investigator describes well the placement of the probe, and to account for possible differences in temperature obtained from different sublingual areas, the same area was used in each subject. Attention to the placement and use of the same probe for each subject are important aspects of controlling factors that could affect the findings. There was no report, however, that the thermometer readings obtained with the single probe were compared with readings from another thermometer. This simple check of reliability of instruments used to measure biophysiologic variables would strengthen the credibility of the findings. The other equipment used to create the independent variable, oxygen administration, included compressed oxygen tanks, a flow meter to establish the desired liter flow per minute, a humidifier, and a nasal cannula for each subject.

The investigator also addressed control of several factors that are known to influence one's temperature; these include gum chewing, ingesting food or fluid, and smoking. Identification and control of other factors that may influence either the independent or the outcome variables are especially critical steps in designing and conducting studies in which biophysiologic variables are measured. How the researcher accounts for these confounding variables must be specified in the research plan and included in the report of the findings. For example, if you did not know that the investigator had had the subjects refrain from eating, drinking, and smoking before and during the experimental procedure, you would have to question the findings reported, because you know these factors influence the dependent variable (oral temperature) of interest. Having or acquiring knowledge about the topic area of the research problem and reading numerous studies relevant to the area will be of tremendous value in helping you to become aware of the potential influencing factors, special characteristics of the equipment used, and the important measurement issues that need to be addressed to ensure credibility of the findings.

In another study, using 40 healthy adult volunteers, the effect on oral temperature of 15-minute periods of oxygen administration by aerosol, venti-mask, or nasal prongs was examined (Hasler & Cohen 1982). This is an example of a counterbalanced design; the effects of each method of oxygen administration was tested on each subject. The sequence of presentation of the oxygen devices is illustrated well by the authors in a table in which this counterbalanced design is shown. Equipment similar to that described in the last example was required to conduct this study. These investigators reported that with a reliability check of the electronic thermometer, there was a range of 0.4° F. Consequently, they decided that for a change in temperature to be considered clinically significant, the observed change in response to the experimental treatment would have to be greater than 0.5° F. This notion illustrates yet another important point in studying biophysiologic variables. Although it may be possible to show statistically significant differences, these differences may, in fact, not be clinically significant. Unless the equipment is tested for reliability and the variation taken into account (as it was in this study), the observed changes could be due to variation in measurement by the instruments used.

Suctioning Suctioning and heel stick (to obtain a blood sample) are environmental stimuli that are part of the routine care of premature infants. Measurement issues are presented for several of these studies.

Norris and colleagues (1982) examined the effects of these procedures on blood oxygen levels in 25 premature infants with respiratory distress syndrome. To conduct this study, no additional equipment or instruments were required; the subjects were hospitalized, and everything that was needed to collect the desired data was already available and being used in the routine care of the infants.

This may be the case for a number of studies in which biophysiologic variables are measured. To measure the dependent variable of blood oxygen level, a transcutaneous oxygen monitor was used. Baseline measures were obtained before the experimental treatments were begun, and rest periods were provided between the treatments. In studies where some experimental treatment is used as the independent variable (in this case, suctioning), the more commonly used research design includes obtaining baseline values for the dependent variable (blood oxygen level) before subjects are given the experimental treatment. Without this baseline measure, it would be difficult or impossible to demonstrate the effects of the treatment, that is, to show change in the outcome variable of interest as a result of the experimental treatment.

Another point to consider when conducting this kind of study is that it is also critical for the experimental treatment to be carried out in some well-defined standard method for each subject. The following are examples of procedural issues that need to be specified:

1. Will different nurses be carrying out the suctioning?

2. Will continuous suctioning or will intermittent suctioning be used?

3. What amount of normal saline (if any) will be instilled before suctioning?

4. For what period of time will suction be applied?

5. Will nurses turn the infant's head in each direction for a different pass of the suction catheter?

6. Will the endotracheal tubes have a side port through which oxygen administration will be continued throughout the suctioning procedure?

All of these possible variations in the independent variable would influence the dependent variable (blood oxygen levels). Other influencing factors are whether hyperoxygenation or hyperinflation is to be included as part of the procedure, and if so, how similarities in delivery will be determined. To avoid this kind of problem, researchers must make decisions about conditions for the experimental treatment and specify precisely how it will be administered to all subjects. Again, this care and precision in the research process will make the findings more credible and will allow others to replicate or to extend the work.

Determining the effects of suctioning is one area in which there have been a number of studies. Most of them have been conducted to determine techniques to decrease tracheobronchial trauma or to prevent a fall in the arterial oxygen tension as a consequence of suctioning. These studies have been conducted on animals as well as on humans of varying ages. When these studies are conducted in adults, if the dependent variable of interest is the arterial oxygen tension, it is necessary to obtain blood samples for blood gas analysis. Although the suction equipment is available and being used clinically, for purposes of research, the type to be used and the precise technique for suctioning need to be specified. Examples of this kind of information are found in the reports of the suctioning studies (Adlkofer & Powaser 1978, Belling, Kelley, & Simon 1978, Skelley, Deeren, & Powaser 1980).

Measurement of *transcutaneous oxygen tension* has also been used to determine the effects of nonnutritive sucking in premature infants (Burroughs et al 1978). This monitor is used clinically, and in the premature infant it has been shown to be reasonably reliable as an indirect measure of blood oxygen levels. Thus, it is possible to design studies to determine the effects of a variety of environmental stimuli or clinical therapeutics, using this piece of equipment to measure a clinically important parameter, oxygen levels. Clinical availability of equipment and the clinical importance of the dependent variable are major considerations in designing a study in which changes in biophysiologic variables are to be quantified.

Sleep Sleep, as a biophysiologic variable, has been examined by nurse investigators primarily as a dependent variable. It has been measured by several different approaches, which need to be considered as you read the research reports. One approach has been to ask the subjects their perception of their sleep; descriptors such as quality and duration, frequency and duration of periods of wakefulness, and identification of factors that facilitate or impede sleep have been included. You should recognize that in such an approach the data collection instrument (whether by interview or by a paper-and-pencil, self-administered technique) is not a standardized instrument; that is, no validity or reliability data are accumulated. There are also acknowledged problems with self-report data. Findings are credible to the extent to which you can rely on the veracity and accuracy of the report given by the subjects.

Another approach to collecting data on sleep is the participant–observer technique. Someone can actually observe the subjects over specified periods of time, or a television camera and recorder can be used. The videotape recording can then be viewed by a panel of expert observers, and the periods of sleep rated. These examples are still indirect and imprecise measures of sleep but they are more objective than the self-report approach. However, you may be more interested in obtaining the subjects' perceptions about the quality of their sleep than in actually documenting the precise minutes and hours of sleep versus the periods of wakefulness.

The more direct measure of sleep is with the use of EEG and EMG recordings. There are EEG and EMG patterns which characterize the various stages of sleep. From these tracings it is possible not only to distinguish periods of sleep from periods of wakefulness but also to determine the stage of sleep and the length of time spent in each stage. The equipment required to obtain this more precise objective measurement of sleep, although rather commonly used for diagnostic purposes, may not be readily available for research purposes. In addition, training and

skill in interpreting the tracings are requisite.

A variety of approaches can be used to measure sleep; they range from indirect, subjective measures to direct, objective measures. Examples are:

- Self-report (from interview or questionnaire)
- Participant observer technique
- Activity rating scale
- Television recordings
- EEG tracings

For example, perceived changes in the sleep-awake patterns three months after cerebral concussion were studied using self-report data from an adapted version of an investigator-developed questionnaire (Parsons & Ver Beek 1982). Effects of noise in intensive care units and number of interruptions to sleep have been studied using the participant observer technique (Walker 1972). An activity scale for recording sleep observations was developed and used by a participant observer to determine the effects of auditory (recording of a heart beat) and kinesthetic (rocker bed) stimulation on general maturation, weight gain, and sleep-awake behavior in premature infants (Barnard 1973). Television recordings were used to assess time for sleep onset (and incidence of regurgitation) in relation to specified feeding practices in newborn infants (unpublished thesis). The relationship between breathing patterns and stability of sleep was determined in six chronic obstructive pulmonary disease patients; the investigator had access to a well-equipped laboratory (Smyth 1980).

The purpose of the study, the research questions, and the state of the art of the measurement techniques should be the primary criteria used in determining the measurement strategies. Practicality, availability, and cost to the investigator and to the subjects also need to be considered in making the selection.

Surgery Hypothermia has been observed to occur in the immediate postoperative period. In this instance surgery and its attendant procedures are the environmental stimuli. However, other factors may influence the frequency, magnitude, and duration of postoperative hypothermia.

For example, the relationship of age, anesthesia, and shivering to rewarming was examined in 198 adult postsurgical patients (Vaughan, Vaughan, & Cork 1981). These are all biophysiologic variables. In this study the outcome variable, body core temperature, was measured with a disposable tympanic membrane sensor that had a battery-operated monitoring unit. The measurement and calibration procedures used are described in the research report. Observations were used to determine the presence or absence of shivering; thus, the shivering data were dichotomous (present or absent). There was considerable variety in the surgical procedures, in the range of duration of anesthesia, and in the characteristics of the study sample.

This, too, represents a study in which the equipment needed to assess the biophysiologic variables was not elaborate. Data were collected by instrumentation (temperature), from the medical record (age, surgical procedure, anesthesia), and from observation (shivering). Data for a variety of variables can be obtained from the medical record and from observation. Collecting data for biophysiologic variables does not have to involve complex equipment or great cost.

Touch   The effects of touch have been studied by nurse researchers. Touch, as an environmental stimulus, or as a therapeutic intervention, is not yet well defined operationally.

In an earlier study the effect of pulse palpation (touch) on cardiac arrhythmia in 62 patients hospitalized in a coro-

nary care unit was examined (Mills et al 1976). The investigators concluded from the findings that autonomic responses to human contact (pulse palpation) can affect the rate of ectopic impulse generation. In 31 of their subjects who exhibited cardiac arrhythmia, ectopic beat frequency changed when the pulse was palpated.

This study required no additional equipment that was not in use for routine care; the subjects were connected already to electrocardiographic monitoring equipment, tracings were available, and pulse palpation was done routinely at least every 4 hours. In evaluating the findings of this study, questions about sample selection, exclusion and inclusion criteria, and sample characteristics (such as medication regimen) and other circumstances occurring in the environment simultaneously during the periods of data collection, all need to be raised. Acquiring extensive knowledge about the topic area will help you to critique the studies (see Chapters 2 and 7).

Touch, in the form of a stroking motion to the side of the face and to the back of the hand, was used as an independent variable in a study of 30 patients who were connected to an intracranial pressure monitoring device (Wallech 1983). A counterbalanced design was used; the subjects were assigned randomly to have either the side of the face or the back of the hand stroked first, followed by a 4-minute period of rest and then stroking (2 minutes) the other site (hand or face). This information is given in an abstract, and no information is given about the subjects, such as type of pathology (head injury versus some other state) or state of consciousness. No data are reported, but the investigator concluded that stroking did lower the intracranial pressure.

Without baseline values of the intracranial pressure and the values obtained during and after the stroking, the magnitude and duration of the decrease in intracranial pressure remain unknown to the reader. More information is needed to evaluate this study, and it would be given in a full report. The study does represent an experimental approach to quantify the effect of touch (stroking) on intracranial pressure. Again, the only extra equipment not part of the patient's routine equipment needed to conduct this study is a stopwatch or clock to time the periods of touch and rest accurately. Data for the dependent variable, intracranial pressure, were obtained from the monitors already being used for evaluation of the patients' clinical progress.

In a more recent study, an attempt was made to differentiate between therapeutic touch and physical touch (Randolph 1984). The effect of these two types of touch on physiologic response to stressful stimuli was evaluated in 60 female college students. They were subjected to a 13-minute silent film depicting a tribal ceremony of an Australian Aboriginal tribe as the stressful stimulus. Within the film "a sequence of operations performed with a sharp stone on the genitals of adolescent boys" was shown (p. 34). Therapeutic touch was given to the experimental group of subjects by eight nurses who had completed a course on therapeutic touch and who had at least a year of experience using the technique. Application of this kind of touch is described in the report. With energy and attention directed to the subject, the subject's abdomen and back were touched with the nurses' hands. For the control group, eight other nurses were used to apply physical touch; this involved light placement of hands on the subject's abdomen and lower back. Physiologic response was operationalized to encompass several measures, including skin conductance, muscle tension, and peripheral skin temperature. These measures of physiologic response were selected as being reflective of central, autonomic, and peripheral nervous system function.

This study required a variety of equipment, which is described in the research report in sufficient detail. A 16-mm film projector to deliver the stressful stimulus, an Autogenic 2000 Feedback Thermograph and a *thermistor* to measure peripheral skin temperature, and an Autogenic 3400 Feedback Dermograph and silver/silver chloride electrodes to measure skin conductance are examples. This kind of specific information about equipment will be useful to those who want to compare findings across studies, offer possible explanations for any differences or similarities found, or design and conduct a study. Although not of great interest to all readers, this kind of information should be included in sufficient detail in research reports, because it is important to those who are intensely interested in the topic area. Reporting of this information makes possible the replication of the study or identification of problems in the instrumentation.

The differences in the physiologic responses of the two groups in this study were not statistically significant. The experimental group (therapeutic touch) did not remain more relaxed than the control group (physical touch). One interesting possibility that might account for the findings is that being touched could also provoke a physiologic response. To account for this possibility, a third group of subjects could have been subjected only to therapeutic touch (not the film) for 13 minutes. When designing a study, it is important to think about what alternative explanations could also influence the findings and to design the study so that the major factors are controlled or studied.

Slow-stroke back massage has been used in combination with guided imagery as a therapeutic intervention for chemotherapy-induced nausea and vomiting in cancer patients. Touch, although variously defined, is an environmental stimulus that has been studied in different populations. In addition to the examples just cited, the effects of touch have been explored using very different biophysiologic measures as the dependent or outcome variables. Within the confines of this chapter, it is possible to include only a few representative studies.

Pain   External or internal environmental conditions may result in pain. Although the sensation of pain is a subjective phenomenon, nurses have been concerned about the relief of pain and the promotion of comfort. Because pain is subjective, it is difficult to quantify precisely. Pain, in the human model, has been measured primarily as the dependent variable. A variety of clinical therapies have been tested as the independent variable, with their effects on pain reduction assessed.

For example, Bafford (1975) used progressive relaxation as an intervention to control pain in open-heart surgery patients. Thirty subjects were assigned to three groups. The dependent variables were the direct pain response, related patient behavior, and mental status disturbance. Direct pain response was operationalized to be the count of medications received for pain, sleep, or tension by each subject (as recorded on their charts) and by self-reports from each subject estimating the amount of pain experienced. A type of visual analog scale was used for this self-report. The subjects drew a horizontal line across a 10-inch vertical line to indicate the total amount of pain they had experienced since surgery. The bottom of the vertical line represented no pain and the top of the line represented the most pain possible. The distance from the bottom of the line to the location of the horizontal line drawn by the subjects was measured; this length was used as the subject's score of total pain experienced since surgery.

Descriptions of the other dependent variables are provided in the report; although they are of interest, they are not included here because they are not specifically related to the measurement of pain. Little difference was found between the three experimental groups on the dependent variables. Several questions could be raised. The extent to which the one experimental group practiced and achieved relaxation is unknown. The extent to which the subjects were able to assess the "total amount" of pain experienced over a 9-day period remains elusive. The extent to which "count" of medications received for sleep and tension (in addition to pain medica-

tions) is reflective of pain is open to debate. These are all examples of issues that readers of research as well as researchers need to address because these factors may influence the findings obtained.

Another study was conducted to determine the effectiveness of a relaxation technique in increasing the comfort level of postoperative patients in their first attempt to get out of bed (Flaherty & Fitzpatrick 1977). Forty-two subjects were assigned to the experimental group (relaxation technique) or to the control group. After their first attempt to get out of bed, self-report pain and distress scales were used to assess the subjects' incisional pain and body distress. The pain and distress scales used had been developed and tested previously by Johnson (1972, 1973). The investigators determined the amount of analgesics used and compared values obtained for blood pressure, pulse, and respiratory rates before surgery and after the first attempt to get out of bed. From the findings obtained, these investigators concluded that use of the relaxation technique to reduce muscular tension did increase the subjects' comfort levels.

Operational definitions for each of the variables, including the relaxation technique, are well defined in the research report. For example, comfort level was assessed from the responses on the pain and distress scales, the total amount of analgesics used in the first 24 hours after surgery, and changes in the vital signs; thus, a composite of measures was used in quantifying the dependent variable, comfort level.

Electrical surface stimulation (ESS) has been used as a therapeutic intervention for the control of pain. It involves low-level controlled electricity being administered through the skin.

In one study the effect of ESS on control of acute postoperative pain and on the prevention of ileus and atelectasis was determined in a group of subjects having abdominal surgery (Menzel & Martinson 1975). From their study of 27 subjects, the investigators concluded that ESS was not effective in reducing postoperative pain nor in preventing the two complications. The group was assigned randomly to the experimental or control group. One transcutaneous electric surface device was designed to operate without giving stimulation; this was used for those assigned to the control group. A double-blind design was used, so neither the subject nor the nurse using the device knew who was receiving the experimental treatment.

In this example the manufacturer of the instrument cooperated with the nurse researchers in providing the device to be used for the control group. A description of how the electric surface stimulator was applied is provided in the report. Measurement of pain was achieved by interviewing the subjects 24 hours after the surgery. Their subjective reports were rated on an ordinal scale (see Chapter 15). The range of possible responses was *none*, *a little*, *some*, *quite a bit*, or *a lot*. The investigators acknowledged the lack of validity and reliability for this instrument.

These studies did not require any elaborate equipment; they did require careful definition of the variables. Most of the data were collected from the chart or from the subjects. In each of these studies the subjects were asked to rate their perception of their pain, and the amount of analgesic used was accounted for. In each example different scales were used for assessing the pain experience. Because pain is a subjective variable, precise quantification in the human model remains problematic. However, pain is a biophysiologic variable of considerable interest to both clinicians and researchers.

Nursing Research and Measurement of Biophysiologic Variables

The studies included in this chapter were selected to illustrate a range of important issues to be considered in reading research reports and in designing and conducting studies that measure biophysiologic variables. To achieve a sense of order in the diverse body of content of these studies, we categorized and presented them within five broad biophysiologic phenomena—feeding alterations, activity and position, patient education outcomes, healing and infection, and environmental stimuli. Comments pertinent to specific problem areas were included to illustrate important factors that need to be considered to strengthen the studies and thus enhance the credibility of the findings.

Many additional examples could have been included; they are so numerous that it is not possible to provide an exhaustive list. Some have been used as the independent variable, whereas others have been studied as the dependent, or outcome, variables. How these variables are measured is diverse because there is a multitude of instruments and equipment available for measurement. Some of the instruments provide indirect measures of the variable; others provide a direct, precise measurement. Determining measurement reliability of the instruments is essential. The biophysiologic phenomena, variables, and instruments included in this chapter were selected because they represent the possible range and reflect the current state of the art of this type of nursing research.

Some biophysiologic variables require subjective assessment, but most can be quantified by some objective measure. For some variables, a battery of several measures is necessary, because there is no single best measure. Quantification of many biophysiologic variables yields interval-level data, and ratio level can be obtained frequently. Biophysiologic variables can be influenced by other factors than experimental treatment, and these other factors need to be identified and accounted for in the research design.

There are many clinical situations in which the instruments or equipment needed for research are already available and being used for monitoring purposes. Extensive knowledge about the problem area and familiarity with the clinical management of the population of interest are invaluable assets for the researcher. It is from this perspective that the most credible research evolves.

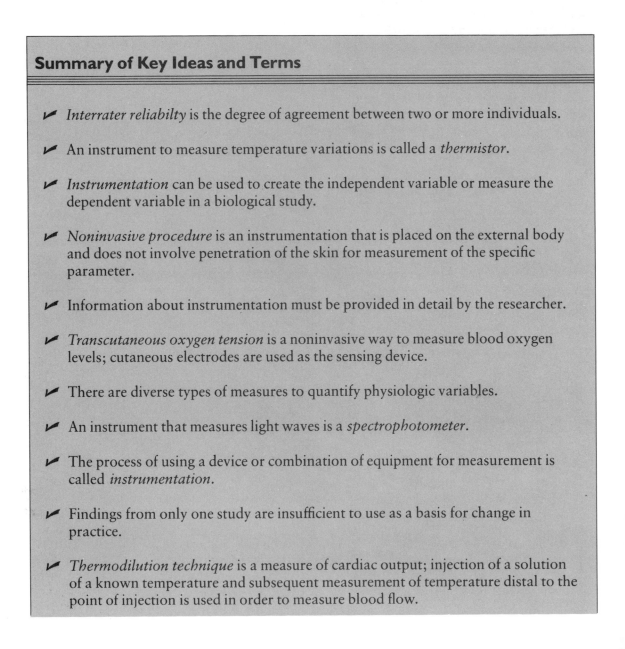

Summary of Key Ideas and Terms

✔ *Interrater reliabilty* is the degree of agreement between two or more individuals.

✔ An instrument to measure temperature variations is called a *thermistor*.

✔ *Instrumentation* can be used to create the independent variable or measure the dependent variable in a biological study.

✔ *Noninvasive procedure* is an instrumentation that is placed on the external body and does not involve penetration of the skin for measurement of the specific parameter.

✔ Information about instrumentation must be provided in detail by the researcher.

✔ *Transcutaneous oxygen tension* is a noninvasive way to measure blood oxygen levels; cutaneous electrodes are used as the sensing device.

✔ There are diverse types of measures to quantify physiologic variables.

✔ An instrument that measures light waves is a *spectrophotometer*.

✔ The process of using a device or combination of equipment for measurement is called *instrumentation*.

✔ Findings from only one study are insufficient to use as a basis for change in practice.

✔ *Thermodilution technique* is a measure of cardiac output; injection of a solution of a known temperature and subsequent measurement of temperature distal to the point of injection is used in order to measure blood flow.

- ✔ A combination of resources helps you to select the most appropriate instrument for your research.

- ✔ The *Kundin wound tool* is an instrument to measure volume of tissue loss in a wound.

- ✔ A *Max Planck respirometer* is a device for measuring respiratory gas consumption.

- ✔ Instrumentation that involves penetration of the skin for measurement of some internal parameter is called *invasive procedure*.

- ✔ An instrument used to shave off various thicknesses of skin is a *dermatome*.

- ✔ *Animal models* use animals as research subjects.

- ✔ Availability, direct or indirect measures, single or multiple measures, sensitivity, validity, reliability, invasive versus noninvasive measures, and levels of data and cost are all considerations in selecting a biophysiologic instrument.

- ✔ Graphic representation of changes in a variable over time is a *waveform*.

- ✔ An *electroencephalogram* (EEG) is a waveform or recording of the electrical activity in the brain.

- ✔ An *electrocardiogram* (ECG) is a waveform or recording of the electrical activity of the heart.

- ✔ The *Douglas bag technique* is a means for measuring respiratory gas consumption by having the individual breathe into a special large bag under standardized conditions.

- ✔ For some biological variables a battery of measures must be used.

- ✔ A *plethysmograph* is a noninvasive instrument to measure flow.

- ✔ An instrument that records electrical activity of muscles is called an *electromyograph*.

- ✔ The guiding force for instrument selection must be the conceptualization of the phenomenon being studied.

> ✔ The instrumentation one uses and how it is used depend on the research question and research design.
>
> ✔ A *treadmill* is a platform covered with a moving walking surface; the speed and angle of the platform can be altered to produce a known physiological demand.

References

Adlkofer R, Powaser M: The effect of endotracheal suctioning on arterial blood gases in patients after cardiac surgery. *Heart Lung* 1978; 7:1011–1014.

Atwood JR, Gill-Rogers BP: Metatheory, methodology, and practicality: Issues in research uses of Roger's science of unitary man. *Nurs Res* 1984; 33:88–91.

Bafford DC: Progressive relaxation as a nursing intervention: A method of controlling pain for open-heart surgery patients. *Commun Nurs Res* 1975; 8:284–290.

Barnard K: The effect of stimulation on the sleep behavior of the premature infant. *Commun Nurs Res* 1973; 6:12–33.

Belling D et al: Use of the swivel adaptor aperture during suctioning to prevent hypoxemia in the mechanically ventilated patient. *Heart Lung* 1978; 7:320–322.

Burroughs A et al: The effect of nonnutritive sucking on transcutaneous oxygen tension in noncrying preterm neonates. *Res Nurs Health* 1978; 1:69–75.

Chulay M, Miller T: The effect of backrest elevation on pulmonary artery and pulmonary capillary wedge pressures in patients after cardiac surgery. *Heart Lung* 1984; 13:138–140.

Cotanch PH: Relaxation training for control of nausea and vomiting in patients receiving chemotherapy. *Cancer Nurs* 1983; 6:277–283.

Dyer ED, Bagnell HK: Local tissue and general temperature changes in dogs produced by temperature applications. *Nurs Res* 1970; 19:37–41.

Erikson R: Oral temperature differences in relation to thermometer technique. *Nurs Res* 1980; 29:157–164.

Flaherty GG, Fitzpatrick JJ: Relaxation technique to increase comfort level of postoperative patients: A preliminary study. *Nurs Res* 1977; 27:352–355.

Foster SB et al: Cardiovascular nursing research: Past, present and future. *Heart Lung* 1984; 13:111–116.

Geden EA: Effects of lifting techniques on energy expenditure: A preliminary investigation. *Nurs Res* 1982; 31:214–218.

Gill BP, Atwood JR: Reciprocity and helicy used to relate mEGF and wound healing. *Nurs Res* 1981; 30:68–72.

Grose BL et al: Effect of backrest position on cardiac output measured by the thermodilution method in acutely ill patients. *Heart Lung* 1981; 10:661–665.

Gruber PA: Changes in cardiac rate associated with the use of the rectal thermometer in the patient with acute myocardial infarction. *Heart Lung* 1974; 3:288–292.

Hanson RL: Effects of administering cold and warmed tube feedings. *Commun Nurs Res* 1973; 6:136–140.

Hasler ME, Cohen JA: The effect of oxygen administration on oral temperature assessment. *Nurs Res* 1982; 31:265–268.

Hathaway D, Geden EA: Energy expenditure during leg exercise programs. *Nurs Res* 1983; 32:147–150.

Heitkemper M et al: Effects of rate and volume of tube feeding in normal human subjects. *Commun Nurs Res* 1977; 10:71–95.

Helton MC et al: The correlation between sleep deprivation and the intensive care unit syndrome. *Heart Lung* 1980; 9:464–468.

Hill BJ: Sensory information, behavioral instructions and coping with sensory alteration surgery. *Nurs Res* 1982; 31:17–21.

Janson-Bjerklie S, Clarke E: The effects of biofeedback

training on bronchial diameter in asthma. *Heart Lung* 1982; 11:200–207.

Johnson JE: Effects of structuring patients' expectations on their reactions to threatening events. *Nurs Res* 1972; 21:499–504.

Johnson JE: Effects of accurate expectations about sensations on the sensory and distress components of pain. *J Pers Soc Psychol* 1973; 27:261–275.

Johnston BL et al: Oxygen consumption and hemodynamic and electrocardiographic responses to bathing in recent post-myocardial infarction patients. *Heart Lung* 1981; 10:666–671.

Kagawa-Busby KS et al: Effects of diet temperature on tolerance of enteral feedings. *Nurs Res* 1980; 29:276–280.

Kennedy GT et al: The effects of lateral body positioning on measurements of pulmonary artery and pulmonary artery wedge pressures. *Heart Lung* 1984; 13:155–158.

Kerr JC et al: A comparison of the effectiveness of two methods of intravenous antibiotic administration. *West J Nurs Res* 1979; 1:101–110.

Kim HS: Use of Rogers' conceptual system research: Comments. *Nurs Res* 1983; 32:89–91.

King I, Tarsitano B: The effect of structured and unstructured pre-operative teaching: A replication. *Nurs Res* 1982; 31:324–329.

Kinney M: The scientific basis for critical care nursing practice: 1972 to 1982. *Heart Lung* 1984; 13:116–123.

Kirchhoff KT: An examination of physiologic basis for "coronary precautions." *Heart Lung* 1981; 10:874–879.

Kirchhoff K: A diffusion survey of coronary precautions. *Nurs Res* 1982; 31:196–201.

Layton P et al: Nutritional assessment of allogeneic bone marrow recipients. *Cancer Nursing* 1981; 4:127–135.

Lim-Levy F: The effect of oxygen inhalation on oral temperature. *Nurs Res* 1982; 31:150–152.

Lindeman CA, Van Aernam BV: Nursing intervention with the presurgical patient—The effects of structured and unstructured preoperative teaching. *Nurs Res* 1971; 20:319–332.

Lindsey AM: Phenomena and physiological variables of relevance to nursing, review of a decade of work: Part I. *West J Nurs Res* 1982; 4:343–364.

Lindsey AM: Phenomena and physiological variables of relevance to nursing, review of a decade of work: Part 2. *West J Nurs Res* 1983; 5:41–63.

Lindsey AM: Research for clinical practice: Physiological phenomena. *Heart Lung* 1984; 13:496–507.

Lindsey AM, et al: Social support as a moderator of health outcomes in post-mastectomy women: A review. *Cancer Nursing* 1981; 4:377–384.

Marshall LA: Patient reaction to sound in an intensive care unit. *Commun Nurs Res* 1972; 5:81–92.

Martinson IM, Anderson SE: Effects of thermal applications on the abdominal temperature of rats. *Res Nurs Health* 1978; 1:123–130.

McCorkle R, Young K: Development of a symptom distress scale. *Cancer Nursing* 1978; 1:373–378.

Measel CP, Anderson GC: Nonnutritive sucking during tube feedings: Effect on clinical course in premature infants. *J Obstet Gyn Neonatal Nurs* 1979; 8:265–272.

Melzack R: The McGill Pain Questionnaire: Major properties and scoring methods. *Pain* 1975; 1:277–299.

Menzel NJ, Martinson IM: Effects of electrical surface stimulation on control of acute postoperative pain and prevention of atelectasis and ileus in patients having abdominal surgery. *Commun Nurs Res* 1975; 8:273–283.

Mills M et al: Effect of pulse palpation on cardiac arrhythmia in coronary care patients. *Nurs Res* 1976; 25:378–382.

Mitchell P: Intracranial hypertension: Implications of research for nursing care. *J Neurosurg Nurs* 1980; 12:145–154.

Mitchell PH et al: Moving the patient in bed: Effects on intracranial pressure. *Nurs Res* 1981; 30:212–218.

Nath C, Rinehart J: Effects of individual and group relaxation therapy on blood pressure in essential hypertensives. *Res Nurs Health* 1979; 2:119–126.

Neal MV: Vestibular stimulation and development of the small premature infant. *Commun Nurs Res* 1977; 8:291–302.

Nichols EG et al: Relationship between incidence of phlebitis and frequency of changing IV tubing and percutaneous site. *Nurs Res* 1983; 32:247–252.

Norris S et al: Nursing procedures and alterations in transcutaneous oxygen tension in premature infants. *Nurs Res* 1982; 31:330–336.

Parsons L, Ver Beek D: Sleep–awake patterns following cerebral concussion. *Nurs Res* 1982; 31:260–264.

Perry JA: Effectiveness of teaching in the rehabilitation of patients with chronic bronchitis and emphysema. *Nurs Res* 1981; 30:219–222.

Pfeiffer E: A short portable mental status questionnaire for the assessment of organic brain deficit in elderly patients. *J Am Geriatr Soc* 1975; 23:433–441.

Porter LS: The impact of physical–physiological activity on infants' growth and development. *Nurs Res* 1972; 21:210–219.

Randolph G: Therapeutic and physical touch: Physiological response to stressful stimuli. *Nurs Res* 1984; 33:33–36.

Roesler LD: A comparison of two treatments of decubitus ulcers: Op-Site and Bard products. *Final Report, Department of Nursing Research, Stanford University Hospital* September 28, 1983.

Schiffman RF: Temperature monitoring in the neonate: A comparison of axillary and rectal temperatures. *Nurs Res* 1982; 31:274–277.

Skelley B et al: The effectiveness of two preoxygenation methods to prevent endotracheal suction-induced hypoxemia. *Heart Lung* 1980; 9:316–323.

Smyth ML: Alterations in respiratory patterns in sleeping subjects with chronic obstructive pulmonary disease. *Commun Nurs Res* 1980; 13:25.

Stotts NA, Cooper DM: *Development of an Instrument to Assess Wounds: Preliminary Stages.* [Unpublished data, 1984.]

Teasdale G, Jennett B: Assessment of coma and impaired consciousness: A practical scale. *Lancet* 1974; 2:81–83.

Vaughan MS et al: Postoperative hypothermia in adults: Relationship of age, anesthesia and shivering to rewarming. *Anesth Analg* 1981; 60:746–751.

Walker BB: The postsurgery heart patient: Amount of uninterrupted time for sleep and rest during the first, second and third postoperative days in a teaching hospital. *Nurs Res* 1972; 21:164–169.

Wallech C: The effect of purposeful touch on intracranial pressure. Abstract. *Proceedings of the American Association of Critical-Care Nurses National Teaching Institute.* Newport Beach, Calif.: American Association of Critical-Care Nurses, 1983, p. 335.

Ward MJ, Lindeman C (editors): *Instruments for Measuring Nursing Practice and Other Health Care Variables.* Vols 1 and 2. Washington, D.C.: U.S. Department of Health, Education, and Welfare, 1978.

Wells N: The effect of relaxation on postoperative muscle tension and pain. *Nurs Res* 1982; 31:236–238.

Williams KR, Walike BC: Effect of the temperature of tube feeding on gastric motility in monkeys. *Nurs Res* 1975; 24:4–9.

Woods NF, Falk SA: Noise stimuli in the acute care area. *Nurs Res* 1974; 23:144–149.

Yoshitake H: Relations between the symptoms and the feelings of fatigue. *Ergonomics* 1971; 14:175–196.

Zook DJ, Yasko JM: Psychologic factors: Their effect on nausea and vomiting experienced by clients receiving chemotherapy. *Oncology Nursing Forum* 1983; 10:76–81.

Further Readings

Carrieri VL et al (Eds.): *Pathophysiological Phenomena in Nursing: Clinical and Theoretical Perspectives.* Philadelphia: Saunders, 1985 (anticipated publication date).

Polit D, Hungler B: *Nursing Research: Principles and Methods, 2nd ed.* Philadelphia: Lippincott, 1983.

Robbins SL, Cotran RS: *Pathologic Basis of Disease.* Philadelphia: Saunders, 1979.

Smith LH, Thier SO: *Pathophysiology: The Biological Principles of Disease.* Philadelphia: Saunders, 1981.

Williams CA (ed.): *Nursing Research and Policy Formation: The Case of Prospective Payment.* Papers of the 1983 Scientific Session. Kansas City, MO: American Academy of Nursing, 1984.

Chapter 13

Strategies of Field Research

Firsthand Knowing Under Natural Conditions

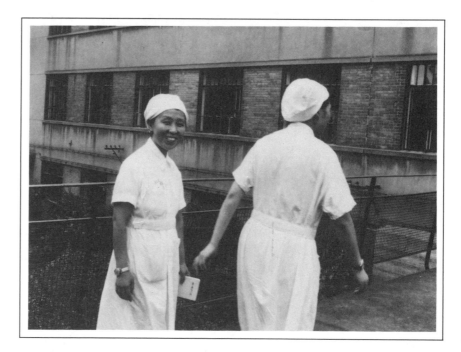

Field research relies on firsthand knowing, under natural conditions. This method requires a nurse researcher to enter an unfamiliar social world and discover its logic.

Chapter Outline

Chapter Objectives

After reading this chapter, the student should be able to:

- Discuss the intellectual roots of field methods
- Explain why nursing science can profit from carefully documented field studies
- Enumerate three characteristics of field research
- Compare and contrast the logic of inquiry in field research with traditional, deductive research
- Describe strategies useful in the five major stages of fieldwork: (1) locating the field, (2) gaining entrée and access, (3) bargaining for a role, (4) collecting and recording data, and (5) leaving the field
- Recognize the advantages and disadvantages of the roles of complete participant, participant as observer, observer as participant, and complete observer
- Demonstrate the ability to solve practical and ethical issues related to each fieldwork stage
- Evaluate the balance in types of data according to the criteria of information adequacy and efficiency
- Formulate a plan for observing based on four guidelines
- Organize observations into the recording system of observational notes (ONs), theoretical notes (TNs), methodological notes (MNs), and personal notes (PNs)
- Comprehend the characteristics of partially structured and unstructured interviews
- List the advantages and disadvantages of interviews vis-à-vis questionnaires
- Pose clarifying questions that reflect active listening
- Distinguish between case histories and case studies as sources of data
- Distinguish between scientific and artistic modes of analyzing qualitative data

In This Chapter . . .

Field methods are data-collection strategies, including observation, interviewing, case studies, case histories, and document review, that rely on "firsthand knowing" under natural conditions. Field research grew out of a combination of traditions in cultural anthropology and the social philosophy of symbolic interactions (see Chapter 1). These traditions have taught us that experience is defined differently in different places. The field worker's philosophy of science is based on the belief that people have not only different customs, language conventions, kinship patterns, religious practices, and expectations of their lives but also different worlds with different realities. Ethnography requires the special skill of entering such an alien world and discovering its own logic. The very best field workers do this kind of science with their hearts as well as their intellects. *The Teachings of Don Juan* is a story by the anthropologist Carlos Cas-

taneda of a Yaqui Indian from Sonora, Mexico—a brujo (medicine man). It describes the five years that these two men spent together, in which Don Juan taught Castaneda the uses of peyote, jimson weed, and other plants in achieving mastery over a nonordinary reality (Castaneda 1968). Although some would reasonably argue that this study and subsequent successful trade books based on it were merely products of the 1960s, timely in topic and style, others believe that it is among the best portrayals of human reality divested of intellectual detachment, eroding jargon, and officiousness. How to use field research methods and to decide whether such a rendering is *true* by scientific as well as pragmatic criteria are the subjects of this chapter. Our emphasis here is on doing fieldwork. Analyzing the data collected is covered in detail in Chapter 14.

Intellectual Roots of Field Research

The Growth of Anthropology

Anthropology, one of the youngest disciplines in the social sciences, gets its name from the Greek words *anthropos*, meaning "man," and *logos*, meaning "study." It can be divided into three branches.

In the later 19th century anthropologists concerned themselves with what is now called *physical anthropology*—the study of human anatomy, physiology, and the biological bases of behavior. A. C. Haddon organized and led the Torres Straits expedition from Britain in 1889 to "find out possible physiological or racial bases for cultural differences in primitive cultures on

islands near Australia and New Guinea." This first "field study" was considered the original purely anthropological expedition. Haddon and his associates concluded, by the way, that "islanders hardly differed from Europeans in their perceptions, and that the differences that were found were personal rather than racial" (Penniman 1965, p. 99).

The second major type of anthropological problem is the study of ancient objects and the remains of former civilizations. The emphasis here is on discovering major lines of development and paths of influence on contemporary society. This branch of anthropology is called *archaeology*.

Ethnology, the third division of anthropology, is concerned with individual human beings as social or cultural actors, thinkers, and communicators rather than exclusively as physical organisms. It focuses on cultures and societies as systems of rules, rights, roles, language customs, and established relationships rather than as physical remains of ancient environments.

Early ethnologists were strongly influenced by a tradition in Europe in the 19th century called sociology, particularly the works of Herbert Spencer, August Comte, Max Weber, George Simmel, and Emile Durkheim. Among these thinkers, culture or society was considered a unit of study in and of itself and was not reducible to its parts or members. Spencer called this concept *civilization*, and Comte called it *social principle*. The word for the idea became *culture* in Germany and the United States, and scholars in England and France called it *society*. From these early thinkers came a philosophic attitude about studying people summarized by Leaf:

It is the idea that the actions of an individual are relative to his cultural surroundings . . . and have to be evaluated in terms of the moral principles and beliefs of his society or culture. . . . One cannot arrive at a proper evaluation of the actions of persons in another culture by imposing the values or beliefs or meanings of one's own culture upon them [1974, p. 28].

Social scientists of the 1940s and 1950s sought a fair-minded, universal research method that would avoid imposing their own values and ideas upon the cultures they studied yet would result in a balanced, comparative analysis. *Ethnology* was dubbed the "whole science of man." Its focus was observable individuals and their setting or environment. Important scientific works of this period included Clyde Kluckhohn's *Navaho Witchcraft*, Ruth Benedict's *The Chrysanthemum and the Sword*, Weber's *The Protestant Ethic and the Spirit of Capitalism*, Claude Lévi-Strauss' *Elementary Structures of Kinship*, and Edmund Leach's *Political Systems of Highland Burma*. In 1943 William Foote

Whyte published a study of an Italian slum society in North Boston that has become a fieldwork classic. In a section he entitled "Reflections on Field Research," Whyte made the following observations about the method he used to produce this important and influential work:

As I carried through the Cornerville study, I was also learning how to do field research. . . . I learned to understand a group by observing how it changed through time. This familiarity gave rise to the ideas in this book. I did not develop these ideas by any strictly logical process. They dawned on me out of what I was seeing, hearing, doing—and feeling. They grew out of an effort to organize a confusing welter of experience. . . . I had to try to get outside of my participating self and struggle again to explain the things that seemed obvious. . . . I was seeking to build a study based upon observed interpersonal events. That to me is the chief methodological and theoretical meaning of *Street Corner Society* [1955, pp. 357–358].

The burgeoning scientific tradition called field research expanded to guide the work of scientists in related disciplines. In the 1960s the psychologist Kenneth Keniston published two brilliant studies of alienated youth and the New Left in American society, *The Uncommitted* and *Young Radicals*. The psychiatrist Robert Coles reported on nonviolent youth in the South in his paper "Serpents and Doves." Howard Becker explained the process of becoming a marijuana user in a monograph called *Outsiders*. In an effort to make the management of dying more rational and compassionate, the medical sociologists Barney Glaser and Anselm Strauss, in collaboration with a team of nurse researchers at the University of California, San Francisco, published their works *Awareness of Dying* (1965) and *Time for Dying* (1968). In the world of physical science the geneticist James D. Watson (1968) revealed the human side of his discovery of the structure of DNA when he expressed a view in *The Double Helix* that science proceeds in a far less logical manner than is imagined by nonscientists. Personalities and human events play major parts in scientific discovery.

Field Research and Nursing

In 1970 the National Commission for the Study of Nursing and Nursing Education put forward as its first recommended priority the study of problems in nursing practice. Scholars and scientists at Yale University defined *nursing practice research* as problems in patient care where either direct or indirect nursing care is given to people and their significant others. They advocated the position that the essence of research is in everyday nursing practice and that the business of nursing research is to examine, describe, define, explain, and predict that practice. Diers summarized the ideas of scholars and scientists: "The closer the relationship between nursing practice and nursing research, the better the research and the better the practice" (1979, p. 5). Research questions about everyday nursing practice are waiting around every corner and down every corridor: "What keeps staff nurses going when they confront the stresses of working in a neonatal intensive care unit?" "How do elderly indigent patients get around with emphysema?" "How do patients manage to live with incurable pain?" "What is the influence of 'high tech' equipment on compassionate nursing care?" "How do nurses provide culturally sensitive postpartum care to Mexican-American mothers?" "How do Arab immigrants define their health care needs?" "What is the nature of usual inpatient treatment in a community mental health center's locked unit?" "How do the chronically ill view their world?" "How can a diabetic diet be best taught to an adolescent patient?" "What can a nurse do to ease the trauma of pain during 'tubbing' of burned children?" "Why do intensive care unit patients feel exhausted?" "Do relaxation techniques assist in the management of hypertension?" "What effects will positioning a patient have on his or her intracranial pressure?" "What's the proper length for insertion of a nasogastric (ng) tube for feeding?"

Finding answers to such questions is the goal of clinical nursing research. The answers can improve patient care. Clinical research generates the knowledge necessary to guide patient-care practices based on science, not trial and error or tradition. It considers the whole patient in relationship to his or her environment. The knowledge gained is valued for the use it may have *in the real world* of decisions, judgments, and human encounters. Given all of this, we are not surprised to learn that research strategies originated by sociologists and anthropologists in their field studies have held considerable interest for nurse researchers.

Characteristics of Field Research

Fieldwork as a mode of scientific inquiry immerses the researcher in processes of day-to-day life that may be as novel as living with an isolated Eskimo band or as tense as spending many months incarcerated with inmates on death row in a maximum security prison. Wherever it may be, "the field" is the social-psychological area where the investigator gathers data to find answers in the central area of inquiry. In a pain study the field might be hospital wards; in a study of face-to-face interaction with disfigured or handicapped persons it might be bureaus or agencies. Field studies have been conducted by nurses in prenatal classes, labor rooms, nursing homes, self-help-group meetings, herbal pharmacies, pot parties, and rock concerts. The features that characterize such studies, whatever their location, are these:

1. The researcher, through face-to-face interviewing or participant observation, is the primary "instrument" for data collection.

2. Data collection and analysis go on in the natural setting. The investigator tries to learn about how variables vary under usual and unusual conditions rather than trying to control all variables except for the few under scrutiny.

3. The logical progression of field research contrasts with more traditional research in the ways summarized in Table 13-1.

4. Field researchers must make particular accommodations to the ethical principles discussed in Chapter 3. They usually conduct their work in close association with the people and situations they study. The potential for conflicts of interest, deception, exploitation, invasion of privacy, inconvenience to the subjects, and loss of confidentiality are all particularly intense. If I learn in a study of prior child abusers and their children that a new incident has occurred, should I report it? Should I make my field notes accessible to the police? What should I tell subjects about such matters from the start? No matter how unobtrusive, field research always pries into the lives of informants, usually with little personal gain to them. It can be used, however, to affirm their rights, interests, and sensitivities, and all informants have the right to know the researcher's aims, to remain anonymous, to refuse to participate, and to withdraw at any time without penalty.

The heart of the fieldwork enterprise, according to the sociologist Herbert Blumer, is "getting close to the people involved in it, seeing it in a variety of situations they meet, noting their problems and observing how they handle them, being party to their conversations and watching their way of life as it flows along" (1969, p. 37). As you can surmise, fieldwork commits the researcher to learning to define the world from the perspective of those being studied and requires that he or she gain as intimate an understanding as possible about their way of life. Methodological techniques in field research include ob-

Table 13-1 Comparison of Traditional Research With Field Research

Traditional Deductive Research	Field Research
Start with hypotheses derived from reading existing literature—for example, independent variable yields dependent variable ($x \rightarrow y$)	Look at the data first. Then come up with your own multiple tentative hypotheses
Study a few propositions	Study many propositions
Proceed through a linear process	Proceed through a multidimensional process resembling a Rubic's cube or a spiral
Comply with precise steps for correct data collection and analysis	Gather data and analyze it simultaneously based on a general principle of being pragmatic and evolving the analytic scheme
Test, confirm, or refute hypotheses	Develop concepts, propositions, and middle-range theories

SOURCE: S. Fagerhaugh. Presentation at Qualitative Research Conference. San Francisco, Calif., 1983.

servation, informal interviews, life histories, document analysis, and other nonintrusive, nonstructured methods. The following section clarifies the procedures and general rules that are available for locating the field, learning how to enter it, maintaining working relationships with subjects, collecting and recording data, and making a smooth exit. Most field researchers would admit, however, that the canons of fieldwork must frequently be bent and twisted to accommodate the particular demands and requirements of the study situation and the personal characteristics of the field worker. The exact recipe for doing field research, as Shaffir, Stebbins, and Turowetz (1980) conclude, can at best only be suggested.

Stages of Fieldwork

Stage 1: Locating the Field

Any place or area of activity can become the field for research on a study question. A bus station where strangers wait aimlessly in one another's presence, a gay bar, the waiting room of an intensive care unit, a city hospital's emergency room, a running track, an Alcoholics Anonymous meeting. You can select a single social situation and expand it to many to acquire contrasts and variations. When Glaser and Strauss studied dying patients, they made observations in emergency rooms, hospice care units, neonatal intensive care units, operating rooms, nursing homes, and elsewhere, to grasp the full range of variation relevant to their emerging concepts *awareness contexts* and *the dying trajectory* (1965, 1968).

Appraising the suitability of the setting or field is a first stage in doing fieldwork. Researchers examine the setting to determine if it will yield data bearing on the purpose or research question that focuses their study. The success of a field study often depends on the attention paid to this preresearch phase. Familiarity with the routines, realities, and structure of the proposed setting facilitate not only the negotiations that follow but also the qualitative data that you can collect.

One nursing doctoral dissertation focused on psychiatric nurses' styles of communicating with psychiatric patients. The investigator was forced to abandon her original hospital unit in favor of another one because the patient population rarely if ever presented the psychotic language patterns that she wished to investigate. This discovery consumed many weeks of negotiation and observation and served as an early source of frustration for her in an already difficult and challenging scientific undertaking.

The importance of background interviewing and document research before a setting is adopted cannot be underestimated when planning a field study.

Stage 2: Gaining Entrée and Access

Field research proceeds by clearing the initial hurdle of getting into the selected setting or situation so that you can observe and talk to people about your research question. Then you must build rapport and trust so that subjects will willingly serve as informants and respondents. Barriers to getting in abound, and success depends on your ability to determine the wisest

Example: Covert Research in "Tearooms"

Humphreys's (1975) research investigated impersonal homosexual encounters in public restrooms (called "tearooms") in St. Louis from 1965 to 1968. The study required Humphreys to assume a phony role as "lookout" in these public facilities. Thus, he began with disguised observation in that he did not make his identity as a social researcher known to the participants. His sampling techniques furthermore involved tracing automobile license numbers in order to track down the names and addresses of the men who engaged in these encounters. When interviewing the respondents at their home, he explained only that they had been chosen as part of a sample of men for a "social health survey" of the community. Respondents were not told the true purpose of the study, and the researcher disguised his appearance so as to avoid recognition. The ethics of such subterfuge have been both criticized and defended in a long list of subsequent publications.

Study subjects did not give informed consent

An example of deception

The ethics of field research are an important consideration

---

approach to the situation and cultivate the various "gatekeepers."

Covert and Overt Research   Problems and strategies for "getting in" are influenced in part by the decision whether to engage in covert or overt field research. The covert approach obviously eliminates the need to explain and justify the research or your presence. Here the investigator poses as an authentic participant in the setting—a diabetic, a hospital worker, a single parent, a drug abuser—to get a look at the social life of the subjects without any influence on them from knowing that they are under study. Such undercover research, although done in the past, is being subjected to serious ethical criticisms.

Degree of Accessibility   Obviously, social situations or settings offer varying degrees of accessibility. On the one hand, you can enter a hospital lobby and observe easily. Observing transactions at the admissions desk, on the other hand, would probably require the permission of the hospital's administration. The operating room could in some cases prove to be completely inaccessible. Hospital board meetings are less accessible for a nurse researcher than unit change-of-shift reports. Intensive care units

(ICUs) are less accessible than well-child clinics. Delivery rooms are less accessible than prenatal classes. All these settings offer opportunities for conducting field research, but the greater the accessibility and the freer the entry to the social situation, the less complicated and time consuming is this stage of the research.

Strategies to Use With "Gatekeepers"   When you elect to conduct overt research in a limited or restricted situation, you must convince those in charge as well as the subjects to cooperate with you. Strategies that have worked for other field researchers include the following:

First, attempt to serve the interests of the research setting in some way through your research. In Hutchinson's study of neonatal intensive care units (NICUs), one director of nurses urged her to study this unit because:

She had never seen so much anger in her life! Nurses were quitting left and right and everyone said they were under a lot of stress. Doctors were blaming the nurses for infants' deaths. People had various explanations; the physical space was small, it was very crowded, there were no windows; the nurses were all suffering from depression and burn-out [1983, Field notes].

Hutchinson's field study was designed to examine and dissect the facts in this nursing care situation so as to discover the unarticulated problems and formulate solutions to them. Thus, the value of her research project influenced her initial acceptance in a positive way.

A second entry strategy might best be to "cultivate" the good will of the subjects by "contouring" one's own behavior to fit in with them. Here, the researcher attempts to present a personal style that enlists the help and support of others. In my own Soteria study (Wilson 1982), the suspicious, slightly antiestablishment, non-professional staff caring for psychotics in an antipsychiatric community found field methods to be more congruent with their own humanistic ideology than questionnaires or psychometric tests. They believed that the latter reduced their reality to a numerical score. How one's research and one's role are defined by others influences the trust and confidence a field researcher depends upon in order to obtain data. And even experienced researchers attest to experiencing feelings of uncertainty and self-doubt that are associated with entering the field. As acceptance increases and anxiety decreases, the quality of the work invariably improves.

The two preceding suggestions not withstanding, nothing seems as important in gaining entrée as a genuine appreciative interest in the subjects. Even the most impressive credentials will only open certain doors (and may even close others). Genuine rapport, in contrast, is established when the subjects accept the investigator for personal qualities rather than formal status, suggesting that research imitates life. A few principles to keep in mind in the interest of achieving rapport include:

1. Reducing social distance and other interpersonal barriers increases trust in the researcher.

2. What you reveal about yourself becomes a factor in establishing the kinds of interaction you establish.

3. There is always a certain amount of risk taking when presenting one's research and self to potential informants.

3. Trying to get into the other person's shoes improves cooperation and the quality of data.

All these principles are illustrated in the field note excerpt below.

R. asks who is going to see my stuff and whether I'm working for the project director, being paid, etc. She expresses concern about everything becoming public knowledge. I explain that I'm writing a dissertation but that I hope the findings will be helpful to Soteria people in explaining and understanding what is going on. I assure her that my findings will be abstract enough to protect specific identities. I feel challenged and uncertain about how to portray my work because I don't know how R. and the rest of the staff feel about the project directors. I tell W. that I won't write things that they ask me not to (i.e., various forms of "making out" like picking up receipts in supermarket for reimbursement). I mention that the management of work through humor interests me. They nod acceptingly at this kind of focus.

Most field workers agree with Schatzman and Strauss when they point out that "entrée is a continuous process of establishing and developing relationships not only with a chief host but with a variety of on-site persons. . . . Successful negotiation through the front door is not always sufficient to open other doors" (1982, p. 22).

Issues that ought to be considered during entry negotiations include:

1. the researcher's right to publish material in his or her own scholarly community, given protection of the subjects' confidentiality

2. the extent of the researcher's freedom of access to documents, people, and situations

3. the expectations the hosts may have of the researcher for performance of work of some kind, copies, or final study reports, formal presentations of findings, and so forth.

Stage 3: Bargaining for a Role

Gold (1958) proposes that a field researcher can opt for any one of four roles, ranging on a continuum from complete participant to complete observer (see Figure 13-1). Between these two extremes are the participant-as-observer and observer-as-participant roles. Schatzman and Strauss (1982) refine these four into six types. The researcher's decision on the nature of his or her role influences how entrée and access are obtained and the kind of data that are collected.

The Complete Participant   In the role of complete participant, the field researcher joins an organization or takes a job in order to learn about the inner workings of a situation. In many such studies the true identity and purpose of the field researcher are not known to those being observed, and "role pretense" is a basic although ethically questionable theme (see Chapter 3). Goffman's classic sociological study on life in a mental hospital, *Asylums* (1961), was based on data he collected while working as an attendant. All complete-participant roles have three potential problems:

1. The investigator may become so self-conscious about revealing his or her true identity that both the participant and observer role performances are hampered.
2. The researcher may "go native" and lose the intellectual distance required to analyze the how and why of study data and instead begin thinking in terms of should or shouldn't, right or wrong.
3. The demands of participation on the investigator for performing work may use time, energy, and flexibility needed for data collection.

Many experts now agree that the combination of these problems along with ethical questions about the propriety of doing "undercover" research outweigh the potential benefit of learning about aspects of behavior that otherwise might not be accessible to the field worker. The exception, of course, might be in the case of research conducted in a free-access setting such as a subway station or supermarket.

The Participant as Observer   Although basically similar to the complete-participant role, the participant-as-observer role differs in that both the field worker and the informants are aware of the research process. The advantage of this role is that the researcher not only watches what others do but also learns from doing it. The major problem of this role is that participants may come to expect the field worker to become more of a colleague and participant than he or she is capable of being without jeopardy to the research. Nurses are particularly vulnerable to these conflicting demands when conducting research in a health care setting where they possess the skills to actively intervene in situations and, in fact, are accustomed to doing so. If a patient asks for a glass of water or help to the bathroom, do you ask her to wait while you call a nurse? Do you suggest she call the nurse herself? Or do you do it and lose data potential?

The Observer as Participant   The role of observer as participant calls for more formal observation and entails less risk of getting overly in-

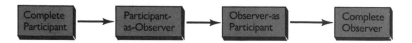

Figure 13-1   Fieldwork role continuum.

volved in the work of the setting. The researcher limits his or her interaction to seeking clarification of events going on. This approach diminishes intrusion, conveys interest, and gets at meaningful data. In some cases, however, brief relations with a greater variety of people over shorter periods of time lead to fundamental misperceptions and misunderstandings of the social worlds under investigation.

The Complete Observer In the role of complete observer the field researcher attempts to observe people in ways that make it unnecessary for them to take him or her into account. Examples include systematic eavesdropping, loitering, bystanding, and spectating in free-access public places. This role also can involve analysis of cultural artifacts and secondary sources such as patients' charts, case histories, or diaries. Obviously, this approach decreases the chances of losing intellectual distance as well as the impact of the investigator's presence on natural conditions in the field. But its drawbacks include the inability of the researcher to collect focused data from informants by interacting with them and the risk of never getting to understand their point of view. Complete observers watching the world go by risk less and are probably less anxious about rejection from others. But they also often wish that they could interrupt and ask questions about the meaning of what is going on. Many studies that begin with a completely passive role—for example, observing from outside the window of a hospital nursery to see how nurses hold infants and how long they allow them to cry—move on to a more active form of involvement by the researcher.

Shaffir and colleagues summarize their ideas concerning the stage of bargaining for a role with a list of questions or issues that most field researchers must thoughtfully answer, whatever the role assumed, based on a sense of pragmatism about what stance will best serve the interests of the research project and based on ethical considerations.

Fundamental Questions in Bargaining for a Role *

Q. How do I identify myself to others in the research setting?

A. Honesty is probably the best policy here. Simply state that you are a nurse doing a study of what it's like to be in this kind of setting or activity (self-help group, diabetic clinic, emergency room, prenatal class). This identification is usually legitimate enough to allow you to stay yet vague enough to keep your focus open and avoid making the subjects self-conscious about their behavior.

Q. After becoming a "regular," how do I avoid being entirely assimilated?

A. Be wise enough to take personal notes (PNs) and write memos on your own impressions, behavior, and feelings during the research process. Periodically withdraw from the field for theoretical reflection to move concrete descriptions to an abstract theoretical level. Be wary of abandoning the excitement of developing your *ideas* about the study setting or situation for the excitement of being *a part* of the setting per se, no matter how interesting it may become for you.

Q. How actively involved can one get as a participant without jeopardizing either the research, the subjects, or one's personal and professional ethics?

A. As you become secure about your acceptance in the study setting, feel free to continue to interpret your role. In a study of juvenile delinquents you may dress like them to keep from standing out, but you should also indicate your preference not to participate in crimes, buy "hot" merchandise, or do drugs. Be as clear and consistent as possible about what you will and will not do, keeping in mind that some of these decisions

* From W. B. Shaffir, R. A. Stebbins, and A. Turowetz, *Fieldwork Experience: Qualitative Approaches to Social Research*, New York: St. Martin's Press, 1980.

will influence the kinds of data that you collect. If you are studying tolerance ranges, cutting points, and the like on the subject of how long nurses will let a patient go before administering a pain medication, giving it yourself will obviously prevent you from obtaining indicators on the research question. But as a nurse and humane individual, you may well be willing to make such a choice.

Dealing with these questions satisfactorily and presenting oneself in field research typically evokes edginess, discomfort, uncertainty, and anxiety in even seasoned field researchers. Sometimes we feel awkward about prying into other people's private lives. Fears of rejection from either the officials of an organization or the day-to-day participants remind us to go through channels, cultivate relationships, contour our appearance, withhold evaluative judgments, and be as unobtrusive and charming as possible.

Finally the absence of a questionnaire, psychometric test, blood-pressure cuff, or other "tool of the research trade" often results in extreme feelings of self-consciousness in the researcher. Recalling his study of Boston's North End, Whyte relates an instance early in his research when he attempted to enter into the small talk of the corner bars by blurting out a string of obscenities and profanities. The gang members looked at him in surprise and said, "You're not supposed to talk like that. That doesn't sound like you" (Whyte 1955, p. 304). Learning the ropes often reveals that study participants realize that the investigator *is* different and that they don't expect the investigator to behave just as they do. Such a discovery can relieve, in part, the burden of feeling self-conscious. The researcher who shows a respect for those being studied and is willing to consider their points of view and rights to confidentiality and privacy has already got a solid basis for becoming attuned to the social world under investigation. Bargaining for a role and learning the ropes are continuous processes that must allow enough flexibility to modify your role and cope with unanticipated developments. Rosalie Wax (1971) suggests that any researcher who feels embarrassed or out of place in unfamiliar circumstances ought to think twice before trying to do participant observation.

Stage 4: Collecting and Recording Data

The objective of field research is to spend an intense period of time in an arena of social interaction and record the ongoing experiences of its participants. This requires that the field researcher gain an understanding about others' ways of perceiving life. Data collection is shaped by the emerging themes and hypotheses that develop in the course of doing qualitative analyses (see Chapter 14). Thus, in most field studies data collection and analysis go on simultaneously.

Data collection begins with the question "What shall I look at?" Douglas (1976, p. 195) suggests that we begin by "casting a wide net." This means talking to all kinds of people and investigating all kinds of settings associated with the phenomenon in question. Polsky says that the initial rule for field researchers is "keep your eyes and ears open but keep your mouth shut" (1969, p. 12). In short, submerge yourself in everyday social life. This initial approach ought not be continued for too long, however, because you run the risk of simply generating an unmanageable explosion of irrelevant data. In Box 13-1 Lopata (1979) gives us a sense of the breadth of data-collection strategies she used to develop her analyses of role modifications and support systems of American urban widows.

Clearly, the initial data-collection principle in a field study is to record everything that might be vaguely or remotely relevant to your unfolding analyses, because you don't know until your focus narrows what might be useful. This process is loosely called "hanging around" (but I discourage using the phrase itself to describe your methodology in a thesis or grant proposal). It seems that observation is particularly arbitrary at the beginning of a field study. As the

---

Box 13-1   Qualitative Data Sources in a Study of American Widows

1. a content analysis of two sets of letters (74) directed to the author in response to a television program and the announcement of her study in the newspaper

2. interviews of half an hour with ten of the letter authors

3. an examination of the literature on aging, grief, divorce, single status, ethnic family construction, and the like with an eye toward their effects on widowhood

4. reinterviews of 35 previously contacted widows, attempting to cover all combinations of living situations

5. interviews with various groups of women to learn about racial and economic factors

6. interviews with mothers and daughters or other kin members with respect to relationship strains

7. attendance at and field notes on meetings of organizations for widows or single women and an analysis of their publications

8. attendance at meetings of groups that by nature attracted widows though did not focus on helping them per se, like the YWCA and church groups

9. attendance at meetings and tours of facilities, interviews with people and reviews of the publications from Home-Delivered Meals, the Mayor's Commission on Senior Citizens, and the like to determine their perceptions of problems of widowhood

10. collections and analyses of diaries and histories of events

11. interviews with friends and relatives of widows focusing observations on the process by which someone is selected to assume responsibility for a widowed mother

SOURCE: H. Z. Lopata, *Women as Widows: Support Systems*. New York: Elsevier, 1979.

---

study progresses, however, you begin to accumulate more detailed information. Hypotheses present themselves, and your analyses and observations become more purposeful and focused. Field researchers often search documents in the exploration phase and then use unstructured interviews to raise specific questions and to supplement data gathered initially from published and archival sources. The interviews allow you to test hypotheses, fill in blank spots, and seek interpretations and clarifications. By unstructured interviews, I mean:

1. stressing the interviewee's definition of the situation

2. encouraging the interviewee to structure the account of the situation

3. letting the interviewee introduce the notions of what he or she considers to be relevant

instead of relying on the investigator's notions of relevance

The major methods of collecting data in the field, including participant observation and interviewing, will be examined in detail later in the chapter (see Appendix C).

Stage 5: Leaving the Field

Although the fieldwork experience is viewed by many as more of a continuous process than a series of separate stages, all agree that a wise field researcher attends to closure and leaving the field at some point in the process. Ultimately, the investigator must gracefully withdraw from the study setting and from most, if not all, of the personal relationships that have for a time been relatively intense. Clearly, if one researcher is insensitive or is viewed unfavorably upon departure from the field, future investigators' efforts to gain entrée and access will be handicapped.

Problems that have developed may need to be addressed, entrée bargains reappraised, and personal relationships resolved. If a nurse has been a complete participant on a hospital unit, he or she may need to redefine this role once the study is completed. The following checklist offers some basic and general guides for leaving the field:

1. Be prepared for some respondents to feel abandoned, misrepresented, or even duped. The transition from personal involvement and intense concern for those in the field to preoccupation with analyses and publication of findings may come as an abrupt shock to some who expected on some level that you would live out your involvement with the study setting. When study subjects become aware of your diminished interest in their life and situation, some may come to feel cheated.

2. Because of the considerations just mentioned, withdraw gradually if at all possible, clearly defining your timetable of diminishing contacts. Junker (1960, p. 11) has called this strategy "easing out."

3. If norms for leaving the situation or setting exist, such as a farewell wine-and-cheese party or an exchange of gifts, allow these norms and customs to facilitate your withdrawal or role redefinition as well. Sometimes, however, there are no formal good-byes, just drifting off and returning intermittently to talk less and less frequently. This alternative, termed "suspended" rather than "terminated" research, leaves room to drift back and resume data collection at a later date.

4. Fulfill the commitments you made in order to gain access and entrée. If you promised a hospital staff a preliminary presentation of your findings once your analysis began to solidify, schedule a date and time to make that presentation as a closure ritual. If you promised to provide a copy of your final report to subjects in recognition of their contributions, do so. But be prepared for some to greet their anonymity with less than enthusiasm and others to feel that confidentiality was only thinly protected.

5. Be prepared to have become so involved and attached that you don't want to make your exit and find yourself thinking up excuses to extend your stay. It is usually advisable to make clear from the outset, to yourself and to others, how long you plan to remain in the field. Even then be prepared to experience some feelings of alienation, guilt, and melancholy when relationships are ended. This is particularly likely when the research project depended a lot on trust and friendship between investigator and respondents or informants.

6. Impersonal, structural factors sometimes offer a convenient (and honest) explanation for terminating a field study relationship. The expiration of a research grant, termination of a visa, completion of a degree, or a geographic move all help the process of easing out without offending setting participants.

Major Methods of Field Research

Fieldwork experts classify the methods for obtaining data in the field into either three or four types, depending upon the particular author's point of view. All agree that Type 1 consists of participant observation, that Type 2 is the interviewing of informants, and that Type 3 involves accumulating countable data through surveys or psychometric tests. (This last type of data collection was the subject of Chapter 11.) Proponents for limiting the types to these three argue that the analysis of documents really represents results or combinations of the three primary types of data collection. For example, documents such as diaries and logs are basically an informant's *written* account of his or her experience and should be treated just like any other evidence of perspectives or occurrences. Other documents, such as hospital staffing patterns, the books of a nursing service department, or the membership rolls of a state nurses' association, are essentially enumerations.

Some authorities, however, choose to categorize as Type 4 the analysis of documents, case studies, case histories, videotapes, and the like, grouping them under the term *unobtrusive*, or *nonreactive*, *methods*. An unobtrusive measure is any method of observation that directly removes the observer from the interactions or events being studied. Archival document analysis such as chart audits, observation of play therapy for disabled children from behind a one-way glass, audio tapes of psychiatric intake interviews, and physical trace analysis that involves the study of signs left behind by people (personal objects the elderly take with them when they move into nursing homes, special toys 2-year-olds bring to the hospital, and the like) all allow researchers to make inferences about people while minimizing the influence that the investigator might have on behavior. For example, just knowing that a field worker is studying nonprofessional behavior among professional staff can have a reactive influence on the people in the field and incur doubt in the investigator about how typical the data collected really are.

Criteria for Balancing Types of Data

Answers to certain kinds of question are most efficiently and accurately obtained with one data-collection method. In making decisions about which strategies you should plan to use as a field worker, two important criteria guide the choice:

1. *information adequacy*—that is, precision and completeness of the data
2. *efficiency*, meaning the cost of obtaining the information

Such criteria notwithstanding, most experienced field researchers also agree that a study's validity is enhanced when you *triangulate* your data-collection methods. Triangulation means that you use several different collection methods to obtain different "slices of data" on the same study question and then cross-check accounts against one another for consistency and comparability. In short, triangulation requires that a researcher examine the study question from as many different perspectives as possible. The sociologist Norman Denzin (1970) also uses the term *triangulation* to refer to:

1. including a wide variety of data sources (individuals, families, groups)
2. involving a variety of investigators working individually and in teams
3. combining a range of theoretical orientations on the same situation—for example, approaching a study of hospice care for dying patients from psychological, biological, and sociocultural theory

Methodological triangulation is, however, the most conventional meaning for the term. In a discussion of nursing studies on the concept of stress, for example, Muhlenkamp (1978) wrote that it was important to use a variety of stress indicators, particularly ones that did not share the same bias and measurement error.

Each of the major types of data-collection strategy used in field research is discussed in the sections that follow, with the exception of Type 3, to which an entire chapter has been devoted (see Chapter 11).

Observation

If the field worker elects to emphasize participant observation in a specific study setting rather than interviews about a social experience, here are some guidelines that are helpful in getting started.

Guidelines for Observing

1. Begin by orienting yourself to what Schatzman and Strauss (1982) call "the various social, spatial and temporal maps of the setting." If you are studying an institution, you may obtain organizational charts, a schedule of meetings and routines, even a blueprint or floor plan. In a study of burn units, you might take notes on the physical layout, routines and emergencies, pacing of work, division of labor, status relationships, treatment ideologies, ideals and values, and problems and concerns.

2. Take a "tour of limited discovery"—a first extensive (not intensive) look at things, persons, and activities that constitute "the site" (Schatzman & Strauss 1982). Don't be concerned about missing things. Underlying patterns will occur over and over. Use this step to identify informants, meet and cultivate people, establish your legitimacy, and figure out what your next steps will be.

3. Selectively sample people, places, events, and any other categories that are suggested by the initial mapping and beginning analysis. Typically, if you are studying a hospital or police system that is on a 24-hour day, you will selectively sample all times of the day, all days of the week, activities such as routines and shifts, and special occasions and events.

4. Decide on locations from which to observe. Select these based on where events and information will come within your line of sight. Sometimes you may follow one person around; at other times you may sit in the corner of a nurses' station or clinic waiting room. Schatzman and Strauss suggest the use of single, multiple, and mobile positioning. *Single positioning* is staying put for a period of time so as to gain a greater familiarity with one station. *Multiple positioning* means moving around the setting to observe in different locations. *Mobile positioning* is the term for actually following someone—a woman in labor, a nursing student, a chemotherapy patient—through the course of a day or an experience. You can maximize your variety of perspectives by seeking out people who you anticipate might have different points of view, such as oldtimers versus newcomers, patients versus staff, or advocates versus critics. Most field researchers learn that they can ultimately listen for what they didn't see. One's continuous presence and repeated visits over a relatively long period result in the regulars telling the researcher what was missed between visits.

You should have been here on Saturday night. It was a really heavy time! We admitted this guy who tried to shoot the governor (from field notes).

Recording Field Notes A field researcher needs a system for remembering observations and, even more importantly, retrieving and analyzing them. If your identity and general purposes are known, you may take notes on a notepad or small clipboard in the presence of participants. Most of the time, field researchers jot a key word or phrase or cue down and then periodically leave the scene briefly to fill in full notes. Some field researchers dictate their observations into a tape recorder and later rely on a transcriber to type them. The danger of the latter approach is that weeks and months of observing can yield a veritable ocean of disorganized data, and its continuous flow can be as overwhelming to a researcher as the original experience of entering the field.

Writing and then typing one's own field notes increase the likelihood that the notes will be legible years later and will include sufficient detail and context to serve as a fund for future analyses, yet not be so voluminous as to be unapproachable. Each researcher tends to develop an individual format and approach for recording field notes. Schatzman and Strauss offer the following model as a starting point.

Observational notes (ONs) are descriptions of events experienced through watching and listening. They contain the who, what, where, and how of a situation and contain as little interpretation as possible. An example of an ON from a field study of a burn unit follows:

ON: The burn unit is laid out with a central nursing station that faces three glassed-in wards. Male and female patients are in the same ward. The treatment room has a big tub shaped so that arms and legs can be spread out. The tub has a whirlpool mechanism. The ratio of staff to patients seems to be one staff member to three patients. Staff members seem to work in groups of two's and three's, and the atmosphere is one of tremendous hustle and bustle.

Theoretical notes (TNs) are purposeful attempts to derive meaning from the observational notes. Here you interpret, infer, conjecture, and hypothesize in order to ultimately build your analytic scheme. A TN from Fagerhaugh and Strauss' (1977) burn study is below: *

TN: There is a cocoon-like effect on the unit. Patients spend weeks and months there. Visitors are limited to the family. There are no mirrors or windows. Four patients could tell me about the day they came into the hospital but *none* knew what day it was today. They state that the days all "run together," that thinking about how long they'd been in didn't matter. It was the excrutiating treatment

---

*This and other quotations from S. Fagerhaugh and A. Strauss, *Politics of Pain Management*, Menlo Park, Calif.: Addison-Wesley, 1977.

pain that consumed them. The pain is absolutely indescribable for its intensity. S said It reduces him to a blubbering baby, something that he never was.

Methodological notes (MNs) are instructions to oneself, critiques of one's tactics, reminders about methodological approaches that might be fruitful.

MN: I decided to spend one day observing the varieties of painful treatments. There seem to be plenty of them! I decide to look for situations in which staff members actually talk about the god-awful pain these people are experiencing instead of the technical matters related to burn management.

Personal notes (PNs) (not a component of the original Schatzman and Strauss format) are notes about one's own reactions and reflections and experiences. Fieldwork relies on the investigator's ability to "take the role of the other" and be introspective. A final illustration from the burn study presents a PN.

PN: I had a somewhat unnerving morning. There's so much pain and misery on the unit yet the lightheartedness of the staff and the lack of pain expression among the patients except during treatments creates in me a sense of horror and awe! My friends and husband don't want to hear about working with burn patients. It's too horrible! I feel isolated and wonder if other nurses avoid the nurses on the burn unit or keep shop talk to superficial social "chit-chat."

After ONs, TNs, MNs, and PNs are recorded, they are customarily typed, paginated, labeled and dated, duplicated, and filed and become the basis for analytic memos (see Chapter 14). Remember to use headings and subheadings for ease of data retrieval and to leave wide margins around the edges for penciled codes.

The development of a good set of field notes not only relieves the investigator of some of the burdens of remembering events but also constitutes a written record of the development of observations and ideas to be used in future publications of the research findings and method.

Interviewing

Interviews depend on the respondents' verbal report about experiences, perceptions, preferences, problems, feelings, attitudes, or whatever other phenomena may be relevant to the study question. Some interviews may be highly structured, in the sense that the wording of each question, the sequence in which they are asked, and the possible responses are planned by developing an interview schedule (a lot like a script). Interviewers are trained to use it. Structured interviews are akin to questionnaires, with the exception that the interviewer and the respondent are in each other's presence when the interview is used.

The next sections of this chapter address the use of partially structured and unstructured interviews, because these two types are generally preferred by nurses doing field research.

Partially Structured Interviews   A *partially structured*, or focused, *interview* begins with at least an outline of topics the investigator intends to cover with each subject; but both the interviewer and the subject are free to deviate from the prepared agenda and introduce thoughts or observations that are particularly relevant to their personal perspective as the conversation unfolds. (See Box 13-2 for a progression of questions for assessing the sexual needs of the aged.) Partially structured interviews offer the interviewer more latitude to move from content area to content area, to follow up on cues suggested by the respondent, and to spend various amounts of time interviewing one subject or another. Focused interviews, however, require that by the end of the interview *all of the predetermined topics or questions have indeed been covered in some sequence, in some form with each interviewee.*

Clinical interviews are basically a subtype of focused interview. They are used when the interviewer is a clinician, the respondent is a patient

---

Box 13-2   *Guidelines for Assessing the Sexual Needs of the Aged*

1. When you were growing up, did people you knew discuss sex and romance?
2. How do you feel about discussing it now?
3. What do you think about romance at this stage in your life?
4. What were you told about sex when you were a child?
5. Do you think it is a very important part of life satisfaction for people of all ages?
6. How important has sexual activity been in your life?
7. What were you told about masturbation?
8. What does sexuality mean to you?
9. Does your present living situation give you opportunities to express your sexuality?
10. What values and morals influence your feelings about sex now?
11. How are your needs of intimacy being met now?

SOURCE: H. Wilson and C. Kneisl, *Psychiatric Nursing*, 2nd ed., Menlo Park, Calif.: Addison-Wesley, 1983.

or client, the circumstances involve a health care problem, and the purpose of the interview is to collect data to formulate a nursing diagnosis or health care problem assessment. Nursing histories, psychiatric intake interviews, and verbal mental status examinations are all used by clinicians to identify problems, make nursing diagnoses, and plan nursing care. Box 13-3 presents an example of a psychosocial clinical interview guide (Wilson & Kneisl 1983, pp. 4–5). Clinical interviews can also provide data that are valuable to nurses conducting research. McCorkle (1977) used such interviews to study the impact of a diagnosis of inoperable lung cancer on a person's attachments and goals as the illness progressed. Data from clinical interviews helped reestablish the subjects' disease state and clarify their perception of their illness as well as to discover the differences and similarities in the quality of living for subjects with terminal cancer. Most researchers who use partially structured interviews believe that they are effective for exploration and hypotheses formulation but not appropriate or practical for hypothesis testing.

Unstructured Interviews The *unstructured interview* may be either spontaneous or scheduled, but its identifying characteristic is that respondents are encouraged to talk about whatever they wish that is relevant to the researcher's interest. Many such interviews begin with very open-ended questions such as: "Tell me some about what it was like when you and your husband first learned that Stephen was retarded?" or "What concerns you most when you think about managing your life, knowing what you do about your illness?" Some unstructured interviews begin by just inviting the interviewee to talk about whatever he or she wishes. The intent of the unstructured interview is to get to the subject's perception of the meanings in his or her world without introducing the investigator's conception of it. In fact, it is the method of choice among field researchers, and most researchers intentionally *avoid* structuring their interviews. Structure limits in advance what top-

ics are important to ask about and often what the possible categories of response from interviewees might be. Unstructured interviews, in contrast, allow the interviewer a great deal of freedom in exploring whatever seems important to the respondent and promote what Brink (1983) calls the likelihood that responses will be spontaneous, self-revealing, and personal.

Advantages of Interviewing Listening to people talk about their perceptions and experiences has a number of important advantages as a data-collection strategy:

1. The invitation to subjects to tell their story face to face to an empathetic person usually gets a better response rate than mailing them an impersonal questionnaire or structured data form.

2. Interviews allow you to collect data from people who either because of their literacy level or some other communication barrier such as paralysis following a stroke, bandages after burns, or immobilizing tubes or traction simply can't write.

3. Interviews are usually more effective in getting at people's complex feelings or perceptions. In describing the burden of implementing the recommended regimen for their diabetic children, interviewed mothers in one nursing study spoke of a period of being overwhelmed as they tried to understand the "whats" and "whys" of food management for their children. One mother told the nurse researcher when describing the tensions of carrying this responsibility, "I felt like I was holding a stick of dynamite."

4. Interviews allow you to clarify responses that you don't understand fully, to probe certain responses in more depth, and to reword and rephrase questions so that they are more easily grasped by the interviewee.

5. Unstructured interviews, particularly, allow you to discover the unexpected. In Lopata's (1979) study of American widows she commented:

Box 13-3 Psychosocial Interview Guide

1. *Physical and Intellectual Factors*
   a. Presence of physical illness and/or disability
   b. Appearance and energy level
   c. Current and potential levels of intellectual functioning
   d. How client sees personal world, translates events around self; client's perceptual abilities
   e. Cause and effect reasoning, ability to focus

2. *Socioeconomic Factors*
   a. Economic factors—level of income, adequacy of subsistence; how this affects life-style, sense of adequacy, self-worth
   b. Employment and attitudes about it
   c. Racial, cultural, and ethnic identification; sense of identity and belonging
   d. Religious identification and link to significant value systems, norms, and practices

3. *Personal Values and Goals*
   a. Presence or absence of congruence between values and their expression in action; meaning of values to individual
   b. Congruence between individual's values and goals and the immediate systems with which client interacts
   c. Congruence between individual's values and assessor's values; meaning of this for intervention process

4. *Adaptive Functioning and Response to Present Involvement*
   a. Manner in which individual presents self to others—grooming, appearance, posture
   b. Emotional tone and change or constancy of levels
   c. Style of communication—verbal and nonverbal; ability to express appropriate emotion, follow train of thought; factors of dissonance, confusion, uncertainty
   d. Symptoms or symptomatic behavior

   e. Quality of relationship individual seeks to establish—direction, purposes, and uses of such relationships for individual
   f. Perception of self
   g. Social roles that are assumed or ascribed; competence in fulfilling these roles
   h. Relational behavior
      - Capacity for intimacy
      - Dependence—independence balance
      - Power and control conflicts
      - Exploitiveness
      - Openness

5. *Developmental Factors*
   a. Role performance equated with life stage
   b. How developmental experiences have been interpreted and used
   c. How individual has dealt with past conflicts, tasks, and problems
   d. Uniqueness of present problem in life experience

SOURCE: H. Wilson and C. Kneisl, *Psychiatric Nursing*, 2nd ed., Menlo Park, Calif.: Addison-Wesley, 1983. Adapted from B. Compton and B. Galloway, *Social Work Processes*, 2nd ed. Homewood, Ill.: Dorsey Press, 1979, pp. 250–251.

My clumsiness with the tape recorder in the exploratory stages of my study proved to be a boon, preventing me from making some of the mistakes of new researchers not familiar with the world of their subjects. I knew what I wanted to ask these women. . . . My reading had filled me with questions and anticipated responses. The mechanical problems of using the recorder and the accompanying non-directed interaction finally forced me to listen to what the widows *wanted to talk about* before I had a chance to ask questions. Their monologues often focused on subjects very different from what I assumed would be important to them. . . . These interviews contributed to my increasing awareness that role modifications and support systems of widows contain a variety of realities which my lack of familiarity with their lives had not anticipated (p. 71).

Interviews when used as part of field studies, although they may be focused on pinpointing the development of one analytic idea or another, are essentially conversations *in situo*, which vary widely in style and type. About their two years of fieldwork in two clinics, twenty wards, and nine hospitals on the politics of pain management study the authors stated:

We did no interviewing that involved asking identical questions of a pre-selected number of people, even when interviewing patients with similar disorders . . . Even pre-arranged interviews followed no particular format, but the interviewer followed through on areas deemed relevant or on leads offered by the interviewee (Fagerhaugh & Strauss 1977, p. 306).

These kinds of interviews are most often done when checking hypotheses developed from extensive field notes or the analysis of case studies. For example, about an interview with one informant the investigators wrote:

Mrs. Noble taught us, rather early in the study to think about unfamiliar technology as a condition that might affect the patient's ability to get the staff to accept her pain as truly legitimate and thus influence the staff's handling of pain-relief tasks. The in-depth, free-response questioning usually used in fieldwork grows not only from the investigator's philosophy of science [See Chapter 1], but also from the fact that the research question at hand is one for which the investigators don't necessarily know the full range of possible responses (Fagerhaugh & Strauss 1977, p. 309).

Disadvantages of Interviewing As you might imagine, such free-response, unstructured interviews also have disadvantages, according to their critics:

1. In nursing studies, particularly, interviewees often expect some sort of direct help as a result of participating in the interview—a solution to their problems or even a complete change in their life. They may assume that the nurse interviewer can put them in touch with some special resources or benefits, unless he or she is careful in addressing with all candor the personal benefits section of the consent process (see Chapter 3).

2. Open-ended, nonstructured, or semistructured interviews are time-consuming procedures for collecting data and similarly time-consuming to analyze word by word, phrase by phrase (see Chapter 14).

3. It is difficult to make conventional quantitative comparisons across interviews in the absence of an interview schedule that assures that all interviewees are asked the same set of questions with the same terminology.

4. If a substantial number of interviews are to be conducted, interviewers must be trained, particularly in the use of clear, nonleading language, the ability to expand or clarify a respondent's initial response, and their listening skills.

5. Subjects may be self-conscious about being recorded on tape or about notes being taken about their replies. Thus, they may edit comments that they would make on an anonymous questionnaire.

Listening: An Essential Research Skill   Listening is perhaps more crucial in unstructured interviews than is the art of questioning. Listening involves an active process of responding to words and body language. Parsons and Sanford (1979), two nurses writing about interpersonal interaction, encourage us to use Egan's (1970) definition: "Listening for our purposes means becoming aware of all the cues that the other emits and this implies an openness to the totality of the communication of the other" (Egan 1970, p. 248).

Effective listening requires the following steps:

1. coding what is said into something that makes sense for you the interviewer
2. interpreting the meaning in the respondent's framework or perspective
3. responding by conveying to the interviewee that she or he is being heard and understood

Some specific strategies for making listening more effective have been developed by Brammer (1973, pp. 81–87) and applied to the research interview. They include:

1. establishing eye contact with the interviewee (The difficulty of accomplishing this *while writing notes* is one of the reasons some field researchers prefer to tape record interviews.)
2. clarifying and checking perceptions by restating a summary of the basic message, asking for a repetition, but not interrupting
3. using clarifying questions that ask for elaboration, examples, and extensions of the original message

Most nurses are well acquainted with the principles of effective communication with pa-

tients (see Wilson & Kneisl 1983, Chapter 6). However, communicating with patients with the major objective of helping them directly is different from interviewing people to obtain data bearing on a research question and an analysis that may not offer them any direct benefit. For some nurse researchers, interviewing for research purposes rather than clinical ones presents something of a barrier. For others, it's an intellectual challenge.

Analysis of Documents, Case Studies, and Case Histories

Documents and Records   Nursing research has tended to use document and record analysis more often than the other types of unobtrusive measure mentioned earlier in this chapter. An agency's perspective often emerges from analysis of statistics, reports of medication errors, nursing notes, policy statements, and procedure manuals. Field researchers realize that through such official documents they learn the agency's interpretation of what is going on or has occurred and what is valued. Sudnow (1967), in studies of birth and death statistics, has commented on some of the ambiguities of relying exclusively on such official documents. His observations suggest that similar organizations processing the same sets of events may not generate comparable data on those events. Variations in delinquency rates, for example, may often really represent only differences in organizational bookkeeping. Because of this possibility, field researchers must always report document analysis as data obtained within a particular situated context. In my qualitative field study of Soteria House, a nonconventional residential care setting for psychotic adults, documents revealed a pattern of limited and partial disclosures based on the audience for which a particular document was intended. The memo on the facing page summarizes my analysis.

Documents such as diaries, books, letters, newspapers, meeting minutes, legal documents, and reports as well as photographs, films, and

Example: Memo on Documents

Self-portrayals of Soteria share two general properties: ambiguity and a tendency toward chameleon-like protective coloration. Keeping Soteria ambiguous . . . limits a potential critic's ability to evaluate its success or failure. Self-portrayals in documents take on different characteristics depending on the audience. A manual called "The Care and Feeding of a Soteria" professes as its purpose: "to provide some examples of how various types of behavior gave rise to problems dealt with at Soteria." Its informal, atheoretical style is almost unrecognizable in a letter written to solicit financial support from federal funding agencies: "Soteria is a residential treatment program for first-episode schizophrenics utilizing a developmental crisis model. Six specifically trained nonprofessional staff work with the resident patients under the supervision of a psychiatrist and a social worker." Here the presentation attempted to link Soteria to the language of conventional, mainstream psychiatry. Professionals at Soteria recognize that to portray Soteria as a "good space" or "high energy" in the rhetoric and ideology of the staff is to risk being dismissed as naive or ostracized as outrageous. Thus to the professional community documents present it as an experimental research project in psychiatric residential care . . . which in my point of view, it is.

Analysis of properties

Limited, variable, and partial disclosures characterized self-portrayals in documents

---

drawings are also used as sources of data. (A complete discussion of the historical study design can be found in Chapter 6. Analysis procedures for documents and records used as data in field studies are described in Chapter 14.)

Case Studies and Case Histories   The case study has a long and valued history in the sphere of clinical practice research. Here the clinician or researcher conducts an in-depth investigation of a patient, a community group or aggregate, or an institution like a hospital or clinic. Some clinicians have used literature, studying Tennessee Williams's *The Glass Menagerie* to learn more about a physical handicap or Eugene O'Neill's *Long Day's Journey Into Night* to learn about destructive family dynamics. Sylvia Plath's poignant novel *The Bell Jar* may be of greater value in learning to understand severe depression than more conventional quantified scientific modes.

Whether fictional or not, case studies offer information that is rich and sometimes difficult to come by. Obviously, Freud developed his psychoanalytic theory and methods primarily from careful case studies conducted in turn-of-

the-century Vienna. Critics of sole reliance on case-study data underscore their lack of generalizability. The methodology for compiling such data is not as rigorously prescribed as that for collecting survey or even participant observation field notes. Some say there is considerable freedom, if not outright ambiguity, in devising the data-collection strategies. The main principle is once again pragmatism in addressing the study question. And, of course, case study data must be analyzed and interpreted according to one of the qualitative analyses presented in Chapter 14.

Glaser and Strauss (1970) distinguish between a case history and a case study. They believe that the goal in a case history is to get the fullest possible story for its own sake. A case study is said to be focused on description, verification, or developing of theory. A case history, on the one hand, provides highly readable imagery that can be explained and interpreted within theory. It is a way of demonstrating how theory can be used to understand human experience. A case study, on the other hand, generally exists for the purpose of comparative analysis and the generation of data and grounded theories. Even though Glaser and Strauss try to emphasize this distinction, they also recognize that for the most part only a thin line distinguishes most case histories from case studies.

When trying to decide which is which, it is important to determine whether theory is being used to place the case within a more general context, as is done with a case history, or whether theory is actually being developed from the comparative analysis of multiple case studies. One of the most famous of case histories is the classic one by Thomas and Znaniecki (1918), which begins with a threefold typology of Polish emigrant men and then offers the personal history of one. Blau (1955) and Crozier (1964), in contrast, used case studies to correct and amplify Max Weber's theory of bureaucracy.

The potential of both case studies and case histories in nursing is wide open if we can resist succumbing to the accusation that such work fails to uphold the canons of desirable science and should therefore be relegated to the categories of journalism or art. To date, nurse authors have made substantial contributions to the professional literature, depicting case histories particularly.

In 1970 two medical sociologists in collaboration with a team of nurses involved in field research published a book entitled *Anguish: A Case History of a Dying Trajectory*. It was the story of a woman's protracted death in the hospital. According to its authors, the case demonstrated two major features; it was of long duration and it moved slowly but steadily downward. In presenting the case history of this lingering trajectory, Glaser and Strauss (1970) told the life story, or biography, of the patient; the story of how a hospital's staff reacted to her slow decline on their turf; the case history of the two nursing students who served as informants for the study; and, finally, the story of a final stage of a research project that had addressed the topic of dying and lasted over five years.

The interweaving of these four substories illustrates the rich fabric, detail, and complex information that a case history can produce. Its authors remind us, however, that case history is not a novel or merely exciting informative description. It is deliberately intended to highlight and explicate theoretical explanations that can be more broadly generalizable.

Do Field Studies Yield Scientific Truth?

In a critique of Wolanin's (1977) study on confusion, Jackson began with the following comment: "Poor research is the art of drawing sufficient conclusions from insufficient data gathered by faulty methodology and inadequate instruments" (1977, p. 76). Field studies in general are open to criticism on these grounds. Overcoming the implicit and explicit criticisms of field research begins with going beyond a strict and narrow conception of what is science. It moves on to developing a research narrative that proves its credibility by explaining through a linear, logical process the problems, methods, and findings. Finally, it acknowledges the responsibility

of the researcher to provide sufficient detail about the steps of the research process to enable a reader to evaluate the results. Table 13-2 summarizes Eisner's (1981) distinctions between studying something in a *scientific* mode and an *artistic* mode. On Eisner's grounds, most field research would be excluded as a valid scientific approach. But as for its ability to inform and enrich nursing practice, even he argues for seeking "a binocular approach" that includes both artistic and scientific approaches. "Looking through one eye never did provide much depth of field" (1981, p. 9).

Others acknowledge that field research is in-

Table 13-2   Scientific and Artistic Ways of Knowing

Criterion	Scientific Approach	Artistic Approach
Forms of representation employed	Formal, literal language	Idiosyncratic and figurative language
Criteria for appraisal	Whether conclusions are supported by the evidence and whether methods bias the conclusions (canons of sampling and test reliability)	How persuasive and informative the personal vision of the author is
Points of focus	Manifest behavior of the individual or group; experimental approach in search of law	The experience of individuals and the meaning their actions have for others; interpretive approach in search of meaning
Nature of generalization	Trends, central tendencies, and statistical differences	Belief that the general resides in the particular
Role of form	Standardization of style	Various styles
Degree of license allowed	Attempt to avoid bias, be objective, and present the facts	Avoidance of a facade of objectivity; selective use of informants; emphasis on what the author needs to say
Interest in prediction and control	Emphasis on prediction, explication, and control of future events	Emphasis on forms of understanding conveyed through the artistic image
Sources of data	Standardized tests and procedures	The investigator's experience of what he or she attends to
Basis for knowing	A positivistic view in which only formal propositions can provide knowledge	Central role of emotion ("To know a rose by its Latin name and yet to miss its fragrance is to miss much of the rose's meaning.")
Ultimate aims	Making true statements about the world—the laws of nature	Creation of images that people will find meaningful; implication that truth is relative, and diverse

SOURCE: E. W. Eisner, "On the Differences Between Scientific and Artistic Approaches to Qualitative Research," *Educational Researcher*, April 1981.

deed a valid approach to the discovery of conceptual models. Some require that a particular analysis procedure be followed if a study is to be judged as credible (see Chapter 14), but all critics emphasize that the reader must be given sufficient data to judge whether a sample was homogeneous and to know the specifics of data collection and analysis. Brink (1975), criticizing Schuster's (1975) privacy study, writes: "I remain puzzled as to how inductive methodologists analyze their data. . . . I would be hard-pressed to duplicate what she did on the basis of the information presented" (p. 177).

We can conclude from Brink's critique, as well as those of many others, that field studies will receive a more favorable regard among nurse researchers when their results are presented with a clear, concise description of the process that led to the findings presented.

Summary of Key Ideas and Terms

🖝 *Field research* is a mode of inquiry that grew out of anthropology and sociology. It relies on firsthand knowing under natural conditions and unstructured data-collection methods in which the investigator is the primary instrument or tool.

🖝 *Field studies* that examine, describe, define, and explain everyday nursing practice and have practical uses can make valuable contributions, particularly to factor-isolating and factor-relating types of clinical nursing research.

🖝 The major characteristics of field studies are:

- *face-to-face interviewing or observation* by the investigator
- *data collection and analysis* of complex sets of variables that go on simultaneously and in the natural setting
- a combination of *inductive and deductive thinking* to yield multiple, complex concepts, propositions, and middle-range theories

🖝 Field research emphasizes data-collection strategies that are designed to learn about the perspective, or world view, of those who are being studied. It includes participant and nonparticipant observation; unstructured interviewing; analysis of documents, case studies, and case histories; and other unobtrusive measures.

🖝 Appraising the field is a strategy for locating a field that is suitable for conducting research on a study question. Any place or set of activities can be considered "the field" for a study.

🖝 Serving the interests of the setting through your study, cultivating relationships, and contouring your presence to avoid being obviously intrusive are useful strategies in the second stage of field studies. Difficulties vary according to whether your research is overt or covert and to the general degree of accessibility of the study setting itself.

🖝 The role of observer can range along a continuum from complete participant to complete observer. Each role has advantages and disadvantages.

🖝 Data collection in field research begins with casting a wide net and initial mapping of the setting to orient yourself to its various social, spatial, and temporal dimensions. Then it is guided by categories and ideas that are emerging in your analysis.

✔ Guidelines for gracefully leaving the field once your data collection is completed include:

- Be prepared for some subjects to feel abandoned or taken advantage of.

- Ease out gradually, based on a timetable of diminishing contacts.

- Take advantage of any typical exit rituals.

- Fulfill any commitments you have made.

✔ *Single*, *multiple*, and *mobile positioning* are all options for observing in a study setting.

✔ One model for recording field notes is to use a system that organizes them into *observational notes* (ONs), *theoretical notes* (TNs), *methodological notes* (MNs), and *personal notes* (PNs).

✔ Partially structured and unstructured interviews are preferred by field researchers, because the emphasis is on freedom in exploring whatever is important to the interviewee and stimulating responses that are spontaneous and revealing.

✔ The advantages that interviews have over written questionnaires include:

- They usually get a better response rate.

- They can be used with people who are unable to read and write.

- They allow for probing and clarification of complex ideas.

- They allow you to discover the unexpected.

✔ Disadvantages of interviews include:

- They do not directly benefit the respondent in most instances.

- They are time consuming.

- It is hard to make quantitative comparisons of respondents.

- Interviewers must be trained.

- Subjects may be self-conscious and concerned about their loss of anonymity.

✔ Effective listening strategies in field research include:

- attending to the respondent by maintaining eye contact

- clarifying and perception checking by restating summaries of the basic message and asking for repetitions

- using clarifying questions that elicit examples and extensions of the original message

✔ Documents such as diaries, books, letters, meeting minutes, legal papers, reports, films, photographs, and nursing notes are all excellent sources of data in field studies.

✔ *Case studies* are used to develop and verify theory; *case histories* are ways of demonstrating how a theory can be used to understand human experiences.

✔ Some critics argue that field methods correspond more to the artistic rather than the scientific mode of inquiry. Others propose that as long as a field study conveys its logic, methods, and findings in sufficient detail, only a narrow conception of science would exclude it as a route to scientific truth.

References

Blau P: *The Dynamics of Bureaucracy.* Chicago: The University of Chicago Press, 1955.

Blumer H: *Symbolic Interactionism.* Englewood Cliffs, N.J.: Prentice-Hall, 1969.

Brammer LM: *The Helping Relationship.* Englewood Cliffs, N.J.: Prentice-Hall, 1973.

Brink PJ: Critique of "Privacy and the hospitalization experience," pp. 172–180 in *Communicating Nursing Research*, Vol. 7. Boulder, Colo.: WICHE, 1975.

Brink P: *Basic Steps in Planning Nursing Research.* North Scituate, Mass.: Duxbury Press, 1983.

Castaneda C: *The Teachings of Don Juan: A Yaqui Way of Knowledge.* New York: Simon and Schuster, 1968.

Crozier M: *The Bureaucratic Phenomenon.* Chicago: The University of Chicago Press, 1964.

Denzin NK: *The Research Act.* Chicago: Aldine, 1970.

Diers D: *Research in Nursing Practice.* Philadelphia: Lippincott, 1979.

Douglas JD: *Investigative Social Research: Individual and Team Field Research.* Beverly Hills, Calif.: Sage, 1976.

Egan G: *Encounter: Group Processes for Interpersonal Growth.* Monterey, Calif.: Brooks/Cole, 1970.

Eisner EW: On the differences between scientific and artistic approaches to qualitative research. *Educational Researcher* April 1981:5–9.

Fagerhaugh S, Strauss A: *Politics of Pain Management.* Menlo Park, Calif.: Addison-Wesley, 1977.

Glaser BG, Strauss A: *Awareness of Dying.* Chicago, Aldine, 1965.

Glaser BG, Strauss A: *Time for Dying.* Chicago, Aldine, 1968.

Glaser BG, Strauss A: *Anguish: A Case History of a Dying Trajectory.* Mill Valley, Calif.: Sociology Press, 1970.

Goffman E: *Asylums.* Garden City, N.Y.: Doubleday, 1961.

Gold RL: Roles in sociological field observations. *Social Forces* March 1958; 36:217–223.

Humphreys L: *Tearoom Trade: Impersonal Sex in Public Places.* Chicago: Aldine, 1975.

Hutchinson SA: Creating meaning out of horror. *Nurs Outlook* 1984:32; 86–90.

Jackson RK: Discussion: Alienation, confusion and disorientation and stress factors—Implications for health care delivery, pp. 76–81 in *Communicating Nursing Research*, Vol. 8. Boulder, Colo.: WICHE, 1977.

Junker BH: *Field Work: an Introduction to the Social Sciences.* Chicago: University of Chicago Press, 1960.

Leaf MJ: *Frontiers of Anthropology*. New York: D. Van Nostrand, 1974.

Lopata HZ: *Women as Widows: Support Systems*. New York: Elsevier, 1979.

McCorkle R: Terminal illness: Human attachments and intended goals, pp. 207–221 in *Communicating Nursing Research*, Vol. 9. Boulder, Colo.: WICHE, 1977.

Muhlenkamp AF: Stress: Conceptualization and measurement for nursing, pp. 74–76 in *Communicating Nursing Research*, Vol. 11. Boulder, Colo.: WICHE, 1978.

Parsons V, Sanford N: *Interpersonal Interaction in Nursing*. Menlo Park, Calif.: Addison-Wesley, 1979.

Penniman TK: *A Hundred Years of Anthropology*. London: Gerald Duckworth, 1965.

Polsky N: *Hustlers, Beats and Others*. Garden City, N.Y.: Doubleday, 1969.

Schatzman L, Strauss A: *Field Research: Strategies for a Natural Sociology*, 2nd ed. Englewood Cliffs, N.J.: Prentice-Hall, 1982.

Schuster EA: Privacy and the hospitalization experience, pp. 153–171 in *Communicating Nursing Research*, Vol. 7. Boulder, Colo.: WICHE, 1975.

Shaffir WB et al: *Fieldwork Experience: Qualitative Approaches to Social Research*. New York: St. Martin's Press, 1980.

Sudnow D: *Passing On: The Social Organization of Dying*. Englewood Cliffs, N.J.: Prentice-Hall, 1967.

Thomas WI, Znaniecki F: *The Polish Peasant in Poland and America*. New York: Knopf, 1918.

Watson JD: *The Double Helix*. New York: New American Library, 1968.

Wax R: *Doing Field Work: Warnings and Advice*. Chicago: University of Chicago Press, 1971.

Whyte WF: *Street Corner Society*. Chicago: University of Chicago Press, 1955.

Wilson HS: *Deinstitutionalized Residential Care for the Mentally Ill: The Soteria House Approach*. New York: Grune & Stratton, 1982.

Wilson HS, Kneisl CR: *Psychiatric Nursing*, 2nd ed. Menlo Park, Calif.: Addison-Wesley, 1983.

Wolanin MO: Confusion study: Use of grounded theory as methodology, pp. 68–75 in *Communicating Nursing Research*. Vol. 8. Boulder, Colo.: WICHE, 1977.

Further Readings

Berger PL: *Invitation to Sociology: A Humanistic Perspective*. Garden City: N.Y.: Doubleday, 1963.

Byerly EL: The nurse researcher as participant observer in a nursing setting, pp. 143–162 in *Transcultural Nursing: A Book of Readings*, Brink PJ (editor). Englewood Cliffs, N.J.: Prentice-Hall, 1976.

Davis MA: Some problems in identity in becoming a nurse researcher. *Nurs Res* 1968; 17:166–168.

Evaneshko V, Kay MA: The ethnoscience research technique. *West J Nurs Res* 1982; 4:49–64.

Garfinkel H: *Studies in Ethnomethodology*. Englewood Cliffs, N.J.: Prentice-Hall, 1967.

Glaser B: *Theoretical Sensitivity: Advances in the Methodology of Grounded Theory*. Mill Valley, Calif.: Sociology Press, 1978.

Glaser B, Strauss A: *The Discovery of Grounded Theory*. Chicago: Aldine, 1967.

Gorenberg B: The research tradition of nursing: An emerging issue. *Nurs Res* 1983; 32:347–349.

Hammond PG (editor): *Sociologists at Work: Essays on the Craft of Social Research*. New York: Basic Books, 1964.

Hutchinson SA: *Survival Practices of Rescue Workers: Hidden Dimensions of Watchful Readiness*. Lanham, MD: University Press of America, 1983.

Jacobson, SF: An insider's guide to field research. *Nurs Outlook* 1978; 26:371–374.

McCall G, Simmons JL (editors): *Issues in Participant Observation*. Reading, Mass.: Addison-Wesley, 1969.

Poulos ES, McCabe GS: The nurse in the role of research observer. *Nurs Res* 1981; 30:357–359.

Schutz A: *The Phenomenology of the Social World*. Chicago: Northwestern University Press, 1967.

Spradley JP: *Participant Observation*. New York: Holt, Rinehart & Winston, 1980.

Strauss A: *Negotiations, Varieties, Contexts, Processes and Social Order*. San Francisco, Ca.: Jossey-Bass, 1979.

Chapter 14

The Craft of Qualitative Analysis

From Observations to Explanations

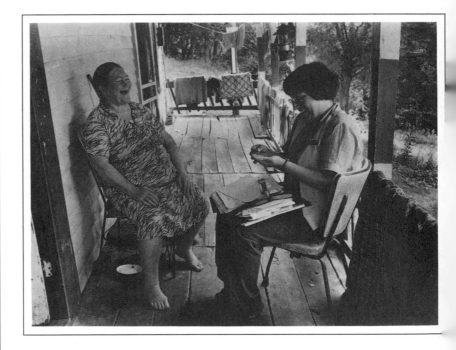

Nurses are experts at understanding the significance of data acquired through observing and talking with patients. We may label this skill as sensitivity, insight, intuition, or perceptiveness. But, in fact, it's all a form of qualitative analysis.

Chapter Outline

Chapter Objectives

After reading this chapter, the student should be able to:

- Define the term *qualitative analysis*
- Explain the qualitative analyst's philosophy of science
- Relate the major purposes of qualitative analysis
- Enumerate the steps involved in labeling, indexing, and filing data in preparation for analysis
- Differentiate among three kinds of data file
- Explain the procedures for four types of qualitative analysis
- Apply these procedures to analyze qualitative data
- Identify criteria appropriate for evaluating the credibility of a grounded theory
- Discuss the relevance of qualitative research to nursing practice and knowledge development in the discipline
- Comprehend the meaning of the terms *theoretical sampling, coding, saturation, basic social process, analytical induction, nominal scale,* and *grounded theory*

In This Chapter . . .

Qualitative analysis is something that you probably do every day in your clinical practice. Each time that you collect information about a patient that is not numerical—not a blood pressure, a temperature, or a laboratory test value—you have to conceptualize, compare, combine, and categorize in order to come up with a clinical interpretation of it. Whenever you use the nursing process to arrive at a nursing diagnosis, you have to make some meaning out of qualitative data. After all, a patient's acuity, adaptive functioning, self-care abilities, support systems, attitude toward health, and so on usually involve more than scores or measurements that can be plotted on a scale and subjected to statistical procedures. One expectant father whom you meet in the labor room is "involved," and a second is "detached." One recovery room patient is "stable," and another is "unstable." One family uses "open" communication, and another engages in "disturbed" communication patterns. Nurses are experts in grasping the significance of data acquired through observing and talking to patients about their subjective, real-world experiences. We may be inclined to call this skill sensitivity, insight, intuition, or perceptiveness, but in fact it involves a form of qualitative analysis.

Despite nurses' familiarity with these analytical operations in clinical practice, the term *qualitative analysis* in the research world is surrounded with definitional disorder. The lexicon of diverse terminology associated with qualitative analysis includes *content analysis*, *descriptive statistics*, *quasi-statistics*, *unstructured methods*, *induction*, *grounded theory*, *discovery*

method, *themes*, *coding*, *categories*, *field methods*, *process analysis*, *hypothesis generating*, *case studies*, *ethnomethodology*, *intersubjectivity*, and *soft science*. Some authorities use the term *qualitative analysis* to talk about the summarizing procedures performed on data that are gathered exclusively through unstructured methods such as participant observation and interviewing. Others view it as an outright misnomer and even a myth, pointing out that statistical operations such as factor analysis (see Chapter 15) are frequently used to categorize nominal or qualitative data. Still others think of it as basically journalism or art, but definitely not science.

This chapter clarifies the varied definitional scene by providing both the consumer and the conductor of qualitative research with a clear understanding of the full array of strategies that can be used when an investigator moves from observations to explanations and from practice to theory. Such an understanding can offer a basis for interpreting, evaluating, and using qualitative research findings in nursing practice and a technology for doing research that not too long ago relied on "immersing oneself in the data" and "having insight" as its major strategies. Topics considered include the qualitative researcher's philosophy of science, strategies for establishing files in preparation for analysis, and examples of four major qualitative analysis procedures. Finally, pointers on evaluating the credibility of a study using qualitative analysis offer you a framework for critiquing and applying your own or someone else's research.

What Is Qualitative Analysis?

Analysis is the separation of data into parts for the purpose of answering a research question and communicating that answer to others. A re-

search report that contained no analysis would be a chronological record of everything that happened during a specified time. Reading this report would be something like watching an Andy Warhol movie in which an actor did nothing but sleep for eight hours or reading a trunkful of computer printouts that typed out the entire data set. By thinking analytically, researchers impose order on a large body of data to answer a study's questions and avoid overwhelming a research consumer with detail when reporting the findings.

In Chapter 15 you will read about descriptive and inferential statistical methods of analyzing data. Such analysis is often called quantitative because data must be collected in or converted to numbers before they can be analyzed. *Qualitative analysis* is the *non*numerical organization and interpretation of data in order to discover patterns, themes, forms, and qualities found in field notes, interview transcripts, open-ended questionnaires, journals, diaries, documents, case studies, and the like.

Classic and Modern Examples

Classic and modern studies in the social sciences have served as prototypes for more contemporary nursing research employing qualitative analysis. These early studies include Anderson's *The Hobo*, Goffman's *Asylums*, Whyte's *Street Corner Society*, Roth's *Timetables*, Becker and colleagues' *Boys in White*, Cavan's *Liquor License*, Olesen and Whittaker's *The Silent Dialogue*, and Glaser and Strauss' *Time for Dying* and *Awareness of Dying* to name but a few. Nurses working in this scientific tradition at a time when our profession was relatively new to the world of research and science had to resist pressures to equate respectable and legitimate science with quantification of data and statistical analysis methods. Yet recognizing as did Berkeley sociologist Herbert Blumer (1969) that "the study of human life calls for a wide range of variables" and that nursing research had to be a basis for improved practice in the real world, a small cadre of nurses has demonstrated the use of qualitative analysis methods in the research liter-

ature. Among their studies are Archibald's "Impact of Parent-Caring on Middle Aged Offspring," Bozett's "Gay Fathers: How They Disclose Homosexuality to Children," Chenitz's "Entry into a Nursing Home as Status Passage," Davis's *Living with Multiple Sclerosis*, Fagerhaugh and Strauss's *Politics of Pain Management*, May's "Three Phases in the Development of Father Involvement in Pregnancy," Quint's "Awareness of Death and the Nurse's Composure," Reif's "Ulcerative Colitis: Strategies for Managing Life," Stern's "Stepfather Families: Integration Around Child Discipline," Hutchinson's *Survival Practices of Rescue Workers: Hidden Dimensions of Watchful Readiness*, and Wilson's study of the Soteria House Approach.

The Qualitative Analyst's Philosophy of Science

Qualitative analysis, like field research (see Chapter 13), is based on the belief that to know *about* people is not enough. Instead, face-to-face knowing is required for the fullest possible comprehension of another's world. Qualitative-research methods aspire to capture what other people and their lives are about without preconceiving the categories into which information will fit. In order to understand others, the qualitative analyst and field researcher try to put themselves in others' shoes to discern how they think, feel, act, and behave. Anthropologists, such as Margaret Mead, have based their research on this notion for decades. In sociology this belief is called "taking the role of the other." It was originally developed by George Herbert Mead and formally named by Herbert Blumer (1969). It is one of the central tenets of a social philosophy called symbolic interactionism. *Symbolic interactionism is a perspective on society and people that emphasizes the need to conduct research in natural settings and to focus on the way people define their reality and construct their actions over time.* Reality, or "the truth," is always viewed as emerging and relative rather than "all out there" waiting to be located and measured with a questionnaire or test. One patient swoons with fear in anticipation of the pain associated with a simple injection. Another dies of cancer never having asked for medication other than aspirin. One person perceives her miscarriage as but one in a long series of signs that she is inadequate. Another person sees her miscarriage as her liberation from an unwanted future.

The symbolic-interactionist philosophy underpinning most qualitative research is based on three simple premises:

1. Human beings act toward things on the basis of the meaning these things have for them.
2. The meaning of things in life is developed from the interactions a person has with others.
3. People handle and modify meaning through an interpretive process.

Qualitative research based on these premises has two main characteristics in common. It concerns itself with the natural everyday world of human group life and thus uses methods of data collection and analysis designed to yield complex and diversified explanations. It also views the research process itself as a form of symbolic interaction, wherein the investigator is the "tool" or "technique" in both data collection and analysis. This notion follows a tradition developed by Alfred Schutz (1967), in which investigators acknowledge that they register not objective fact but rather "intersubjectivity," "*verstehen*," or "subjective interpretation." Based on these ideas, researchers carefully examine their own perspective and interactions as both a source of data and as an analytic strategy. Validity, accordingly, comes from clarity about one's perspective and its influence on the study, not distance, objectivity, and control of variables. Corbin describes her awareness of how her nursing background began to influence her

analysis of data in a study of high-risk pregnant mothers with serious illnesses: *

Initially I was convinced that the pregnant women's strategies for controlling the risk would intensify with the severity of risk. I expected the woman with lupus, for example, to use highly controlling strategies because her illness created a more severe risk than some of the others. I faced the fact that I had to reformulate this proposition when it didn't hold up in the data. The strategies didn't vary consistently with what I, a nurse clinician, assessed as "high risk." Instead it had to do with the mother's own calculations or definitions of her risk severity based on cues of different types. My analysis began to fit the data when I went back into the field and began to sample for this. I ended up with an analytic scheme called *Protective Governing* that included all the ways these women control their illness and their treatment to try to govern the outcome of their pregnancy.

Visually, hypotheses are molecular, rather than the linear linking of a few variables. Swanson's (1980) study of men's perception of their role in family planning revealed that each respondent understood or perceived a contraceptive regimen differently, based on his own information and previous sexual practices. Qualitative methods allowed her to construct explanations that went far beyond the frequency and distribution of the simple variable *contraceptive use* found in most of the literature in her field.

Purposes of Qualitative Analysis

When a study involves open-ended, nonnumerical data, collected through formal or informal

*From J. Corbin, "Coding Data," in *Qualitative Research in Nursing: From Practice to Grounded Theory*, W. C. Chenitz and J. Swanson (editors), Menlo Park, Calif.: Addison-Wesley, 1985.

interviewing, participant observation, documents, diaries, and case studies, the researcher is faced sooner or later with the challenge of making sense of this mass of heterogeneous data in relationship to the study's central questions. In Lofland's words, "The researcher of a qualitative—humanistic bent . . . seeks neither purely novelistic reportage nor purely abstract conceptualizing. . . . The aim is judiciously to combine them, providing the vividness of 'what it is like' and an appropriate degree of economy and clarity" (1971, p. 7). You as an intelligent reader of this kind of research must similarly be prepared to evaluate the credibility of a study's findings when they are based on qualitative data. If a study purports to test hypotheses, establish causal relations, summarize numerical patterns, or demonstrate statistical significance according to the laws of probability, the quantitative methods to be discussed in Chapter 15 should be used. If a study has different purposes and raises different questions, however, particularly questions about people's experiences under natural conditions, qualitative methods will be used to analyze the data. The major purposes that can be served by using qualitative techniques are the following: exploration and description, accounting for and illustrating quantitative findings, discovery and explanation, and extension of theory.

Exploration and Description Sometimes a research study is designed to look for answers to questions in a field where a great deal of scientific work has already been done. A nurse conducting a study about early childhood development and the differential responses to hospitalization based on a child's developmental level would be one example. In this instance the investigator would build his or her study on prior work in the area, perhaps by measuring variables that others have reported as important or using instruments or findings developed by others. If a researcher is tackling a study question about which very little is known, however, and the study is intended to gain insight about a particular group of patients or health conditions, data that are collected may be analyzed to present descriptive and exploratory findings. In this second kind of research the investigator tries to collect and present rich and diverse accounts of findings so that any promising leads and ideas can be developed. Questions would include "What is going on?" "How does something work?" "What is important here?" "What variations exist?"

Throughout history important scientific advances have begun with careful observation and description of the nature of events as they occurred. Examples include Darwin's theory of evolution, Einstein's theory of relativity, Freud's psychoanalytic theory, and the discovery of penicillin, to name a few. Analyzing qualitative data for the purpose of description allows you to accurately and even insightfully characterize an event, a patient population, a process, or a setting. Dickoff and James (1968), scholars formerly at Yale University School of Nursing, call this factor-isolating research.

According to Schatzman and Strauss (1982), description can be done in one of two ways. First, the analyst may use categories or organizational schemes that already exist in the literature of a discipline and simply find classes or cases in the data that correspond to the classification scheme taken from the literature. This is called *straight description*. Describing a unit's patient population by diagnosis or social class would be an example. In the second instance, the analyst attempts to think up novel classes or categories suggested by an active inspecting of the data. This is called *analytic description*. May's (1980) typology of detachment and involvement styles of first-time fathers is an example of the originality that characterizes analytic description.

Accounting for and Illustrating Quantitative Findings. Qualitative anecdotes are often used to answer "why" and "how" questions associated with quantitative study findings. For example, Mosher and Menn (1978) conducted a longitudinal comparative-outcome study of two modes of residential treatment for first-break schizophrenics. They relied on standardized scales like the Ward Atmosphere Scale and a global psychopathology rating before and after treatment to collect data about the settings and patients. Their two-year follow-up study findings supported the effectiveness of the experimental setting (Soteria House). My own qualitative field study was used by them to explain how the Soteria approach worked (Wilson 1982). My theory of *infracontrolling* explained how social order was possible under the conditions of espoused freedom at Soteria House. My concepts of *presencing*, *fairing*, and *limiting intrusion* explained how patients, staff, and outsiders are managed.

Discovery and Explanation Sometimes a researcher wants to go beyond even abstract analytic description to discover in the data core patterns, variables, and categories that provide the basis for developing and then validating hypotheses about relationships. Once relationships are discovered, the analyst attempts to weave what

Example: Norris' Study of Restlessness

Norris, in a clinical study entitled "Restlessness: A Nursing Phenomenon in Search of Meaning," traced the behavioral manifestations of restlessness and related her observations to a theory of rhythmicity. She began with questions like "Who is restless?" "When does it occur?" "How do people experience restlessness?" "How does it differ from rest?" She concluded her study with what she described as a sense of urgency "for all nurses who are at the bedside to observe and describe nursing events until nurses wherever and however they work have the data they need to recognize and assign meaning to the phenomena of nursing" [Norris 1975].

The research questions

The value of describing and explaining nursing phenomena.

Example: Swanson's Study of Men's Roles in Family Planning

Swanson's study of men's perceptions of their role in family planning represents an example of research done in an area that prior to her work was largely limited to counting men and their preferred method of birth control. Swanson used in-depth interviews and fieldwork to go beyond anecdotes and description toward theory development [Swanson 1980].

Interviews as a field method

Anecdotes as a basis for generating a theory grounded in data

Example: Fagerhaugh's Study of Getting Around With Emphysema

Fagerhaugh's study of elderly indigents with advanced emphysema is one example of a grounded theory conducted by a nurse researcher. She explained how these patients juggled and balanced their time, energy, and money to achieve physical mobility and sociability. The outcome of her qualitative study was a diagram or model that linked the categories in relation to one another and explained how the patients in her study "got around with emphysema" (see Figure 14-1). She described her model as analogous to a Rubik's cube that has to be written up linearly [Fagerhaugh 1973].

Key concepts in an explanatory scheme

Visual model of a grounded theory (sometimes called a conceptual map)

Schatzman and Strauss (1982) call "these key linkages" into an explanatory scheme sometimes termed a paradigm, conceptual map, model, or grounded substantive theory (see Chapter 10).

The analyst attempting to develop a grounded theory uses a method of constant comparison and coding to develop a complex explanation of conditions, consequences, strategies, phases, stages, ranges, and other relationships among the classes of variable discovered in the data.

Extension of Theory Sometimes a researcher has developed a theoretical explanation under one set of conditions and wants to extend it, refine it, or even move it from a middle-range *substantive theory* that explains something under a specific set of conditions to a *grand, or formal, theory* that explains how something occurs under a great variety of conditions. In such a study, questions might include: "Is the original substantive theory correct?" "Does it fit other circumstances?" "Are there additional categories or relationships?" Glaser and Strauss' (1971) theory of *status passages* to explain transitions that dying patients experience has been extended to explain a wide variety of situations.

Table 14-1 summarizes some distinctions associated with the four major purposes of qualitative analysis.

Table 14-1 Purposes of Qualitative Analysis

Purpose	Research Questions	Methods	Outcomes
1. *Exploration and description*	**1.** What is going on? **2.** How does it work? **3.** What is important here? **4.** What variations exist?	**1.** Straight description using categories from existing literature **2.** Analytic description generating novel categories from data **3.** Content analysis **4.** Quasi-statistics	**1.** Case studies **2.** Ethnographies **3.** Frequency reports **4.** Descriptive narrative **5.** Typologies **6.** Cross-tabulations
2. *Accounting for and illustrating quantitative findings*	**1.** How did something occur? **2.** Why did something occur? **3.** What are the characteristics, conditions, and consequences involved?	**1.** Analytic induction	**1.** Anecdotes **2.** Grounded substantive theory
3. *Discovery and Explanation*	**1.** What is the basic social psychological process here (BSP)?	**1.** Constant comparison	**1.** Grounded substantive theory **2.** Paradigms **3.** Conceptual maps
4. *Extension of theory*	**1.** Is the original substantive theory correct? **2.** Does it fit other circumstances? **3.** Are there additional categories or relationships?	**1.** Comparative analysis **2.** Content analysis	**1.** Formal theory

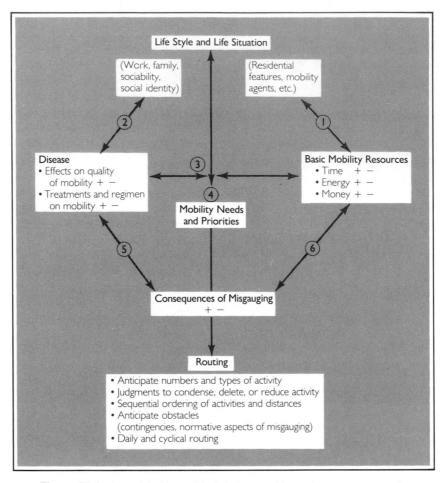

Figure 14-1 A model of how elderly indigents with emphysema get around. Adapted from S. Fagerhaugh (1973). Reprinted with permission.

Preparing Qualitative Data for Analysis

Just as the quantitative researcher must develop a code book, must key-punch data onto cards, and perhaps must enter them into a computer's memory and storage units, the qualitative analyst must develop a system for keeping track of data and the analysis process and retrieving them as needed. Hundreds of hours of field notes and typescripts of interviews can fill endless

cardboard boxes and create a sea of chaotic paper if left lying in piles on the livingroom floor.

Observational research produces an immense amount of detailed description. The records of field notes and interviews in a classic study of medical school education called *Boys in White* occupied 5000 single-spaced typed pages. The qualitative analyst faces the task of analyzing a diverse and seemingly unsystematic mass of data usually collected over many months or even years of fieldwork. One technical problem is being sure that all 5000 pages of evidence are considered each time a related analytic idea or proposition is advanced. To avoid searching through all 5000 pages of notes over and over again, qualitative analysts develop a system for labeling, indexing, filing, sorting, and retrieving their field notes, documents, and interview transcripts.

Code numbers can be assigned to them that refer to the major topics under which a given episode or item might be considered. Entries can then be reassembled by code number so that all items might be considered and all observations on given topics can be located in one place. Each entry is put into as many conceptual categories as it might represent. Finally, the analyst establishes a set of differentiated files. The following steps offer guidelines for indexing and filing data in preparation for analysis.

Steps in Labeling, Indexing, and Filing Data

1. Transcribe all handwritten field notes, taped interviews, and documents onto 8½ × 11 typing paper, doubled spaced. Leave wide margins, especially on the right-hand side of the paper, where you will later write codes.

2. Label each page with identifying information—for example: "Friday, May 13, 1983, Observation in City Hospital. Neonatal Intensive Care Unit, 7 A.M.–3 P.M. First Day in the Field, p. 1." Be certain to use code names or numbers to protect the confidentiality of respondents and settings. A typical typed, labeled field note appears in Box 14-1.

3. Make at least three duplicate sets of your data. Keep one complete set locked up in a safe place apart from your original. Make the third set so that you can cut it up and file information if needed in separate files. (As Chapter 16 suggests, the manual system for sorting and retrieving files described here may well be replaced using a personal computer to accomplish the same goals. A printout of your data should be kept in a safe place, because a power outage always poses the risk of your work being erased.) McCall recommends typing field notes onto ditto spirit, mimeograph, or other inexpensive duplicating masters. Then you can make whatever number of copies you need to have maximum flexibility in manipulating the materials (McCall & Simmons 1969).

4. Establish files. The goal of a filing system is to get your data out of the sheer chronological narrative of your field notes into a flexible storage, ordering, and retrieval format. Some qualitative analysts file their material in file folders and keep them in metal file cabinets, reserving different drawers for different types of file. Others use hanging files with metal "ears" that slide on rails in file drawers. Another possibility is to use boxes like the kind that hold 5000 sheets of ream-wrapped typing paper and can be purchased empty in bulk from wholesale paper dealers. you can use a three-hole punch and keep your notes in three-ring binders. Whatever physical setup you use, you need at least to establish three types of file and be prepared to disassemble copies of your notes for the purpose of cutting them up and refiling them into various categories. If you are limited in the number of copies you can make, you can cross-reference to information in other files by entering a cross-reference page in a file.

Types of File

Organizational Files One file must be kept to keep track of people, documents, places, organizations, phone numbers, and so on. In this file you put material under the most pragmatic category. For example, the interview transcript for a particular patient would be filed under his or her code number or code name. Field notes collected

---

Box 14-1   Sample Field Note With Label

H. Wilson   Friday 9:45 A.M.
Soteria I Study   12:45 P.M.
Feb. 9, 1973   Visit #5

Situation: I arrive at House 15 min. before weekly meeting is to begin. *There's no sign of its beginning on time.* T. and C. are up but D. is asleep in livingroom, H. is in shower, T. and M. are out, and S. is using the phone re: his Real Estate Business stuff. A. hasn't yet arrived.

ON T., H., S., and I sit around kitchen table drinking coffee. T. talks constantly. Asks S. how Kingsley Hall got their money. H. answers with the joke that the residents "work really hard." *They are all in the basement turning our Kinsley Hall souvenirs.* S. says the residents pay and the staff volunteer.

ON A. arrives. I tell her things are going well . . . that I have some germs of ideas. I ask about papers written about S. She suggests that I come up to MRI to see all written documents from various periods in the past year. Ex. A newsletter type thing that was done in the beginning and staff's journals.

ON At 10:30 their meeting still hasn't started. M. and T. come back. They've been to Welfare and T. had a traumatic time because she had to fill out forms about her "disability." T. asks M. to take her out for breakfast and then to Jack LaLaine's gym. M. tells A. she'll do the former thing but doesn't think that latter will be very good for T. and *just doesn't want to be part of it.* A. says she thinks it might be fun but A. doesn't try to convince M. to change her mind. H. agrees to take T. after breakfast.

TN The staff seem permitted to make decisions about patients based on their own personal feelings. This is legitimate at Soteria and unusual in conventional psychiatric treatment.

ON A. begins the meeting without saying, "Well, let's get started, etc." She inquires if there have been any more problems with the police about drugs. Apparently the police had been snooping around the House. T. tells about being stopped by the police with B. and using the occasion to reassure the police that S. was clean. He mentions as an aside that the police asked him what he did (occupation) and he jokingly responded, "*I'm crazy.*"

TN Despite the normalizing that goes on about mental illness in the house there are occasions when it is brought into awareness through contacts with the outside. T.'s experience is one example. While sitting at the table another occurred when C. asked what kind of place S. was called. "A home for the mentally disabled." S. *normalizes* by calling it "a board and care house." C. asked because she was filling out a form. (Welfare?)

---

in different settings would be grouped together under the code name of the setting. The sociologist John Lofland (1971) calls these organizational files "mundane files," because they help you keep prosaic matters straight. They make it easier to locate something that happened months in the past, precluding a search through chronological notes or analytic files that might take

hours. See Box 14-2 for a sample page from an organizational file.

Analytic Files   Files are crucial stimulants to the analytic process itself. The aim is to set up as many separate folders as you have codes or categories developing in your analysis. It doesn't matter if every category you begin with even-

---

Box 14-2   *Sample Page From an Organizational File (Wilson, 1974)*

List of Documents Used in Study Analysis

Community Alternatives for Treatment of Schizophrenia. Research proposal submitted to the U.S. Department of Health, Education, and Welfare, to expand Soteria House, May 1, 1973, to April 30, 1978.

Community Alternatives for Treatment of Schizophrenia. Research proposal submitted to the U.S. Department of Health, Education, and Welfare, to continue Soteria House from Nov. 1, 1974, to Nov. 1, 1979. (Submitted January 31, 1974)

Copes-Scale Profile for Soteria House Staff. Handout prepared by Soteria House professionals for National Institute of Mental Health site visit.

Essential Therapeutic Ingredients of Soteria. Outline prepared by research project staff for site visit, April 8, 1974.

IMPS Profile Sheet for Combined Rates Male and Female Acute Patients. Graph comparing Soteria House patients with control group.

Mosher, L. R. *New Treatment for Schizophrenia: Does It Work?* Paper presented at the meeting of the American Orthopsychiatric Association, held at San Francisco, May 1974.

————, and Others. *Indigenous Nonprofessionals as Primary Therapists for Acute Schizophrenia.* Paper presented at the Eightieth Annual Con-

vention of the American Psychological Association, held at Honolulu, Hawaii, September 1972.

————. *Schizophrenia and Crisis Theory.* Paper presented at the Annual Meeting of American Orthopsychiatric Association, Detroit, April 1972.

Research Design to Evaluate Psychosocial Treatments of Schizophrenia. Paper delivered at the Fourth International Symposium on the Psychotherapy of Schizophrenia. Turku, Finland, August 1971.

Soteria House. *The Care and Feeding of a Soteria: Our First Manual.* San Jose. The House. December 1972.

---

tually becomes a part of your explanatory scheme in the long run. The important points are

1. Continually think about your data in terms of the categories or concepts they may eventually serve as indicators for.
2. Keep track of accumulating theoretical notes (TNs) (see Chapter 13) as they occur to you.
3. Summarize TNs and associated anecdotes or episodes in your data in a growing set of analytic memos. (I will talk more about these memos later in this chapter.)

In any case, analytic files are where you keep track of your emerging analytic scheme and the data related to it. Additional pieces of informa-

tion can be added to each of your existing file folders, or new files can be started as your ideas for categories expand. Most importantly, remind yourself that your analytic files represent your emergent coding scheme, encouraging you to develop ideas about the clinical reality represented in your field work. They are flexible, collapsible, expandable, and stimulating and help you avoid getting too engrossed in the details of your data or becoming too closely involved with the setting for your study.

Methodological Files   Lofland (1971) calls methodological files his "fieldwork files," because in them you accumulate descriptions of *how* you conducted the research itself. These files allow you to bring together the methodological notes (MNs) and personal notes (PNs) (see Chapter 13) from your field notes and give you the basis for writing up your account of the methods used in your study. Reflections on methodological problems, such as gaining entry into a study setting or winning the trust of an informant, can also become valuable articles in and of themselves once your research is complete. After completing my own qualitative study of Soteria House, I published an article in *Nursing Research* using part of my analysis to illustrate the method of discovering theory with the constant comparison method. On the problem of recording field notes openly I wrote:

My problems with recording were more interpersonal than technical. The decision to take notes in full view of the interactants was in part a consequence of the structure of the Soteria setting and in part a conse-

quence of my attempt to avoid the social psychological risks of secretive behavior on my part. Unlike a hospital, a sixteen room house full of people offered little opportunity for slipping off to a cafeteria or restroom to record from memory [Wilson 1982, p. 109].

The system for filing qualitative data just described may well undergo a major transformation in the near future as more field researchers elect to substitute a small personal computer, diskette storage, and printer for the file folders and cardboard boxes cluttering their offices. The computer's capabilities to duplicate, to move whole sections of material around, and to store volumes of information in a small toaster-sized space may well make the cut-and-paste, file-folder operation traditionally used by qualitative researchers obsolete (see Chapter 16).

How to Analyze Qualitative Data

Data gathered through fieldwork methods can occasionally be collected in a standardized form and transformed into statistical data. An observational checklist of a psychiatric unit's dominant philosophy might be an example. But usually the qualitative data we have been discussing are not collected in a form that meets the assumptions of statistical tests. Consequently, some critics of this kind of research question the scientific merit of conclusions drawn from qualitative data because they are often presented to readers with the comment, "We have gone over our data and find that they support this conclusion." Consumers of this excuse for methodology find it difficult to accept the findings without being told what exactly that "going over" consisted of. They feel uncomfortable in the position of having to accept research conclusions on faith.

This section considers four major procedures for systematically making sense out of transcrip-

tions of open-ended interviews, field notes, and documents. These are (1) converting qualitative data to quantitative data, (2) doing a content analysis, (3) analytic induction, and (4) discovering grounded theory.

Converting Qualitative Data to Quantitative Data

In some studies, particularly those whose purpose is exclusively descriptive, an investigator elects to report the frequency and distribution of categories assigned to the data or to correlate their frequency or distribution with some other variables. In these cases the study reports some numerical conclusions but not with the precision evident in most statistical studies. For this reason Becker (1958) calls such an attempt an application of *quasi-statistics*. The essential objective of quasi-statistics is to decide if the concepts or categories in your analysis represent typical and widespread patterns distributed in the data, thereby giving the analytic scheme more credibility. The analysts who blend quantitative methods with qualitative work usually engage in three processes in order to conclude that their final analysis is likely to be an accurate representation of the data or to descriptively depict the frequency and distribution of analytic categories. These processes are:

1. searching for *negative cases* in order to reformulate propositions that don't account for them (*Negative cases* are bits of data that run counter to your propositions.)
2. counting numbers of cases (not necessarily subjects) in each category and, where possible, running descriptive statistics that give you information about the frequency with which certain themes are supported in the data
3. constructing scales for nominal data

A scale for nominal data consists of a number of discrete, mutually exclusive categories of a variable. Data are then summarized in terms of the percentage of subjects in each of the categories. Sometimes numbers are assigned to represent different categories. The number *1* might repre-

sent married, *2* single, *3* divorced or separated, and *4* widowed for the variable *marital status*. The numbers are merely labels that serve as a short-hand method of reporting data. They, in and of themselves, have no other quantitative meaning. In some instances, investigators correlate nominal data by cross-tabulating them with other variables. (See Table 14-2).

The limitations of basing an analysis of qualitative data exclusively on converting the data to some quantified form are probably obvious to you.

• Although searching for negative cases might force revisions in your analysis, there are no hard-and-fast rules to guide you in answering questions such as "How long should I look?" "How many negative cases are too many?"
• The generation of analytic descriptions depends in part on the theoretical sensitivity of the analyst. Field research is designed to allow for the flexibility and creativity required to develop classes, categories, and propositions that are grounded in observational data. There is no guarantee that two analysts working independently with the same data will necessarily achieve the same results. Counting the number of incidents that appear in observational data collected using purposeful rather than probability sampling methods (see Chap-

Table 14-2   Cross-Tabulation of Marital Status and Number of Depressive Symptoms Among a Nursing Home Population

Marital Status	Percentage	Mean Number of Depressive Symptoms ($T = 20$)
Married	22%	5
Single	18%	12
Divorced or separated	30%	15
Widowed	30%	8
	100%	

ter 9) seems rather like an exercise in "number mystification," particularly given the other characteristics of qualitative analysis.

- Scales for nominal data are sorting devices that might help an analyst group subjects into pigeonholes. But because there is no underlying continuum for the scale that links the categories together, they may be more confining than helpful to the rich portrayal of findings that a qualitative analyst seeks.

Doing a Content Analysis

One of the earliest specific procedures for analyzing unstructured qualitative data is called a *content analysis*. It is one way of categorizing verbal or behavioral data, and it shares with the other procedures in this section a requirement for analytic thinking and creativity in the researcher. The first studies that used the method of content analysis simply counted words or their synonyms when analyzing an interview or a document. If, for example, you were studying sexist stereotypes in journal recruitment advertisements for nursing positions you would do the following:

1. Make a list of all the relevant terms that reflected sexist stereotypes.
2. Read a randomly selected sample of recruitment ads from journals.
3. Count the frequency with which each of the key indicators (terms) appeared in the data.

Later content analysis studies coded for latent feeling tone (akin to connotation) as well as the actual appearance of the terms themselves. Both of these types of content analysis were the prototypes for the two types used in contemporary nursing research: (1) *semantic content analysis* and (2) *feeling tone, or inferred, content analysis*. Some authorities differentiate these two types by making a distinction between content analysis done at the obvious, or manifest, level

and content analysis at the implication, or latent, level. Semantic content analysis, simply coding and counting responses in a transcription, is an example of manifest content analysis. Feeling content analysis is an example of latent content analysis. Because in the latter the researcher goes beyond what was said directly to infer the meaning of something, research consumers usually require more evidence of a study's validity. Some studies involve both manifest and latent analyses.

Steps Involved in a Content Analysis The basic techniques for a content analysis are three: (1) deciding what the unit of analysis will be, (2) borrowing or developing the set of categories, and (3) developing the rationale and illustrations to guide the coding of data into categories.

1. *Deciding on the unit of analysis.* Deciding on the unit of analysis simply means deciding whether to use a whole response or to break down responses into separate words, phrases, or sentences.

2. *Borrowing or developing the set of categories.* If your study is concerned with concepts imported from an existing theory, you can set up your classifications in advance and then merely read through your data, code them into the existing categories, and ultimately report the frequency with which responses appeared in the various categories. For example, if you wanted to study a tentative classification system for psychosocial nursing diagnoses such as that published in the 1982 *Standards of Psychiatric Nursing Practice and Professional Performance*, you might read a large sample of nursing notes and code the nursing problem statement into one of the categories listed in Box 14-3. If however, you discovered in the course of your research that statements of nursing problems rather frequently fell outside of the preestablished categories, you would need to devise a set of categories based on themes appearing in the data. Ultimately, you would want to formulate a set of

---

Box 14-3   Tentative Nursing Diagnoses

1. self-care limitations or impaired functioning whose general etiology is mental and emotional distress, deficits in the ways significant systems are functioning, and internal psychic or developmental issues

2. emotional stress or crisis components of illness, pain, self-concept changes, and life-process changes

3. emotional problems related to daily experiences, such as anxiety, aggression, loss, loneliness, and grief

4. physical symptoms that occur simultaneously with altered psychic functioning, such as altered intestinal functioning and anorexia

5. alterations in thinking, perceiving, symbolizing, communicating, and decision-making abilities

6. impaired abilities to relate to others

7. behaviors and mental states that indicate the client is a danger to self or others or is gravely disabled

---

categories sufficiently detailed and mutually exclusive to allow you to code all of the notes in your sample. Researchers who use this method of analyzing qualitative data are quick to point out that it is complex, time consuming, and sometimes quite difficult.

3. *Developing the rationale and illustrations to guide coding of data into categories.* The coding of data into categories requires that the analyst or coder make a judgment on the right category for every response or unit of analysis. It is important to define the categories as fully and clearly as you can. Typical examples from the data help to illustrate the

properties a response should have if it is to be coded into a particular category. In my own master's thesis, focusing on the meaning of rock 'n' roll dancing to delinquent adolescents in an urban ghetto, I coded interview responses into one of the categories in Box 14-4 and then asked an independent judge to code the same data (Kelly 1968). Instructions for each were as precise as I could make them. For example, to code a response as an indicator of "creativity" it had to (1) reflect that the teenager thought kids had "made up" the current dances themselves, (2) report that the respondent had made up a dance once, and (3) include

---

Box 14-4   Categories for Coding Responses on the Meaning of Current Dances

1. conformity to peer-group expectations

2. means of creative expression

3. indicator of adolescents' search for identity

4. route to success, status, and prestige

5. form of socialized sexual and aggressive impulses

6. outlet for rebellion against adult authority

SOURCE: Kelly, H. S., "The Meaning of Current Dance Forms to Adolescent Girls: An Exploratory Study," *Nursing Research*, November/December 1968, 17:513–519.

an illustrative example of an experience of creating a dance. If someone other than the primary investigator in a study is to code the data, coders must be well trained and have opportunities to practice coding data into categories with supervision or discussion among a team of researchers.

The "Unfolding Tributary" Method of Evolving Categories Some content analysts apply what might be called the "unfolding tributary" method of extracting categories from the data rather than borrowing them from existing theory. This method proceeds systematically from two broad categories to more specific ones. If diagrammed, the process might look something like the decision trees nurses use in clinical practice (see Figure 14-2).

For example, if you decided to study hospitalized patients' awareness of and attitude toward the part that nursing services had played in their recovery from surgery, you might begin by coding your interview data in one of two major categories:

1. mentioned nursing services

2. did not mention nursing services

You would then reread the interview data and separate the data coded initially as having mentioned nursing services (a semantic content analysis) into more precise feeling-tone codes:

1. mentioned nursing services positively

2. mentioned nursing services negatively

3. mentioned nursing services neutrally

This branching evolution can continue until the researcher has achieved a degree of precision that adequately summarizes the meaning discovered in the qualitative data in relation to the original study question. Cross-tabulations might then be run correlating the frequencies of responses in these nominal categories with other data of interest. For example, if an investigator suspected that the elderly patients were more likely to express positive awareness of the role nursing had played in their hospital experience, frequencies in this content analysis code could be cross-tabulated by age group (see Table 14-3).

Table 14-3   Cross-Tabulation of Positive Awareness of Role of Nursing in Recovering, by Age

Positive Awareness Frequency	Age of Patient
1%	1–6 years
3%	7–13 years
2%	14–20 years
10%	21–30 years
12%	31–50 years
34%	51–65 years
38%	66 years and older
$T = 100\%$	

Depressed Mood (guilt, agitation, lethargy, etc.)

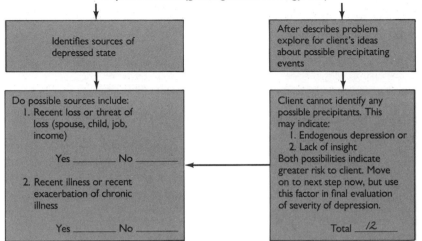

Identifies sources of depressed state	After describes problem explore for client's ideas about possible precipitating events

| Do possible sources include:
I. Recent loss or threat of loss (spouse, child, job, income)

Yes _____ No _____

2. Recent illness or recent exacerbation of chronic illness

Yes _____ No _____ | Client cannot identify any possible precipitants. This may indicate:
I. Endogenous depression or
2. Lack of insight
Both possibilities indicate greater risk to client. Move on to next step now, but use this factor in final evaluation of severity of depression.

Total _12_ |

Ask client to confirm or deny the following: Yes/No

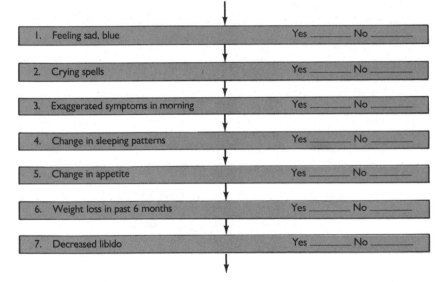

I.	Feeling sad, blue	Yes _____ No _____
2.	Crying spells	Yes _____ No _____
3.	Exaggerated symptoms in morning	Yes _____ No _____
4.	Change in sleeping patterns	Yes _____ No _____
5.	Change in appetite	Yes _____ No _____
6.	Weight loss in past 6 months	Yes _____ No _____
7.	Decreased libido	Yes _____ No _____

Figure 14-2   One page of a decision tree for depression. Adapted from M. Orsolits and M. Morphy (1982). Reprinted with permission.

A careful reading of the case illustration on page 412 not only gives you a sense of how qualitative data analyzed using a form of content analysis is presented in published research reports. It also allows you to tease out the indicators that were used to code a response into one of the four categories of orientation.

Reliability and Validity of Content Analysis
Content analysis, although ostensibly rigorous in its procedure and certainly arduous in its conduct, is still accused by its critics of being prone to problems of validity and reliability. Some of the critical questions directed toward studies that use content analysis are the following:

Example Evaluation of a Nursing Program: An Illustration of Content Analysis

In the late 1970s a team of educational and nursing researchers completed an evaluation study of the first bachelor of science program for RN's accredited by the National League for Nursing, at Sonoma State University in California. The task required that the team analyze qualitative responses to some open-ended questions collected during entry interviews with successive classes of students. In this case data were coded into four categories that reflected the students' attitudes toward their intended role vis-à-vis the profession of nursing. The four concepts, or categories were (1) traditional, (2) academic, (3) leadership, and (4) frontiering. The findings were reported in the following way in the study's final report, giving you an idea of how the results of content analyses appear in a published document.

Frequency of cases

Over one third (35%) of the students were categorized as predominantly *traditional* in their outlook, seeking to maintain or to further their positions in nursing but without volunteering any particular dissatisfactions with the hospital as a practice setting. One responded, "My husband and I separated and I began to think of my profession as a life-term career." Another said, "The handwriting is on the wall, if one wants to work in nursing, you need that degree!"

Traditional orientations as one category

Far fewer entering students indicated an *academic* orientation, but those that did (11%) were so categorized because they spoke of scholastic aspirations, usually including plans for graduate school and a career in teaching and/or research. For example: "At the age of 32 and with family responsibilities I couldn't pursue my interests. Now my children are no longer dependent on me and I want variety, mobility, and intellectual stimulation. I'd like to prepare myself to teach and do research in nursing."

Academic orientation was one category

A somewhat larger group (24%) had a clear *leadership* orientation and came back to school seeking avenues to power and status. One respondent whose long range objective was the presidency of the American Nurses' Association stated, "I'm convinced that change evolves from the top. To elicit change, you have to be involved at the top!"

Leadership orientation was one category

The most intriguing of the orientations is the one that earned the label, *frontiering*. More than 4 out of every 16 entering students were so categorized. Their responses in the interviews reflected an interest in non-traditional positions and careers, a questioning of established health care delivery and a willingness to pioneer or even create new and autonomous nursing roles. Many looked forward to functioning as independent practitioners, particularly in remote rural areas. Others hoped to "set up new programs, develop new ideas for health care in the community, participate in the management of an out-patient health service organization, set up programs for mental health and nutrition, to improve the current system, to be creative, innovative and constructive." One respondent characterized his intended role as "to joust with the system." *

Frontiering orientation was one category

Indicators for coding data into the frontiering category

---

*From M. W. Searight, et al., *Demonstration Study of a Second Step Nursing Program*. Rohnert Park, Calif.: Sonoma State College, unpublished Final Report, 1978.

1. How personal and idiosyncratic are the categories?

2. Would another researcher independently come up with the same ones?

3. How clear are the instructions for placing a response into a code?

4. How reliable is the coding?

5. What checks did the researcher include on the reliability and thoroughness of coding?

6. Do the categories have at least face validity (see Chapter 11)?

7. What kind of evidence is presented to establish face validity?

8. Do the content analysis categories meet other necessary criteria such as homogeneity, inclusiveness, usefulness, mutual exclusiveness, and clarity and specificity?

   • *Homogeneity* means that all categories are variations of the same thing. Are all the categories on similar levels of abstraction?

   • *Inclusiveness* means that the categories include every possible aspect of the variable without reverting to a catchall category such as *mixed* or *miscellaneous*.

   • *Usefulness* means that each category serves a purpose and relates to an important question under study. Proliferating too many categories detracts from a category's usefulness.

   • *Mutual exclusiveness* means that the categories are separate and independent. If responses can reasonably be coded into more than one place, the reliability of the coding is suspect.

   • *Clarity* and *specificity* simply mean that the categories are stated in clear, direct terms that other people can understand.

Ultimate validity for your content analysis relies on:

• your ability to develop a rationale for your categories

• your ability to define the categories

• your ability to show how the categories are appropriate to your data

• your ability to illustrate the fit with which the data can be coded into the categories

• your ability to demonstrate relevance of the categories to the research question

Analytic Induction

Analytic induction and a cluster of approaches resembling it depart from the two methods discussed previously in this chapter, in that reliance on frequency and the hope of quantifying qualitative data, even using scales for nominal data is no longer the key to discovering the truth. Instead, the analyst attempts to search for concepts and propositions in the data that apply to all cases of a question under analysis. This approach assumes the careful consideration of all analytic evidence, the intensive analysis of individual cases, and the comparison of cases to one another. According to Norman Denzin (1970), a sociologist whose name has become linked with this method in the social science literature, analytic induction involves the following steps:

1. Formulate a rough definition of the phenomenon to be explained. What is the study problem?

2. Based on files of qualitative data, formulate concepts and hypothetical explanations about what is going on (e.g., identify general categories).

3. Examine cases in the data to see if emerging propositions fit the facts.

4. Search for negative cases, and reformulate your hypotheses based on them.

5. Continue this process until a universal pattern of relationships or set of propositions is identified, explained, and supported with data.

6. Compare with other groups or conditions to

develop an even more abstract and generalizable explanatory scheme.

Some Practical Questions

Q. How does an analyst using the induction method arrive at the classes, categories, or concepts?

A. If you don't use classes, concepts, or constructs from existing literature, like assessing, planning, problem identifying, goal setting, evaluation, implementing or power structure, communication network or decision linkages, you must come up with original concepts by reading and thinking about the data. According to Schatzman and Strauss (1982) you have succeeded in devising a category when you can identify its properties or characteristics, know its boundaries, and can give it a name.

Lofland suggests "interrogating" your data according to three beginning research questions:

1. What are the characteristics of what is going on here? What forms does it assume? What variations can I find out about?

2. What are the conditions that preceded its occurrence, and what variations exist in them?

3. What are the consequences of a social phenomenon I can find here?

He believes that almost all qualitative analyses using a variation of analytic induction can be reduced to attempts to answer these three basic questions (Lofland 1971). He goes on to offer six *units of analysis*, ranging from microscopic to macroscopic, that can help you begin to classify your data:

1. acts—action in a situation that is temporary and brief

2. activities—action of major duration in a setting, consuming people's involvement as well as time

3. meanings—the verbal productions of participants that direct action

4. participation—people's involvement in or adaptation to the setting under study

5. relationships—interactions among different people

6. settings—the entire setting under analysis

Q. Once I can divide my data into Lofland's categories and maybe even find a novel name for what I observe in each category, then what?

A. Within each of Lofland's six units, a researcher can conduct either a static analysis or a phase (or sequence) analysis. This distinction is similar to that between a photograph of the phenomenon under study and a motion picture that captures processes evolving over time.

Typologies often result from *static analysis* of the six units of analysis. If, for example, we look at Alvin Gouldner's (1958) analysis of the different "types" employed in college teaching we find that he identifies:

1. *cosmopolitans*—those low on loyalty to the employing organization but high on commitment to specialized skills and likely to use an outside reference group orientation. These are further divided into:

    • the outsiders
    • the empire builders

2. *locals*—those high on loyalty to the employing institution, low on commitment to specialized skills, and likely to use an interior reference group orientation. They were further subdivided into:

    • the dedicated
    • the true bureaucrat
    • the homeguard
    • the elders

An illustration of *phase analysis* can be found in Fred Davis's (1968) stages experienced by nursing students who are undergoing what he named *doctrinal conversion*—a social-psychological process whereby students come to exchange their own lay views and images of the nursing profession for those that the profession ascribes to itself. He identified this status passage as consisting of six stages:

1. initial innocence
2. labeled recognition of incongruity
3. psyching out
4. role simulation
5. provisional internalization
6. stable internalization

Q. Once you establish classes and relationships, how do you use the data?

A. Once classes, subclasses, and relationships are discovered, specific vignettes in the data are coded as indicators of them in order to further develop their properties and ultimately formulate an overall integrative scheme. Unfortunately, "hearing" meaning in the data is a major difficulty for many researchers who try to work with qualitative data. Data, as Schatzman and Strauss (1982) suggest, "do not leap off the page to speak for themselves" and fall into some insightful interpretive scheme. Every investigator must either eventually confront his or her own ability to make some sense out of notebooks full of field notes and hear their meaning in a complex explanatory analysis or revert to simple or analytic description to salvage the study. Even crude typologies in which types are defined but not related to one another represent movement from completely unordered data to more refined categories.

Validity and Reliability Just as quantifying qualitative data and doing a content analysis can be questioned for their reliability and validity, so can analytic induction. Critics ask: "Can the observations made in one setting with one population be generalized to others?" "Do observations represent real differences, or are they merely the artifacts of the observer's biases?" "How honest and reliable are informants and respondents?"

When it comes to answering the first question about generalizability, the researcher must demonstrate that the case or cases studied are representative of the class of units to which he or she wants to generalize the findings. This is accomplished by carefully specifying the conceptual conditions under which observations were made and propositions were advanced. In answering the second objection, the investigator must introspectively examine his or her own perspective and indications in the data that it colored either what was seen or how data were interpreted. Anecdotes about PNs in the research report often emphasize these efforts. Finally, when you try to evaluate the credibility of informants, you can ask yourself some questions about them:

1. Do the informants have reason to lie or conceal what they think is the truth?
2. Does vanity or expediency lead them to misstate the facts?
3. Are they firsthand witnesses to the occurrence?
4. Are feelings about issues likely to lead to an alteration in the story line?

An alternative strategy for dealing with questions about credibility is to accept the philosophical position that an individual's statements and descriptions of events are indications of his or her personal reality and unique perspective and should be studied and interpreted as such. Here you view each datum as valuable in and of itself but with respect to different conclusions. For example, instead of learning what the quality of nursing care is like on a particular unit, you might find out what people think good nursing care ought to consist of.

Discovering Grounded Theory

The most highly evolved and explicitly codified method for developing categories and propositions about their relationships from qualitative data is called the *discovery of grounded theory*. According to Glaser (1978), one of the method's originators: "The grounded theory method offers a rigorous, orderly guide to theory development that at each stage is closely integrated with a method of social research. Generating theory and doing social research are two parts of the same process" (p. 2).

Basic Assumptions Developing theory from qualitative data using Glaser and Strauss's discovery method (1967) rests on a set of basic assumptions:

1. *One goal of a theory or analytic explanation is that it have "grab."* "Grab" means that a theory is interesting and useful. To achieve this, theories must fit, be relevant to, and work to explain, predict, and be modified by the social phenomena under study. Therefore, data are not forced or selected to fit preconceived theories. Instead of testing a few hypotheses deduced from existing theory, data are used to develop a rich, dense, complex explanatory or analytic scheme.

2. *Unlike verificational research, in which data collection and analysis are viewed in a linear way—that is, as separate, consecutive steps—data collection and analysis go on simultaneously.* The concepts and propositions that emerge from the data direct subsequent data collection. Although this process is sometimes called "an inductive approach" because it starts with the more specific and moves to the more abstract, it actually reflects both inductive and deductive thinking at various points.

3. *The grounded theory method is transcending.* Substantive theory developed in one area of study always has the potential for transcending a particular setting and being extended to a wide variety of circumstances. An example is the discovery of a process like "fairing," used by nonprofessional staff members to manage their work in Soteria House, where conventional administrative controls were muted and denied. This process could be extended to analyze the distribution of labor in a family where sex-role stereotypes, job assignments, and the like were absent. It is also transcending of other theories. It does not confront or refute existing theories but incorporates them as part of the data base for the analysis. It also transcends scholarly disciplines and can be as useful to nursing as to sociology. The possibilities, according to Glaser, are limited only by the analyst's capabilities.

4. *Despite the diversity that characterizes qualitative data, the grounded theory approach presumes the possibility of discovering fundamental patterns in all of social life.* These patterns are called core variables, or *basic social processes* (BSPs), and they account for most of the variations characterizing an interaction under study. Hutchinson found after spending months on three neonatal intensive care units that the nurses had to cope with a social-psychological problem of dealing with the horror associated with the deformities, death, and even some of the treatments of the newborns. The BSP, or core variable, she explicated in her theory was called *creating meaning*. It explained how, given the conditions and problems in a NICU, the nurses created meaning and obtained satisfaction from their work. When nurses failed to make some kind of meaning of their work world, they experienced burnout, depression, and low morale (Hutchinson 1984).

5. *Generating grounded theory takes time and the ability to think conceptually.* It takes time for ideas to develop about the data, and the analyst must be sensitive to pacing the study to provide for the creativity and energy it requires.

The final product of a grounded approach to qualitative analysis is a theoretical explanation that:

- fits the substantive area under study
- is sufficiently *dense* (accounts for a great deal of variation) and abstract to generalize to diverse situations
- allows for partial control over structures and processes in daily situations such as nursing practice

There are seven steps in developing a grounded theory: the research problem, reviewing the literature, sampling, coding, memoing, discovering the overriding analytic scheme, and sorting memos to produce an outline.

Step 1: The Research Problem For the purposes of writing a funding proposal or for a thesis or dissertation proposal review, the grounded theorist explains that the specific study problem will emerge from the data but that initially the research asks: "What are the basic social and psychological processes that explain interaction in a particular setting or under certain conditions?" This initial sensitizing question is supplanted with a grounded one in the final research report.

Unlike most deductive, theory-verifying research, a grounded theory begins without a highly focused research problem. A major requirement for a grounded theory is the discovery of a core variable, or BSP, that explains what is going on, but this conceptualization earns its way into the study by being grounded in the data. The analyst spends a considerable time in the field mapping out its relevant dimensions before a specific researchable problem is discovered. My experiences suggest that at least 50 hours of fieldwork precede one's ability to articulate a grounded study problem, the explanation of which becomes the core variable in the analysis. In my study of Soteria House, I began by asking the grounded theorist's initial questions:

1. What is it?
2. What are its properties?
3. How did it come to be and what is it becoming?

4. Under what conditions and with what strategies and consequences does it work?
5. What is the main story line here?

From data bearing on these questions I wrote the following TN:

> Soteria House has a noncontrol system as contrasted with the conventional system in mental hospitals. I've seen a conscious effort to mute and deny elaborate control structures like formal authority lines, a hierarchial division of labor, organizational ideology, schedules, therapies, medications, locked doors, uniforms, etc. An ethic that emphasizes freedom, spontaneity and individuality and opposes established psychiatric practices predominates. In doing away with traditional controls, problems of social order are not eliminated [Wilson, unpublished field notes].

The specific research problem that emerged from these notes became: "In the absence of conventional, elaborate psychiatric control structures, *how are problems of social control solved*" (p. 103)?

Step 2: Reviewing the Literature The sociologist Anselm Strauss once commented, "Be aware of the wisdom of questioning received wisdom!" Theory-verifying and hypothesis-testing studies require that we read related literature to get the fullest coverage possible, from which we can then synthesize our theoretical framework (see Chapter 10), operationalize concepts, and perhaps import an existing measurement tool. We then collect data relevant to the concepts in our framework. In some cases, if the fit is poor, we make adjustments to fit the data to the framework as necessary.

When discovering grounded theory, you collect data in the field before reviewing literature. In Glaser's words, "It's hard enough to generate one's own ideas without the 'rich' detailment provided by literature in the same field" (1978, p. 31). Once the analytic scheme emerges, the grounded theorist reads other studies to discover how his or her work fits with existing research and what contribution it has made. Reviewing other literature is done for correspondence, comparative analysis, and integration into a discipline's body of knowledge—not as a study's starting point or as an attempt to launch oneself to scholarly fame. This attitude about reading is not meant to ignore the fact that ideas are built on other ideas or to be antiacademic and antischolarly. But protecting one's theoretical sensitivity and originality in interpreting data is of prime importance with this mode of inquiry.

Step 3: Sampling   Again, grounded theory contrasts with theory-verifying research when it comes to sampling procedures. Instead of aiming at a predetermined probability (random) sample (see Chapter 9), grounded theory uses a purposeful method called *theoretical sampling*. Theoretical sampling rethinks statistical sampling standards in order to address interactive research questions. Theoretical samples are judged by the quality of the theory that emerges, whereas statistical samples are judged by their conformity to the rules of probability sampling theory. The analyst who uses theoretical sampling looks for variation, for situations that provide new properties of a process. A comparison between theoretical sampling and statistical sampling is summarized in Table 14-4.

Step 4: Coding   Collecting, coding, and analyzing data go on simultaneously from the first day that a grounded theorist enters the field. Coding is the process of conceptualizing the underlying patterns in a set of empirical indicators. Instead of deciding on *operational definitions* (see Chapter 4) of important concepts in advance of collecting data, the grounded theorist reads through each incident, phrase, line, paragraph, episode, anecdote, or statement in the data, line by line, and asks: "What concept is this datum an indicator of?" "What is actually happening in the data?" "What are these data a study of?" This is simply a more systematic and codified way of noticing the patterns in your clinical practice. Glaser calls it *concept specification* instead of concept definition.

Three major types of code are substantive, selective, and theoretical.

Substantive, or open, codes are words that you find in the data that capture "what is going on." They are often words used by participants themselves. They are the terms used to describe:

1. dimensions
2. properties
3. conditions

Table 14-4   Comparison of Theoretical Sampling and Statistical Sampling Approaches

Item	Theoretical Sampling	Statistical Sampling
Purpose	To discover concepts, hypotheses, and their inter-relationships—that is, theory. The magnitude of the relationships may be, but is not necessarily, part of the hypotheses	To obtain accurate evidence on distributions of people among categories to be used in descriptions or verifications
Adequacy	Judged on how wisely and diversely the analysts have chosen groups for insight into the full range of categories according to the type of theory—formal or substantive—they wish to develop. Inadequate sampling is characterized by a theory that is thin and not well integrated and by many obvious, unexplained exceptions	Judgment is based on techniques of random and stratified sampling used in relation to the social structure of a group or groups sampled
Closure	Must be learned. Data collection for a grounded-theory study stops when new categories and their related aspects stop appearing in the data	Data collection must continue until the predetermined sample size is achieved

4. strategies

5. consequences

Among the long list of substantive codes I wrote in the margins of my Soteria House study field notes were: *insulating*, *appeasing*, *being with*, and *low profiling* (see Appendix C). Substantive codes allow you to move in your data from descriptive excerpts to a higher level of abstraction—concepts and constructs. In this way substantive codes "earn their way" into your theory. The grounded theorist then does not assume the face value relevance of any conventional variable like sex, race, or social class until it emerges as relevant in the data.

Open substantive coding both verifies and saturates individual codes. You can verify that patterns corresponding to your codes exist in the data by actively seeking variations and constantly comparing each incident with existing ones to become confident that your set of codes captures the major conceptual variations that exist under a certain set of circumstances. At this stage of your analysis it is important not to go for premature closure on your substantive codes. Proliferate them as they appear, but always look for (1) their relationship to one another and (2) their relation to a possible core variable, or BSP.

Technically, the mechanics of substantive coding are:

1. Read through the data, line by line, and write the code in the margin of the field note next to the indicator.

2. Construct a "laundry list" of substantive codes. Swanson found in her study of men's role in contraception that men reported getting information about contraception in a long list of ways. They:

   • read magazines
   • listened to the radio
   • watched television
   • talked to others
   • saw films
   • read pamphlets

Once her list stopped growing and codes were just being repeated, she moved on to the second type of coding operation, called selective coding.

Selective coding requires that the analyst note what is similar and what is different about the codes on the list and cluster codes to create *categories* that relate to one another. For example, one code in the list for how men get information about contraception was through talking to others. She then selectively coded data about talking with others into:

• public talking
• private talking
• professional talking
• same-sex talking
• cross-sex talking

Once possible variations on a core variable are identified, the analyst selectively codes for the full *range*, *variations*, and *properties* of the category. For example, for cross-sex talking, Swanson interviewed people who engaged in only partial disclosures about contraception and people who had extensive conversations about it. These data allowed her to compare "truncated talk" with "full-range talk" by beginning the third type of coding, theoretical coding. The step of selective coding is necessary in order to move from the more concrete list of open codes to a more abstract, parsimonious set of categories. Once your process of theoretical sampling stops generating new categories, *saturation* has been reached. *Saturation of categories* means that the major recurring patterns have been discovered. Deciding when you have reached saturation requires that you know the difference between a new event on a descriptive level and a genuinely new conceptual dimension.

Theoretical coding involves figuring out how the substantive categories are related to one another. You accomplish this step by formulating propositions about relationships and actively verifying the proposed relationship in your data.

The theoretical codes must earn their way into the analysis as well. Glaser (1978) identifies the following "families of theoretical codes":

1. the six Cs (causes, contexts, contingencies, consequences, covariances, and conditions)

2. process (stages, phases, passages, transitions, careers, orderings, trajectories, sequences, cycles)

3. degrees (limits, ranges, intensity, amount, boundaries, rank, averages, grades, criteria)

4. dimensions (elements, facets, properties, segments, aspects, sections)

5. types (kinds, styles, classes, genres)

6. strategies (tactics, mechanisms, techniques, plays, procedures)

7. interactions (reciprocity, covariance, interdependency)

8. identity/self (self-image, self-concept, self-worth, self-evaluation, self-realization)

9. cutting points (boundaries, breaking points, benchmarks, tolerance levels, turning points)

10. culture (norms, values, beliefs, rules)

11. consensus (agreements, contracts, definitions of the situation, opinions, conformity)

12. mainline (social control, recruitment, socialization, status passage, stratification, social mobility)

13. ordering (temporal, conceptual)

14. units (group, nation, organization, social world, society, family role, status)

In my study of conventional inpatient psychiatric treatment under the community mental health movement I discovered a highly prescriptive structure of policy, regulations, and standards that transformed the old state hospital warehouse into a similarly bureaucratized *clearinghouse*. Here treatment consisted primarily of a *dispatching* process, in which patients were screened, patched together with medication, stamped with a diagnostic label, sorted into a legal category, and disbursed back into an unwelcoming community. Obviously the *dispatching* analysis is an example of relating categories as stages in a people-processing operation (Wilson 1985).

Step 5: Memoing   Writing up analytic memos of your ideas about how the data, codes, categories, and relationships will eventually be integrated into a core explanatory scheme is a critical component of the grounded theory method. The analyst's goal is to develop theoretical ideas about his or her data that, once sorted, provide the basis for writing up the final integrative scheme (see Appendix C). The source for memos is TNs written during the process of constantly comparing indicator with indicator, and then indicator with concept.

A memo can be a sentence, a paragraph, or a few pages. Memos help your developing theory in five ways:

1. They require that you move your thinking about the data to a conceptual level.

2. They summarize the properties of each category so that you can begin to construct operational definitions.

3. They summarize propositions about relationships between categories and their properties.

4. They begin to integrate categories with clusters of other categories.

5. They relate your analysis to other theories.

Memos allow you to escape the self-imposed tyranny of writing well at this stage and provide the freedom to capture ideas. Your objective is to get an idea down on paper and not worry about perfect prose.

Rules for memoing, according to Glaser (1978), include:

1. Keep memos separate from data, but cross-reference them to useful illustrations in the data.

2. Always interrupt data collection or coding to write a memo when an idea occurs to you.

3. Modify existing memos as your ideas are modified.

4. Keep a list of your substantive codes. Write memos on each one on the list.

5. If too many memos on two different codes are similar, collapse the two codes into one.

6. Keep memos conceptual.

7. Write up one idea at a time and one idea per memo.

8. Keep memos flexible so that they can be sorted in a variety of sequences.

9. Label each memo with the code or codes it describes.

You will ultimately end up with hundreds of pages of memos, moving from specific codes to categories to relationships among categories and finally to a dense analytic scheme that accounts for all major patterns of behavior. A grounded theory is a molecular rather than a linear set of relationships. Most analysts try to diagram this complex set of interrelationships when they write up their final analysis (for an example, see Figure 14-1).

Step 6: Discovering the Overriding Analytic Scheme Arriving at a final integrative scheme means that you have discovered, through the constant comparison method and the techniques described, a core category. This analytic scheme accounts for most of the patterns of behavior in the area under study and integrates and interrelates a dense array of other subcategories and propositions. You discover it by searching through your data, codes, and memos looking for the main theme, or "story line," that explains the problem going on in the data. Some of the criteria suggested by Glaser (1978) for recognizing the core category in your analysis are these:

1. It must be central. You can easily relate all other codes, categories, and relationships to it.

2. It must recur frequently in the data—that is, be relatively stable and pervasive.

3. It must make sense to the people in the study setting.

4. It must allow for a "dense" explanation by incorporating a lot of descriptive variation.

5. It can be any one of the types of theoretical code.

Examples of core categories that were also BSPs include *cultivating, defaulting, centering, becoming, dispatching, infracontrolling, covering, balancing the mandates, protective governing,* and the like.

Step 7: Sorting Memos to Produce an Outline Sorting memos puts the data back together again in a coherent story. It integrates all the main ideas into a scheme. Technically, the analyst sorts all memos by codes:

1. specifying conditions, contexts, strategies, consequences, and interrelationships as recorded in the memo fund

2. linking up illustrative examples from the analytic data files

3. incorporating relevant memos on related literature

The outcome of memo sorting is a theoretical outline on which the final research report is based. In my Soteria House study, it looked like this (Wilson 1982):

Infracontrolling: Social Order Under Conditions of Freedom in an Antipsychiatric Community

I. "Presencing": Control of Resident Patients
   A. Mere presence
   B. Monitoring
   C. Intervening
      1. Active strategies
      2. Passive strategies

II. "Fairing": Management of Staff Work
  A. Establishing a fairing code
  B. Unfairing
  C. Restoring
III. Limiting Intrusion: Control of Outsiders
  A. Minimizing approachability
    1. Situational positioning
    2. Partial disclosure
  B. Deflecting
  C. Disengaging

Once memos are sorted, the grounded theorist writes the report, moving from the more general proposition to specific illustrations and including quotations and vignettes that make it plausible. The theory constitutes the study's "findings." Because it is grounded in data, it has relevance to the real world of nursing education, administration, and practice.

Evaluating the Credibility of a Grounded Theory

The aims and methods of discovering grounded theory are quite different from the aims and methods of theory-verification research. The criteria for critiquing a grounded theory and evaluating its credibility differ accordingly.

Some critics dismiss studies that use the methods described as invalid, unreliable, and too subjective. Others relegate this method to a form of "artistic" rather than "scientific" inquiring, based on a definition of scientific research as "inquiries that use formal instruments as the primary basis for data collection, transform the data collected into numerical indices of one kind or another, and attempt to generalize to some universe beyond itself" (Eisner 1981, p. 5).

The canons of quantitative analysis on issues like sampling, coding, reliability, validity, indicators, frequency distributions, hypothesis construction, and presentation of evidence must be replaced by alternative criteria when judging the credibility of qualitative research and grounded theory analysis.

Five Basic Criteria

Five criteria suggested by Glaser and Strauss (1966) represent the generic elements of the grounded theory method itself.

1. joint collection, coding, and analysis of data to promote maximum variation and verification in the data

2. systematic choice and study of several comparative groups that allow for the full generality and meaning of each category in the analysis

3. trust in the researcher's own credible knowledge, based on having lived with partial analyses and tested them every step of the way and having had firsthand, face-to-face knowledge

4. a presentation of findings that includes clear statements of description to illustrate the analytic framework

5. confirmation by participants in the social world under investigation

Secondary Criteria

A good grounded theory, according to nurse scientists who work to develop them:

- results from formulating and discarding hypotheses if they are not supported by data
- has included a look for contradictory occurrences

- is based on a variety of *slices of data*, direct observations, interviews, and document analysis
- can transcend the substantive area and have broader relevance
- specifies the conditions under which it was developed and to which it can be generalized
- fits the data
- works to explain the variations in behavior in a given area and to predict what can occur when conditions change
- is relevant and comprehensible to people in the study setting
- is modifiable, dense, and integrated into a tight analytic framework

May (1985) suggests that the consumer ask the following questions when evaluating the credibility of a grounded theory.

1. *The research question.* Is it too narrow? Has the original question been supplanted with one grounded in data? Does it focus on exclusively psychological variables or social-interactional ones?
2. *Data sources.* Are multiple slices of data from a variety of sources (field notes, interviews, documents) used as the basis for analyses? Is the data base sufficient to capture all the range and variation in codes and categories?
3. *The literature.* Does the study include correspondence with, but not overreliance on, related literature?
4. *The analytic scheme.* Is it clear, plausible, and well integrated?
5. *Relevance to the real world of practice.* Will it make a difference?

Pitfalls of Grounded Theory

It must be obvious by now that developing a grounded theory is not a simplistic process. There are two primary pitfalls, premature closure and failing to find a core variable to integrate the analysis.

1. Premature closure refers to ending theoretical sampling and coding before the full range and variation for codes and categories have been discovered. This often occurs when an investigator is under the time constraints associated with a thesis or dissertation deadline.
2. A second significant pitfall occurs if a core variable, or BSP, does not surface. The question then becomes how to salvage the study. Writing the report as an analytic description is one option. The study may then be more exploratory and descriptive but still offer directions for further research.

Applications to Nursing Practice

Clinical nurses have only recently begun to rely significantly on reports of research findings to answer their questions. Heretofore they tended to turn to authority, tradition, and trial and error when deciding whether to warm an infant's formula or to oxygenate before, in between, or after suctioning (see Chapter 1). Much of nursing practice was a combination of folk healing traditions and technology. Nursing has operated at the "preparadigmatic" phase of developing theories in the discipline (Meleis et al 1980). As its unique perspective has become clearer, Goldman's challenge has become more compelling: "It is up to us to accept strange and difficult ideas and to abandon the complacency of converting all that is novel into clichés of the familiar" (1980, p. 14).

The methods of qualitative analysis discussed in this chapter, and the discovery of grounded theory in particular, offer nursing one approach for developing much-needed middle-range theories for practice (see Chapter 10) while capitalizing on the observational sensitivity of practicing nurses. Nursing needs modes of inquiry and analysis that offer the freedom to explore on a conceptual level the richness of human experience, with all its variation. Nursing care requires an understanding of people in complex, changing social contexts. Its scope of practice encompasses people of all ages, social classes, developmental levels, and degrees of wellness and illness who are engaged in all sorts of psychological, physical, and social processes. Nurses apply and synthesize knowledge from physical, social, and medical sciences as well as the humanities to form their knowledge base. They recognize that theirs is a complex and diversified professional domain. They need research methods that are rigorous and that allow them to predict causes and outcomes. But they also need analytic methods that allow them to define, describe, and explain the real practice world of nursing to themselves and others. Grounded theory methods enable nurses to ask: "How can we become more sure of what we already know?" and "How can we know that which is not known?" instead of "How can we measure variables that we already know from a model or theoretical framework" (Swanson & Chenitz 1982, p. 242)?

Different research and analytic approaches need not compete with one another. No one entrenched philosophical stance or pet method in and of itself will lead to theoretical advances in nursing. True discoveries in nursing will probably come only from analytic pluralism. The qualitative methods and procedures described in this chapter represent one set of legitimate approaches for understanding certain kinds of research question about everyday nursing practice—one way of moving from observations to explanations and from practice to theory.

Summary of Key Ideas and Terms

✔ *Analysis* is the separation of data into parts for the purpose of answering a research question.

✔ *Qualitative analysis*, a controversial process, is the nonnumerical organization and interpretation of data in order to discover patterns, themes, forms, and qualities found in unstructured data.

✔ The philosophy of science on which qualitative research is based is called *symbolic interactionism*. Implications of this philosophy for research are:

• Research should be conducted in the natural setting.

• Reality and truth are emerging and relative, depending on the way people define them.

- The research process itself is a source of data and analytic ideas.

✔ Four major purposes of qualitative analysis are:

  - exploration and description

  - accounting for and illustrating quantitative findings

  - discovery and explanation

  - extension of theory

✔ *Substantive theory* is a middle-range theory that explains something under a specific set of conditions

✔ *Formal theory* is a grand theory that explains how something occurs under a great variety of circumstances.

✔ *Cognitive maps* are visual models or diagrams of categories and relationships in the analysis.

✔ *Straight description* uses categories imported from existing literature to organize data.

✔ *Analytic description* involves devising novel categories suggested to the analyst by "interrogating" the data to organize it.

✔ Preparing qualitative data for analysis involves duplicating field notes and interview transcripts, labeling them, and establishing organizational, methodological, and analytic files.

✔ Four major procedures for analyzing qualitative data are:

  - converting to quantitative data

  - doing a content analysis

  - analytic induction

  - discovery of grounded theory

✔ Six units of analysis for analytic induction are:

  - acts

  - activities

  - meanings

- participation
- relationships
- setting

✔ *Grounded theories* begin with five questions:

- "What is it?"
- "What are its properties?"
- "How did it come to be, and what is it becoming?"
- "Under what conditions and with what strategies does it work?"
- "What is the main story line here?"

✔ Tasks in creating a grounded theory include:

- discovering the problem
- integrating literature
- theoretical sampling
- open coding
- selective coding
- theoretical coding
- memoing
- memo sorting
- discovering a core variable through constant comparisons
- developing an outline
- writing the theory

Some go on simultaneously.

✔ BSPs (basic social processes) serve as one type of core variable to explain most of the variations in behavior in the situation under study.

✔ *Saturation of codes and categories* occurs when no new conceptual patterns or properties emerge in the data. It tells you when to stop collecting data.

✔ Grounded theories must be evaluated for their credibility by research consumers who use alternative scientific canons.

> ✔ The potential for nursing of qualitative analysis in general, and grounded theory in particular, is as an alternative to importing existing theory from other disciplines but instead developing nursing theory from observations of nursing practice.

References

Becker HS: Problems of inference and proof in participant observation. *Am Soc Rev* December 1958; 23:652–660.

Blumer H: *Symbolic Interactionism.* Englewood Cliffs, N.J.: Prentice-Hall, 1969.

Corbin J: Coding data. In *Qualitative Research in Nursing: From Practice to Grounded Theory,* Chenitz W C, Swanson J (editors). Menlo Park, Calif.: Addison-Wesley, 1985.

Davis F: Professional socialization as subjective experience: The process of doctrinal conversion among student nurses, pp. 235–251 in *Institutions and Persons,* Becker H et al (editors). Chicago: Aldine, 1968.

Denzin NK: *The Research Act.* Chicago: Aldine, 1970.

Dickoff J, James P: A theory of theories. *Nurs Res* September/October 1968; 17:197–203.

Eisner E: On the differences between scientific and artistic approaches to qualitative research. *Educational Research* April 1981:5–9.

Fagerhaugh S: Getting around with emphysema. *Am J Nurs* January 1973; 73:94–99.

Glaser BG: *Theoretical Sensitivity.* Mill Valley, Calif.: Sociology Press, 1978.

Glaser BG, Strauss AL: The purpose and credibility of qualitative research. *Nurs Res* Winter 1966; 15:56:61.

Glaser BG, Strauss AL: *The Discovery of Grounded Theory: Strategies for Qualitative Research.* Chicago: Aldine, 1967.

Glaser BG, Strauss, AL: *Status Passage.* Chicago: Aldine, 1971.

Goldman I: Boas on the Kuakiutl: The ethnographic tradition. Sarah Lawrence College: Essays from the Faculty. 4:5–23, 1980.

Gouldner A: Cosmopolitans and locals: Toward an analysis of latent social roles—2. *Administrative Science Quarterly* March 1958; 2:444–480.

Hutchinson S: *Survival Practices of Rescue Workers: Hidden Dimensions of Watchful Readiness.* Lanham, MD.: University Press of America, 1983.

Hutchinson S: Creating meaning out of horror. *Nurs Outlook* 1984: 32:86–90.

Kelly HS: The meaning of current dance forms to adolescent girls: An exploratory study. *Nurs Res* November/December 1968; 17:513–519.

Lofland J: *Analyzing Social Settings.* Belmont, Calif.: Wadsworth, 1971.

May KA: A typology of detachment and involvement styles adopted during pregnancy by first time expectant fathers. *West J Nurs Res* 1980; 2:445–461.

May, KA: Writing the grounded theory study. In *Qualitative Research in Nursing: From Practice to Grounded Theory,* Chenitz WC, Swanson J (editors) Menlo Park, Calif.: Addison-Wesley, 1985.

McCall G, Simmons JL (editors): *Issues in Participant Observation: A Text and Reader.* Reading, Mass.: Addison-Wesley, 1969.

Meleis A et al: Toward scholarliness in doctoral dissertations: An analytic model. *Res Nurs Health* 1980; 3:115–124.

Mosher LR, Menn A: Community residential treatment for schizophrenia: Two-year follow-up. *Hosp Comm Psychiatry* 1978; 29:715–723.

Norris CM: Restlessness: A nursing phenomenon in search of meaning. *Nurs Outlook* February 1975; 23:103–107.

Orsolits M, Morphy M: A depression algorithm for psychiatric emergencies. *J Psychiatric Treatment Eval* April 1982; 4:137–145.

Schatzman L, Strauss AL: *Field Research.* Englewood Cliffs, N.J.: Prentice-Hall, 1982.

Schutz A: *The Phenomenology of the Social World.* Evanston, Ill.: Northwestern University Press, 1967.

Searight MW et al: *Demonstration Study of a Second Step Nursing Program.* Rohnert Park, Calif.: Sonoma State University, unpublished report, 1978.

Standards of Psychiatric and Mental Health Nursing Practice. Kansas City, Missouri: American Nurses' Association, 1982.

Swanson JM: *Men's Sexual and Contraceptive Work Biographies and the Management of Contraception.* Paper presented at the 108th annual meeting of the American Public Health Association, Detroit, October 21, 1980.

Swanson J, Chenitz C: Why qualitative research in nursing? *Nurs Outlook* 1982; 30:241–245.

Wilson HS: Limiting intrusion—Social control of outsiders in a healing community: An illustration of qualitative comparative analysis. *Nurs Res* March/April 1977; 26:103–111.

Wilson HS: *Deinstitutionalized Residential Care for the Mentally Disordered: The Soteria House Approach.* New York: Grune and Stratton, 1982.

Wilson HS: Dispatching: Usual Hospital Treatment in the USA's Community mental health system. In *Qualitative Researching Nursing: From Practice to Grounded Theory*, Chenitz WC, Swanson J (editors). Menlo Park, Calif.: Addison-Wesley, 1985.

Further Readings

Archibald P: Impact of parent-caring on middle aged offspring. *J Gerontol Nurs* 1980; 6:78–85.

Bogdan R, Taylor JJ: *Introduction to Qualitative Research Methods.* New York: Wiley, 1975.

Bozett FW: Gay fathers: How they disclose their homosexuality to their children. *Family Relations* 1980; 29:173–179.

Broadhead R: Qualitative analysis in evaluation research: Problems and promises. *Symbolic Interaction* 1980; 3:23–40.

Chenitz WC: Entry into a nursing home as status passage: A theory to guide nursing practice. *Geriatr Nurs* 1983; 4:92–97.

Davis MZ: *Living with Multiple Sclerosis.* Springfield, Ill.: Charles C Thomas, 1973.

Fagerhaugh SY, Strauss AL: *Politics of Pain Management: Staff–Patient Interaction.* Reading, Mass.: Addison-Wesley, 1977.

Fuller SS: Holistic man and the science and practice of nursing. *Nurs Outlook* 1978; 26:700–704.

Glaser B, Strauss AL: *Time for Dying.* Chicago: Aldine, 1968.

Goodwin LD, Goodwin WL: Qualitative *vs.* quantitative research or qualitative *and* quantitative research? *Nurs Res* 1984; 33:378–380.

Hammond PE, Pillemer DB: Numbers and narrative: Combining their strengths in research reviews. *Harvard Educational Review* 1982; 52:1–26.

May KA: Three phases in the development of father involvement in pregnancy. *Nurs Res* 1982; 31:337–342.

Oiler C: The phenomenological approach in nursing research. *Nurs Res* 1982; 31:178–181.

Quint JC: Awareness of death and the nurse's composure. *Nurs Res* 1966; 15:49–55.

Reif L: Ulcerative colitis: Strategies for managing life. *Am J Nurs* 1973; 73:261–264.

Sims LN: The grounded theory approach in nursing research. *Nurs Res* 1981; 30:357–359.

Stern PN: Grounded theory methodology: Its uses and processes. *Image* 1980; 12:20–23.

Stern PN: Stepfather families: Integration around child discipline. *Issues in Mental Health Nursing* 1978; 1:50–56.

Strauss AL et al: *Psychiatric Ideologies and Institutions.* Chicago: Aldine, 1964.

Strauss AL, Glaser BG: *Chronic Illness and the Quality of Life.* St. Louis: CV Mosby, 1975.

Whyte WH: *Street Corner Society.* Chicago: University of Chicago Press, 1955.

Chapter 15

Applying Statistics to Quantitative Analysis

Sifting the Probable From the False

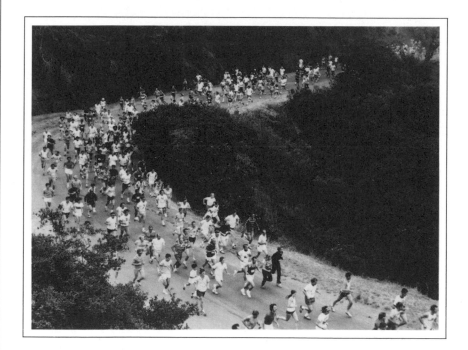

Reports of nursing research in recent years reflect a general trend toward accelerated statistical savvy in the use of both descriptive and inferential techniques.

Chapter Outline

Chapter Objectives

After reading this chapter, the student should be able to:

- comprehend the concept of scientific scales of measurement
- compare and contrast scales for nominal, ordinal, ratio, and interval data
- differentiate between descriptive and inferential statistics
- explain the processes for calculating frequency distributions; measures of central tendency, including the mode, median, and mean; measures of variability, including the range, the interquartile range, and the standard deviation; and measures of contingency and correlation
- interpret descriptive statistics from graphic presentations in research articles
- explain the logic and language associated with inferential statistics
- perform the four steps needed to test hypotheses using inferential statistics
- determine whether parametric or nonparametric statistics are appropriate in a nursing study
- compare and contrast appropriate use and interpretations of *t* tests and analyses of variance (ANOVA)
- interpret an *F* ratio from an ANOVA summary table
- discuss nonparametric statistical procedures, particularly the chi-square
- apply the guidelines for choosing a statistical procedure in determining whether published nursing studies have employed statistics correctly and in planning one's own study
- recognize when advanced multivariate statistics are required

In This Chapter . . .

This chapter examines quantitative analysis procedures and statistical tools. It is not a substitute for a course in statistics or a good statistics textbook. Instead, it presents the information you'll need as a responsible reader and conductor of nursing research to interpret, evaluate, base decisions upon, and add to the expanding body of numerical data that is important to improving nursing practice. Does biofeedback training reduce respiratory rates among patients with chronic obstructive pulmonary disease? If you increase the frequency of IV tubing changes and percutaneous site changes, can you reduce the incidence of phlebitis? Is it possible to quantify nursing-care needs in a home health service? Understanding what statistical concepts mean, matching analysis procedure to study purpose and design, and knowing the correct procedures for their use are critical to applying nursing research findings on such questions to practice, planning sound research in the first place, and analyzing quantitative data that are collected.

In this era of pocket calculators and personal computers a reasonable degree of competence in the field of statistics need not involve complete mastery of all complex derivation computations. Once you know what statistics are appropriate, can interpret their meaning, can translate them into words, and can arrive at logical conclusions based on them, you probably need not become involved in elaborate mathematical calculations. A computer program can do them for you (see Chapter 16). Studying statistics in relation to nursing research should not become a matter of calculated tedium, fear, or trepidation. Nor should you shy away from this topic because you think of statistics as anathema to nurses who are dedicated to discovering the truth through case studies and field research. Unless you can interpret statistics and know the worth of the data and conclusions presented, you risk basing your practice decisions, and the health care decisions of patients who consult with you, on poor information.

This chapter introduces you to the statistical concepts and operations used in much of contemporary nursing research. They are presented in the context of varied examples and are offered in the hope that being able to think statistically will sharpen your ability to think critically about nursing research. The kind of statistical knowledge that this chapter emphasizes will help you sustain a healthy attitude of skepticism when you read in the local newspaper that "a high proportion of women who take birth control pills have strokes" or that "compulsive jogging is just like anorexia nervosa." Furthermore, it will instruct you in the various considerations necessary to avoid inadvertently using statistics yourself that mislead others. Although reports of nursing research in recent years reflect a general trend toward increased statistical savvy, incidents of incorrect use of statistical tests, failure to meet statistical test assumptions, failure to attend to power analysis to determine an adequate sample size (see Chapter 9), misinterpretation of results, and what Reid (1983) calls "galloping alpha rates" still occur. If you, as a reader of research, are able to detect the misuse of statistics, you have gained important knowledge with which to decide if an investigator's conclusions are justified.

In the pages that follow, statistics are covered as both a collection of numerical facts that are expressed in terms that describe and summarize quantitative data and as tools for going beyond description to use results as a basis for speculation and prediction. Thus, both *descriptive statistics*, which organize, summarize, and present information in a usable, understandable form, and *inferential statistics*, which are concerned with making inferences about populations based on samples taken from them, get full treatment.

We begin with the concept *measurement*, which we've indirectly discussed in earlier chapters (see Chapters 6, 11, and 12). A great deal about measurement is familiar to most of us—the number of cubic centimeters in a vial, a patient's pulse rate or blood pressure, the amount of urine excreted over a 24-hour period. But nursing research is also concerned with less directly and precisely measureable phenomena. We will talk more about scales for measuring variables such as a patient's self-esteem, intelligence, stress response, disorientation, support system, and the like. The various ways of measuring and scales for levels of data provide a backdrop against which the major descriptive statistics, measures of central tendency and variance, inferential statistics, and the concept of multivariate statistics are examined.

Some say that the element of *uncertainty* sets statistics apart from other areas of applied mathematics. In arithmetic, algebra, and geometry, conclusions can actually be proven. In statistics, the ultimate aim is only to show that something is either *more* or *less likely* to occur. Systematically knowing even that much more about the outcomes of nursing interventions, however, is to advance the scientific basis for practice far beyond trial and error or the authority of tradition. Statistics are valuable tools for analyzing numerical data to answer certain research questions relevant to nursing practice and building the knowledge base for the discipline.

Measurement Scales

Before doing your own research or even reading intelligently about research done by others, you need to start with an understanding of the concept *scientific measurement*. We all engage in informal measuring every day. The well-baby clinic was busy that day, or it wasn't. The operating room schedule was full or pretty full. A patient's wound is healing quickly or slowly. *Measurement in research, however, can be distinguished from casual day-to-day measuring by certain specific characteristics.* Many of these have been alluded to in earlier chapters on validity and reliability (see Chapter 7) and of course on data collection itself (see Chapters 11, 12, and 13). In short, measurement processes in research should:

- be explicit enough so that other observers could use them and come up with the same measures
- be applicable to more than one individual
- occur according to a well-specified, reasonable set of rules for assigning numbers to represent the qualities or attributes being measured
- attempt to isolate one attribute at a time in complex concepts like *quality of care* or *creativity*
- correspond as precisely as possible to the reality being measured
- reflect the researcher's awareness that most of the time one can only tap a small percentage of the possible data relevant to the attribute being measured
- be at the highest level possible given the phenomena being measured

A visually oriented person might summarize the definition of *scientific measurement* like this:

Measurement = actual value + or − error

The types, sources and ways to minimize error were discussed in Chapter 7. This chapter's focus is on measurements that approach actual values of phenomena important in nursing studies.

Measurement involves the process of assigning numerical values to concepts under investigation. *Statistics* allow you to analyze those numerical values. (The major methods of analyzing *qualitative* data were explained in Chapter 14.) When an investigator spells out how something is to be quantitatively measured, he or she is in fact operationally defining and quantifying the study's key concepts or variables. Intelligence may be "a score" on a standard IQ test like the Stanford-Binet Intelligence Test. A patient's preoccupation with body diseases might be measured using his or her score on some of the 550 items of the Minnesota Multiphasic Personality Inventory (MMPI). Postoperative recovery rate might be measured by the number of hours that elapse before a child returns to preoperative eating, sleeping, playing, and communicating patterns when split-screen videotapes of the child are shown to a panel of expert judges. These operations, called data collection, were considered in Chapters 11, 12 and 13. Most authorities are quick to point out, however, that it is not really possible to measure something itself. Rather, *one measures the attributes or qualities about something that vary.* You can't measure a female per se, but you can measure her height, weight, political attitudes, or self-esteem. These varying characteristics or attributes of something are called a study's variables (see Chapters 4, 6, and 9). The clearer and more credible your process of transforming concepts or variables into measurements is, the more likely you are going to be convinced that your measurement reflects actual value rather than error.

Let's illustrate this process by imagining that we are interested in conducting a study of psychiatric nurses' beliefs about mental illness. We could collect data on this variable by interviewing a sample of nurses and use qualitative analysis methods. Or we could administer the *Beliefs About Mental Illness Inventory*, which contains items like those depicted in Box 15-1. Our subjects' reponses could then be transformed into scores or measures by developing a system of assigning numbers to the responses. Interpretation of the results would then have to be done according to the proper uses of scales of measurement. Knowing what kind of scale you are dealing with influences which statistical procedures can be used to analyze your data.

Defining a Scale of Measurement

A scale of measurement specifies all the possible values a given measurement might have. What really defines a scale of measurement is the complete set of potential measurement categories, not just the ones into which your subjects fall. Of course, measures can be crude or precise, ranging from only a few possible values to a larger number of them.

All measurement scales do have to have *at least two different possible measurement categories, or values.* In our example, for instance, we could score the psychiatric nurses who take our *Beliefs About Mental Illness Inventory* as simply "positive" or "negative." We could even score the intensity of the belief as "strong" or "weak." The actual system for scoring data generated using this particular instrument involves assign-

---

Box 15-1   *Beliefs About Mental Illness Inventory Items*

Examples of a 2-Choice Scale

Beliefs About Mental Illness

Positive   Negative
(+) ----------------------------- or ----------------------------   (−)

Strong (1)----------------------------- or -----------------------------Weak (0)

ing numbers to responses. Totals for various items are then added to determine whether or not the subject's dominant beliefs reflect the following:

- authoritarianism
- benevolence
- a mental hygiene ideology
- social restrictiveness
- interpersonal etiology orientation

There are four levels of measurement and whatever the scale of measurement it should, in addition to having at least two possible values, *be exhaustive*. This means that you can assign some number to each respondent in your study. For example, it would be inadequate to measure the clinical specialization backgrounds of Registry nurses in your city by specifying only *OB–PEDS* and *MED–SURG* on your scale. You would at least have to add the category *Other* to be exhaustive.

Finally, measures along any scale of measurement should be *mutually exclusive*. If you are measuring the consciousness level of intensive care unit (ICU) patients, you can't put the same patient into both the "conscious" and the "unconscious" category at the same time. If you ever find yourself in doubt about the appropriate category, consider the possibility that your scale needs to be more precise and discriminating by providing, for example, a graded series of options between fully conscious and fully uncon-

scious. Decisions about scaling must be made at a study's outset, however, so that all subjects will be measured with the same scale, using the same measurement rules. Knowing from the start the scale you intend to use also influences what statistics you will be able to employ to analyze your data. And knowing this keeps you straight about what kinds of question your study will and will not be able to address since statistical procedures must be appropriate for a study's purpose and level of data.

Types of Measurement Scale

Scales for Nominal Data The most primitive and least precise measurement scale from a traditional scientific perspective is called a nominal scale—a scale for nominal data. *Nominal* (or "naming") *scales* arbitrarily assign some number to represent the categories into which an attribute or quality can be sorted. Measuring the sex of patients who develop lung cancer in the United States by labeling each as male or female and assigning numbers so that 1 = male and 2 = female is an example of a very simple nominal scale, or code, with two possible measurement categories. Sorting patients according to their blood type or nursing diagnosis and assigning numbers to a longer list of categories are other examples of creating nominal scales (see Box 15-2). The numbers themselves have no real meaning except as *a convenient code*. There is no implication of equal-sized steps between the

---

Box 15-2   Nursing Diagnoses for Psychiatric Patients

1.00   Self-care limitations
1.10   Emotional stress or crisis
1.20   Emotional problems related to daily living
1.30   Physical symptoms which occur with altered psychic functioning
1.40   Alterations in thinking, perceiving, communications and decision-making abilities
1.50   Behaviors and mental states that indicate the client is a danger to self or others or gravely disabled

numbers or of any inherent ordering of the categories in relation to one another. All we can conclude from nominal scales is that data sorted into different categories are nonequivalent. Nominal scales are nevertheless considered examples of scientific measurement, because two rules apply in the assignment of numbers: (1) all responses that are sorted into the same qualitative category are given the same number, and (2) no two categories can be assigned the same number.

The value of transforming qualitative, categorical data into nominal scales was covered in Chapter 14. Clearly you can perform crosstabulations with other numerical data, calculate frequencies, and communicate more efficiently with a computer if variables are expressed in numerical terms. The chi-square statistic discussed later in this chapter is also appropriate for nominal data. But don't be fooled into assuming that research results that have transformed qualitative categories into nominal scales have somehow invested the numbers themselves with any more meaning or order than that of convenient labels.

Scales for Ordinal Data *Ordinal scales*, or scales for ordinal data, are "ordering" scales. Numbers that are assigned to data according to ordinal scales have the characteristic of ordered categories. We can't assume, however, that the numbers along the scale represent the same amount or change in the variable from one point to the next. An ordinal scale allows you to rate or rank "low," "medium," and "high," but it doesn't tell you anything about the *distance between* low and medium or medium and high. In short, although you can rate a variable on an ordinal scale, your measurement categories *can-*

not be presented or treated as having equidistant intervals, even though the numbers you assign to the ratings might suggest it. You can ask parents, for example, to rate their hospitalized children on a 5-point scale where 1 = *not at all regressed* to 5 = *extremely regressed*. Even though the raters use the numbers from 1 to 5 to make the ratings, there is no guarantee that the intervals between the numbers are equidistant in the same way that measures of weight or time are. It might take only a few behavioral changes to alter a rating from 2 (slightly regressed) to 3 (moderately regressed), yet a dramatic change in activity might be necessary to alter the rating from 4 (very regressed) to 5 (extremely regressed) (see Figure 15-1). Because the numbers are assigned without the assurance of equidistant intervals, most experts agree that any statistical procedures that involve adding them, subtracting them, or taking their average are inappropriate. Frequency counts, percentages, and a few limited statistical operations explored later in this chapter can be used with ordinal scales.

What you *can* assume with an ordinal scale like this one is that 5 is more regressed than 4, that 4 is more than 3, that 3 is more than 2, and that 2 is more than 1. Therefore, it's easy to see at least that ordinal scales are more precise quantitative tools than nominal scales. Obviously, being able to say that an attribute is *different in degree and direction* conveys more information than just saying that two attributes are in two different categories. Many nursing research studies that investigate attitudes use self-developed and standardized Thurstone and Likert scales (see Chapter 11). Although ordinal scales are considered higher level measurements for the purpose of statistical analysis, sensitive

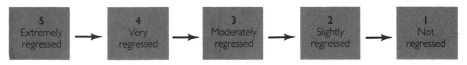

Figure 15-1 Example of ordinal scale for *regression* where 5 > 4 > 3 > 2 > 1.

and systematic categorization is still a preferred analysis if the study question is well matched to this approach.

A Scale for Interval Data   An *interval scale*, or scale for interval data, consists of potential measurement categories that, as in an ordinal scale, have an inherent order; but in addition, the possible measures along an interval scale are *equidistant* from one another. This characteristic allows researchers to make statements about the *actual differences* between measures rather than just saying that something has more or less of an attribute than something else. Studies in the nursing literature concerned with the impact of preoperative care on postoperative patient outcomes might employ ordinal scales that simply rated a patient's overall postoperative course as having "more" or "fewer" complications. An interval scale that plots temperature elevations indicative of infection clearly offers more precise information on the study question. *Investigators, therefore, prefer to use interval scales whenever possible, because they not only provide more precise information but also permit the adding and subtracting of measures and the use of more sophisticated statistics that require taking a mean of measures.* Most standardized psychological tests used in nursing research studies are based on interval scales. Blood pressure readings represent another example of an interval scale. A reading of $^{150}/_{90}$ is higher than a reading of $^{140}/_{90}$, and a reading of $^{140}/_{90}$ is higher than a reading of $^{120}/_{90}$. Furthermore, an interval scale assumes that the differences between systolic readings of 140 and 130 and 120 are essentially equivalent.

It's a good idea to point out, however, that even with interval scales where measurement rules indicate that differences have the same meaning, the meaning of a difference when it comes to clinical application may be a distinctively different one. For example, a hypertensive diet designed for two clients with blood pressure readings of $^{130}/_{90}$ and $^{120}/_{80}$ might be different, while a second plan for two other clients with blood pressures of $^{160}/_{100}$ and $^{150}/_{100}$ might be

very similar. The first comparison reflects the difference between an elevated blood pressure and one that is normal, from a clinical point of view. Both readings in the second case are clinically hypertensive.

A final point on the subject of the interval scale is that, although it is considered to be a higher-level scale than either nominal or ordinal, it does not have what is called *an absolute zero point*. Zero on interval scales is arbitrary. Almost all authors on this subject use the Fahrenheit and Celsius thermometers for measuring temperature to illustrate this idea. Both are interval scales; the Celsius uses an arbitrary zero point of 0, and the Fahrenheit scale has an arbitrary zero point of 32. Neither point, however, really signifies the total lack of heat (see Figure 15-2). In sum, the interval scale has neither a real zero point nor the ability to provide information on the absolute magnitude of an attribute for any particular object.

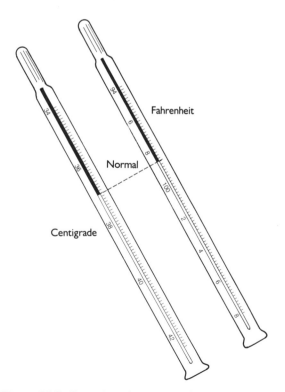

Figure 15-2   Illustration of two types of thermometers.

A Scale for Ratio Data   Because a *ratio scale*, or scale for ratio, level data, has (1) rank ordering of measures, (2) equal intervals between them, and (3) an absolute zero point, it is considered to be the highest level of measurement scale for the purpose of applying statistical analysis procedures. These qualities allow the scale to communicate the maximum and most precise information and also make its data amenable to the most powerful and sophisticated statistical analyses. Examples of ratio scales used in nursing studies include time, length, and weight. Scores of zero on these measures really do represent the absence of the attribute being measured.

Sitzman and her colleagues' (1983) study of "Biofeedback Training to Reduce Respiratory Rates in Patients With Chronic Obstructive Pulmonary Disease" used chest gauges attached to polygraphs that led to control circuitry and a computer to analyze respiratory rates and other variables. These data constituted ratio-level measurements and would have permitted the use of complex statistics, including those that test for statistical differences between groups, had the sample been large enough. Brooten et al's (1983) study of four treatments to prevent and control breast pain and engorgement in nonnursing mothers measured chest circumferences as one attribute of the dependent variable. Because these measures met the requirements for ratio scales, she was able to use a two-way analysis of variance (ANOVA) to analyze her data (see Table 15-10). Hayter's (1983) study of "Sleep Behaviors of Older Persons" included numbers of hours of awake time after sleep onset and total time asleep in bed among the variables measured. Again, because time is a ratio-scaled measurement, Hayter was able to use statistical analysis procedures that might not have been appropriate with the other types of scales we've discussed.

Combining Scales   Some studies incorporate several or all of the four scales and levels of data just examined.

Mercer and her colleagues' (1983) research on a sample of 294 first-time mothers looked at the relationship of a wide variety of psychosocial variables and perinatal variables on perception of childbirth. Her research team used an ordinal scale of 1 to 5 to measure the dependent variable *perception of childbirth*, where 1 = negative and 5 = positive. *Use of medications during labor* was recorded on a nominal scale where yes = 1 and no = 0. *Length of labor*, however, was measured on a ratio scale by the number of hours from the beginning of the first to the end of the third stage of labor. Other variables, such as *length of pregnancy* and *infant's weight in grams*, also constituted ratio scales. The authors accomplished their data analysis using Duncan's new multiple range test, which incorporates multiple comparisons after a significant *F* ratio. (These tests will be explained later in this chapter.)

The important point to remember is that, because ratio scales do have an absolute zero, all statistical procedures and arithmetic operations are appropriate with them. Ratio scales do tend, however, to *dominate among the physical and biological measures* and are rarely used when measuring more abstract psychosocial qualities. Most quantitative researchers prefer working at the highest level of measurement and tend to operationalize their study variables so as to increase their ability to do so.

Quantitative Analysis Using Statistics

Analyzing quantitative (or numerical) research data begins, as the first part of this chapter has suggested, by recognizing measurements of variables under study as one of the four major levels of data. As emphasized earlier, knowing the level of measurement involved in a study informs decisions about what statistical procedures can be used to analyze the data and answer the research question at hand.

Planning Ahead

It is important to mention that a researcher should plan how his or her data are to be analyzed. As should be clear from the discussion of scales, some statistical procedures require that data be collected in a particular way. Furthermore, the assumptions of some statistical tests require equal numbers in all groups of data (for example, equal numbers of control and experimental patients). If you intend to rely on computer-assisted data analysis, you should know whether the program you intend to use reads blanks but not zeros, or vice versa, and formulate your data collection operations to account for this (see Chapter 16). It is probably wise to consult a statistician who can handle statistical questions, a computer analyst who can address questions related to a particular system or statistical package, or both early in your study planning phase to anticipate potential problems. Many experts urge that you actually think through your analysis to the extent of setting up what they call dummy tables, or dummy analysis forms, to ensure that you will know how to handle the data once it is in. A *dummy table* is simply a table without the numbers on it. Figure 15-3 illustrates a sample dummy table for a study on postoperative infection. Once data have been collected, statistical-analysis procedures constitute the initial tools that are used to interpret or make meaning out of the findings in relation to the study's theoretical framework and its specific research problem.

Specific analysis procedures depend not only on the research question and the type of data collected but also on the study design. Even if hypotheses are being tested, most investigators also attempt to analyze the data that may not relate just to the study hypotheses in the hope that some unanticipated insight may emerge.

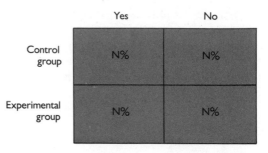

Figure 15-3 Sample dummy table. Frequency of postoperative infection.

Most analysts also examine data on possible intervening variables. For example, in an outcome study of experimental and control patient groups where the independent variable is *mode of teaching preoperative patients to cough, turn, and deep-breathe* and the dependent variable is *the incidence of postoperative pneumonia*, analytic procedures would very probably include a comparison of the characteristics of the two study groups themselves to demonstrate that they were not significantly different, either physiologically or psychosocially, to begin with.

Categories of Statistical Test

The goal of analysis is ultimately to summarize your data in ways that will allow you to answer your research question. Although hundreds of statistical techniques are used to analyze data, they are usually classified in one of two categories.

Descriptive statistics, on the one hand, are those methods that summarize or describe the characteristics of the data from your sample. Examples of descriptive statistics include frequencies, measures of central tendency, measures of variance, and correlations.

Inferential statistics, on the other hand, go beyond mere description to make inferences about a whole population based on sample data. Inferential analysis tests for significant relationships among variables or finds statistical support for confirming or refuting hypotheses. An analysis plan for quantitative data may include both, depending on a study's purpose. Specifics of each are taken up in sections that follow. Advanced multivariate statistical operations are summarized in Table 15-11.

Descriptive Statistics

Descriptive analysis includes a range of possible statistical operations from crude to precise methods of summarization for an entire data set. The choice depends first, of course, on your study question and then on the level of measurement at which you collected your data. Let's imagine that a school nurse has administered a battery of assessment tests to a group of elementary schoolchildren (visual, hearing, intelligence, personality inventories, health histories, and physical exams). What are some of the strategies available for transforming this vast array of numerical data into some useful and meaningful form? She or he could:

1. rearrange the various scores by how often they occurred so as to get an overall picture of the data set

2. construct tables, graphs, and figures to permit visualization of the data

3. convert raw scores to other types of score such as percentile ranks, standard scores, or grades

4. calculate averages on each important variable to learn something about the typical status of the group

5. figure out the ranges or dispersion of scores and ratings in relation to the central point

6. look for relationships or correlations between two or more different measurements

All of the methods in the list above represent various kinds of descriptive statistics. Let's look at them in a bit more detail.

Frequency Distributions

A *frequency distribution* represents one way of organizing a mass of what might appear at first to be overwhelming and chaotic information. It involves systematically arranging numerical values from the lowest to the highest and then counting the number of times each value appeared in the data. A frequency distribution lets you quickly see what the lowest and highest scores were, where most of the scores tended to cluster, and, in fact, what the most commonly obtained score was (see Table 15-1). The construction of frequency distributions and frequency tables is really a rather simple process. If

Table 15-1   Frequency Distribution of Test Scores (*n* = 55)

Raw Score	Frequency
28	1
27	1
26	2
25	5
24	5
23	9
22	10
21	5
20	6
19	4
18	3
17	3
16	0
15	1

you are working with an extremely large number of measures, a computer program can construct frequency tables for you automatically (see Chapter 16). The steps for constructing a frequency distribution manually are as follows:

1. Find the lowest and highest scores or numbers in the data set for which you want to construct a frequency distribution.

2. Decide what the class interval will be and how many classes you will have. These are commonly called the Xs. Arrange them from lowest to highest value. Be sure that the classes of observation are mutually exclusive and exhaustive.

3. Construct a table that has columns for (a) each class, (b) the tally, or count, of how often the class appeared in the data, and (c) a frequency (a percentage).

4. Read through your raw data sequentially, and make a mark in the count column using the familiar method of four vertical lines and then a slash for the fifth occurrence (卌).

5. Add up all the frequencies, called the fs, and put the total number for each class in the *frequency* column. The sum of the numbers in that column ought to equal the total size of your sample ($\Sigma f = n$).

6. Complete the percentage column by dividing each frequency by the total number of data items and multiply by 100 ($\% = 100 \times f/n$).

Graphic Displays   Many research studies that you read may display frequency data in *histograms* or *frequency polygons*. These are simply ways of displaying in graphic form the same information contained in a frequency table. In Figure 15-4 you can see that the vertical axis contains the frequency totals, with a zero at the bottom and the highest frequency at the top. The horizontal axis contains the classes of totals, with the lowest value on the left and the highest value on the right . Next, bars are drawn in the shape of rectangles over each class of score with a height equal to the frequency of that particular class. Some researchers and consumers believe that such visual depictions of frequency information are easier and quicker to read than a table.

In the case of frequency polygons, dots connected by straight lines are used instead of bars to show the number of times that a class occurs. See Figure 15-5 for a frequency polygon based on hypothetical data.

The following example illustrates how you might organize and summarize measurements you've collected using the method of creating a frequency distribution.

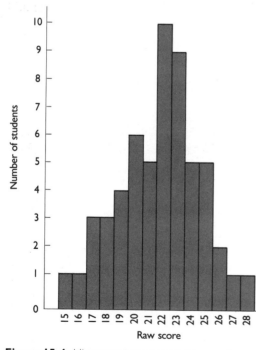

Figure 15-4   Histogram based on text scores from Table 15-1.

Imagine that you have recently taken a position as a clinical nurse III in an educational facility for mentally retarded children. As part of your responsibilities you intend to plan and implement a health teaching curriculum for the chil-

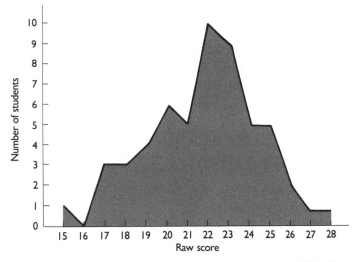

Figure 15-5 Frequency polygon based on test scores from Table 15-1.

dren in your care. You also believe that systematic assessment and clinical research are crucial to the development of your new role. You decide to begin by getting some sort of assessment of the intellectual capacities of the center's resident population. According to the sampling principles presented in Chapter 9, you go to the records and pull out a random sample of 45 patients. You write down their IQ scores on a piece of paper and end up with results that look pretty much like Table 15-2.

As you mull over these figures, it becomes obvious that you really can't make much sense out of them unless you organize them in some systematic way. You decide to list all the scores from lowest to highest and put a slash mark beside each score every time it occurs. The number of slash marks then represents the frequency of occurrence of each score. By this kind of grouping you can get a picture of the distribution of IQ scores for the retarded children you hope to teach (see Table 15-3). In this way you have achieved a manageable array of scores to help you target your health teaching curriculum to meet learner needs and abilities.

Frequency Distributions for Different Types of Data Scale If the data or scores you are working with are interval level and you have too many different scores or classes (usually more than 10) to make for a frequency table that is easy to read, you can combine measurements into bigger cate-

gories, because the measurements are ordered and equidistant.

If the data and scores you are working with are ordinal level, you can combine measurement categories into bigger classes but must not add raw scores together.

If you are constructing frequency distribu-

Table 15-2   IQ Scores of Educational Center Children ($n = 45$)

x	f	x	f	x	f
104		81		79	
83		69		70	
66		53		69	
78		58		65	
35		50		67	
50		61		75	
55		80		79	
100		54		78	
68		85		77	
47		63		61	
60		62		61	
60		61		60	
55		60		55	
58		59		54	
61		58		50	

Table 15-3 Frequency of IQ Scores of Educational Center Children

x	f	x	f	x	f
104	I	65	I		
100	I	63	I		
85	I	62	I		
83	I	61	IIII		
81	I	60	IIII		
80	I	59	I		
79	II	58	III		
78	II	55	III		
77	I	54	II		
75	I	53	I		
70	I	50	III		
69	II	47	I		
68	I	35	I		
67	I				
66	I				

tions for nominal data, you can tabulate the number of subjects assigned to each class and the proportion of the total sample assigned to each category, so that you can compare one frequency distribution with another in a way that makes sense. The only difference is that you *cannot* place the classes or scale values in any order, because nominal data scales have no inherent order.

Measures of Central Tendency

Comparing whole frequency distributions offers one way of making some kind of order out of an array of numerical data. But it can also be somewhat awkward when you have several groups or conditions to take into account. In many cases a group pattern is of less importance than some statistic that can summarize a whole distribution in a single number. Whenever a researcher is interested in questions like "What is a typical degree of nausea in the first trimester of pregnancy?" or "What is the APGAR score of most babies born at home birth centers?" or "What is the average length of hospital stay for open heart surgery patients?" the researcher is raising questions of central tendency. There are several measures of central tendency, and deciding which one to use depends on:

1. the scale on which a variable was measured
2. the shape of the frequency distribution
3. the purpose for which you want to report it

Central refers to a middle value, and *tendency* refers to the general trend of the numbers.

Distribution Shapes Frequency distributions are usually characterized as either symmetrical or nonsymmetrical (also called skewed). *Symmetrical distributions* are shaped so that if divided into halves, the halves could be folded over on each other and fit almost exactly (see Figure 15-6). *Skewed distributions* have off-center peaks or humps and longer tails in one direction or another. If the longer tail points to the right, it is called *positively skewed*; if the longer tail points to the left, it is called *negatively skewed*.

Frequency distributions can answer a lot of different questions: "What is the most frequently occurring class of scores?" "What is the distribution in a pattern of scores?" "How close does the distribution approximate a normal curve?"

An example of data that would appear as a skewed frequency distribution is the age at which American women complete menopause, because the majority of subjects would be located in the later half of life. (See Figure 15-7 for examples of skewed distributions.)

Distributions are also characterized by the modality of their shape. A *unimodal distribution* has only one high point, and a *bimodal* or *multimodal* shape has two or more (see Figures 15-8 and 15-9). The most common type of symmetrical, unimodal curve is called a *normal curve*. A *normal distribution*, or *normal curve*, is bell-shaped with the greatest frequency at the center. As you move away from the center, the

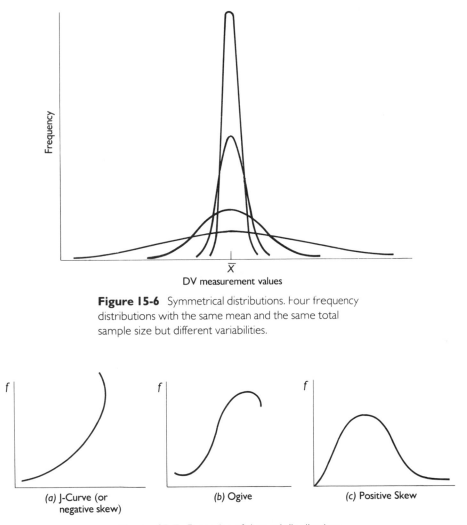

Figure 15-6 Symmetrical distributions. Four frequency distributions with the same mean and the same total sample size but different variabilities.

(a) J-Curve (or negative skew)

(b) Ogive

(c) Positive Skew

Figure 15-7 Examples of skewed distributions.

frequencies become smaller and smaller. (See Figure 15-10; we will talk more about normal curves as this chapter progresses.)

The Mode For a frequency distribution of data from a nominal scale, the mode is the only measure of central tendency that makes sense. Calculations of the mean and median, discussed in the sections that follow, require equidistant categories or ordered categories. Neither of

these, as you recall from the first part of this chapter, is possible with a nominal scale. The *mode* is simply the category, or class, that has the highest frequency. In the case of a symmetrical distribution with a single peak, the mode will be the same value as the median or the mean (if you can calculate them). As Polit and Hungler (1983, p. 477) write, "The mode, in other words, identifies the most 'popular' score.'" Uses of modes in further statistical

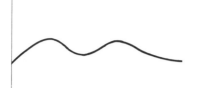

Figure 15-8 A bimodal curve.

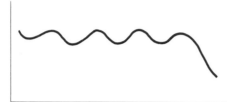

Figure 15-9 A multimodal curve.

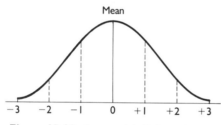

Figure 15-10 A normal, bell-shaped, curve.

analyses are, however, very limited. You figure out a mode simply by looking at, or "inspecting," the frequency distribution into which you have ordered your data. Computer programs can also do this task for you (see Chapter 16).

The Median The *median* is the measure that corresponds to the middle score, because it lies at the midpoint of the distribution and divides the scores into halves. When your data are based on an ordinal scale, the median is an appropriate measure of central tendency. The median is that point that divides the scores you have obtained

exactly in half. Another way of saying this is that the median is the score at the 50th percentile. exactly in half. Another way of saying this is that the median is the score at the 50th percentile. One major characteristic of the median is its insensitivity to extreme scores. This can work as a limitation or an advantage, depending on a study's objectives. In the set of scores 1 3 4 11 96, the median is 4. This is true even though the data set contains one extreme score of 96. It is important that the median address the average position of a distribution of numbers, not the value of the scores themselves.

The Mean The *mean (arithmetic mean)* of a set of measurements is simply the sum of the values divided by the total number of subjects. Stated in algebraic form it looks like this:

$$\bar{X} = \frac{X_1 + X_2 + \cdots X_n}{N} = \frac{\Sigma X}{N}$$

where $\bar{X}$ = the mean
N = the number of scores
Σ = the mathematical verb directing us to sum all the measurements

This measure of central tendency, also called the *average*, is the most widely used one in statistical tests of significance. Most researchers attest that of all the measures of central tendency, *the mean is the most stable, the most sensitive to extreme scores, and the most reliable.* That means that if you calculated means of different samples drawn from the same population, they would fluctuate or vary less than modes or medians. Because calculating the mean involves the addition of different values or categories, *the mean can only be properly calculated for intervally scaled data,* because categories must be ordered and equidistant. Whether the mean is necessarily the best statistic to describe intervally scaled measures depends on whether the frequency distribution is *symmetrical* and *unimodal.* Skewed distributions will have means that lie below the distribution's peak, and the mean for a bimodal distribution may fall between the two humps and not be very representative of actual values.

Of course, the primary basis for a decision to use the mode, median, or mean as a measure of central tendency is the nature of your study question. If you want to know what a typical well baby weighs at a certain age, the median is the best statistic. If you want to know if two groups of patients receiving different nursing care for dicubiti are different on an attribute, you need to use the mean. If you want to know what the self-care ability of the majority of a nursing home population is, you go for the mode. Because most nursing studies that intend to fully describe the data and that involve an array of scores or numbers use computer technology to print out and perform calculations on their data, you'll find that when possible, all three measures of central tendency are usually reported. (See Fig-

ure 15-11 for illustrations of measures of central tendency in normal and skewed distributions.)

Measures of Variability

The purpose of describing the central tendencies of data is to describe the ways subjects group together. The *variance*, in contrast, examines the dispersion, or how the measures are distributed. If the scores in a data set are very similar, there is very little variability. Two sets of data with bell-shaped distributions and the same sample size and same mean could, however, be very different in terms of the set spread or distribution of the measurements (see Figure 15-8).

Most authorities agree that to fully describe a distribution of measures, you need to include measures of variability that reflect the extent to which scores are different from or similar to one another. *The most common measures of vari-*

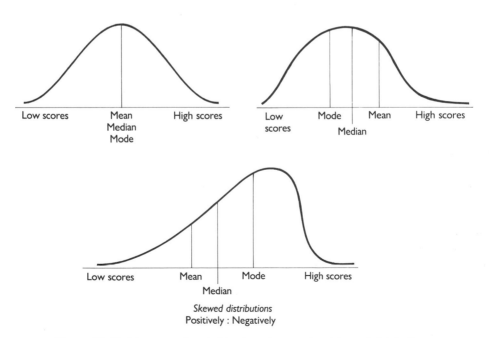

Figure 15-11 Measures of central tendency in normal and skewed distributions.

ability are the range, the interquartile range, and the standard deviation. These measures express the degree of dispersion of scores around the measures of central tendency. Many investigators believe that the standard deviation is the most useful measure of dispersion in descriptive statistics, because it captures the degree to which individual scores in a frequency distribution deviate from one another. Let's start with the range.

The Range The *range* is the simplest measure of dispersion. It defines the difference between the smallest and largest numbers in the distribution. You compute it by subtracting the lowest score from the highest (Total range = the largest $X-$ the smallest X). Table 15-4 lists a sample of hypothetical APGAR scores for newborn infants in a rural community hospital. Their range is $7 - 4 = 3$.

One of the obvious advantages of reporting the range is that it is easy to compute, but its disadvantages tend to outweigh this advantage. For one thing, it is considered a comparatively unstable statistic. One additional extreme score can change it. The APGAR score range of a second sample of babies born in the same rural

community hospital, for example, might tend to fluctuate a lot. The range also doesn't take into account variations in scores between extremes and thus is customarily reported along with other measures of variance. If you relied exclusively on the range, a change in one individual score, the lowest or the highest, could alter the entire range figure drastically. To correct for this last problem the *interquartile range* or *semiquartile range* is often used as the measure of variability.

The Interquartile Range The *interquartile range* is based on middle cases rather than extreme scores. It is more stable than just the range. It is found by lining up the measurements in order of size and then dividing the array into quarters. The range of scores that includes the middle 50% of the scores is the interquartile range, that is, the range between the scores composing the lowest quartile, or quarter, and the highest quartile. Where Q is the symbol for quartile, the formula for obtaining the interquartile range is:

$$\text{Interquartile range} = Q_3 - Q_1$$

where Q_1 = the category in and below which one-quarter of the scores fall

Q_3 = the category in and below which three-quarters of the scores fall

The semiquartile range is one-half of the range of scores within which 50% of the scores lie and is obtained by dividing the interquartile range by 2. The addition of deviant cases at either extreme leaves the interquartile (and semiquartile) range virtually unchanged. The interquartile range is rarely reported in nursing research.

Table 15-4   Sample of Hypothetical APGAR Scores for Newborn Infants in a Rural Community Hospital

7	5	6
5	6	6
7	4	6
7	5	5
6	6	4
6	7	5
6	7	7
5	6	7
7	6	6
6	5	5

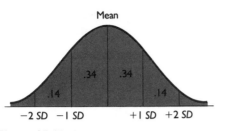

Figure 15-12 Bell-shaped curve and standard deviations.

The Standard Deviation   One way to define a *standard deviation* is as an average of the deviations from the mean. It is the most widely used measure of variability when the frequency distribution approximates a normal curve. The bell-shaped, or normal, curve (originally called the Gaussian curve, after Carl Friedrich Gauss, its discoverer) has certain characteristics that distinguish it:

- In a normal curve, the mean, median, and mode are equal to zero.

- Most of the scores or measurement values cluster together to form the mode, median, and mean.

- A smaller number of scores has values on either extreme of the curve.

- It is symmetric and unimodal.

- There are approximately three standard deviations above and below the mean (68% of all values fall within one standard deviation on either side of the mean, 95% of all values fall within two standard deviations from the mean, and 99.87% fall within three standard deviations from the mean (see Figure 15-12).

- When you calculate the mean for a group of measures, you have the basis for calculating how much each individual measure deviates from the mean.

- Deviations for each individual score from the mean fall one-half on the positive side of the curve and one-half on the negative side, resulting in a summated score of 0. Therefore, each number should be squared to eliminate the negative signs. *Standard* refers to the fact that the standard deviation indicates a group's average spread of scores or values around their mean. *Deviation* indicates how much each score is scattered from the mean.

Standard deviation of a population is found by the formula:

$$ SD = \sqrt{\frac{\Sigma X^2}{N - 1}} $$

and thus is equal to the square root of the variance. The standard deviation, like the mean, takes into consideration all the scores or values in a distribution. It tells how variable the scores in a data set are. If, for example, we compared anxiety-scale scores for two samples of patients, each from a different culture, we might find that both distributions had a mean of 35. But when we calculated the standard deviation, we would discover that one had a standard deviation of 4 and the other a standard deviation of 9. We could immediately conclude that although the means were the same, the first sample was more homogeneous on the variable measured by anxiety score.

In summary, if you do not use a computer to calculate it, you can follow this step-by-step procedure to calculate a standard deviation:

1. Calculate the mean of all your measurements or scores.

2. Find the difference between each individual score value and the mean.

3. Square each deviation.

4. Add up all the squared deviations, and divide by the total number of values to get the mean or averaged squared deviation.

5. Take the square root of the average squared deviation to obtain the standard deviation.

It is not difficult to conclude that using the computer to accomplish such calculations, particularly when the number of scores or values in your data set is huge (for example, a national survey of all members of the American Nurses' Association), is dazzling in its ability to save you time and eliminate arithmetic errors (see Chapter 16). In reporting standard deviations, authors may use the abbreviation *SD*, the symbol *S*, or the Greek symbol σ.

Standard scores, represented by the small letter *z*, tell us how many standard deviations away from the mean a particular raw score is. Many intelligence and achievement tests use standard scores with a preestablished mean and standard deviation. The formula for computing the standard score is:

$$z = \frac{(X - \bar{X})}{SD}$$

where *z* = standard score
  X = an individual score
  $\bar{X}$ = mean score
  SD = standard deviation

The *z* score can be looked up in a table to find out how much of the distribution would lie below and above the corresponding raw score. In this way you can use the *z* score to determine the *percentile* of any particular raw score (for example, the percentage of values equal to or less than that score). When a researcher reports an individual test score, it is sometimes more meaningful to give a *z* score or a percentile than to give just the raw score. From a *z* score it is possible to express one person's test performance in relation to the whole group. Another value of the *z* score is its ability to compare scores on two different tests.

Measures of Contingency and Correlation

Contingency Tables   Many nursing studies are not just *factor-isolating*, or one-variable, studies. Most of the time we are asking more complicated questions about the interrelationships among variables. "Is there a difference in the morbidity rates of people from different socioeconomic backgrounds?" "Is there a relationship between the incidence of AIDS (acquired immune deficiency symdrome) and sexual practices?" "Do men and women have different attitudes about receiving intimate bodily care from male nurses than they do from female nurses?" All of the questions above have a few things in common:

1. They deal with two or more categories (usually nominal or ordinal scales with only a few levels, or ranks).

2. The data consist of frequency counts that are tabulated and slotted into the appropriate cells of a table.

3. Answers to our research questions require that we cross-tabulate frequencies of the two variables under investigation.

The method for answering such questions is to construct what is called a contingency table. A *contingency table* is a two-dimensional frequency distribution in which the frequencies of two variables are cross-tabulated.

If you were trying to determine whether reminiscence or remotivation groups were selected at different rates by clients 70 years of age and older versus those less than 70 years old, you could construct a simple contingency table by placing one variable (*age*) along the vertical axis and the other (*type of support group*) along the horizontal axis. You would then tabulate the number of subjects belonging in each cell of the table and compute percentages (see Table 15-5). A reader can then see at a glance that patients 70 years or older preferred the reminiscence group and patients under the age of 70 preferred the remotivation group.

Measures of Correlation A lot of aspects in our daily lives are influenced by predictions that scientists have made based on associations or correlations between variables. For example, if you are an obese, city-dwelling, unmarried, cigarette-smoking man with a family history of heart disease, you may pay more for health insurance no matter what your own health record may be. This typical policy is based on strong correlations between heart attack rates and these variables. A correlation addresses the question of to what extent two variables are related to each other. For example: "To what extent is cigarette smoking related to the incidence of lung cancer and emphysema?" "To what extent is a diet high in saturated fat related to gall bladder disease?" "To what extent is a positive attitude toward labor and delivery related to the presence of one's mate in the labor and delivery rooms?" These questions are answered by calculating a statistic, or index, that expresses the magnitude or degree of relationship. There are two types of correlations between variables: (1) positive correlations and (2) negative correlations. Statistics of correlation theoretically vary between 0, indicating no correlation, and ±1, indicating a perfect correlation. Plus and minus signs in the case of ordinal, interval, or ratio data also indicate whether the correlation is positive or negative. Many (but not all) correlation statistics are represented by the letter r.

If a nurse weighed and measured all patients on an inpatient psychiatric unit and found that the tallest people weighed the most and the shortest people the least, we could say that a positive correlation existed between height and weight for this sample. A positive correlation is also called *a direct relationship* between the two variables. A negative correlation is called an *inverse relationship*.

The graphic, or visual, presentation of a correlation between two variables is called a *scatter diagram*, or *scatter plot*. Each dot, *X*, or point represents the position of a subject on the *X* and *Y* axis variables. A scatter diagram can reflect both the direction (positive or negative) and the approximate magnitude of a correlation. The more the dots resemble a straight line, the higher the correlation. When you can know a person's position on one variable because you know his or her position on the second, the correlation is called a "perfect correlation." A perfect cor-

Table 15-5 Sample Contingency Table for Age-Type Group Preference (*n* = 60)

	Reminiscence		Remotivation	
	Group	Percentage	Group	Percentage
70 years or over	40	66	20	33
Under 70 years	20	33	40	66

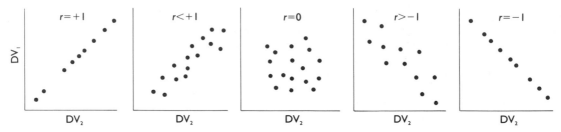

Figure 15-13 Sample scatter diagrams for different degrees of correlation between DVs.

relation (negative or positive) is depicted on a scatter diagram by a sloped straight line (see Figure 15-13).

The *sign* of a correlation, either a plus or a minus, conveys the nature of the relationship of two variables measured by a correlation coefficient symbolized by *r*. The *size* of a correlation is expressed by the numbers. They indicate the strength of the correlation. The closer the coefficient is to either +1 or −1, the higher, or stronger, the correlation is. The closer the correlation, or *r* number, is to 0, the lower, or weaker, the relationship is. Table 15-6 illustrates some examples of correlation coefficients. A correlation that is published without a plus or minus sign is usually interpreted as positive; that is, *r* = .66 means *r* = +.66.

The two most common correlation statistics are the *Pearson product–moment correlation* (or Pearson *r*) and the *Spearman rho*. The first is a parametric technique that requires continuous data such as weight, height, and time. The second is a nonparametric technique that requires only rank-order scales. Because the Spearman correlation technique involves ranks, statisticians usually refer to it as the rank-order correlation technique. Both can be calculated by hand according to mathematical formulas, but most investigators use a computer to calculate and

Table 15-6   Sample Correlation Coefficients

+.99, +.90 +.88	High positive correlation
+.33, +.29 +.39	Low positive correlation
.00, +.12, −.01	No systematic correlation
−.19 −.33, −.25	Low negative correlation
−.93, −.77, −.80	High negative correlation

print out these descriptive statistics (see Chapter 16).

Perfect correlations are rarely found in nursing studies. If you read about or conduct a study about psychosocial correlations and the *r* = +.50 or +.60 or +.70, you could consider the relationship between the variables under investigation to be in a very positive direction. High correlations are more likely to be found when a study focuses on physiologic variables rather than psychosocial ones (see Chapter 12). Remember, however, that a high correlation or even a perfect one does not indicate causation between the two variables. High IQs may be correlated to height, but neither definitely causes the other in the statistical sense of causation.

Inferential Statistics

In the preceeding section of this chapter you learned that one approach for analyzing quantitative data is to use descriptive statistics such as measures of central tendency, variation, and correlation to summarize the data set. Many nursing studies, however, are conducted for purposes that go beyond merely reporting characteristics of a particular sample of data. The investigators want to at least report something about the descriptive characteristics of the population from which the sample was drawn. *Inferential statistics* are the statistical techniques that researchers use to generalize from the characteristics of a sample to the larger, unmeasured population from which that sample was drawn. (Certain correlational procedures are also used as inferential statistics when an alpha level is reported.)

Inferring From a Sample to a Population

Suppose you wanted to know the average length of hospital stay for organ transplant patients in the United States. On the one hand, you could track every single patient admitted to an American hospital for this procedure, but your approach would be costly and time consuming. If, on the other hand, you used the principles and procedures of inferential statistics, you could select a representative random sample from the population, calculate its mean length of hospital stay, and then make an inference about the mean length of hospital stay for the entire population. (See Chapter 9 to review the meaning of representative and random samples.) *Remember that inferential statistics are based on the assumption that the investigator has taken a random sample from the population.* You ought to find the sampling procedure reported in a journal article in one of the forms presented in Box 15-3.

Sampling Errors

Even when you infer characteristics of a population from a properly selected random and representative sample, there is always some chance that the actual mean of the population will be slightly different from the means suggested in samples drawn from it. Remember that statistics are not about certainty but rather about likelihood of something being true. If you calculated the mean for several different samples drawn from the same population, it would be unlikely that they would all have identical means. The fluctuation of a statistic from one sample to another is called *sampling error*. Hypothetically, if

---

Box 15-3   Hypothetical Journal Excerpts Reporting on the Random Sampling Procedure

Twenty-five male and 25 female participants in prenatal classes were randomly selected from a population of 100 class members.

or

Twenty-five male and 25 female participants in a rural community health center's prenatal classes were randomly selected from a 100-member population by putting their names in an alphabetical list by first name, assigning consecutive numbers, and then selecting the sample using a table of random numbers.

you plotted a frequency polygon of the means of all the possible samples that could be drawn from the population, you would end up with what is called a *sampling distribution of the mean* and could then calculate the mean of the population based on the distribution of means in the frequency polygon. This notion, however, is really a theoretical one, because it requires you to draw an infinite number of samples. Theoretically, though, statisticians tell us that the sampling distributions of means tend to follow a normal, or bell-shaped, curve. Therefore, you can calculate the standard deviation of a sampling distribution and reasonably assume that 68% of all the sample means fall between $+1$ and -1 standard deviations from the population's actual mean. The standard deviation of a theoretical frequency distribution of means of samples is called the *standard error of the mean*. The smaller the standard error, obviously, the more accurate a sample mean is as a reflection of a population mean.

Calculating the Standard Error of the Mean

Inferring characteristics of a population from just one random sample can be computed using the following formula to calculate the standard error of the mean. The calculations can be done by hand calculator or, more often, by computer program.

$$s_{\bar{x}} = \frac{SD}{\sqrt{n}}$$

where SD = the standard deviation of the sample

n = the sample size

$s_{\bar{x}}$ = the standard error of the mean

The important point about all this is that you can increase the accuracy of your estimate of a population's mean *by increasing the size of the sample* on which you calculate the standard de-

viation. When you read a study critique or discussion of limitation and a small sample size is mentioned, you now know that it can be because the accuracy of generalizing from the sample to the population is statistically questionable (see Chapter 9).

Testing Hypotheses

Estimating the parameters of a population from a sample is one of the major uses for inferential statistics. *Testing hypotheses* is the other. Usually a researcher uses inferential statistics to compare two or more groups to find out if the corresponding populations are similar. Hathaway and Geden (1983), in a study of energy expenditure during three types of exercise program, were able to use an inferential statistical procedure called *analysis of variance* (ANOVA) to demonstrate that for oxygen consumption and heart rate the groups *were not similar*. In fact, for these two dependent variables, the isometric and active exercise programs were significantly more demanding than the passive or rest programs. Statistical procedures provide investigators with the means for deciding whether a study's outcomes reflect true population difference or whether an apparent difference is due only to chance and not likely to happen again.

The General Logic of Inferential Statistical Tests

All inferential statistical tests are built around the assumption that *chance* is the only thing that produces variation between groups. Based on a mathematical model, statisticians can calculate the probability that a statistical test will take a certain value if only chance is operating. Most tests are designed so that the larger the statistic, the lower the probability that it was produced by sampling error, chance, unsystematic variation, or random error. So that researchers who use statistics don't have to keep recalculating the chance probabilities of different statistical tests over and over again, these values are available in tables. Most tables are set up to give you probabilities such as 1 in 20 (.05), 1 in 100 (.01), or 1 in 1000 (.001) according to different sample sizes, because, as we saw earlier, sample size is an important factor in calculating the accuracy of estimates. (See Chapter 9 on "power analysis.")

Most inferential statistics let you reject the possibility that the results of a study are strictly due to chance whenever your statistical value is larger than what you find in the table (called the critical value). The confidence level listed in the table tells you how sure you can be about rejecting the idea that the difference between two groups was not due to chance.

Hanson and Chater (1983) studied role selection by nurses, examining the relationship between interest in management roles and certain personality, demographic, and career background characteristics of 122 female nurses. The authors used a multivariate analysis of variance (MANOVA). It showed that at a .05 confidence level, 7 of the 11 scales of the vocational preference inventory differentiated the management from nonmanagement groups (a distinction that was based on their scores on the business management scale of the Strong-Campbell Interest Inventory). Their findings allowed them to conclude that those who exhibited managerial interests were more practical minded, sociable, conforming, dominant, and expressive and had more occupational interests than those who did not exhibit such interest. Differences between the two groups on the 19 demographic and career background variables were not statistically significant.

Steps in Using Inferential Statistics to Test Hypotheses

Step 1: State the Null Hypothesis The rules of statistical hypothesis testing are based on what at first seems like strange logic. They allow you to reject the idea that any difference between groups that you find is due to chance or error, rather than allowing you to prove that there is a

real relationship between the variables that you are studying. They allow you to sift the probable from the false. The initial step in testing a hypothesis is to set up a null hypothesis. The *null hypothesis* is a statement that no difference exists between the populations being compared (see Chapter 9). This is essentially a statement that explains a study's results as being due *only* to chance factors or sampling error. The results of our statistical test will then be stated in terms of the probability that the null hypothesis is false. The hypothesis, or opposite of the null hypothesis, is sometimes called the *alternate hypothesis* in research articles. If testing the null hypothesis shows that there is no difference, the hypothesis, or alternative hypothesis, indicates that there *is a difference* between groups being studied that is not due to chance alone.

In formulaic terms the null hypothesis (H_0) predicts that the population mean for one group $A(m_A)$ is the same as the population mean for group $B(m_B)$:

$$H_0 = m_A = m_B$$

Using a stratified random sample of 130 patients from three hospital units, Nichols, Barstow, and Cooper (1983) tested the relationship between frequency of changing IV tubing and percutaneous sites and the incidence of phlebitis. They found that there were no significant differences in rates of phlebitis whether tubings were changed every 24 or 48 hours or whether sites were changed every 48 or 72 hours. Their null hypotheses were stated as follows:

Null Hypotheses:

There will be no difference in the incidence of phlebitis between the three treatment groups.

Group 1: IV tubing changed every 24 hours, percutaneous site changed every 48 hours.

Group 2: IV tubing changed every 24 hours, percutaneous site changed every 72 hours.

Group 3: IV tubing changed every 48 hours, percutaneous site changed every 72 hours.

Step 2: Select a Level of Significance   The level of significance is a probability that tells you how unlikely the sample data must be before you can reject the null hypothesis. In other words, when you reject a null hypothesis, you need to know what the chances are that you are making a mistake in doing so. There are two kinds of mistake that you can make. A *Type I error* is committed when you conclude that the null hypothesis is false when it is really true. That is, you conclude that the difference is not due to chance when in fact it is. Type I errors are also called *alpha errors*. Reid (1983) comments that the most prevalent statistical problems in the nursing literature that reflect the lack of protection against Type I errors are:

1. initial use of a *t* test to compare more than one set of means

2. use of the *t* test for comparison of Pearson correlation coefficients

3. use of univariate statistical tests when multivariate statistical procedures are more appropriate (see Table 15-11).

Type II errors occur when you conclude that the differences between groups were due to chance when in fact the independent variable, or experimental treatment, had indeed had an effect on the dependent variable. Type II errors are also called *beta errors*.

For most studies, a level of significance of $p = .05$ (a 1 in 20 chance of being wrong) is the maximum risk investigators are willing to accept for making a Type I error. A level of .01 (1 in 100 chance of being wrong) or .001 (1 in 1000 chance of being wrong) means that the likelihood that you are mistaken in rejecting the null hypothesis is lower and the significance of your results is greater. When you read a research report in a journal article, the level of statistical significance is sometimes called the *level of probability*. Finally, the .95 *level of confidence* refers to the same thing as the .05 level of significance, except it is stated backwards. As should be clear from the preceding discussion, the harder a researcher tries to lower the risk of committing a Type I error, the greater the risk of committing a Type II error. In other words, if you use strict criteria to reject the null hypotheses, you increase the chance that you accept a false one. The best balance forces a thoughtful investigator to consider in advance all the important measurement, scaling, sampling, and statistical considerations important to this issue.

Step 3: Look Up a Test's Significance in a Table   In addition to knowing the name of the test performed, you need two bits of information to look up the statistical significance or critical value of a calculated statistic in a table, be it a z table, t table, f table, or χ^2 table. These bits of information are the *degrees of freedom*, which is a value related to the size and number of samples being tested (often $df = n - 1$) and the confidence level (.01, .05, or .001) of the test statistic for whatever degree of freedom you decide on. The *critical value* for a specified degree of freedom and confidence level is the value of the test statistic that your calculated statistic would need to be less than in order to accept the null hypothesis. You find the critical value in statistical tables (see end papers of this book).

Step 4: Choose the Right Statistical Test   Most statistical tests used in hypothesis testing by nurse researchers are classified into two types: *parametric* statistics and *nonparametric* statistics. Parametric tests have three important requirements:

1. They involve the estimation of at least one parameter.

2. They require measurements on *at least an interval-level measurement scale*.

3. They involve the assumption that the variables are normally distributed (according to a bell-shaped curve) in the population, suggesting that *a sample size of at least 20 scores per cell is essential*. Parametric tests are considered to be more powerful and therefore are preferred by most nurse re-

searchers who are analyzing numerical data. *t* tests and analysis of variance (ANOVA) are discussed in the pages that follow.

If the assumptions for parametric tests cannot be met, the second type of statistic is used. The nonparametric statistic is not based on the same assumptions, but instead it:

1. can be used with nominal and ordinal measurements

2. can be used when the sample size is small and there is no way to assume that the scores follow a bell-shaped curve or normal distribution

---

Putt (1977) studied the effects of noise on fatigue in healthy middle-aged adults. The term *fatigue* was defined to include an identifiable set of body processes that underlie complex relations between the organism (person) and the environment, with an orientation toward demands of some sort being made on the organism. Putt studied a sample of 60 healthy adults to look at whether *rest* as a nursing intervention made any difference in perception of energy expenditure after performance of a psychomotor test. She also studied whether a noisy background made a difference. She used *t* tests of group means for effects on each of the two variables under investigation. Although Donaldson (1977) presented a strong critique of some of the Putt study's conceptual underpinning, the study did illustrate the basic and most familiar parametric procedure for testing the differences in group means—the *t* test. Most nurse researchers elect to call upon the computer to calculate *t* tests on their data (see Chapter 16).

The *t* Test

When you use *t* tests, you have to decide whether you need to be sensitive to differences in either direction (greater or less). The *one-tailed t test* is sensitive to differences in only one direction.

When the direction of difference between populations is unknown to the researcher, it makes more sense to use a two-tailed test. For example, in testing a specific group intervention program against a placebo (or just a spontaneously informal group exchange), you wouldn't know which direction of difference was significant and therefore might choose a two-tailed test. When you want to reject the null hypothesis for any difference in means, be it positive or negative, you use a nondirectional two-tailed *t* test.

t **Test for Paired Samples**   In either a *within-subjects design* or a *matched-groups design* (see Chapter 6), a score in one situation can be paired with a score in another. In a within-subjects pretest and posttest design, you have a prescore and postscore for each respondent. You can then figure out the effect of a nursing intervention by testing whether you have statistically significant differences between the pretest and posttest mean scores. In a matched-groups design, a score in one situation can be paired with a score in another, and you can figure out the effect of intervention by estimating the difference for each pair. This statistic is often used in nursing studies that don't have control or experimental groups but rely instead on comparing values or scores of a sample from before an intervention (biofeedback training, for instance) with scores from after the intervention. The procedure involves comparing the pretest and posttest measures using an equation for paired-measure *t* tests and then comparing the computed value of *t* with the *t* values in a table. For this kind of *t* test, the degrees of freedom are equal to the number of pairs minus 1 ($df = n - 1$). Before you actually do the calculations, be sure you are using the correct *t* formula for the study. These formulas can be found in a good statistics book or by consulting a statistical consultant.

Advantages and Disadvantages of a One-Tailed *t* Test   The major advantage of a one-tailed *t* test is that a smaller difference between the means of two groups will be statistically significant. But its disadvantage is that if there is a large negative effect of the independent variable, you have to redo the experiment to deal with the unexpected outcome. You are not supposed to change your hypotheses after the fact to cover results that are the opposite of what you expected. Therefore, it makes sense to use one-tailed t tests when you have good reason to expect the direction of a relationship or when you don't care about a result that goes in the opposite direction. Good reporting requires that you explain whether you've done a two-tailed or one-tailed test and the rationale for doing so.

In certain situations when the study involves a very small sample or the distribution of scores does not even approximate a bell-shaped curve, a few nonparametric statistical tests can be used to calculate the differences between groups. Two of them are summarized in Table 15-7. If you are using computer software to test your hypotheses (see Chapter 16), you need only select the statistical operation and give the command.

Analysis of Variance

A one-way *analysis of variance* (abbreviated ANOVA) is an inferential statistical procedure that has about the same purpose as a t test, that is, to compare the mean scores of two groups. The difference between an ANOVA and a t test is that the t test is used for comparing two groups, whereas a one-way ANOVA can be used to compare two or more groups. Because the ANOVA can be used with a greater number of groups, it is considered to be a more versatile statistical procedure. Also, because ANOVA alternative hypotheses do not state a direction, you don't have to worry about making one-tailed or two-tailed comparisons, as you do with the t test.

Calculating the f Ratio   Using an ANOVA involves calculating what is called the F ratio and then checking the value of that statistic against a table of F values for its statistical significance. Calculating an analysis of variance consists of obtaining two independent estimates of variance. One is based on the variability between groups (between-group variance, or s^2B), and the other is based on the variability within groups (within-group variance, or s^2W). If the between-group variance is large relative to the within-group variance, the F ratio is large, and the null hypothesis is rejected. If the between-group variance is small relative to the within-group variance, the F ratio will be small, and the null hypothesis will be more likely to be accepted.

A basic concept in calculating the F ratio in ANOVA is *the sum of squares*. The formula for analysis of variance divides the total sum of squares into the within-group sum of squares and the between-group sum of squares. To obtain variance estimates from these two numbers,

Table 15-7   Nonparametric Statistical Tests

Name	Purpose	Rationale for Use
Mann-Whitney U test	Nonparametric test for determining difference between means of two samples	Tends to be more powerful than others because it "throws away fewer variables"
	Requires ordinal level data and independent samples	
Wilcoxon matched pairs signed-rank test	Involves taking the difference between a pair of scores and ranking the absolute difference	Is very simple to compute
	Requires ordinal level measures within and between groups	

you divide each by the appropriate degrees of freedom (usually the number of groups minus 1, or $n - 1$). The final operation with ANOVA is calculating the actual F ratio to determine whether the two or more variance estimates could have been drawn from the same population. If not, then you can conclude that the experimental treatments produced a significant difference between the means. The formula for the F ratio is the between-group variance estimate divided by the within-group variance estimate, or:

$$F = \frac{s^2 B}{s^2 W}$$

where: F = F ratio
$s^2 B$ = between-group sum of squares
$s^2 W$ = within-group sum of squares.

There are a lot of different analysis of variance tests, and learning about all of them requires either the help of a statistical consultant, a more advanced statistics course, or both. We can, however, consider two kinds of ANOVAs in this chapter—the analysis for a single independent variable design and the analysis for the effects of two or more independent variables on a dependent variable. The latter type is often called a *multifactor ANOVA*.

When a study examines dependent variables from more than two conditions—for example, Norris and her colleagues' (1982) study of the effects of three nursing procedures (suctioning, repositioning, and a heel stick) on blood oxygen levels in premature infants—the researchers need some way to determine whether variation of the sample means was too large to be accounted for by repeated random sampling from one population. Rephrased in the opposite terms, researchers need some way of knowing if the independent variables, or experimental conditons, had differential effects on the dependent variable. In the Norris study the investigators wanted to know if the effects of the three routine nursing procedures differentially affected the blood oxygen levels in sick premature infants (DV = transcutaneous oxygen mea-

sured with a TcpO$_2$ monitor). They used an ANOVA to compare variances of the sample means with an estimate of the variance of the population of 25 babies who weighed less than or equal to 1900 grams at birth and were diagnosed with respiratory distress syndrome in a neonatal intensive care unit.

The population variance is estimated by combining the variances of the individual samples. If the variance of the means is close in value to the estimated population variance, then the researchers assume that all the means come from samples of the same population. If the variance of the means is larger than the estimated population variance (as if the case in the Norris study), then the researchers conclude that at least some of the means come from different populations. This finding indicates that the independent variables are having a real differential effect on the dependent variable. Norris and her associates found that TcpO$_2$ was decreased significantly during suctioning and repositioning of the babies but not during the heel stick and that the three nursing procedures had different degrees of change. Suctioning elicited the greatest decrease in TcpO$_2$, followed by repositioning and then heel stick. These results suggested that the type of procedure determined the sick infants' response. F ratios of $F = 27.01$, $p .0001$, for suctioning and $F = 8.01$, $p .001$, for positioning were calculated. ANOVA of the TcpO$_2$ trends during heel stick indicated that this condition did not differ significantly from the estimated population mean (p. 333).

Interpreting F Ratios From an ANOVA Summary Table It is harder to calculate F ratios than t values, and therefore most contemporary nursing research studies use computer programs to do the actual calculations. The results are usually presented in a summary table. To help you understand how ANOVA works and to practice comprehending presentations of ANOVA findings, let's decipher a hypothetical table.

Table 15-8 has five columns: *source, df, SS* (for sum of squares), *MS* (for mean square), and F. Under the first column are the names for the three rows. The first row is the name of the independent variable, in this case, *test forms for a nursing theory exam*. Another common name for the first row is *between-group*. The second row is usually labeled *within-group* or *error term*, and the third row is labeled *total*.

Table 15-8   ANOVA Summary Table for Experiment Comparing Different Item Arrangements

Source	df	SS	MS	F
Test forms (IV)	2	16	8	4
Between group (error)	15	30	2	
Total	17	46		

The numbers in the column labeled *df* (degrees of freedom) are computed by subtracting 1 from the number of different groups involved in the study. There were three groups in the hypothetical study for this table, just as the Norris study of premature infants had three groups, so the test form source of the between-group row has 2 degrees of freedom. The degrees of freedom allow us to find the critical value for a test statistic in a table at a particular probability of the null hypothesis being true. To get the total *df* the researcher simply subtracted 1 from the total number of subjects, resulting in a 17. To get the within-group *df*, simply subtract the *df* in the first row from the total, yielding 17 − 2, or 15.

The various sums of squares (*SS*) are calculated using a relatively complex formula. But in reading a table like this or in constructing one, remember that the bottom number in the column, or total *SS*, should be equal to the sum of the other two *SS*. Most *SS* in reported nursing studies contain a decimal point, so the numbers in the hypothetical table are fictitious for ease of understanding.

The values in the column for the mean square (*MS*) are found by dividing the *SS* by the *df* found in the same row. There are only two values in the *MS* column, and if an author puts one in the *total* row, he or she has made a mistake.

The most important number is the single value in the *F* column, because it is this value when compared with the critical values for *F* in a statistical table like the one simulated in Table 15-9 that permits you to reach a decision about accepting or rejecting a study's null hypothesis. The investigator looks up the between-group *df* (2) and the within-group *df* (15) at the approxi-mate alpha level to find the critical value for *F*. If the *F* ratio that has been calculated is *larger* than the critical value at the appropriate place on the *F* table, then there is a statistically significant difference between the sample means. You can then conclude that the null hypothesis (that the groups are from the same population) should be rejected and that there is indeed a difference at a specified level of certainty that can be attributed to the different treatments, interventions, or procedures that make up the study's independent variable. Authors of research articles will often emphasize this finding in their report by putting an asterisk next to the calculated *F* value in the summary table and indicate under the table the level of significance, for example, $p = .05$. Some *F* tables give critical values for two levels of significance in the same table by listing the higher level in parentheses or a different-sized type.

Follow-Up Multiple Comparison Tests   If you conduct a study using a one-way ANOVA to compare three groups and obtain an *F* ratio that is significant enough to reject the null hypothesis of equal means, you still don't know which of the means are different from the others. A number of statistical tests called *multiple comparisons*, or *post hoc comparisons*, exist to help the investigator locate exactly where the significant differences lie after a significant overall *F* ratio has been obtained. These techniques are named after the people who developed them and include:

- Fisher's LSD
- Duncan's new multiple range test
- Newman-Keuls

Table 15-9 Critical Values for F

df Within-Groups for	df for Between-Groups					
	2	4	6	8	10	20
5	5.89 (13.4)	5.29 (11.5)	5.05 (10.8)	4.92 (10.4)	4.87 (10.2)	4.66 (9.65)
10	4.20 (7.66)	3.58 (6.09)	3.32 (5.49)	3.17 (5.16)	3.07 (4.95)	2.87 (4.51)
15	3.78 (6.46)	3.16 (4.99)	2.89 (4.42)	2.74 (4.10)	2.65 (3.90)	2.43 (3.46)
20	3.59 (5.95)	2.97 (4.53)	2.70 (3.97)	2.55 (3.66)	2.45 (3.47)	2.22 (3.04)
40	3.33 (5.28)	2.71 (3.93)	2.44 (3.39)	2.28 (3.09)	2.17 (2.90)	1.94 (2.47)
120	3.17 (4.89)	2.55 (3.58)	2.28 (3.06)	2.12 (2.76)	2.00 (2.57)	1.75 (2.13)

- Turkey's HSD
- Scheffe's test

Why Not Just Do Repeated t Tests? Although these multiple comparison procedures are a lot like applying several t tests to the data following a significant F ratio, they differ in one important way—they don't increase the probability of getting a significant result by chance alone. If you used multiple t tests at the .05 level of significance, by the time you made three t test comparisons of two means at a time, as a group the significance level would be at the .14 level. The multiple comparison procedures mentioned above adjust the level of significance to reduce the influence of chance due to having more than just one comparison. A *liberal* multiple comparison test will find a significant difference between means that are relatively close together. the Fisher's LSD is the most liberal of the tests mentioned above. A *conservative* comparison test will work only when the means are far apart. Of the comparison tests listed above, Scheffe's is the most conservative. Those of you reading or writing about multiple comparison results may not find these reported in tables but rather will find the results of multiple comparisons reported in the text of a research article.

Two-Way Analysis of Variance The nursing studies that would use a one-way ANOVA to analyze collected data are those that measure the effects of one independent variable on two or more conditions that make up the dependent variable. Suppose you want to study the best way to teach nursing students and set up a design that looks at both *attributes of the learners* and *a specific instructional strategy or treatment*. In this study, you are dealing with the effects of interaction between the *two different independent variables* on a dependent variable (*successful learning*). Obviously, such a study involves testing more than one hypothesis. You are interested in testing for both the effects of the independent variables and also for the effects of the interaction between the two independent variables. The analytic technique called for in studies with these characteristics is a *two-way*, or *multifactor*, *analysis of variance* (see Table 15-11). The advantage of this statistical technique is that it allows you to study more complex and interactive questions. An illustration of the use of a two-way ANOVA is presented below.

Loustau (1977) reported a study that investigated an attribute-by-treatment interaction between two variables that she thought might be relevant to effective individualization of instruction. The attribute measure was the nursing student's preference for internal versus external control; the treatment variable was exposure to either an overt or covert approach to a programmed instruction task. Her study tested for five hypotheses:

1. Internally oriented subjects would perform equally well on a programmed instruction task under overt and covert response conditions, whereas externally oriented subjects would perform better under overt response conditions.

2. Subjects who responded overtly to the programmed instruction task would spend more time on the task than subjects who responded covertly to the task.

3. Subjects who responded overtly to the programmed instruction task would spend less time on the postlearning measures.

4. Subjects who responded overtly to the task would obtain higher scores on the postlearning measures that required constructed responses.

5. There would be no difference between the performance of the overt and covert responders on recognition or multiple-choice tests.

Her sample consisted of 102 women nursing students from her associate degree nursing program, and she used a two-way ANOVA to test each hypothesis. The results for hypothesis #2 is presented in Table 15-10 as an illustration. This study failed to support an internal–external by overt–covert technique interaction. However, the issue of amount of time spent suggested areas for further research and raised the practical implication for educators that a time-consuming educational activity appears not to improve scores on postmeasures.

Nonparametric Statistical Tests

The statistical tests of inference that we have discussed thus far all rely on two important assumptions: (1) that the population distribution from which the samples were drawn conforms to a normal, or bell-shaped, probability curve and (2) that the data collected are interval- or ratio-level scales of measurement. Many nursing studies, however, focus on variables that don't conform to these two assumptions. A study that ranked patients in terms of their cooperativeness with a health care regimen would be an example.

Table 15-10   Summary for 2 × 2 Analysis of Variance for Internal–External Preference and the Overt–Covert Treatment

Dependent Measure: Time (min) on Programmed Instruction Task	Internal Overt	Internal Covert	External Overt	External Covert
Number	25	25	25	25
Mean	140.4	79.9	119.6	72.5
Source	SS	df	MS	F
Internal–external	4,970.25	1	4,970.25	4.15*
Overt–covert	72,307.21	1	72,307.21	60.36†
Internal–external × overt–covert	1,122.21	1	1,122.21	.94
Within (error)	115,000.00	96	1,197.92	

Note: $F \leq 3.95$; significant at the .05 level.
*$p < .05$.
†$p < .01$.

The data would be ordinal, not interval or ratio, data and would not necessarily be distributed according to a bell-shaped curve. Clearly, parametric statistics would not apply, and the investigator would have to choose a statistical test appropriate to the data.

Nonparametric tests are those statistical tests that make no assumptions about the shape of the population distribution, and they are therefore called distribution-free tests. Different nonparametric statistical tests have been devised for few-category and many-category situations as well as for different designs. Some of the tests for ordinal data have a version for small samples (fewer than 20) and one for large samples. For analysis of data involving nominal, ordinal, or nonnormally distributed interval dependent variable scales, you'll need to refer to a good nonparametric statistics book. One classic is Siegal's (1956) *Nonparametric Statistics for the Behavioral Sciences.* Remember when choosing a statistical test or when reading about the choice another researcher has made that using parmetric statistics when they don't apply can lead to mistaken conclusions. But using nonparametric statistics when parametric statistics were appropriate can mean that a less powerful test has been used, and the significance of data can easily be underestimated.

Hints for Using Nonparametric Procedures Saslow (1982) offers the following hints for doing nonparametric statistical tests.* These suggestions hold for parametric tests as well.

1. If you are unfamiliar with a particular test, read the introductory material carefully to see whether the test is right for your study.

2. If you decide to use the test, work through at least one example that is close to your study situation.

3. Be sure you understand the instructions for using a particular table for the test. There are many different formats for statistical tables, even for the same test.

4. Remember that selecting the correct statistical test for your data is more important than being able to do the actual calculations. These can be done by calling upon the computer (see Chapter 16).

The Chi-Square for Nominal Data The chi-square (χ^2) is one of the most frequently used nonparametric statistics reported in the nursing research literature. This test can be used when your data are nominally scaled and you are interested in the number of responses, objects, or people that fall in two or more categories. The chi-square is calculated from the differences between observed frequencies and the frequencies expected under the conditions of the null hypothesis. Sometimes it has been called the "goodness of fit" statistic. *Goodness of fit* refers to whether a significant difference exists between an observed number and an expected number of classes or scores that fall into the nominal categories set out by the investigator. The expected number is what you would expect by chance or according to the null hypothesis. When the discrepancy is large between what turns up in your data and what you would expect to occur by chance, the chi-square statistic will be large. If it exceeds the critical value in a chi-square table, taking into account its degrees of freedom, you can reject the null hypothesis and accept the alternative hypothesis.

The chi-square test is relatively easy to do, with only a few things to watch out for, according to Saslow (1982):*

1. Be sure to set up your null hypothesis correctly so that you know what you are rejecting. Whether you want a large or small difference depends on your research question.

2. If your sample size is too small, you might have to use a variation of the chi-square test

*SOURCE: Based on C. A. Saslow, *Basic Research Methods,* Reading, Mass.: Addison-Wesley, 1982, p. 246.

*SOURCE: Based on C. A. Saslow, *Basic Research Methods,* Reading, Mass.: Addison-Wesley, 1982.

(the smallest expected frequency must be 5 or more).

3. If your degrees of freedom are small (equal to 1), you will have to use a correction factor. (This involves subtracting one-half from each difference score before squaring.)

Let's look at how the chi-square was used in a study of the effects of electrical surface stimulation on the prevention of atelectasis in experimental and control patients having abdominal surgery.

Menzel and Martinson (1977) focused on the effectiveness of electrical surface stimulation in controlling postoperative pain. But they were also interested in seeing whether the use of electrical stimulation near surgical wounds could alleviate the postoperative complication of atelectasis. A double-blind study of 27 adults who had had large abdominal incisions was conducted, and the patients were randomly assigned to experimental and control groups. The parameter of the presence or absence of atelectasis during the first 48 postoperative hours (nominal data) was included, based on the assumption that if patients were getting relief for their incisional pain from the electrical stimulation, they would then be better able to turn, cough, and hyperventilate, thereby preventing the accumulation of infiltrate in their lungs. Their findings on this parameter using the chi-square test showed that the day-1 and day-2 combined percentages for the experimental and control patient groups revealed no significant difference at the p .05 level. Usually you determine that each group has a 50% chance of being in the category. After the observed numbers are obtained, a formula is used to calculate an χ^2 statistic, or you use a computer software package to calculate it for you.

To recapitulate:

- Chi-square is an inferential statistic that can be used with nominally scaled dependent variables (*yes* or *no*, *presence* or *absence*).

- A one-way chi-square test compares an observed frequency with the frequency expected by chance.

- The degrees of freedom for a one-way chi-square are the number of dependent variable categories minus 1.

- A two-way chi-square test can determine whether the frequency distributions of two variables are independent of each other.

- When there is only 1 degree of freedom for chi-square, a correction factor must be added to the chi-square formula.

- The chi-square test requires that there be a minimum expected frequency of 5 in any category. Meeting this requirement can involve combining categories or measuring larger samples.

- For repeated measures of the same subjects on the same dependent variable, a special variant of the chi-square test is needed, the McNemar or Cochran Q test (Siegal 1956, pp. 63, 161).

Guidelines for Choosing the Right Statistical Test

Choosing the correct descriptive or inferential statistical operation to use in your study involves knowing the answers to a few important questions:

1. You need to know on what level of scale the data for a dependent variable was measured.

2. You need to know whether you are working with a normal, or bell-shaped, distribution.

3. You need to know the details of your study design.

4. You need to understand your research question or hypotheses.

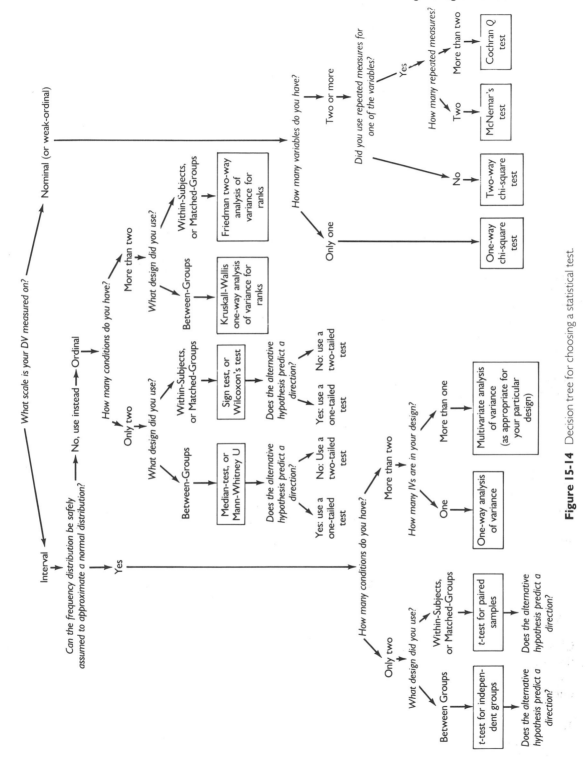

Figure 15-14 Decision tree for choosing a statistical test.

Saslow (1982) offers the decision tree in Figure 15-14 for choosing a statistical test correctly or for determining whether studies that you read in the research literature have employed statistical tools according to the rules. An investigator must sometimes consider using multivariate or more advanced and complex statistical procedures. This occurs when a study is intended to untangle relationships among three or more variables. These procedures include multiple

Table 15-11   Multivariate (Advanced) Statistical Procedures*

Name of Procedure	What Is It?	When Is It Used?
Multiple regression	A way of making predictions by understanding the effects of two or more IVs on a DV. Also called multiple correlation	When the DV is interval level data, you have two or more IVs and you want to know how much the IVs correlate with the DV
Stepwise multiple regression	A method in which all potential predictors can be considered simultaneously to see which combination has the greatest predictive power	When you have many IVs and want to know which set is most powerful in predicting the DV
Path analysis	A method of untangling the relative contributions of various IVs to the variance in a DV	To determine which of a number of IVs is the most influential predictor
Analysis of covariance (ANCOVA)	A combination of analysis of variance and regression that tests the significance of group means after first adjusting scores on the DV to eliminate effects of covariance	If an experimental design is not possible and you want to adjust or control statistically for differences between treatment and comparative groups
Factor analysis	A statistical means for condensing or combining many variables into smaller numbers that are interrelated	Used to reduce a large set of variables into a smaller set of unified concepts
Discriminant analysis	An alternative to multiple regression when the criterion variable (DV) is at the nominal rather than interval level of measurement	Used to predict membership in a category or group based on measure of the IVs.
Canonical correlation	A test that analyzes the relationship of a set of IVs with a set of DVs	Answers the same questions that a multiple regression does except here you have multiple DVs as well
Multivariate analysis of variance (MANOVA)	A test that does for ANOVA what CANON does for multiple regression. Extends ANOVA to two or more DVs	Lets you answer ANOVA questions when you have multiple DVs

*Refer to statistical textbooks or seek statistical consultation to apply these tests to your data.

correlation regressions (simultaneous, stepwise, and hierarchical), analysis of covariance, factor analysis, and discriminant analysis. (The purpose and conditions for some of them are presented in Table 15-11). Once again, the value of specialized statistical consultation and computer resources can't be underestimated if your research or the research that you read involves such advanced procedures.

Summary of Key Ideas and Terms

- If as a reader or doer of nursing research you are able to detect the misuse of *statistics*, you have gained an important knowledge with which to evaluate a study's findings.

- Statistics are analytic tools that allow you to show that something is more or less likely to occur according to the laws of chance or probability.

- *Measurement* is a process of assigning numerical values to concepts under investigation and is equivalent to actual value plus or minus error.

- *Scientific measurement* involves measuring the attributes or qualities of a phenomenon called a variable.

- A *measurement scale* specifies all the potential measurement divisions into which a variable might fall and includes at least two categories that are exhaustive and mutually exclusive.

- The types of measurement scale or levels of data are *nominal*, or naming; *ordinal*, or ordering; *interval*, in which possible measurements are equidistant from one another; and *ratio*, which is the highest level of scale for data with rank ordering, equal intervals, and an absolute zero point.

- Knowing the kind of measurement scale and level of data you are working with informs decisions about which statistical operations are appropriate.

- It is a good idea to consult a statistician, a computer analyst, or both early in a study's planning phase in order to anticipate how to best analyze your data.

- Statistical tests fall into two major categories. *Descriptive statistics* summarize the characteristics of data in a sample. *Inferential statistics* allow you to make inferences about a whole population from sample data and to test hypotheses.

✔ Frequency distributions presented in tables, figures called histograms, and polygons; measures of central tendency such as the mode, median, and mean; measures of variability such as the range, the interquartile range, and the standard deviation; and measures of correlation are the primary techniques of descriptive statistics that allow you to describe a data set.

✔ The formulas and assumptions about scale level for any statistical test should be looked up carefully in a statistics book.

✔ All inferential statistics are based on the assumption that the investigator has taken a random sample from the population, and you can improve the estimates about a population by increasing the sample size.

✔ The logic behind all inferential statistics is that chance is what produces variation among groups. The statistical test is designed to reject this assumption and conclude with a specified level of certainty that differences between dependent variables are due to the independent variable.

✔ The *critical value* is the size of a number in a statistical table that your calculated number must exceed to reject the explanation that differences are due to chance.

✔ The main steps in using inferential statistics to test hypotheses are:

  • State the null hypothesis (a statement that asserts that differences are due only to chance).

  • Select a level of statistical significance (the probability that tells you how unlikely the sample data must be to reject the null hypothesis).

  • Look up a test significance in the appropriate table to find the critical value for the degrees of freedom and confidence level you decide upon (.01, .05, 001).

  • Choose the right test for your study questions and type of data.

✔ If your sample size is larger than 20 scores per cell, if your variables are normally distributed (a bell-shaped curve), and if the measurement scale is at least an interval level, you can use more powerful parametric, rather than nonparametric, tests to test hypotheses..

✔ *Analysis of variance* (ANOVA) is an inferential statistical procedure that can be used to compare two or more groups by calculating what is called an F ratio.

✔ *Multiple comparison tests* are preferable to doing multiple t tests, because the significance level need not be adjusted upwards.

> 🡆 The *chi-square* is one of the most frequently used nonparametric statistics for testing hypotheses with nominal data, but it must be modified if the sample size is small and the degrees of freedom are as low as 1.
>
> 🡆 Advanced statistics such as multiple correlation regression, analysis of covariance, factor analysis, and discriminant analysis can be used when a study is trying to untangle complex relationships among three or more variables.

References

Brooten DA et al: A comparison of four treatments to prevent and control breast pain and engorgement in nonnursing mothers. *Nurs Res* July/August 1983; 32:225–229.

Diers D: *Research in Nursing Practice*. New York: Lippincott, 1979.

Donaldson SK: Critique: Effects of noise on fatigue in healthy middle-aged adults. *Commun Nurs Res* 1977; 8:35–40.

Hanson HA, Chater SS: Role selection by nurses: Managerial interests and personal attributes. *Nurs Res* January/February 1983; 32:48–52.

Hathaway D, Geden E: Energy expenditure during leg exercise programs. *Nurs Res* May/June 1983; 32:147–150.

Hayter J: Sleep behaviors of older persons. *Nurs Res* July/August 1983; 32:242–246.

Loustau A: Interaction between internal–external preference and response to an overt or covert treatment in a programmed instruction task among nursing students. *Commun Nurs Res* 1977; 9:273–283.

Menzel NJ, Martinson IM: Effects of electrical surface stimulation on control of acute postoperative pain and prevention of atelectasis and ileus in patients having abdominal surgery. *Commun Nurs Res* 1977; 8:273–283.

Mercer RT et al: Relationship of psychosocial and perinatal variables to perception of childbirth. *Nurs Res* July/August 1983; 32:202–207.

Nichols EG et al: Relationship between incidence of phlebitis and frequency of changing IV tubing and percutaneous site. *Nurs Res* July/August 1983; 32:247–252.

Norris S et al: Nursing procedures and alterations in transcutaneous oxygen tension in premature infants. *Nurs Res* November/December 1982; 31:330–336.

Polit D, Hungler B: *Nursing Research*, 2nd ed. Philadelphia: Lippincott, 1983.

Putt AM: Effects of noise on fatigue in healthy middle-aged adults. *Commun Nurs Res* 1977; 8:24–34.

Reid BJ: Potential sources of type I error and possible solutions to avoid a "galloping" alpha rate. *Nurs Res* May/June 1983; 32:190.

Saslow CA: *Basic Research Methods*. Reading, Mass.: Addison-Wesley, 1982.

Siegal S: *Nonparametric Statistics for the Behavioral Sciences*. New York: McGraw-Hill, 1956.

Sitzman J et al: Biofeedback training for reduced respiratory rate in chronic obstructive pulmonary disease: A preliminary study. *Nurs Res* July/August 1983; 32:218–223.

Further Readings

Armstrong G: Parametric statistics and ordinal data: A pervasive misconception. *Nurs Res* 1981; 30:60–62.

Burlington RS, May DC Jr: *Handbook of Probability and Statistics*. Sandusky, Ohio: Handbook Publishers, 1953.

Campbell DT, Stanley JC: *Experimental and Quasi Experimental Designs for Research*. Chicago: Rand McNally, 1963.

Churchman CW, Ratosh P (editors): *Measurement: Definitions and Theories*. New York: Wiley, 1963.

Cohen J, Cohen P: *Applied Multiple Regressions:*

Correlation Analyses for Behavioral Sciences. New York: Halsted Press, 1975.

Harris RJ: *A Primer of Multivariate Statistics*. New York: Academic Press, 1974.

Huck SW et al: *Reading Statistics and Research*. New York: Harper & Row, 1974.

Jacobscn, BS: Know thy data. *Nurs Res* July/August 1981; 30:254–255.

Kerlinger FN: *Foundations of Behavioral Research*, 2nd ed. New York: Holt, Rinehart & Winston, 1973.

Nunnaly JC: *Psychometric Theory*. New York: McGraw-Hill, 1978.

Philips JS, Thompson RF: *Statistics for Nurses*. New York: Macmillan, 1967.

Shaw ME, Wright JM: *Scales for the Measurement of Attitudes*. New York: McGraw-Hill, 1967.

Sokal RR, Rohlf FJ: *Biometry: The Principles and Practice of Statistics in Biological Research*. San Francisco: Freeman, 1969.

Triola M: *Elementary Statistics*, 2nd ed. Menlo Park, Calif.: Addison-Wesley, 1983.

Winer BJ: *Statistical Principles in Experimental Designs*. New York: McGraw-Hill, 1969.

Chapter 16

Computers and Data Processing in Nursing Research

Hardware, Software, and People

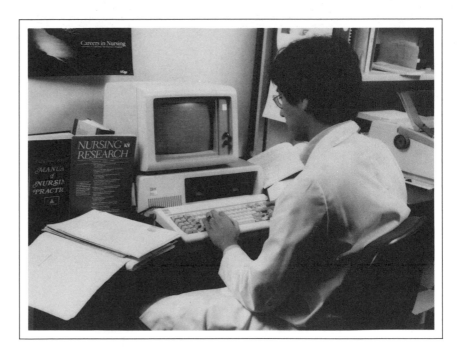

There are many good reasons for becoming computer literate when conducting nursing research. Computers are fast, don't make mistakes, can do tedious jobs, can cope with the information deluge, can increase productivity, and can reduce costs.

Chapter Outline

Chapter Objectives

After reading this chapter, the student should be able to:

- Explain the most frequently used computer terminology
- Collect information about local computer resources that will be helpful in getting acquainted with the system
- Identify the four variables that differentiate microcomputers from mainframe computers
- List the ways of inputting and outputting data on a computer
- Discuss the steps for inputting data to the computer using keypunch cards
- Compare and contrast the advantages and disadvantages of keypunching versus keyboard as computer input devices
- Describe the functions of the two parts of a computer's central processing unit
- Compare and contrast the advantages and disadvantages of different means for secondary storage
- Explain how using a software program can make manuscript preparation quicker and easier
- Follow a procedure for using *CMS* to run SAS jobs on nursing research data
- Name statistical procedures that can be performed on research data using the SPSS software program
- Describe the steps that are usually involved when analyzing research data on a computer
- Evaluate at least one microcomputer using the six factors to consider suggested in this chapter
- Estimate a budget for computer-related services and costs in a research project
- Recognize the roles of various computer resource persons

In This Chapter . . .

This chapter introduces you to the equipment, people, and language you need to appreciate the power, fascination, and excitement that applying the computer to nursing research can provide. There are five good reasons for trying to become "computer literate" and avoiding computer phobia:

1. Computers are fast.
2. Computers rarely make mistakes.
3. Computers can do boring or tedious jobs.
4. Computers can cope with the information deluge.
5. Computers can increase productivity and reduce costs.

The What and How of a Computer

The main use of a computer is to process large amounts of data rapidly. This function is the basis of the term *data processing*. Once data are processed, they are called *information*. Computers can process both *numerical data* such as age, weight, height, blood pressure, test scores, or diagnostic codes and *alphanumeric data* such as letters, punctuation, names, and addresses. The time in which a computer can execute an instruction is usually measured in less than a *millisecond* (a thousandth of a second). Some computers can execute an instruction in *microseconds* (a millionth of a second), and the *nanosecond* range is approachable (a billionth of a second).

A computer system consists of three areas designed to process data into usable information: *input*, *processing*, and *output*; they are backed by a fourth, *storage*, for keeping data. *Hardware* refers to the computer parts you can touch—the equipment in the system that stores, processes, and controls information. These units are related in the system as illustrated in Figure 16-1. *Software* is another word for the *programs* that instruct a computer what to do.

All computers are made of chips of silicon, a nonmetallic substance found in sand, rocks, and clay. A typical *silicon chip* is 1/8 of an inch square. You can get 16 of them on a fingernail. In bright light a chip shimmers like a soap bubble. It can accomplish the same work today that 30 years ago required a 30-ton computer housed in a warehouse the size of a football field.

Silicon is used for chips because it is a semiconductor; that is, it will conduct an electric current when it has chemicals shot into its lattice-like crystalline structure. Patterned on the silicon base are minuscule switches, joined by wires etched from thin films of metal. These are complete, or *integrated*, electronic *circuits*. Under a microscope, the chips's intricate terrain looks uncannily like the streets, plazas, and buildings of a giant metropolis viewed from miles up. The circuits (electrical switches) are turned off or on according to a *binary system*. The binary system is a yes–no "two-state system" that turns the circuit switches on or off through combinations of ones and zeros that represent data. One switch inside the circuit is called a *binary digit*, or *bit*. A single chip holds 3000 or 4000 bits. A group of eight bits that stands either for zero or one is called a *byte* (see Figure 16-2). The eight bits on one byte can be arranged in 256 different ways to represent complicated data. Figure 16-2 illustrates how a byte, by turning off and on like a lightbulb, represents the numerical code for the letter *A* to the computer. The number of combinations in one byte is more than enough to represent each letter, number, and punctuation mark in this chapter.

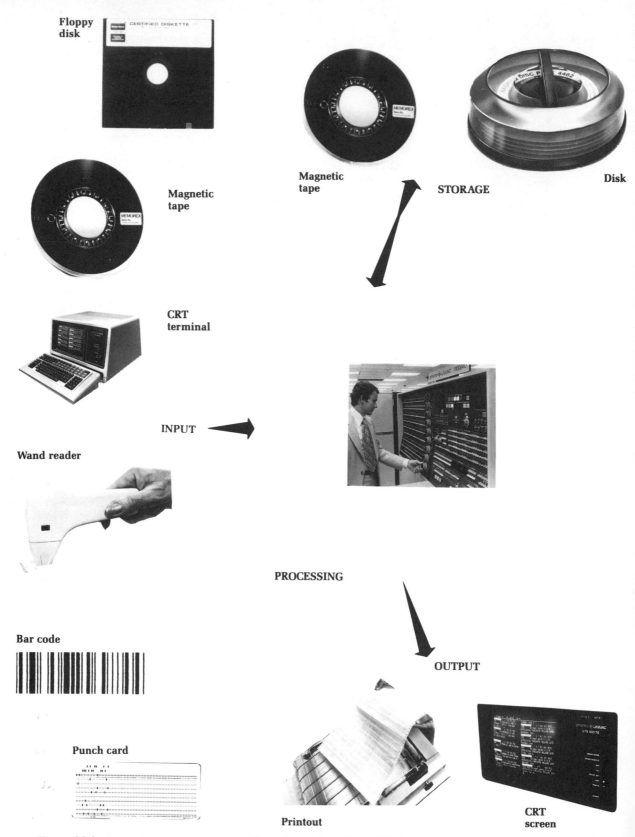

Floppy disk

Magnetic tape

Magnetic tape

STORAGE

Disk

CRT terminal

INPUT

Wand reader

PROCESSING

Bar code

OUTPUT

Punch card

Printout

CRT screen

Figure 16-1 A complete computer system. (From Capron & Williams, 1984).

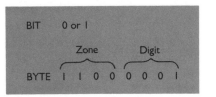

Figure 16-2 The byte shows the letter "A" in computer code.

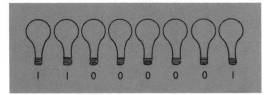

Figure 16-3 The bit as a lightbulb flashing on and off.

Learning About Your Computer Center

Most contemporary universities and hospitals (as well as banks and businesses) own or lease a large, million-dollar *mainframe* computer with terminals located in different places and connected to the computer by telephone links. Early mainframe computers were made from vacuum tubes about the size of lightbulbs and required a space the size of an airplane hangar in which to house them. If you intend to use the contemporary descendant located in the computer center at your institution, the following categories of information will help you get acquainted:

- Building, room number, and telephone number where computer is located
- Type and description of computer systems available to you
- Hours when computer center is open
- Staff members and consultants available
- Introductory computer courses, workshops, and contact person
- Computer languages in use
- Location of terminals
- Availability and location of users' manuals
- Steps to get a user's I.D. number
- Programs available in your computer library
- Location of keypunch machines, sorters, etc.

Most institutions also have a *minicomputer* about the size of a refrigerator and a number of *microcomputers* (also called *personal* or *business computers*) located in offices throughout the building. The main differences between the three main types of computer is their power as reflected in

1. speed
2. cost
3. amount of storage
4. number of users who can simultaneously share the machine

Otherwise, all three do about the same things.

Taking a Tour of the Hardware

Hardware refers to the machines in the computer system that store, process, and control information. The primary parts are *input devices*, *the central processing unit*, *output devices*, and *external storage devices*.

Input Devices   Input devices put data into a form that the computer can recognize. The ways of entering data into a computer are:

1. a card reader, into which keypunch cards are put
2. the keyboard of a terminal, on which data are typed
3. a machine that reads data off of floppy disks (to be explained later in the chapter)

4. a magnetic ink character reader (*MICR*), which reads (for example) numbers on a personal check

5. an *optical scanner*, which recognizes optical marks like those used on the answer sheet of a computer-scored test

6. a wand, which recognizes optical characters (for example, that which is found attached to the cash register of a department store)

7. a light pen for altering data directly on a CRT (cathode ray tube) screen

Voice input units are in the process of development, and Apple has adopted the *"mouse,"* or pointer, for its newest computer. We will be considering more closely the two most common input devices used in nursing research—the card reader and the terminal keyboard.

Keypunch cards contain small holes that represent data and can be read by a card reader. These cards contain 80 vertical columns and 12 rows (see Figure 16-4). Each single column may contain a punch representing the numbers from zero to nine. Usually rows zero to nine are printed on the card, and the top few rows are used for identifying information. Data are coded on the card through a process called *keypunching*. A keypunch machine is a lot like a typewriter, except that it is used to punch holes into the columns of the card. After a deck has been keypunched, it can be taken to another machine, called a verifier, which checks that the holes in the cards are correct by comparing the originally punched data with rekeyed data.

Researchers prepare their data for keypunching by plotting out a *code book* to designate which columns will contain which data (see Table 16-1). Figure 16-4 illustrates how descriptive data on students enrolled in a nursing course are translated into numbers that can be punched into specific columns of a card. The system you see here is called a *fixed-column format*, because the values for each variable you are studying are located in the same column for every case or subject. When the data for one subject require more than one card, the variables must be entered on the same card for all members of the sample. For example, if David Bowie's age is punched in columns 6 and 7 of the third card, every other respondent's age would also occupy columns 6 and 7 of the third card in their case. Figure 16-5 shows three examples of cases organized in a fixed-column format. In the first example, there is only one card per case or subject. In the second, there are two cards per subject, and in the third, four cards per case. There is no fixed limit to the number of cards a case may contain, and blank spaces need not be included between variables on a card. They make it easier for you to read the cards, but the computer doesn't need them.

Once punched, the set of cards, or *deck*, is then placed into a *card reader*. This machine sends the data on the cards onto the computer by translating the holes into electrical impulses. Then it returns the cards on the opposite side of the card reader in the card stacker. Proper reading of your cards won't occur unless you put them in correctly. Some readers require that you put the print side face up, and others require it face down. A card reader can process from 600 to 2000 cards per minute. The time that elapses between turning your deck of computer cards into the computer center and receiving your output is called *turnaround time*. Turnaround time is usually a reflection of how busy the computer center staff is at the time you submit your data. Experienced computer center users suggest that it's wise to find out when the slow times are to decrease your turnaround time.

If large amounts of data need to be processed, most investigators hire a professional keypunching service. It is not impossible, however, to learn to keypunch your own cards. The following eight steps offer a beginning guide:

1. Turn on the keypunch machine.
2. Turn on *print* and *autofeed* switches.
3. Make sure the cards in the hopper have no punches on them.

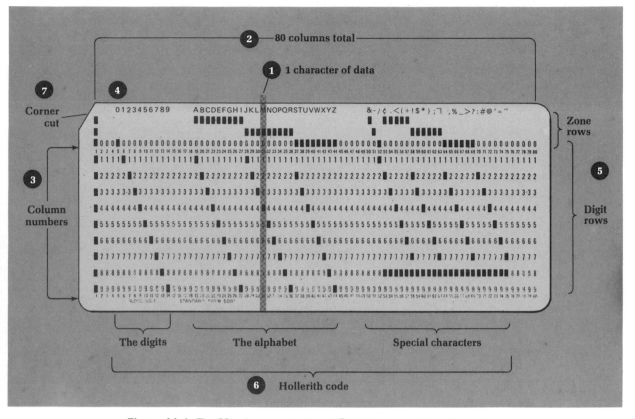

Figure 16-4 The 80-column punched card. Data is incorporated on the card as follows: (1) One character of data is represented by the punches in one column. (2) There are 80 columns on the card. (3) The column numbers are indicated in two places on the card. (4) As holes are punched in the card, the symbol reproduced is typed across the top of the form. (5) There are 12 rows. (6) Data is represented on the card using Hollerith code. (7) The corner cut is to aid in getting the cards to face in the proper direction. (From Capron and Williams, 1984.)

4. Place the cards in the hopper according to directions (usually facing forward with the nine edge down).

5. Press the *feed* button twice.

6. Keypunch your data.

7. Press the *Rel* (release) key to advance the next card for key punching.

8. Continue until all cards are completed.

If an error is made in keypunching, a new card will have to be typed to replace the one with the error on it, and your entire deck will have to be reread by the card reader to put it into the computer correctly.

Because they are sturdy, cards are fairly economical to store and use. But cards are also heavy and bulky. They take up a lot of space and are hard to carry around. They are also easy to drop or lose on a cluttered desk.

The keyboard of a computer terminal looks a lot like a typewriter's except that it has several extra keys (see Figure 16-6). It allows you to type data into the computer for processing. The com-

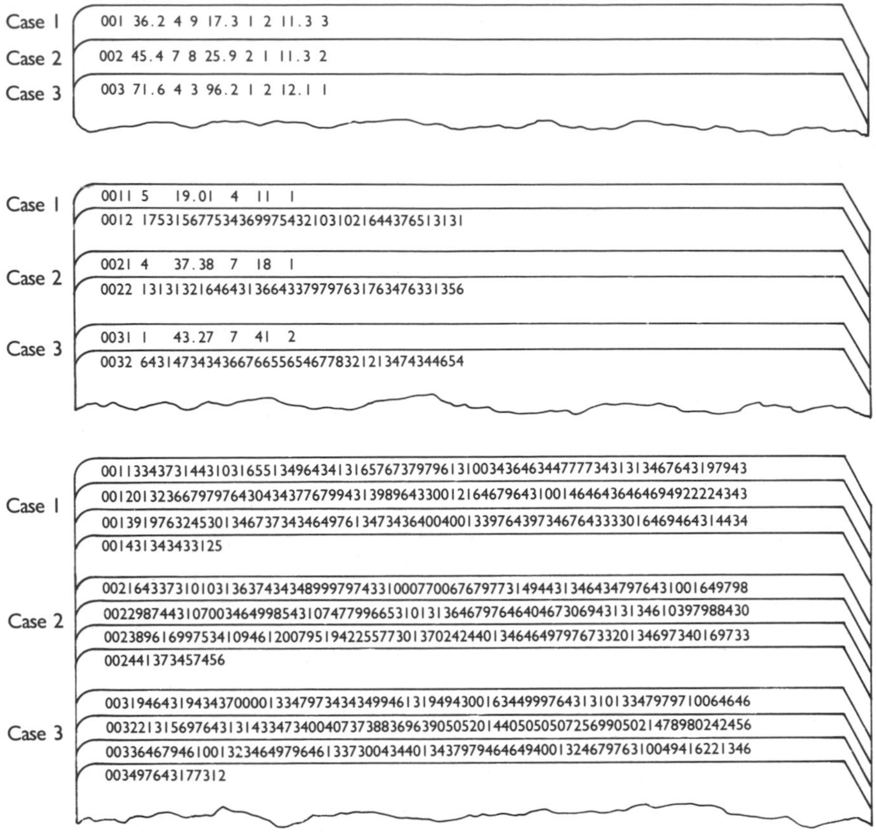

Case 1   001 36.2 4 9 17.3 1 2 11.3 3
Case 2   002 45.4 7 8 25.9 2 1 11.3 2
Case 3   003 71.6 4 3 96.2 1 2 12.1 1

Case 1   0011 5   19.01   4   11   1
          0012 1753156775343699754321031021644376513131

Case 2   0021 4   37.38   7   18   1
          0022 131313216464313664337979763176347633 1356

Case 3   0031 1   43.27   7   41   2
          0032 6431473434366766556546778321213474344654

Case 1
   0011334373144310316551349643413165767379796131003436463447777343131346764319 7943
   00120132366797976430434377679943139896433001216467964310014646436464694922224343
   001391976324530134673734346497613473436400400133976439734676433330164 69464314434
   001431343433125

Case 2
   0021643373101031363743434899979743310007700676797731494431346434797643100 1649798
   0022987443107003464998543107477996653101313464679764640467306943131346 10397988430
   00238961699753410946120079519422557730137024244013464649797673320134697340169733
   002441373457456

Case 3
   00319464319434370000133479734343499461319494300163449997643131013347979710064646
   003221315697643131433473400407373883696390505201440505050725699050214 78980242456
   0033646794610013234649796461337300434401343797946464940013246797631004941 6221346
   003497643177312

Figure 16-5 Cards in a fixed-column format.

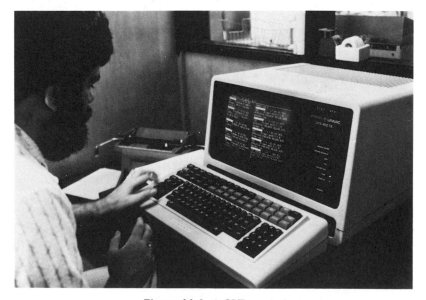

Figure 16-6 A CRT terminal.

puter also interacts with you, the user, by displaying instructions and responses on a screen called a *cathode ray tube* (CRT). This kind of two-way communication between user and computer is referred to as the *interactive mode.* Keyboards can be used to type data onto tape or disks (also called diskettes and *floppy disks*). Floppy disks look like a 45-rpm record and are encased in a heavy paper jacket (see Figure 16-7). Key-to-tape and key-to-disk methods of data input have advantages over keypunching cards; the process is quieter, and you have more control, because you can correct errors on the screen before entering the data.

There are these other advantages:

1. Tape and disks can be reused for different data, whereas punched cards cannot.

2. Records need not be limited to 80 columns.

3. Input is faster, because key-to-tape or disk is electronic, not mechanical.

4. Productivity is increased. Key strokes per hour can go up to 18,000 with a disk.

Output Devices Output transforms data into information and can appear as printing on paper (printouts), spreadsheets (a particular form of printout), color graphics, electronic signals, and sounds (see Figure 16-8).

A *printer* is a machine that produces *hard copy,* or printouts (unlike soft copy, which is output displayed on the screen). There are two types of printers, *impact printers*, which work much like a typewriter by physically striking paper, and *nonimpact printers*, which use heat, lasers, or sensitized paper. Impact printers include:

• *character printers,* which print character by character across the page from one margin to the other. The daisy wheel, consisting of a removable wheel with a set of spokes containing a raised character, is an example.

• *line printers,* which assemble all characters in a line at one time and print them out simulta-

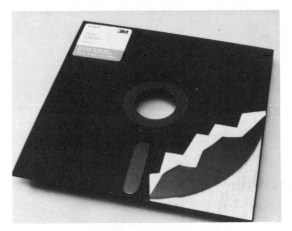

Figure 16-7 5¼ inch floppy disk.

neously. The printing can form either a solid character of *letter-quality print* or a *dot-matrix character,* which constructs a character by activating a matrix of pens that produces the shape of the character. Dot-matrix printers are both faster and cheaper than letter-quality printers.

Nonimpact printers have fewer moving parts and are quicker and faster. They include:

• *electrostatic printers,* which supply an electrical charge through the pens into the paper in the shape of the character. When passing through ink the particles stick to the charged areas of the paper producing a visible image

• *electrothermal printers,* which essentially burn the images onto the paper. You may have to buy special paper for them, and in some cases the print fades from the page over time

• *laser printers,* which reflect laser beams off of a rotating disk that contains the characters and onto the paper

• *xerographic printers,* which are a lot like photocopiers. They involve electrical transfer onto a photoconductive surface, to which ink is then applied.

1ANALYSIS OF NATIONAL PSYCHO-SOCIAL PROGRAM DESCRIPTION

FILE   NONAME   (CREATION DATE = 11/03/81)

0NATFAC
-

CATEGORY LABEL	CODE	ABSOLUTE FREQ	RELATIVE FREQ (PCT)	ADJUSTED FREQ (PCT)	CUM FREQ (PCT)
0CMHC	1.	1	6.3	6.7	6.7
0SMF	2.	1	6.3	6.7	13.3
0RESID RX FACIL	3.	3	18.8	20.0	33.3
0HALF WAY HOUSE	4.	1	6.3	6.7	40.0
0COMMUNAL GROUP HOME	6.	8	50.0	53.3	93.3
0WORKING FARM	7.	1	6.3	6.7	100.0
0	99.	1	6.3	MISSING	100.0
		------	------	------	
	TOTAL	16	100.0	100.0	

1ANALYSIS OF NATIONAL PSYCHO-SOCIAL PROGRAM DESCRIPTION

FILE   NONAME   (CREATION DATE = 11/03/81)

0NATFAC
-     CODE
          I
    1. ****** (1)
          I   CMHC
          I
          I
    2. ****** (1)
          I   SMF
          I

    3. *************** (3)
          I   RESID RX FACIL
          I
          I
    4. ****** (1)
          I   HALF WAY HOUSE
          I
          I
    6. *** (8)
          I   COMMUNAL GROUP HOME
          I
          I
    7. ****** (1)
          I   WORKING FARM
          I
          I
   99.   · (1)
 (MISSING) I
          I
          I.........I.........I.........I.........I.........I
          0   2   4   6   8   10
          FREQUENCY
0
 VALID CASES   15   MISSING CASES   1
1ANALYSIS OF NATIONAL PSYCHO-SOCIAL PROGRAM DESCRIPTION

FILE   NONAME   (CREATION DATE = 11/03/81)

Figure 16-8 Sample printout.

- *ink-jet printers*, which spray ink through an electronic field that deflects the ink and produces dot-matrix characters

For real on-line time transactions, when you are interacting with a computer, a computer *terminal*, or CRT, is best used for output as well as input. CRTs produce two major forms of output–alphanumeric and graphic. Alphanumeric terminals look like small television screens and display numbers and characters that include punctuation and dollar signs. Word processors display letters in both upper and lower case and are a type of alphanumeric terminal. Graphics terminals display colorful graphs, maps, and charts, sometimes in spectacular color. Most graphic terminals can also display alphanumeric data, but few alphanumeric terminals can also do color graphics.

As computer technology advances, additional forms of output become available. Other output devices include:

- computer output microfilm, called *microfiche*, which allows a lot of printed material to be presented in a small space
- graphics plotted on paper, using either flatbed plotters or drum plotters
- photographic graphics
- robots
- voice output devices

The Central Processing Unit (CPU)   The central processing unit is the part of the computer that corresponds to the brain (see Figure 16-9). Its function is to keep track of what is happening and execute a program that processes your data. It consists of two parts: (1) a control unit, which takes care of operating the machinery, and (2) an arithmetical–logical unit (ALU), which computes all the calculations that can be performed at hundreds of thousands per second by running an operating program. The control unit acts as an orchestra leader directing other parts of the system to execute program instructions. The

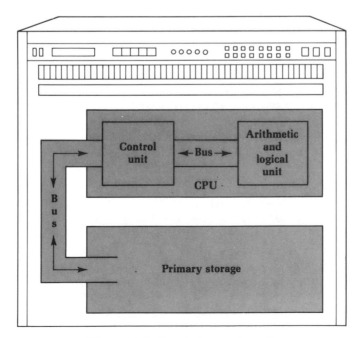

Figure 16-9 A central processing unit.

ALU controls arithmetical operations or mathematical calculations and logical operations.

Operations a computer can perform on your data include:

- calculations. A computer can add, subtract, divide, multiply 1 million problems in a second! These calculations are commonly called "number crunching."
- rearrangements. A computer can put your data into alphabetical or a numerical order.
- reading input. A computer can read 100,000 characters each minute.
- writing data onto an output unit. A computer can print out 260,000 characters each minute.
- storage. A computer can store data in its own temporary memory or transfer it to an external storage device.

There are two types of processing. *Batch processing* of your data, on the one hand, is a technique in which transactions are collected into groups, or batches, to be processed. One advantage of batch processing is that it is usually less expensive than other types of processing because it is more efficient. One disadvantage is that you have to wait for your data to be processed. *Direct access* (also called interactive) *processing*, on the other hand, is a technique for processing transactions in any order they occur. *Real-time processing* is a common form of direct access processing. It requires that your terminal be *on line*—that is, directly connected to the computer. The first advantage of real-time processing is that you don't have to wait. The second advantage is that you can continuously update your data. *Time sharing* is a system in which two or more computer users can share the use of a central computer and, because of the computer's speed, can receive simultaneous responses.

Storage The *primary storage unit* is also called main storage, internal storage, or *random access memory* (RAM), and it temporarily holds data and instructions for processing while a program is being run. A *secondary storage device* allows data to be stored outside the computer on magnetic tape, magnetic disk, or mass storage. External, secondary storage is necessary because the storage inside the computer is only temporary. Auxiliary, or secondary, storage devices allow you to store data in a far more enduring, space-saving, and convenient way than using volumes of files or shelves of boxes of keypunched card decks. The ability to store a great deal of data in a small space is one of the computer's most impressive capabilities. Characteristics of secondary storage include:

1. economy—because you save space and time in filing and retrieving data
2. reliability—because others can't tamper with or remove your data
3. convenience—because endless hours of searching through file cabinets and notebooks can be eliminated

The major types of secondary storage are (1) magnetic tape, (2) magnetic disk, and (3) mass storage.

Magnetic tape looks a lot like the tape we use on reel-to-reel tape recorders. It's about half an inch wide and is wound on a reel that's 10½ inches in diameter (see Figure 16-10). The tape has an iron oxide coating that can be magnetized. The most common length of a reel of tape is 2400 feet, and the amount of data on the tape is the number of bytes per inch or characters per inch. A customary storage capacity or density is 1600 bits per inch (bpi). High-density tape is now 6250 bpi. A magnetic tape unit can either read data onto or retrieve data from the magnetic tape, using an electromagnet that reads the magnetized areas on the tape, converts them to electrical impulses, and sends them on to the processor. Data on tape are stored sequentially. This means that your records are written onto the tape one after another. So, if you want to read case 33 of a data set, you must bypass all the preceeding cases. Capron and Williams (1984)

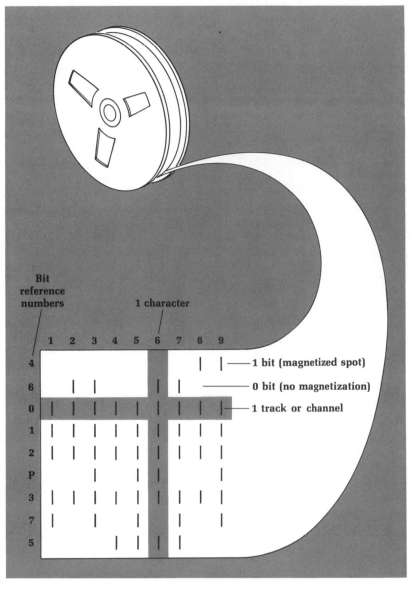

Figure 16-10 How data are represented on magnetic tape.

cite the following advantages of magnetic tape for storing your research data:

- It is compact. One 2400-foot reel of tape at 1600 bpi can hold as much as 240 boxes of punched cards, and at 2000 cards per box these boxes would completely fill a closet!
- It is reusable. Data on tape can be erased.
- It is relatively inexpensive. A 2400-foot reel of tape costs less than $15.

Despite its advantages, it still has at least two drawbacks:

- It is vulnerable to physical damage from heat, dust, stretching, and tearing.
- It is sequentially organized, and you may have to read the contents of an entire file in order to add, delete, or revise one particular record.

Magnetic disk storage is a second form of external, or auxiliary, storage. A magnetic disk is a metal platter coated with ferrous oxide that looks something like a long-playing stereo record but is usually 14 inches in diameter. Disks are grouped together in a disk pack that looks like stereo records on a spindle. Data can be retrieved much more quickly from a disk than from a tape, because the disk pack rotates over the read–write mechanism 40 times each second. Data are recorded as magnetic spots on the tracks on the surface of the disk. Disk capacity ranges from a low of 250,000 characters on a small, one-record disk to a high of 200 million on a modern disk pack. With disk storage you can go directly to the data you want at any point on the disk. This ability is called *direct access storage*. The most obvious disadvantage of using disk storage is the cost. One disk pack typically costs $300 or more. The disk storage unit can cost thousands more. Also, confidentiality may be a problem, because unauthorized persons can access your data. *Diskettes*, or floppy disks, as we have seen, are magnetically coded disks used in personal computers. They can be double-sided and hold up to half a million characters. One diskette can hold a 200-300-page term paper and costs only about four dollars.

Mass storage is the third form of secondary storage. It allows you to store large amounts of data that might have been collected, for example, in a national survey of health care needs or resources. Mass storage devices consist of honeycomblike structures that contain magnetic tapes. When data are needed a mechanical arm retrieves the cartridge from the cell and transfers the data on it to a magnetic disk. The whole process takes just 3 to 8 seconds. Some computer experts think the future of storage lies with bubble memory, because with these futuristic devices that consist of a chip coated with magnetic film, data do not disappear when the power goes off.

Software

A computer's hardware is no better than the software used with it. Software is the programs that make hardware do what you want it to do. The process of writing the series of instructions that tells the computer what to execute is called *programming*, and the person who does it is called a *programmer*. In the early days of computers a program was entered directly by punching the programming code onto cards with a card punch. These were then read into the computer, using the same card reader that would read your deck of cards containing the data set. As technology improved, computer users began to transmit instructions to the computer using an interactive system that allowed them to carry on a dialogue with the computer by typing at a terminal. Since the advent of the terminal, data sets that used to exist on cards in a card deck are now called *files*, and each lane or collection of related data items on a file is called a *record*. A *"card image record"* is still 80 characters long, corresponding to the 80 columns on a punch card.

The programs that run on big computers work like a series of Chinese boxes. While one program is running, another program is running within that program. Some programs run all the time. For example, the operating system is always translating commands from you so that the control program can handle the computer's machinery. Other programs run only when invoked by the computer user.

Programming Languages At present there are about 150 programming languages in use for communicating with and instructing the computer. Some have colorful names like Hearsay and Jovial. The most commonly used ones, however, are FORTRAN (Formula Translation), COBOL (Common Business Oriented Language), PL/1 (Programming Language One), and BASIC (Beginners' All-Purpose Symbolic Instruction Code). Pascal (named after the mathematician Blaise Pascal) and RGLII (Report Generation Language) are two others. Languages are called lower level if they are more like the language the computer uses (the binary system of zeroes and ones). Languages are called higher level if they are more like the languages people use. Following are a few illustrations of frequently used programs.

Word Processing Programs Word "processing" to most writers sounds at first like a nasty and uncreative thing to do to a word. But typing this chapter on a computer means I can simply delete mistakes electronically, stick in an idea I just thought of, move whole chunks of material to another part of the chapter with just a press of a few buttons, correct the spelling of a word throughout the whole chapter, run a thesaurus program that can provide half a dozen synonyms, check my spelling against a dictionary program, count the numbers in the chapter, and do automatic footnoting and indexing. With a special box called a *modem* (modulator–demodulator) that connects my computer to my telephone line, I can do library research or access

major data bases via the computer on numerous topics without leaving home. When I've finished writing, I press a few more buttons, and my printer prints out the manuscript in less than 1 minute per page with margins even and pages numbered.

A typical word processing program offers the following list of abilities:

- You can "word wrap." That means when you come to the end of a line, the next letter automatically begins at the start of the following line; words aren't broken.
- You can search for and replace a name or misspelled word everywhere it appears.
- You can justify margins.
- You can move pieces of the text.
- You can type over existing print.
- You can edit the portion of your paper that's displayed on the screen.
- You can view comprehensive instructions on typical computer problems without the need to refer to the manual.

The Statistical Analysis System Statistical Analysis System (SAS) is a package of programs for analyzing research data (see Chapter 15). The *Statistical Package for the Social Sciences (SPSS)* and the *Biomedical Statistical Software Package (BMDP)* are other statistical application packages. To analyze your research data by computer, you have to tell the computer what to do. The *Conversational Monitoring System (CMS)* is an interactive system that allows you to give commands to the computer that are acted on or responded to immediately. As you will recall, the interactive mode is different from batch processing, in which you give the computer your program and your data keypunched on cards and then wait until your job is executed. The interactive mode is much faster and gives you much more control over what the computer does. The following section represents one illustration of a typical procedure for using statistical programs on research data that is specific to CMS. Others are quite similar.

Using CMS to run SAS Jobs on Your Data

Step 1: Find an available computer terminal. Two of the keyboard keys are particularly important to you. The ENTER key is usually located in the same place as the carriage return key on an electric typewriter; the location of the BREAK, or ATTENTION, key varies. Until ENTER is pressed, your command is not sent to the computer. The function of the BREAK key is to be able to interrupt the computer in whatever it is processing and tell it to stop, thereby saving time and money.

Step 2: Logging on is how you gain access to a computer so that you can use it. To log on, you have to have a valid account number with the computer center, a user identification number (*USERID*), and a *password*. You get the USERID from your computer center, and you specify your own password at the time you make your application for a USERID. The password protects you from having someone else use your account without authorization. For your research course work on the computer, you will probably be given your instructor's USERID and password.

Step 3: Turn the machine on, and press ENTER. The computer will respond ENTER-CLASS.

Step 4: You then enter a number and press ENTER again. This number tells the computer which computer you want to use. After a few seconds the terminal will read: SELECT SYSTEM OR ?

Step 5: You enter the letters CMS. The system will then print: ENTER USERID.

Step 6: You enter your CMS USERID. Similarly, the computer will ask for your password. Once you have given your password and pressed ENTER, you are in the CMS Chinese box. If the information is valid, the computer will next type: READY or R, indicating that CMS is ready for your first command.

Step 7: To run any program in CMS you enter the name of the program followed by the file that contains the directions for using the program. If you wanted to view your results at your screen you would enter the word LISTING at the prompt "Type file name." If you decide that you want your output printed on paper, you can enter the PRINT command, which sends a copy of your file to a high speed printer where it is printed out. If you decide you no longer need a file on your disk, you can get rid of it with an ERASE command.

Step 8: When you have finished analyzing your data, you can quit by typing: LOGOFF. Be sure to log off when you are through, because if you walk away, you are charged for being connected to the computer. Remember, turning off a hardware terminal will *not* log you off! Box 16-1 offers you a sample session in which you are interacting with CMS at your terminal.

System Crashes Occasionally, the computer system will *crash* while you are logged on. This means that the computer is "down," or no longer running. The telling sympton is a lack of response to anything you do at your terminal. In most cases, you will be automatically logged off. Be prepared to cope with frustration, because there is nothing you can do about it if a system crash occurs.

Box 16-1   Sample Session Interacting With CMS on Your Terminal

ENTER CLASS	*(your prompt from the port selector)*
1 ⟨cr⟩	*(1 indicates you have a typewriter style terminal)*
SELECT SYSTEM OR ?	
.cms ⟨cr⟩	*(ask for cms here)*
ENTER USERID	
.cmsuser ⟨cr⟩	*(type your userid and press ⟨cr⟩)*
ENTER PASSWORD:	
.SSSSSSS ⟨cr⟩	*(enter your password and press ⟨cr⟩)*
LOGON AT 20:41:28 PST TUESDAY 09/22/81	
PUT8104C	
⟨**cr**⟩	*(enter a ⟨cr⟩ only)*
Y (19E) R/O	
R; T=0.19/0.33 20:41:36	*(you are now logged on to CMS)*
.⟨**cr**⟩	
CMS	
logoff ⟨cr⟩	*(this is the command to leave CMS)*
CONNECT=00:00:18 VIRTCPU=000:00.32 TOTCPU=000:00.82	
SESSION USE=$.07, TO DATE=$1753.45	
LOGOFF AT 20:41:49 PCT FRIDAY 9/22/81	

Research Applications of the Computer

Computers are used by nurse researchers to clean data (that is, to find keypunching errors, implausible responses, and missing data), compute the statistical procedures discussed in Chapter 15, and conduct literature searches. If you decide to use computer programs to compute statistical analysis procedures or store your research data, you ought to consult user's manuals, guides, and references to learn all the appropriate commands and computer languages. SAS can:

• create an SAS data set (that is, all the scores obtained by all the subjects in your sample) and print it out for you (see Box 16-2).

• do statistical operations or procedures (PROCS) on that data set (see, for example, the multivariate statistical procedures in Chapter 15).

Although scientists agree that SAS is probably the most powerful statistical package available, it does not have a very complete selection of nonparametric statistics (see Chapter 15), nor does it have good capacity for doing scale reliability. Some of the programs that are available with SPSS include:

1. descriptive statistics
2. frequency distributions

Box 16-2   Norbeck Data File Printout

FILE: NORBECK   DATA   A   UNIV. OF CALIFORNIA, SAN FRANCISCO

```
0011110440490500410530480450430 2333333332220000000000000 10040100000000054
00123026282523272423252727                          35555335333
0021110500510430450470460350430 2233324438800000000000000 00000000000000000
00222928282828252224122929                          33555444244
0031100400440380300350260340330 2222333333000000000000000 00000000000000000
00322615182421271427152600          5434444425
0041150750750740740740730730480 2222222213333330000000000 10000100000000013
00423030303030303030302930303026          333333333333334
0051241110780560651200751170850 2222223222333332222222222 10020100000000034
0052273015223023261521191918172122141530202323191919 5544444433332223333444444
0061080280300290210170130330270 1222233500000000000000000 10010100000000023
00622920202421070611          55531134
0071080380390370330280260350270 1223223500000000000000000 10010101000000033
00723020202930302418          55513314
0081060250220210220300230280220 1222240000000000000000000 00000000000000000
00822720252923210          555241
0091241111110840771200601160770 1222233333333333233343333 10000100000000012
0092302727272928232223262223222220222323222021212121 5554454444333344222311111
0101040200180200140200200020013 2233000000000000000000000 10000100000000013
010228282828          4423
```

SOURCE: Jane Norbeck, School of Nursing, University of California at San Francisco.

---

3. cross-tabulations
4. *t* test
5. correlations
6. scatter diagrams
7. multiple regressions
8. analysis of variances
9. factor analysis

See Box 16-3 for an example of an SPSS file printout.

Data Cleaning and Beyond

Before using a statistical package to analyze quantitative data, however, you should be sure that your data are "clean." *Data cleaning*, or finding the errors in your data, is one of the most unpopular parts of data analysis, because most people find it tedious and boring. But it can mean the difference between an otherwise fine study and disaster. Poor quality data yield poor quality results—thus the expression "garbage in, garbage out," or GIGO. The usual method for data cleaning is to run frequencies for all the scores on each item and then inspect them for the appearance of anything that is not plausible. For instance, if the possible range of scores is 1 to 5 and two cases have a 6, a keypunching error has probably been made. Once data are clean, the investigator usually asks the computer to obtain descriptive statistics or marginals on it, including measures of central tendency (mean,

Box 16-3   Norbeck SPSS File Printout

FILE: NORBECK   SPSS   A   UNIV. OF CALIFORNIA, SAN FRANCISCO

EDIT	
RUN NAME	CREATION OF NORBECK SPSSFILE FROM RAW DATA
FILE NAME	NORBECK
DATA LIST	FIXED(2)/1 IDNO 1-3 CARDNO 4 NOLISTED 5-6 AFFECT1 AFFECT2 AFFIRM3 AFFIRM4 AID5 AID6 DURATION FREQCON 7-30 SOURCE1 TO SOURCE24 32-55 LOSS LOSS1 57-58 LOSS2 TO LOSS5 59-66 LOSS6 TO LOSS9 67-70 LOSSNO 71-72 LOSSAMT 73 /2 PERSON1 TO PERSON24 5-52 CONTAC1 TO CONTAC24 54-77
INPUT MEDIUM	DISK
RECODE	IDNO TO CONTAC24 (BLANK=-1)
MISSING VALUES	IDNO TO CONTAC24 (-1)
VAR LABELS	IDNO SUBJECT NUMBER/CARDNO CARD NUMBER/NOLISTED NUMBER LISTED IN NETWORK/DURATION DURATION OF RELATIONSHIP/ FREQCON FREQUENCY OF CONTACT/LOSS RECENT LOSS/ LOSS1 LOSS SPOUSE OR PARTNER/LOSS2 LOSS FAMILY OR RELATIVES/ LOSS3 LOSS FRIENDS/LOSS4 LOSS WORK OR SCHOOL ASSOCIATES/ LOSS5 LOSS NEIGHBORS/LOSS6 LOSS HEALTH CARE PROVIDERS/ LOSS7 LOSS COUNSELOR OR THERAPIST/LOSS8 LOSS MINISTER, PRIEST,RABBI/LOSS9 LOSS OTHER/ LOSSNO NUMBER LOSS/LOSSAMT AMOUNT OF SUPPORT LOST
VALUE LABELS	SOURCE1 TO SOURCE24 (0)NONE (1)SPOUSE OR PARTNER (2)FAMILY OR RELATIVES (3)FRIENDS (4)WORK OR SCHOOL ASSOCIATES (5)NEIGHBORS (6)HEALTH CARE PROVIDERS (7)COUNSELOR OR THERAPIST (8)MINISTER,PRIEST,RABBI (9)OTHER/ LOSS (0)NO (1)YES/ LOSSAMT (1)NONE (2)A LITTLE (3)MODERATE (4)QUITE A BIT (5)A GREAT DEAL/ CONTAC1 TO CONTAC24 (1)DAILY (2)WEEKLY (3)MONTHLY (4)A FEW TIMES A YEAR (5)ONCE A YEAR OR LESS
COMPUTE	AFFECT=AFFECT1+AFFECT2
COMPUTE	AFFIRM=AFFIRM3+AFFIRM4
COMPUTE	AID=AID5+AID6
COMPUTE	TLFUNCT=AFFECT+AFFIRM+AID
COMPUTE	TLNETWRK=NOLISTED+DURATION+FREQCON
COMPUTE	TLLOSS=LOSS+LOSSNO+LOSSAMT
ASSIGN MISSING	AFFECT TO TLLOSS(-1)
SAVE FILE	

SOURCE: Jane Norbeck, School of Nursing, University of California at San Francisco.

Table 16-1   Computer Code Book for Scoring the Norbeck Social Support Questionnaire (NSSQ)

Column	Variable Name	Variable Label	Value Label
1-3	IDNO	Subject Number	—
4	CARDNO	Card Number	—
5-6	NOLISTED	Number Listed in Network	—
7-9	AFFECT1	Affect Question 1	—
12-12	AFFECT2	Affect Question 2	—
13-15	AFFIRM3	Affirmation Question 3	—
16-18	AFFIRM4	Affirmation Question 4	—
19-21	AID5	Aid Question 5	—
22-24	AID6	Aid Question 6	—
25-27	DURATION	Duration of Relationship Question 7	—
28-30	FREQCON	Frequency of Contact Question 8	—
32	SOURCE1	Source Category	
33	SOURCE2	Source Category	
34	SOURCE3	Source Category	
35	SOURCE4	Source Category	
36	SOURCE5	Source Category	
37	SOURCE6	Source Category	
38	SOURCE7	Source Category	
39	SOURCE8	Source Category	0 = none
40	SOURCE9	Source Category	1 = spouse or partner
41	SOURCE10	Source Category	2 = family or relatives
42	SOURCE11	Source Category	3 = friends
43	SOURCE12	Source Category	4 = work or school associates
44	SOURCE13	Source Category	5 = neighbors
45	SOURCE14	Source Category	6 = health care providers
46	SOURCE15	Source Category	7 = counselor or therapist
47	SOURCE16	Source Category	8 = minister/priest/rabbi
48	SOURCE17	Source Category	9 = other
49	SOURCE18	Source Category	
50	SOURCE19	Source Category	
51	SOURCE20	Source Category	
52	SOURCE21	Source Category	
53	SOURCE22	Source Category	
54	SOURCE23	Source Category	
55	SOURCE24	Source Category	
57	LOSS	Recent Loss Question 9	0 = no, 1 = yes
58	LOSS1	Loss Spouse or Partner	—
59-60	LOSS2	Loss Family or Relatives	—
61-62	LOSS3	Loss Friends	—
63-64	LOSS4	Loss Work or School Associates	—
65-66	LOSS5	Loss Neighbors	—
67	LOSS6	Loss Health Care Providers	—
68	LOSS7	Loss Counselor or Therapist	—

Table 16-1   Computer Code Book for Scoring the Norbeck Social Support Questionnaire (NSSQ) (continued)

Column	Variable Name	Variable Label	Value Label
69	LOSS8	Loss Minister/Priest/Rabbi —	
70	LOSS9	Loss Other —	
71-72	LOSSNO	Number Lost —	
73	LOSSAMT	Amount of Support Lost	0 = none
			1 = a little
			2 = moderate
			3 = quite a bit
			4 = a great deal
1-3	IDNO	Subject Number	—
4	CARDNO	Card Number	—
5-6	PERSON1	Person Total Functional	—
7-8	PERSON2	Person Total Functional	—
9-10	PERSON3	Person Total Functional	—
11-12	PERSON4	Person Total Functional	—
13-14	PERSON5	Person Total Functional	—
15-16	PERSON6	Person Total Functional	—
17-18	PERSON7	Person Total Functional	—
19-20	PERSON8	Person Total Functional	—
21-22	PERSON9	Person Total Functional	—
23-24	PERSON10	Person Total Functional	—
25-26	PERSON11	Person Total Functional	—
27-28	PERSON12	Person Total Functional	—
29-30	PERSON13	Person Total Functional	—
31-32	PERSON14	Person Total Functional	—
33-34	PERSON15	Person Total Functional	—
35-36	PERSON16	Person Total Functional	—
37-38	PERSON17	Person Total Functional	—
39-40	PERSON18	Person Total Functional	—
41-42	PERSON19	Person Total Functional	—
43-44	PERSON20	Person Total Functional	—
45-46	PERSON21	Person Total Functional	—
47-48	PERSON22	Person Total Functional	—
49-50	PERSON23	Person Total Functional	—
51-52	PERSON24	Person Total Functional	—
54	CONTAC1	Individual Contact	
55	CONTAC2	Individual Contact	
56	CONTAC3	Individual Contact	5 = daily
57	CONTAC4	Individual Contact	4 = weekly
58	CONTAC5	Individual Contact	3 = monthly
59	CONTAC6	Individual Contact	2 = a few times a year
60	CONTAC7	Individual Contact	1 = once a year or less
61	CONTAC8	Individual Contact	

continued

Table 16-1   Computer Code Book for Scoring the Norbeck Social Support Questionnaire (NSSQ) (continued)

Column	Variable Name	Variable Label	Value Label
62	CONTAC9	Individual Contact	
63	CONTAC10	Individual Contact	
64	CONTAC11	Individual Contact	
65	CONTAC12	Individual Contact	
66	CONTAC13	Individual Contact	
67	CONTAC14	Individual Contact	
68	CONTAC15	Individual Contact	5 = daily
69	CONTAC16	Individual Contact	4 = weekly
70	CONTAC17	Individual Contact	3 = monthly
71	CONTAC18	Individual Contact	2 = a few times a year
72	CONTAC19	Individual Contact	1 = once a year or less
73	CONTAC20	Individual Contact	
74	CONTAC21	Individual Contact	
75	CONTAC22	Individual Contact	
76	CONTAC23	Individual Contact	
77	CONTAC24	Individual Contact	

SOURCE: Copyright 1980 by Jane Norbeck. School of Nursing, University of California at San Francisco.

mode, and median) and measures of distribution (standard deviations, variance, and range) (see Chapter 15). In addition to descriptive statistics, most researchers ask for a list of all the data elements for each subject on a printout to be used for reference in the future.

Steps in Using a Computer on Data

Once data are cleaned, running any program or procedure on your research data will invariably involve six key steps:

1. You have to prepare your data for input into the computer, using a code book and either keypunch cards or the keyboard (see Table 16-1).
2. You will have to enter your data into the computer using your USERID and PASSWORD.
3. You will have to define your data to the statistical package you intend to use.
4. You will have to transform your data to create any new variables that you want to study.
5. You will have to run statistical procedures.
6. You will have to store your data on tape, cards, or disk or transfer them to a diskette.

Conducting a Computerized Literature Search

You are certainly aware of the value of knowing how to use the library to search the literature related to your research project (see Chapter 9). You should also know about the benefits of using the computer to search the literature. Computerized literature searches represent another major application of technology in the research process. The most frequently used computerized bibliographic service among health professionals is called *MEDLINE* (the National Library of Medicine's *Index Medicus* data base.) This system and *MEDLARS* (Medical Literature Analysis and Retrieval System) were initiated by the National Library of Medicine in 1971. Over 2700 journals are indexed in these systems. A Medline bibliography, for example, provides full journal citation including authors, article, title of journal, volume, issue, number of pages, and date. Nursing journals included in the *International Nursing Index* are available through this source.

To use the Medline search you have to select search terms that are likely to yield references that are relevant to your topic. In most cases you will be able to request such a computerized literature search through your health science library for a fee of about $30. If you are ever ambitious enough to compile a comprehensive bibliography on a topic of interest or are assigned to do so in a course, the most conscientious and scholarly approach would be to begin with a computerized search of the literature. Otherwise, it's tempting to make expedient and convenient rather than comprehensive choices (for example, including only those journals in your local School of Nursing library), a practice not recommended to the readers of this text.

Buying Your Own Personal Computer

A decision to buy a personal computer (microprocessor) should be made cautiously. The fear of being left out in the cold or the desire to be the first among equals in your research class is propelling many of us into computer stores. But once aboard, the new owner of a computer may find to his/her dismay that the eleusian light that surrounds computer equipped scientists in many of the magazine ads doesn't come with the machine! If you decide to buy a microcomputer you'll probably want to get the following standard microcomputer components:

• A keyboard
• A computer processor
• A display screen
• At least two disk drives
• A memory device
• A dot matrix or letter quality printer

If you do decide to shop for a computer let the following rules guide you:

1. "Software dictates hardware." Find the software you want, usually in the form of a 5¼ inch floppy disk, and then study the machines that run it.

2. Never betray your primary use. If you have decided you can justify the price of a computer for a particular purpose—let's say word processing—don't be distracted by secondary uses like graphics.

3. Don't buy anything until you see it work. The proverbial road test you'd demand before springing for a new car is doubly important here.

The new generation of true 16-bit personal computers is by and large a stunning rack of hardware. Each seems to have hitched its wagon to a particular and often unique capability. One is portable and another is able to make the quality charts and graphs heretofore limited to costly machines. To sum up, here are six factors to think about as you look for a personal computer.

Factors to Consider
When Buying a Personal Computer

1. **Memory** Remember, memory is measured in kilobytes (K) and megabytes (mbs). We usually figure that one K contains 1000 bytes (actually there are 1024, but even computer buffs don't quibble over 24 bytes). In 1 mb, there are 1 million letters or about a 420-page paperback. The size of your computer's memory limits what programs you can use. The internal memory of a computer has two phases—*Read Only Memory* (*ROM*) and *Random Access Memory* (*RAM*). ROM is permanent memory and contains the computer's operating systems software and assembly language. The RAM loses its contents when the power is turned off and so is called volatile working memory. When you plug in a program, its instructions are dumped into the RAM. A complex statistical program will require considerable RAM capacity. Most experts suggest that you get a minimum of 128K of RAM for analyzing research data.

2. **External Memory or Storage** Storage of data outside the computer itself is usually done on tape cassettes, floppy disks, hard disks, or video disks. Storage is also measured in kilobytes. Floppy disks file information as a series of magnetic traces. Their principal use is to store programs and feed them into your computer. You should be wary about using cassettes to store important data. Not only are they easily damaged, but they operate serially so you must wind and rewind to locate specific files. Most desktop or personal computers come with a diskette drive that holds two floppy disks—a storage disk, and an applications program disk. One diskette can store about 1 million bytes depending on size and quality.

3. **Display** This is what pops up on your screen. It can be color or monochrome (usually green or amber) and its capacity is figured by the number of characters or columns per line. The *resolution* of your display (that is, how clear and easy it is to read) is determined by the number of picture elements (pixels) it has. The more there are of them, the sharper the letters.

4. **The Keyboard** You should choose your keyboard carefully. Some are springy, some are spongy. Some keys don't move mechanically. Cheap keyboard feels mushy. Find one that gives a nice crisp sensation.

5. **Interfaces** These are the places where you attach *peripherals* such as printers or disk drives to your computer through the Input/Output (I/O) ports. The more I/O ports your computer has, the more peripherals you can use.

6. **Documentation** Documentation is the computer term for the manuals, instructions, and guides that come with your hardware and software. Read them carefully and try out some procedures before you buy. Instruction manuals that are difficult to understand can be a quick way of ruling out some computers.

Computer Costs for Research

If by choice, necessity, or virtue of the size of your data base you intend to use an institution's computer resources, you should anticipate the costs that will be involved. Three primary sources of costs related to computer-based data analysis include:

1. data coding and input
2. analysis costs (CPU and consultant time)
3. data storage on a magnetic medium

Writing proposals to obtain funding for your research will be easier if you are familiar with these costs and include them in your budget (see Chapter 8).

Data Coding and Input Costs*

The usual method of transferring data to coding sheets and keypunching them onto cards is rather costly. Coding assistance generally costs $5 to 7 per hour, and keypunched cards approximately 20 to 30¢ each if verified (i.e., 100 cases with 50 variables might cost in the range of $50 to 75). This cost can be reduced if the keypunching can be done directly from the data sheets. Keypunching is the most accurate method for large data sets with many variables, particularly if they have a number of different values (integer, decimal, alpha, etc.) in the same data set.

A less expensive method for data input comprised of only a few variables is direct entry, using a terminal or microcomputer. The costs include the research assistant's time for inputting the data, and $1.00 per hour connect time for CMS or UNIX (i.e., 100 cases with 50 variables would cost approximately $20). The charge for connect time is almost eliminated using a microcomputer, because entry can be done and verified by the microcomputer, then it can be connected and uploaded to the mainframe system. This requires a training session for the data entry person. For longitudinal studies, data entry programs can be written for the microcomputers.

* SOURCE: Adapted from Computer Resources, University of California School of Nursing, San Francisco, 1983.

Data Analysis Costs

These generally involve the use of one or more of the major statistical packages available on the computer center mainframe system (SPSS, SAS, BMDP, etc.). Estimating computer costs for analysis largely depends on whether the project calls for a specific single analysis or an exploratory approach. Secondary analyses fall into the exploratory category, usually involving a series of computer runs through the data.

For single analysis on a relatively small number of cases and variables (e.g., a t test on two groups of twenty subjects on two different variables) a hand calculator can be used. It is useful to have the data keypunched or entered onto computer tape in case other analyses are needed. The keypunching for this example would cost about $15.00.

A large-scale project will involve a number of computer runs to clean the data, test preliminary hypotheses, specify subsamples, debug the programs, and run the various statistical analyses. The total cost would be in the range of $100 for: storage, CPU, and print charges for a final printout of each of the analyses listed. Note that a ratio of about 10 to 1 for final cost versus single run cost is a good estimator for a project involving a number of different computational analyses (crosstabs, regressions, ANOVAs, etc.). This is not a good formula for analyses with a large number of cases and complex statistical procedures (factor analysis, multivariate procedures). In general, those analyses are expensive, often costing several hundred dollars when done with complex data sets.

Note also the difference in cost between the statistical packages. There is often a considerable difference for the same analysis, due to different computational procedures used in the computer. *The best resource for the choice of statistical package is a data analysis consultant.*

A cost-cutting method, which can be used for expensive analyses, is the processing of large computer runs during night and weekend hours, when the cost is reduced by 80%. This can be a very significant saving, although it requires more attention by a programmer who is familiar with the computer system, in order to schedule delayed program execution. A recent School of Nursing dissertation required a factor analysis costing almost $100 per run at regular rates. Weekend runs saved the project a large amount, with only a small delay in the amount of time required for the full analysis.

The final factor involved in project analysis costs is the cost of the statistical consultant. Consultation is based on a per-hour charge. Most projects should include at least 1 to 2 hours of consultation for initial planning and at least 2 to 4 hours for data analysis. This should be increased if the consultant is to do the actual programming and if multiple analyses are planned. A typical project might involve several hours of consultant time spread over a number of days or weeks, as successive analyses are per-formed. Invariably, unforeseen problems arise during data analysis for large research projects, which add to the consultant time. *In general, at least 2 to 4 consultant hours should be included in grant proposals, and frequently more is advisable.*

Data Storage Costs

Tapes are the least costly method of storage. A standard 2400-foot tape is more than sufficient for storage of all raw data, statistical programs, and computer system files until they are needed for future analysis.

On-line CMS minidisk storage is approximately $10 per month for most situations. Because of the expense, this is not recommended for long-term storage unless easy and immediate access to the raw data and statistical programs is needed at all times.

Computer People

Computer people include data entry people, computer operators, librarians, programmers, and system analysts. If you are a novice with no prior computer experience, you should turn to the experts for consultation and assistance.

- *Data entry people* put data on cards, disks, or tape for processing.
- *Computer operators* monitor the console, review procedures, and keep peripheral equipment such as printers running.

- *Librarians* are in charge of cataloging processed disks and tapes and keeping them secure.
- *Computer programmers* design, write, test, and implement programs.
- *System analysts* know about programming but have broader responsibilities that include planning and designing whole systems of programs, based on a clear understanding of users' requirements.

Summary of Key Ideas and Terms

- American Standard Code for Information Interchange (ASCII, pronounced "asky") is a standard code that assigns specific bit patterns to the alphanumeric characters on your keyboard. Example: the letter *E* is coded as "1000101."

- Beginner's All-Purpose Symbolic Instruction Code (BASIC) is the most popular personal computer language. Some other languages include Pascal, Ada, Logo, C, FORTRAN (Formula Translation), and COBOL (Common Business Oriented Language).

- *Baud* refers to speed of data transmission rate of a modem.

- Board or card is a rectangular (usually green) piece of hardware inside the computer that the chips and circuits are mounted on. Several boards can be attached to a chassis called a mother-board. Well-designed boards are said to have good architecture.

- To *boot* is to load a program into a computer.

- Any defect or malfunction in hardware or software is called a *bug*.

- Control Program for Microcomputers (CPM) is a popular disk operating system for 8-bit machines.

- The speed of a printer is measured in characters per second (cps).

- Cathode ray tube (CRT) is the screen on the computer, also called a monitor. The more pixels—individual points of light—it has, the easier it is on the eyes.

- Documentation is the printed information available for software and hardware. With any luck, these manuals are user-friendly—that is, easy to understand. Hardware that's designed with human comfort in mind is *ergonomic*.

- The typefaces on a *dot-matrix printer* are composed of tiny dots. A *letter-quality printer* uses either a daisy wheel or thimble mechanism to make typewriterlike typefaces.

- *Dual processors* are systems or boards that have two 8-bit chips, which "access" 8 bits of information at a time. Most software on the market is written for dual processors, but they support a maximum RAM of only 64K. The newer 16-bit processors are faster and can handle up to 1 megabyte of RAM.

✔ Input–output (I/O) devices can be hooked up to your computer, such as a printer or a modem that connects to your telephone line. These are called *peripherals*.

✔ A personal microcomputer that works as a stand-alone machine is an *intelligent terminal*. A dumb terminal is one of many terminals hooked up to a giant mainframe computer.

✔ MegaHertz (MHZ) refers to the speed of microprocessors in millions of cycles per second. When the performances of the two different machines are compared, the test is a benchmark.

✔ A computer system consists of three areas: input, processing, and output; they are backed by a fourth area—storing data.

✔ Operations that a computer can perform on data include calculations, rearrangements, input, output, and storage.

✔ Statistical Analysis System (SAS), the Statistical Package for the Social Sciences (SPSS), and Biomedical Statistical Package (BMDP) are the major software programs used to compute statistical analyses of nursing research data.

✔ Finding errors in data by "data cleaning" can mean the difference between a good and poor analysis.

✔ Nurse researchers also use the computer to conduct literature searches.

✔ Consultation with resource people in your computer center will help you achieve a realistic estimate of computer costs involved in conducting a research study.

✔ Buying a personal computer should be done thoughtfully, keeping in mind the purposes that it will serve.

References

Capron HL, Williams BK: *Computers and Data Processing*, 2nd ed. Menlo Park, Calif.: Benjamin/Cummings, 1984.

Computer Resources. University of California School of Nursing, San Francisco, 1983.

Further Readings

Abrams MD, Stein PG: *Computer Hardware and Software—An Interdisciplinary Introduction.* Reading, Mass.: Addison-Wesley, 1976.

Banks PM, Doupnik JR: *Introduction to Computer Science.* New York: Wiley, 1976.

Boraiko AA: The chip: Electronic mini-marvel that is changing your life. *National Geographic* October 1982; 162:421–476.

Edmunds L: Teaching nurses to use computers. *Nurse Educator* Autumn 1982; 7:32–38.

French N, Parrett, T: Information is power. *Savvy* November 1982: 54–79.

Hedberg A: Choosing the best computer for you. *Money* November 1982: 68–117.

Jacobsen BS: Know thy data. *Nurs Res* 1981; 30:254–255.

McElmurry BJ, Newcomb BJ: Clarification of the database concept. *Nurs Res* 1981; 30:155.

Nie NH et al: *Statistical Package for the Social Sciences.* New York: McGraw-Hill, 1975.

Stern R, Stern N: *Principles of Data Processing*, 2nd ed. New York: Wiley, 1975.

Van Gelder L: A few systems. *Ms* February 1983: 37–42.

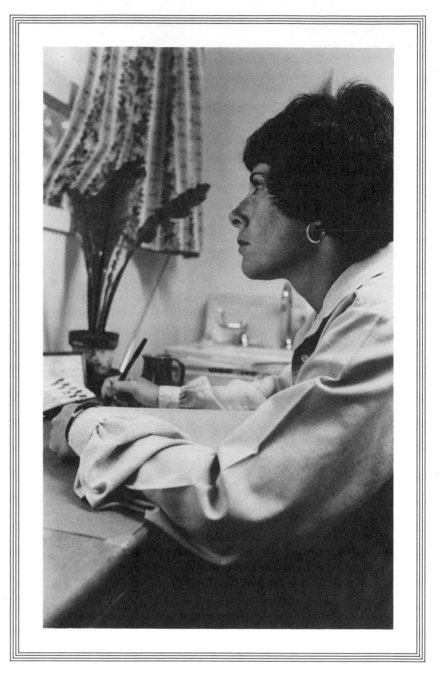

"Why publish? Because the future of the profession depends on it."

M. M. Styles (1978)

4

Scholarly and Intellectual Craftsmanship in Nursing

Chapter 17

Disseminating Research

The Scholar's Commitment

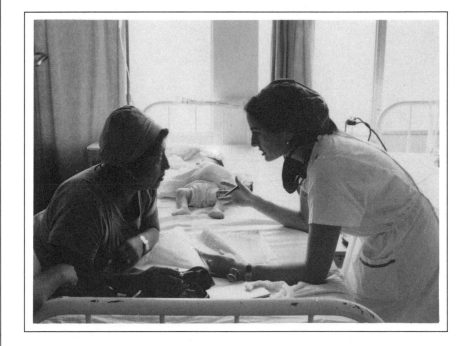

Preparing a scientific speech or a scholarly article is not an easy task. They involve thinking and communicating, clearly and effectively. And both are essential, if we are to build a scientific basis for nursing practice.

Chapter Outline

Objectives

After reading this chapter, the student should be able to:

- Compare and contrast oral presentations with journal writing or book writing as options for disseminating research findings
- Organize and execute journal articles, theses and dissertations, or speech scripts according to basic assumptions that promote a clear, readable style
- Choose words with precision, avoiding ambiguity, jargon, and unnecessary words
- Assemble essential writing aids
- Plan for effective use of visual aids in a professional speech
- Formulate strategies for effective speaking delivery
- Anticipate techniques for fielding questions when giving a talk
- Evaluate his or her own oral presentations as well as those of others
- Design a focused and organized outline for a research paper
- Take steps to avoid rejection of an article by journal editors
- Write a good query letter
- Evaluate issues that arise when two or more authors collaborate
- Compose concise, specific, informative, and interesting article titles and leads
- Work quotations into manuscripts smoothly
- Differentiate plagiarism from paraphrasing
- Prepare tables and figures according to accepted guidelines
- Apply accepted criteria for writing the sections of a research report
- Discuss initial considerations in negotiating with a publisher to publish a book
- Advocate the value of disseminating research through writing and speaking

In This Chapter . . .

The only way the information produced through your scientific work can contribute to the emerging body of knowledge in nursing or become part of the basis for making clinical decisions is for you to report your results, your methods, and your conclusions to others. You can do this by writing a thesis or dissertation, a book, a journal article, or a technical report or by giving a talk at a professional meeting. This chapter will suggest rules, techniques, and illustrations for making your scientific writing and speaking clearer and better. Preparing a formal speech and producing scholarly writing are not easy. Thinking effectively and clearly can be laborious. When you sit down to write, you may need an act of will to push yourself over the gap between you and the page. Having specific skills will certainly help you do that.

This chapter encourages you to view writing (including the preparation of a script for a speech) as involving a three-step process:

1. *prewriting*, when you gather together your materials, take notes, and put your ideas into some beginning form or structure such as a detailed outline

2. *writing*, when you sharpen the tone and style in which you express your thoughts by writing a first draft

3. *rewriting*, when you edit and try to get the most coherent expression that you can, keeping the development of your ideas clear and organized

Guidelines for writing and speaking that you will encounter in this chapter are based on the simple premise that dealing with the theoretical or scientific in your writing and speaking need not work against the goal of communicating your thoughts clearly. As Mirin (1981) suggests, the purpose of scientific writing is communication, not art, "but the basic principles of good writing apply to all writing" (p. 2).

This chapter takes you from start to finish through the steps and considerations involved in either preparing and publishing a manuscript based on your research or planning and presenting a talk in a professional or other forum. It not only considers some of the subtleties of the social psychology required in disseminating research but also addresses questions as specific as "How do I find potential outlets for my work?" "What makes a good query letter?" "What is the general format for a thesis? a scientific article?" "What goes into each section?" "How do I work quotations in smoothly?" "What are the characteristics of effective figures and tables?" "What makes for a good delivery in an oral presentation?" "What are the criteria for quality visual aids?" "What bugs journal editors?" "How do I go about getting a book published?" "What about authorship and copyrights?"

When Styles (1978) was asked why nurses should write for publication, she replied, "Because the future of the profession depends on it" (p. 28). Unless nurses publish, the body of knowledge unique to nursing cannot grow and develop.

Options for Disseminating Research

Two major options exist for disseminating your research results, procedures, and insights. You can write about them, or you can talk about them. Most of us realize that many scholars do

both. Saslow (1982) points out that the advantage of speeches at professional or scientific meetings is that they *promptly inform* an audience about your work even while it's in progress and prompt others to tell you what they think. Articles, books, technical reports, theses, and the like both serve as a *more permanent and complete record* of your work and are also *available to a wider audience.*

A talk obviously has the advantage of obtaining reactions from an interested audience that can stimulate your own thinking about your research. For example, long before I succeeded in having a paper published in the scientific literature about bridging the gap between standard psychiatric diagnostic nomenclature and the nursing diagnosis movement, I had delivered numerous presentations and speeches on it that helped me refine my emerging ideas. Talks can

range from relatively informal presentations in classes for colleagues as part of a colloquium series to formal presentations before a professional organization. In the latter case you must first locate a "call for abstracts" that gives you the guidelines and length limitations for an abstract (see Box 17-1). Next, you have to submit one. And finally, if your abstract is accepted by the program planning committee, you will be scheduled on the program for what is usually a 15- to 30-minute oral presentation.

Written reports of your scientific work create a resource for a much broader audience, but the publication schedules of most professional journals may mean that a year passes before your

---

Box 17-1   American Nurses' Association Council of Nurse Researchers

Guide for Abstract Preparation

Abstracts are to be submitted in duplicate, typewritten and single-spaced on the forms provided. Both pages of the presentation application are to be completed.

Abstracts to be considered for paper presentations and symposia must be of completed research—completed as of the date the abstract is submitted. All abstracts for a specific symposium must be submitted together. Also, the organizer (moderator) for the symposium must submit a face sheet for the presentation application which includes the name, address, and telephone number of the symposium organizer, titles of all abstracts, and a brief summary (100 words) of the overall symposium. Poster presentations may be of either completed or ongoing research.

The summary of the research (250–300 words and must not exceed space provided in the presentation application) is to include:

1. the purpose of the study
2. the design
3. a description of the subjects, including sample size
4. methods of data collection
5. methods of data analysis
6. major findings
7. major conclusions

The investigator who is invited to present a paper at this nursing research meeting will be asked to provide one copy of the paper at ANA 30 days prior to the conference date.

Paper presentations will be limited to one presenter per paper although coauthors of the paper will be acknowledged in

the conference program. Multiple authors may participate in the poster presentations. All presenters will be expected to register for the conference in accordance with the registration procedures established for the conference. Presenters will *not* be reimbursed for expenses for attending the conference.

All paper presenters, primary poster presenters, and symposium organizers must be members of the ANA Council of Nurse Researchers.

Presentation applications should be sent to:

Research and Policy Analysis Department
American Nurses' Association
2420 Pershing Road
Kansas City,
   Missouri   64108
Attention: Dorothy Young

SOURCE: American Nurses' Association, Council of Nurse Researchers, 1982.

findings are available to a nursing readership. Publishing a book or monograph based on your research takes even longer, with approximately 10 months or so required by the publisher for the production phase after you have handed over the completed manuscript. Although the full-length research article (see Chapter 2) is the most common outlet that nurse researchers use for publishing a written account of their work, brief reports, letters to the editor, and abstracts also permit publication of aspects of your research that don't require a full-scale presenta-tion. Of course, written accounts of your scientific work can also take the form of technical progress and final reports required by funding agencies. You may also write a thesis or dissertation, a scholarly treatise in which you present detailed evidence of scientific knowledge and expertise. (Sample guidelines appear in Box 17-2.) Before discussing the three main means for disseminating your ideas—the speech, the journal article, and the book—let's consider a few general assumptions basic to all writing or speaking about your research.

General Guidelines for Presentations

Awareness of certain key principles is basic to preparing any written or oral presentation of your research.

1. Write for Strangers

Don't assume that your audience or readers know what you are talking about or that they will take the time or the energy to make sense of what you are saying. Writing *for* somebody (your audience), and *as* somebody (from a point of view), is what makes writing worth reading and speeches worth hearing. A writer who can achieve the appropriate relationship to his or her audience has mastered the art of creating the proper tone. Achieving an appropriate tone represents taking a big step toward the kind of clear and ordered thinking and writing that defines good scientific work. Remember that the worth of a talk or article is measured by what the audience or reader carries away, not by what the speaker or author puts out. If you present findings about nursing strategies that can decrease the pain associated with intramuscular injections to a general nursing audience in esoteric and obscure terms that require highly specialized knowledge, you severely limit those whom your work will reach. In the case of a general nursing audience, "plain English has a lot to recommend it" (Saslow 1982, p. 325). In the case of an audience of nurse researchers be wary of making the tone condescending, overly emotional, or so technical that the important points are lost.

2. Get Off to a Good Start

Some writers and speakers find it easier to get started on a research report by getting some ideas on paper quickly, even in outline form, believing that they can always edit and polish the word choice and grammar later. Others construct their manuscripts or speeches like a brick wall, needing to feel that one section is perfect before building on it or developing from it. Some authors schedule their writing projects in big blocks of intense time that might involve writing 3000 words or 15 pages or 15 hours each day. Others chip away at an article or speech in 2-hour time slots early in the morning before going to work, late into the night, or between children's naps. Olson (1972) offers these strategies for getting started:

Box 17-2   Dissertation/Thesis Guidelines

A. *Chapter Outline*

1. Introduction: The study problem
   A. Introduction to problem and subproblems (What led you to choose this problem?)
   B. Statement of the problem
   C. Purpose(s) of the study
   D. Need for the study (significance)

2. Literature review and conceptual framework
   A. Overview of relevant research directly related to your problem
   B. Conceptual or theoretical framework (discussion of theoretical framework underlying study and operational description of concepts) (A and B may be reversed)
   C. Assumptions
   D. Research questions and/or hypotheses
   E. Definition of terms

3. Methodology
   A. Research design
   B. Description of research setting (if relevant)
   C. Sample
      1. Human subjects assurance
      2. Nature and size of sample
      3. Criteria for sample selection
   D. Data collection methods
      1. Techniques (observation, interview, instruments, chart audit)
      2. Instruments or apparatus
         a. Description
         b. Reliability and validity
   E. Procedure
   F. Data analysis

4. Results
   A. Preliminary analyses, if relevant (sample characteristics, data reduction techniques)
   B. Analysis of hypotheses or research questions
   C. Other findings

5. Discussion
   A. Meaning of findings in relation to hypotheses or research questions
   B. Significance
   C. Limitations
   D. Implications for nursing
   E. Future research

Box 17-2   (continued)

B. *Standard Format for Dissertation Organization*
Every page must be numbered (including illustrative material) and appear in the order indicated below:

Title page	Not numbered
Copyright page (optional)	Not numbered
Abstract	Numbered with separate pagination (1,2,3)
Preliminary material (dedication, acknowledgments, table of contents, list of tables, list of figures)	Numbered with lower-case roman numerals (i, ii, iii, iv)
Main body of text (chapters with tables and figures incorporated at the appropriate point in the text)	Numbered with arabic numerals
References	Numbered with arabic numerals continued from text
Appendixes	Numbered with arabic numerals continued from references

Logical subcategories under each chapter heading should be developed, following the hierarchy for heading types outlined on page 32 of the APA Manual. Detailed guidelines for developing tables and figures are presented on pp. 43–55 of the APA Manual.

C. *Format for Copyright Page and Abstract Page*

1. Copyright page

TITLE OF DISSERTATION (ALL CAPS)
Copyright © 19xx (year)
by
(Your name as it appears on the title page)

2. Abstract

TITLE OF DISSERTATION (ALL CAPS)
Jane Doe, R.N., Ph.D.
University of the United States, 19xx (year)
(triple space)
Text of abstract (double space) . . . . , etc.

1. Find a place in which to write, and guard it with your life. Words abhor crowds.

2. Write regularly; don't wait for the crack of the whip (or the pressure of an organization's or publisher's deadline).

3. Tell your story once, and tell it on paper.

4. Whenever possible, write about subjects that truly interest you. Bored writers produce bored readers.

5. Remember that getting started is half the battle.

3. Pay Attention to Writing Style

The aim of research reporting is to communicate fully, precisely, and clearly. A well-written manuscript should leave no doubt about what you did, why you did it, what you found, and what your findings imply. Most journals expect authors to use a standard outline format for research articles (see Box 17-3). One of the main reasons for this preference is so that readers can locate aspects of the article quickly and evaluate them without having to plow through all the details. Generally, poetic rhythms, stream of consciousness, personal or original use of words, and entertainment are not encouraged in scientific reporting. Writing according to the standards of scientific writing, however, does not mean that style and technique are irrelevant. They are just as important in scholarly and scientific writing as they are in creative writing. In fact, as Saslow (1982) says, "It takes a good deal of ingenuity to be clear and precise without being dull and repetitive" (p. 328). Although a number of authorities continue to preach that

---

Box 17-3   Typical Format for a Research Report

I. Front Matter
   A. Title page
      1. Title of study
      2. Authors' names
      3. Date

II. Table of Contents
   A. Chapters
   B. Bibliography
   C. Appendixes

III. Sections of the Paper
   A. The research problem
      1. Introduction to the problem
      2. Significance of the problem
      3. Purpose of the study
      4. Scope of the study
   B. Review of the literature (Divide into subheadings as necessary)

C. Conceptual or theoretical framework (Divide into subheadings as necessary)
D. Methodology
      1. Design
      2. Definition of variables
      3. Sampling
      4. Setting
      5. Extraneous variables
E. Data collection
      1. Method and rationale
      2. Results of pilot study
      3. Reliability and validity
F. Data analysis
      1. Method and rationale

G. Results
      1. Presentation of tables and graphs
      2. Interpretation of results
H. Discussion
      1. Summary
      2. Conclusions
      3. Implications for nursing
      4. Recommendations for further study and limitations

Appendixes
   Copy of consent form
   Copy of instruments
   Copy of tally or code sheets
   Correspondence

without exception scientific reports must use the third person and passive voice ("It was found by the investigators that . . ." instead of "We found that . . ."), this old rule is giving way to generally agreed-upon standards of good writing. The so-called "objective" third person and passive voice are no guarantee that the research itself was objective and met the standards of validity and reliability. Lewis, former editor of *Nursing Outlook*, charges that the syndrome of pretentious prose in nursing literature puts unnecessary obstacles between the writer and the reader, makes readers dig for meaning, and impairs communication in a profession that needs a free and comprehensible exchange of ideas and findings on so many subjects. She illustrates her point by referring to an array of phrases scattered throughout nursing manuscripts, and we can add our own: a burgeoning mandate, a plethora of logistics, a conceptually meaningful wholeness, finalization of the implementation of the program, operationalize, in terms of, with reference to, the fact of the matter is, as to whether, and so on. Trust your own voice. Try to avoid affectations and hackneyed expressions. It's easy to fall into a formal, stilted style and forget that your real goal is *logical and lucid language*. Make your writing lean, direct, and specific.

4. Organize

The approach of many novice writers when they sit down to write is what some experts have called "the buckshot approach." This involves scattering your presentation and ideas as diffusely as you can and hoping that you'll hit some of the audience with some of your points, some of the time. The result is disjointed, incoherent writing. The way to avoid this approach is not necessarily, however, to report on your study in exactly the same time sequence as it was conducted, nor to rely on the old standby of "an Introduction, a Body, and a Conclusion." In-

stead, you must, first, *let your thoughts dictate your words*, and second, *develop your paragraphs and sentences by looking backward and thinking of yourself as adding to what you've already done*. This is called organizing your writing according to a *generative rhetoric*, in which you are clear about the focus of your paragraph and about developing and refining what has come before. Once a topic is introduced, subsequent sentences should make the logical support of or development of that topic clear. Subheadings take up more space in a manuscript, but they help to keep the writer from wandering off the topic and help to make the manuscript clear and orderly for the reader as well. A well-organized speech or article should carry the listener or reader smoothly from one topic to another. This is usually handled by designing paragraphs that are neither one sentence long nor lengthy and rambling. Each paragraph should begin with a topic sentence that provides for its focus, and the rest of the paragraph should be related to development of that topic. As you move from one paragraph to the next, you should provide your reader with logical transitions.

5. Avoid Jargon

Because the goal of scientific speaking and writing is clear and precise communication, the words you choose should mean exactly what you intend. Colloquial expressions, pompous circumlocutions, ambiguity and hackneyed clichés are rarely effective ways to convey meaning. Too much writing in nursing literature seems indifferent to meaning. Begin by omitting unnecessary, extraneous words. Strunk and White (1972) and others offer the following rules for vigorous, concise word usage:

• Choose a suitable design or format, and stick to it.

Box 17-4   Examples of Writing Sparely

Wordy or Formal Usage	Concise Substitute	Wordy or Formal Usage	Concise Substitute
acquire	get	continue on	continue
add an additional	add	despite the fact that	although
any and all	any (or) all	during the course of	during
as to why	why	each and every one	each
at the present time	now	for the reason that	because
be acquainted with	know	in a manner similar to	like
commence	start	in all probability	probably

SOURCE: Adapted from R. B. Ward, "Fog and How to Fight It," in *Practical Technical Writing*, New York: Knopf, 1968, pp. 27–28.

- Make the paragraph the unit of composition, and use it to keep the development of your ideas orderly.
- Use the active voice rather than the passive voice.
- Put statements in a positive rather than negative form.
- Use definite, specific, concrete language.
- Omit needless words, including those illustrated in Box 17-4.
- Avoid the verb form *to be* and its variations like *there are* as much as possible. Select vivid, forceful verbs.
- Substitute a simple, familiar word for two complex, obscure ones.

Finally, remember that scientific writing requires an extraordinary attention to consistency and precision in the choice of words. Once a concept or variable is defined in a particular way, substituting synonyms or approximations is less acceptable in research writing than in other expository forms. For example, in reporting a study of social support and self-care among the chronically mentally ill, it would not be acceptable to casually substitute *social network* or *support system* for the concept *sources of social support* unless you defined them to mean precisely the same thing from the start.

6. Read Widely and Use Writing Aids

Most good writers and speakers like to read. They read for ideas, for style, for information, and to avoid duplicating the work of others. In Lewis's words, "In a profession constantly seeking new knowledge or at least seeking to build on and expand existing knowledge, we can't afford to keep on inventing or rediscovering the same old wheel." Reading keeps you informed of what others are doing in your area of research. Reading what is published in a particular journal alerts you to the publisher's preferences about length limitations, tone, placement of footnotes, references, use of illustrations and tables, and the characteristics of the readership. Reading can help you overcome obstacles presented by the need to include carefully and correctly prepared bibliographies, footnotes, tables, figures, and other mechanical details. All writers and speakers should compile, read, and refer to the following writing aids.

- a good style manual, such as Turabian's (1973) *Manual for Writers*, that covers such subjects as spelling and punctuation, capitalization, underlining, quotations, footnotes, bibliographies, tables, illustrations, abbreviations, and numbers as well as the parts of term papers, theses, and dissertations. *Publication Manual* of the American Psychological Association (1983), Linton's (1972) *A Simplified Style Manual*, and the little classic on this subject, Strunk and White's (1972) *Elements of Style* are additional examples.
- a good general dictionary. Although there is no such thing as *the* dictionary, there is a difference between a dictionary that is newly compiled and kept up to date by experts working with a recent accumulation of recorded word usages and a dictionary that is patched together from older word books. The following ones are good choices: *American College Dictionary*, revised edition (Random House), *American Heritage Dictionary of the English Language* (Houghton Mifflin), *Random House Dictionary of the English Language*, *Webster's New World Dictionary of the American Language* (World), and *Webster's New Collegiate Dictionary* (Merriam).
- a historical dictionary. *The Oxford English Dictionary*, in 12 volumes and a supplement, is the greatest storehouse of information about English words. It traces the various forms of each word and its various senses, with dates and quotations from other writers to illustrate each sense.
- a specialized nursing dictionary. The McGraw-Hill *Nursing Dictionary* (1979) is a current and relatively comprehensive choice.
- indexes for locating health science literature and computerized data bases (see Chapter 2). Most good libraries provide a variety of services for locating information already available in health science literature. Your library may be able to obtain copies of articles or books through an interlibrary loan system when the source you seek is not part of its own collection. You may also find that your library has special collections and microfilm files and will conduct computer searches. *Consult your reference librarian regularly.*
- a medical dictionary. Taber's (1981) and Dorland's (1981) are two useful ones.

Reading for the pure joy of it is probably a habit for most writers. But reading manuscript and publication guidelines, articles and books that reflect the state of the art in your area of interest, and resources that represent helpful tools is a professional obligation. Reading does not guarantee that you will become a good writer any more than exposure to fine paintings means you will become an artist. But reading is probably the most valuable formative influence on a writer.

Giving a Talk at a Professional Meeting

Before you ever see your research in print, it's highly likely that you will take the opportunity to present it in part or in full to an audience at a professional or scientific meeting.

Organization

The organization of a report of research findings in a journal customarily follows the format

---

Box 17-5   Ways of Developing Ideas

1. Conjunction (chronology; spatial description): "The stages of wound healing are as follows."

2. Disjunction (separation; mutually exclusive alternatives; comparison and contrast): "Group strategies that are helpful in fostering a client's ability to work through the death of a parent differ for preschoolers and adolescents."

3. Concession (acknowledgment and additional line of thought): "Though the statistical significance of results in this research was inconclusive, the clinical significance leads us to the following suggestions."

4. Condition (interdependent relations): "If the public image of nursing improves and becomes more realistic, we can expect the following shifts in third-party reimbursement policies."

---

presented in Box 17-3, leaving results and discussion to the end. Many speakers, however, start their talk by calling attention to their findings and then follow with supporting evidence and essential methodological and statistical details. Beginning in this way catches the interest and attention of your audience, and including appropriate evidence convinces them that your research was carried out in a competent manner. At the end you can again summarize your findings. Ideas about your findings can be developed in a number of ways. Box 17-5 offers four possibilities.

Visual Aids

Most oral presentations are improved by the use of slides, overhead transparencies, and handouts. Here are some guidelines for preparing these materials.

1. Allow enough lead time for their production.
2. Keep them simple. It's probably a good idea to seek consultation from your institution's media resource department for specifics about just how many lines can effectively go on a single slide or transparency.
3. Make sure they are designed so that your audience can understand them. Remember that tables and graphs often contain printed headings or labels and that an audience must be able to read them from the back of the room. Don't try to cram too much information onto one visual, use extra-large type for labels, and be sure that any symbols or line drawings are clear and distinct.

Delivery

Don't read your paper. It's boring. The result of reading a speech or other oral presentation is often to deliver too much information too fast, because you are unable when busily reading your paper to pick up visual cues from your audience that it isn't following or would love some elaboration or an illustration.

On the other hand, don't count on being extemporaneously fluent. Write out, at minimum, a beginning and closing statement and a detailed outline on a set of notes to which you can refer if your mind goes blank due to performance anxiety. Keep to the sequence and order of your notes, glancing at them as you need to. Avoid the temptation to jump back to revisit an idea that you missed. Don't staple pages together. Turning them by page flipping can be distracting to others.

If you have mistimed the length of your speech or paper and have to omit a section to keep within your allotted time, do so smoothly and unobtrusively without worrying out loud about "running out of time" or talking about all the sections you are having to leave out. Making these blunders only costs you your stage presence, makes the audience feel cheated, and results in the impression that you were poorly organized or poorly prepared.

Never begin a speech or presentation by discrediting your qualifications on the subject at hand, your speaking ability, or your composure by saying, "I'm really nervous" or "I don't know why my work on this topic was selected" or "I despise speaking before audiences." Begin instead with an acknowledgment of the significance of the occasion, a clever anecdote, or some other opening line that piques the interest of the audience.

Always make notes on your script or outline to indicate the place where you intend to use transparencies or slides. This allows you to direct the audience's attention to them even if you can't see the screen from where you are speaking. It also allows you to ask for them from whoever may be operating the equipment. It's not a bad idea to have at least two copies of your referenced script so that your audio–visual assistant can read along with your presentation and anticipate technical matters.

Rehearse, preferably in front of a mirror and with a clock. Practicing your speech makes it familiar and smooth. Timing it allows you to be realistic about how long it takes to deliver various sections of it. A typed page generally takes 2 or 3 minutes to present, so a 30-minute speech should be around 12 pages. Practice also decreases the likelihood that nervousness will cause you to make automatic gestures that may be distracting to your audience. Practicing on the same day as your presentation is a particularly good idea.

Talk to your audience. Use eye contact, timing, and other speaking strategies such as inserted examples or asides to humanize your presentation. Look around the room at responsive members of the audience for signs of positive

feedback, expressions of boredom and fatigue, or messages that you aren't being clear—or even heard. Knowing as much as possible about your audience's composition is always helpful in choosing the right tone and level.

Control the setting for your speech. Arrive in the room at least 30 to 45 minutes before your session to check out the functioning of your audio–visual equipment, to identify the presence of any unforeseen problems such as a fixed podium that's taller than you are, and to make other adjustments. Be certain that your transparency projector is properly focused and that the remote control for the slide projector is hooked up and works. Plan for someone to dim the house lights, and establish how you will cue him or her. If you find yourself in a highly formal convention center or hotel ballroom that seats 500 and only 30 people turn up for your presentation, anticipate strategies that you can use to decrease the distance and formality of your presentation. You might exchange your podium microphone for one that will allow you to move around, come down off the stage into the front of the room, and show your own transparencies or slides.

Fielding Questions

When the moment for your speech arrives, you may feel well organized, well prepared, and well rehearsed. But the prospect of fielding questions or criticisms from your audience—or of encountering total silence as a response to your paper—may be intimidating. You may fear having to think on your feet about new issues or being verbally attacked. A few hints to help you deal with these concerns follow:

- Distribute index cards to those arriving for your speech, and ask them to identify one burning issue they would like to have discussed. Glancing through these suggestions can alert you to topics that might be raised during a question-and-answer period. These questions can also offer material if your later offer to respond to verbal questions is met with silence.

- Plant a few relevant and significant questions with your associates and colleagues in the audience so as to break the ice and make it a bit easier for others to stand up and speak publicly if they wish to.
- Repeat or paraphrase questions that are asked, so that everyone in the room can hear them, so that they will be picked up if your speech is being taped, and so that you will have a little extra time to organize your response.
- If you are unable to answer a question, offer to send references or resource materials later or to talk personally with the questioner during a break.

Speaking is thinking out loud. It requires planning and practice. Because it is impossible to present as much detail in a typical talk as you can present in a research article or, certainly, in a thesis or dissertation, the success of a talk often depends on your ability to select the five or so major points that ought to be emphasized and developed. Saslow (1982) likens deciding what to include in a speech to getting ready for a back-packing trip. You lay out everything that is "essential" and then throw half of it away because otherwise your pack will be too heavy to carry. If you aren't selective about the ideas in your talk, you'll be leaving in too much extra baggage. Conveying too much information in a talk is one of the major pitfalls that you must learn to avoid. The other is assuming that the audience can understand aspects of the presentation that are overly complex or poorly presented.

Scientific Speeches

In any scientific presentation of research findings you should cover the following areas:

1. Describe the research subjects and the sampling procedures in enough detail that the audience realizes how far your findings can be generalized.

2. If your design is at all complicated, be sure to make clear how many subjects were assigned to which group using which assignment method. (A handout or transparency can be useful here.)

3. Be sure that your audience has a clear idea of the amount and variety of data your findings are based on. For instance, in a field study be sure that you report how many hours of participation you employed, how many interviews you conducted and with whom, and the full list of documents you reviewed.

4. If you used statistical analysis procedures, specify the test used and other technical information such as the level of significance.

5. Mention any limitations or assumptions that might have bearing on the interpretation of your findings, to assure the audience of your objectivity and honesty.

Guidelines for Evaluating a Talk

Saslow (1982) offers the following overall set of questions to use when evaluating any oral presentation, including your own: *

1. What were the major findings or conclusions? (They should have been mentioned at least twice.)

2. Were you given enough evidence to have faith in the conclusions?

   a. Did the speaker present enough of the method so that you understood approximately what was done?

   b. Were the results presented in a form you could readily grasp?

   c. Did the speaker report the statistical analysis necessary to establish that the results weren't due to chance factors?

* SOURCE: Based on C. A. Saslow, *Basic Research Methods*, Reading, Mass.: Addison-Wesley, 1982, p. 377.

d. Did the speaker make a clear, logical argument why the results supported the conclusions?

3. Did the speaker give you the information that would allow you to generalize from the results, such as:

 a. type and number of subjects and other subject characteristics?

 b. duration of training of subjects (if appropriate)?

 c. any peculiar conditions of the setting for the study that might not be reproducible elsewhere?

 d. information about potential experimenter bias or subject attitude effects?

4. Did the speaker relate the findings to any wider field of research or application?

5. Did the speaker lose you at any point by:

 a. using jargon or self-defined terms?

 b. drowning you in detail?

 c. presenting information too rapidly?

 d. failing to emphasize the important points and distinguish them clearly from less important information?

 e. distracting you with personal mannerisms?

6. Was the talk interesting?

Writing a Journal Article

Whether you are writing a book, a thesis, a technical report for a funding agency, or a journal article, you will go through a three-stage process: prewriting, writing, and rewriting. This section will deal primarily with how these stages apply to the writing of a journal article.

Prewriting

"Prewriting" is discovering what you have to say about your subject, finding the perspective from which to treat it, and doing all the organizational tasks required before making a deliberate effort to produce a first draft. For a scientific writer, it may include hours of brooding over the results of statistical analyses on computer printouts. Or it may involve returning to the library to take more notes. It usually encompasses targeting a journal or publishing house, obtaining its instructions to authors, sampling some previously published work, sorting out issues of authorship, and drafting a letter of inquiry. Prewriting also involves identifying your subject, deciding on a direction or purpose for your manuscript, and developing your purpose, intent, or direction into an outline of what you want to say about it. The framework of developmental questions in Box 17-6 offers an informal start for an outline of a research journal article. The typical format for a journal article in Box 17-3 and the criteria for a research critique in Chapter 7 are additional resources you can use in developing an outline.

A theoretical analysis or a methodological paper requires that you employ other strategies for developing a topic. These may be exploration, argumentation, or comparison and contrast. The questions in Box 17-7 can provide a start.

Choosing a Journal   It's always possible for you to write your article and then shop for an outlet for it. But journals differ in their length limitations, citation systems, audiences, and circulation. Most authorities agree, therefore, that it's a good idea to *think about where you might publish your manuscript before you even write it* to avoid having to make major revisions in tone,

---

Box 17-6 Questions That Your Outline Should Answer

1. What is the general area of your research problem?
2. Why is studying this area important to nursing?
3. What previous work (theoretical and empirical) has been done that is related to your research?
4. What did prior literature suggest needed to be done next?
5. How does your work respond to this need?
6. What, specifically, did you do?
7. What were your results?
8. What did you expect?
9. What is the broader meaning of your investigation?
10. What needs to be done from here?

Box 17-7 Questions That Aid in Developing a Paper

1. What does my topic mean?
2. What are its characteristics or properties?
3. What are its parts, types, or forms?
4. How is it done?
5. What are the conditions for it or causes of it?
6. What are the outcomes or consequences of doing or using it?
7. How does it compare with something else?
8. What is the present status of knowledge about it?
9. What is its value?
10. What is my personal response to it?
11. What case or arguments can be made against it?
12. How can my topic be summarized?

---

style, and format. It might surprise you to know that McCloskey's 1982 list of 50 American journals (excluding state nurses' association publications) that represented publishing opportunities in nursing had been expanded by Mirin (1981) to 749. Box 17-8 identifies major categories and examples of nursing journals.

Selecting a journal depends on the readership to whom you want to communicate your ideas. Before deciding on several and ranking them in order of your preferred outlet, be sure to read several issues of the journal to:

- get a sense of the tone and style its editors prefer
- get a feeling for the audience that reads it
- determine whether the time from submission to publication is acceptable to you
- judge whether your work will be timely and of interest to the editors

Reasons for Rejection From the start, you should keep in mind that the chief reasons for rejection of manuscripts, either by journal editors, advisory boards, or official *referees* (anonymous peers who review your manuscript), are:

1. The subject of your manuscript is not relevant to the journal's readership.
2. The article is poorly written.
3. The central idea, or "little logic" (see Chapter 2), of your article is not unique.

There are many criteria used by referees, reviewers, editorial board members, and editors to evaluate an article for publication.

Box 17-8   Major Categories of Nursing Journal

Journal Category	Example	Circulation
General nursing	American Journal of Nursing	350,000
	Nursing '85	500,000
	RN	205,000
Speciality nursing	Cardiovascular Nursing	120,000
	Heart & Lung	57,000
	MCN	25,000
	Supervisor Nurse	80,000
	Journal of Nursing Administration	17,000
Research nursing	Nursing Research	8,000
	Advances in Nursing Science	3,019
	Research in Nursing and Health	1,000
	Western Journal for Nursing Research	700

More detailed reasons that articles are rejected by nursing publishers, according to McCloskey (1982), are:

1. The subject was recently covered or is already scheduled for a future issue.
2. The article is too technical for the journal.
3. The content is inaccurate or undocumented.
4. The work is based on a poor research design or faulty methodology.
5. Nursing concerns are not highlighted.
6. The content is unimportant.
7. The article is too much like a speech or term paper and would be difficult to change.
8. The conclusion is unwarranted by the data as presented.
9. The idea was previously published elsewhere.
10. The idea is badly presented.

Advice From Journal Editors Nursing journal editors also offered prospective authors some words of advice in the McCloskey survey (1982):

- Manuscripts must be well organized, look neat, be double-spaced on good-quality bond paper, and have 1-inch margins throughout.
- Specifications for manuscripts are available from journals. Get them and follow them.
- Start with a literature review so you won't reinvent the wheel.
- Outline before you write.
- If what you say is controversial, document your sources and recognize opposing points of view.
- Ask colleagues, mentors, and friends to critique your manuscript before you submit it.
- Write in a straightforward style, using the active voice when possible. Avoid sounding pompous or pedantic.
- Keep information concise, relevant, up to date, and accurate.
- Double-check all your figures and totals.
- Provide your name, title, credentials, address, phone number, and organizational affiliation.

Editorial Policies Most nursing journals include their editorial policy in each issue. From it you can learn exactly what kinds of article a journal wants to publish, what materials should accompany any submission (such as a short biographical sketch or a full résumé), how articles are to be prepared and submitted, and to whom. Some journals such as the *American Journal of Nursing* invite or solicit manuscripts from qualified experts. Others restrict acceptance of manuscripts to unsolicited ones that have been favorably reviewed by a panel of referees according to specific guidelines. Some journals include both. Understanding the editorial policy of a journal prepares you to write the kind of article the journal wants to receive and publish. Kolin and Kolin (1980) differentiate most published nursing articles into five categories:

1. the case study
2. the research article
3. the article on procedures, processes, and techniques
4. the historical article
5. the article on a current topic

Matching the article you intend to write with the right outlet is an essential step toward success in getting published.

The Query Letter   Whereas articles solicited by a journal editor have close to a 100% chance of being published, unsolicited manuscripts must be designed to compete to be seen in print. Writing a letter of inquiry (called a query letter) to the editor of the journal you have decided to aim for is one technique that can increase the likelihood that your unsolicited manuscript will be accepted.

A query letter asks whether an editor of a journal is interested in reviewing your manuscript for publication consideration. Both editors and authors know that a well-written query letter can save them both time and effort, not to mention postage. Although a few journals discourage query letters, desiring instead to review the entire unsolicited manuscript, the majority prefer them.

It is proper to simultaneously mail off several query letters about the same piece of work to a number of different editors. If the responses are all encouraging, the author can then pick and choose. But it is definitely not considered good etiquette to send out copies of full manuscripts to several editors simultaneously. The unwritten code between editors and authors is that an author awaits a decision from one journal before trying another one. One way to alienate editors is to create circumstances in which they have devoted a great deal of time and effort to the review process and accepted your manuscript, only to learn that you have agreed to have it appear somewhere else. Editors don't seem to object to what Mirin (1981, p. 10) calls "mass query mailing," but you must realize that if several journals indicate interest, it's only polite to write back to some of them to let them know that your paper is going elsewhere. Composing a query letter is part of the prewriting, developmental stage, because a note from the editor indicating interest in reviewing the manuscript may also contain some developmental suggestions that can save hours of revision time later. Another reason for writing your query letters early in the manuscript preparation process is that knowing that a publisher or editor is interested in your work is a terrific source of motivation and inspiration, particularly when contrasted with the impact of spending months writing a long article only to have it repeatedly returned to you with a rejection slip.

Mirin (1981) recommends that a query letter be divided into four parts:

1. a lead paragraph or two that catches the editor's interest and lures him or her into reading on
2. a paragraph that tells what the article will be about, what direction it will take, and what it will offer the reader
3. some facts, observations, or other citations that back up your basic premise and offer your credentials for writing the piece

4. two final paragraphs in which you make a strong statement designed to convince the editor that this is an article that he or she should publish and ask if the editor is interested in reviewing the manuscript for publication consideration

A sample of a query letter appears in Box 17-9.

The Question of Authorship Finding the right outlet for your journal article is certainly one of the most critical prewriting details. In the case of work that has multiple authors, determining from the start the order in which names should appear for credit and what responsibilities each should assume is also important. Neither of these decisions should be made frivolously. The dated convention of resolving the decision of author sequence according to alphabetical order of last names is all but obsolete. If the article is chiefly your work, it will matter a lot to you later if you don't get the visibility, credit, and acknowledgment you deserve, especially because journal article publishing rarely involves any financial reward except for a token payment in relatively rare instances. McCloskey (1982) and others agree that the best and fairest way to allocate credit is that the person who assumed most of the work should also get most of the credit.

Writing

Prewriting and writing overlap. Even so, certain considerations tend to present themselves in the context of composing your first draft. Keep in mind that even with the most careful job of prewriting, most well-written manuscripts go through several drafts before the content and organization represent the very best you can do with your topic in the time you have available. Several of the problems encountered in the writing phase are presented in the sections that follow.

Deciding on a Title Aim for a title that is concise, specific, and informative. The title should tell accurately and clearly what the paper is about. Linton (1972) points out that the title you choose may mean the difference between recognition and oblivion for your article: "You are providing the first index to your paper when you write its title and the precision of your title may seriously affect the availability to science of your contribution" (p. 41). Although it's important to avoid unnecessary words that increase the length of your title without adding to descriptive accuracy and completeness, the APA *Publication Manual* (1983) acknowledges that as many as 15 words may be necessary to avoid being overly cryptic. Stay away from pretentiousness, triteness, clichés, and jargon. But a catchy title can generally be acceptable to the audience or readership of the journal if it still serves as an accurate guide to the work you are reporting. Box 17-10 offers some sample titles in poor and improved forms.

A good title should be short but explanatory. You can accomplish this goal by building key information such as your study variables and subjects into the title and avoiding excess padding and unnecessary words. Avoid the tendency to select a title that merely represents one part of your article. Instead try for one that represents the focus and intention of the entire paper.

Writing the Lead Some journals require that you write a several-sentence lead section that can be boxed or put in boldface type at the opening of your article. In the absence of an official lead, consider your first sentences or paragraphs as the lead of your paper. The way you begin your paper shares one important characteristic with your title; it must arouse the readers' attention and interest and inspire them to read on. A lead also sets the tone of the article and limits the article's scope so that the readers know from the beginning what to expect. A lot of writers leave the composition of this very important part of an article until last. Once a manuscript is completed, you have a better idea of its tone and coverage anyway. Kolin and Kolin (1980) identify the following alternatives for leads, depend-

Box 17-9   Sample Query Letter

June 11, 1984

Dr. Shirley Smoyak, Editor
Journal of Psychosocial Nursing
SLACK Incorporated
6900 Grove Road
Thorofare, New Jersey 08086

Dear Dr. Smoyak:

Within two years, "DRG's" and "Prospective Payment" are going to reshape the management of in-patient psychiatric care. In the May, 1984, issue of *Hospital and Community Psychiatry*, authorities in the field urged that psychiatry's extension be devoted to studying ways of estimating resource use and classifications of psychiatric clients. Nursing, whose unique contribution to the interdisciplinary mental health team is observation and management of basic needs among inpatients on a 24-hour-a-day basis, can offer an informed perspective on how psychiatry can participate in a prospective payment system without endangering the quality of patient care. Classification systems are needed to bridge the gap between standard psychiatric diagnostic categories (DSM-III) and what has become known as the "Nursing Diagnosis Movement."

Our article, *The Nursing Adaptation Evaluation* (NSGAE), offers a proposed VI Axis of DSM-III and provides categories for a functional assessment of psychiatric patients useful to planning, documenting, and evaluating the effects of nursing care on hospitalized psychiatric clients. The computer processable numerical code system incorporates the patient's highest level of adaptive functioning in the areas of *Nutrition*, *Solitude and Social Interaction*, *Grooming (and Hygiene)*, *Activity (and Rest)*, and *Elimination* in the past year, and his or her current overall level of adaptive functioning or self-care ability in separate ratings of adaptive functioning in the five basic need areas respectively. Our proposed Axis VI for DSM-IV is based on descriptive criteria, can provide practical guidelines for nursing and interdisciplinary treatment planning, and is currently being systematically evaluated in six clinical settings.

While the list of nursing diagnoses accepted for testing by the "NANDA" group very likely has an important future in the evaluation of a nursing diagnosis taxonomy, many psychosocial nurses attest to the need for a classification system that has interdisciplinary meaning and utility for the particular treatment planning requirements for psychiatric nursing care. We believe that our article introducing the Nursing Adaptation Evaluation (NSGAE) as a proposed Axis VI for DSM-IV responds to those needs and offers an empirical approach worthy of wider study.

If you are interested in receiving our manuscript for publication consideration, we can immediately send it to you for review upon notification.

Sincerely,

Holly Skodol Wilson, RN, PhD
Professor

cc: Eileen Morrison
    Lucy Fisher
    Patricia Underwood

HSW/b

Box 17-10   Sample Titles

Poor	Improved
Now They Can Choose: A Study of Health Beliefs Among Chinese-Americans Who Have Cancer	Health Beliefs About Treatment Among Chinese-American Cancer Patients (eliminates unnecessary words)
Pain Assessment: An Exploratory Study	Behavioral Indicators of Pain in Preschool Children During Burn Debridement (adds specificity and key features such as population and study conditions)
An Interpretative Study of the Nature of the Therapeutic Touch Process	Expectations, Beliefs, and Physical Sensations Experienced by Patients During Therapeutic Touch Treatments (increases specificity and clarity)
Prechemotherapy Patient Education: It's Affect on Patterns of Nausea and Vomitting	Prechemotherapy Patient Education: Its Effect on Patterns of Nausea and Vomiting (corrects misuse of *it's* for *its*, *affect* for *effect*, and picks up spelling error in *vomiting* by proofreading)
Who Seeks Help: A Longitudinal Study	Arthritis in the Elderly: Patterns of Disability and Coping (incorporates key variables, increasing the chance of the articles being properly indexed)

---

ing on the type of journal and, of course, the type of article you have written:

1. a simple, clear, and straightforward statement of purpose often used in scientific journals

2. a dramatic, eye-catching use of statistics

3. a client anecdote or history that arouses human interest

4. a personal experience with which readers are likely to identify

5. a definition that orients readers to the topic

6. a question or several questions, with the implication that readers probably have or should have asked them of themselves

7. a comparison or contrast that whets the readers' appetite for more information

8. a historical summary to place the topic in

context and interest the readers in getting more current information

Leads often must be written and rewritten many times before you are satisfied. Although you may not craft the opening sentences 50 times, as Plato was supposed to have done when he wrote *The Republic*, you should ideally attempt to write a lead or opening that provokes interest, is direct and concise, and makes promises that you fulfill in your article.

Writing Your Rough Draft   The following guidelines will help you get started on the first draft of your article:

1. Decide on an environment that is conducive to writing, preferably one where your resource materials are easily available, one that is free of tempting or annoying distrac-

tions, and one where you don't mind spending some concentrated time. Some writers who prepare their manuscripts on a word processor obviously write where their computer is located.

2. Fill up those white pages. Get something down on paper, and worry about editing and revising later. Follow the topics on your outline, and develop them.

3. Leave three spaces between lines, whether you write in longhand or type, so that you have room for changes and additions.

4. Number your pages and paragraphs so that you can move them around if doing so would improve your organization.

5. Decide what you intend to present in tables or graphs, and flag the pages on which you want them to appear. (Follow the guidelines presented later in this chapter for constructing tables and figures.)

6. Be prepared to cut and paste if you are not working on a word processor or to edit what you've written if you are. Both these strategies help you avoid having to rewrite or retype material when you reorganize it.

7. If at all possible set aside your first draft for at least a few days before rewriting it. A research paper for a course, a thesis, or an article should never be submitted "hot off the typewriter."

8. Ask a friend, colleague, or teacher to critique a later draft, and consider their suggestions before writing your final rendition.

9. Proofread for typographical errors, spelling errors, missing words, awkward sentences, and redundancies.

10. Keep at least one copy for your own files.

It is beyond the scope of this chapter to discuss the technical aspects of grammatical uses and style for scientific writing. For questions about tense, punctuation, parallel sentence construction, word usage, paragraphing, shaping sentences, and spelling, refer to Strunk and White's (1972) *The Elements of Style*, Linton's (1972) *A Simplified Style Manual*, Perrin and Ebbitt's (1972) *Writer's Guide and Index to English*, Kolin and Kolin's (1980) *Professional Writing for Nurses in Education, Practice and Research*, Mirin's (1981) *The Nurse's Guide to Writing for Publication*, or Tornquist's (1985) *From Proposal to Publication: The Nurse Researcher's Guide to Writing*. The following guidelines, however, will help you write your draft in a clear and organized way:

1. Eliminate all unnecessary, dull, and trite words.

2. Use active verb forms.

3. Check the order of paragraphs and sentences to be certain that each paragraph contains a topic sentence, that sentences build upon each other, that effective transitions move the reader between paragraphs, and that the order of ideas and the supporting evidence is clear and effective.

4. Consider your tone in light of your topic, your intended audience, and the type of journal to which you are submitting the article. Make sure your language is consistent with your intended tone.

5. Aim for versatility and variety in your writing. Don't overuse words or sentence structures. Without variety, your writing will be dull.

6. Above all, you must be clear. In Mirin's (1981) words, "Clarity doesn't make style but there can be no style without it and clarity means order. Without order, you cannot communicate" (p. 44).

Working Quotations in Smoothly   If you want your paper to read smoothly, you can't just drop quotations with a thud into your paragraph. You need to introduce a quotation with phrases such as:

- "As Lindsey discovered . . ."
- "In Hutchinson's words . . ."
- "According to Norbeck . . ."
- "Stotts observed that . . ."

Generally speaking, extensive quoting isn't done in scientific articles. Three circumstances provide a rationale for using quotations:

1. The material is authoritative and convincing evidence in support of your thesis.
2. The statement is phrased exactly the way it should be expressed.
3. The idea is controversial, and you want to assure your readers about it.

Plagiarism and Paraphrasing *Plagiarism* means to steal and pass off the work of another as one's own. It usually results from bad paraphrasing or improper referencing. Both paraphrasing that merely substitutes a few word changes for those of the original author and forgetting to use quotation marks and a reference citation are technically considered plagiarism, even if you somehow hypnotize yourself into thinking that those really were your own words to express your own ideas. The only safe way to paraphrase is to read the original over several times and then write your conception of what you've read *without looking at the original*. In other words, when paraphrasing, keep the source book closed.

Preparing Tables and Figures Complex results that involve numbers are often presented in tables and figures in a research article reporting findings. Descriptive statistics such as sample size, means, measures of variability, and the like are clearer and less cumbersome when presented this way. Keep in mind, however, that most journals will discourage excessive use of them and that tables and figures that are numbered separately should be on separate pages at the end of your manuscript. You should also note on the page where you want them to appear, something

like *[insert Table 1 about here]*. An illustration that is not a table is called a figure. Pictures of equipment and graphs are examples of figures.

Good tables have the following characteristics:

1. All tables should have a clear, explanatory title and a number at the top.
2. A table should be comprehensible without any additional explanation. It should stand by itself.
3. A good table should not be overly complicated, and an intelligent reader should be able to figure it out without too much effort. If it's too complicated, put some of the information into a second table.
4. Tables shouldn't duplicate information presented in another form.

Good figures have these characteristics:

1. A figure should have its title or caption at the bottom instead of the top of the page.
2. Like tables, figures should not need additional explanation.
3. In the case of a graph, the axes (x = horizontal and y = vertical) should be labeled.
4. Figures should be used when you want to visually depict change over time or to make a more immediate and dramatic impact on the reader.
5. All figures and tables should be referred to explicitly in the text of your article.
6. No more than four curves should appear on any given figure.
7. It's not necessary to give the total possible range on a grid if none of your data has extreme values.
8. The dependent variable is customarily plotted on the x axis, and the independent variable is plotted on the y axis.

9. Include a legend, or caption, that accompanies the figure and explains it.

10. Figures should not be larger than 8½ × 11 inches when they are submitted for publication.

11. You must get permission to reprint a table or figure that was created by someone else. Consult one of the manuals of style for precise details on how to reference sources for tables and figures and on referencing in general.

Once you have written your first draft, you are ready to move into the final stage of composition, one in which you will pare and prune. Good writing springs not from formulas but from creative activity, clear thinking, and a personal commitment to involvement and self-criticism.

Rewriting

When you've finished your first draft, put it aside for a while, ask someone else to take a look at it, and read it again with the proverbial blue editorial pencil in your hand. Use the four following sets of guidelines (Saslow 1982) in combination with Chapter 7 of this text to evaluate the sections of your research report and the quality of its style.*

Criteria for a Good Introduction   The title, lead, and introduction make an important first impression on your reader. Saslow suggests that the standards on which an introduction should be based include the following:

1. Is the general area of the research clearly introduced, and do you make a case for why more knowledge is needed in the area?

* SOURCE: Based on C. A Saslow, *Basic Research Methods*, Reading, Mass.: Addison-Wesley, 1982, pp. 344–359.

2. Have you summarized the present state of knowledge in the area?

3. Have you built a case for why your approach in the study is a reasonable one?

4. Are sources for facts, ideas, and speculations given and referenced?

5. Is the specific problem for the study clearly stated before proceeding to the methods section?

Criteria for a Good Methods Section

1. Is it clear who your subjects were and how many of them you used as data sources?

2. Are all the data-collection tools and instruments in your research described with enough detail so that someone else could replicate your study? Have you provided sources of any specific tests, figures to illustrate laboratory equipment, and the like?

3. Have you described your study design clearly, including the independent and dependent variables, how subjects were assigned to groups, and so on?

4. Have you sufficiently described procedures such as instructions to subjects and other techniques you used to control extraneous variables so that your reader can evaluate any possible alternative explanations for your results?

Criteria for a Good Results Section

1. Have you described all the preliminary steps used to prepare your data for analysis?

2. Is the section well organized according to initial hypotheses or research questions?

3. Are descriptions and inferential statistics given to back up findings derived from quantitative data, and are analytic methods for qualitative data discussed? Is the statistical test named, and is it appropriate for the level of measurement and study question? Have

you included the calculated test statistic, degrees of freedom, and significance level for inferential statistical tests?

4. Are the necessary tables and figures included? Are they in the proper format, clearly titled or captioned, easy to interpret, and able to stand alone?

Criteria for a Good Discussion Section

1. Are the results clearly summarized and emphasized?

2. Have you explained instances when your results differ from what you expected?

3. Have you discussed the relationship of your findings to the results of others?

4. Have you considered any effects that design or procedural limitations might have had on your findings?

5. Have you made your interpretations of your results clear?

6. Have you included any possible alternative interpretations?

7. Have you suggested ideas for future research or the application of your findings?

Box 17-11 offers you a final checklist for all research papers, whether they be reports of find-

---

Box 17-11   Final Checklist for Papers

1. Do you have a single, controlling idea you want to communicate? (To make your paper really clear, state this idea in the form of a thesis statement, and include it in your first or second paragraph.)

2. Does everything in your paper pertain to that idea? If something doesn't, either find a way to connect it clearly or omit it.

3. Have you organized your essay into clear sections and arranged them in the most logical and effective order?

4. Do you have plenty of supporting evidence to back up your ideas? Don't be afraid to draw upon your own experience; it's the most valid evidence of all. Be Specific!

5. Are your paragraphs well developed? Most good paragraphs consist of at least five sentences that are themselves well focused and packed with essential information.

6. Are your paragraphs themselves well-organized? Each paragraph should have some sort of controlling idea, expressed in the topic sentence.

7. Do you have smooth transitions between paragraphs and sentences?

8. Do you have an interesting introduction, one that will grab your readers and make them want to read on?

9. Have you concluded your essay effectively?

10. Is your essay mechanically correct? Read your last draft and final version aloud; often you will catch errors that your eye might skim over.

11. Look up any words you're not sure how to spell; don't just guess and hope for the best. Also check the meaning of any word you're slightly unsure of.

12. Have you varied your sentence structure? Make sure your sentences aren't too short and choppy. Although an occasional short sentence is effective, more than a couple in a row have the stylistic interest of a Dick and Jane workbook. Practice joining sentences to connect ideas and establish logical relationships between them.

ings or other analytic, methodological, or conceptual essays.

When you are ready to make that trip to the post office to submit your article, reread the journal's information to contributors. Doing so will ensure that you:

- know whether to double- or triple-space the typing
- know how large the margins should be
- know how many copies to send
- know what information you should include about yourself
- know whether you should include an abstract
- know the name and correct address of the editor to whom you are sending your manuscript
- know approximately how long it will take for your article to go through the review process

Postwriting

Reviewers or referees may take from two weeks to two months to make their recommendations about your manuscript to the journal editor. In the meantime, you'll probably receive a postcard acknowledging that your manuscript was received. After that postcard, patience is essential.

If your article is accepted, the editor will probably congratulate you in a letter and let you know when you can expect to receive proofs for proofreading. Be prepared for editors to expect you to be prompt with this task. Sometimes, acceptance for publication in a journal is conditional on making changes specified by the reviewers or editor. You as an author can always decline and send it elsewhere if you disagree with the changes requested. But if you do, you should officially withdraw it from the first journal.

If your manuscript is rejected, most editors will return it to you. The possibility of rejection always exists, and unless you can conclude with certainty that the editor is totally lacking in taste, sensitivity, and vision, you ought to try to determine why it was rejected and to grow from the experience. Editors do miss opportunities and make mistakes. Don't let a rejection from one journal keep you from submitting your article somewhere else if you still believe in its value.

Writing a Book

In most cases authors of books, be they monographs presenting research findings in detail or textbooks like this one, are people who have established themselves as authors through their contributions to the professional literature. When you attempt to write a book, you must be equally clear about your idea, your audience, and the form in which you intend to present your work as when you write a journal article (Kolin & Kolin 1980). Writing a book, however, expands manyfold the amount of time and energy involved. Publishers estimate that it takes an author about 2 years to produce a text or reference book and then another 10 to 12 months to go through the production process. Figure 17-1 illustrates the phases of the book production process.

Approaching a Publisher: The Prospectus

Getting a book published requires that you form a partnership with a publishing company unless you intend to print, market, and distribute your book on your own (an idea that I'd discourage

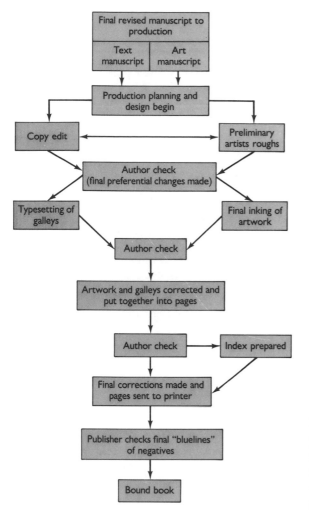

Figure 17-1 The production of a book.

as such it should at least address the following questions:

1. Why do you intend to write this book, and what need will it fill?

2. What is the level of the book, and what audience will be interested in it?

3. What are the main features of the contents and organization of the book?

4. How can the reader use the book to its best advantage?

5. Are there supplementary materials such as software or a student workbook?

6. If this is a revised edition of a previously published book, what is the essence of the revision, and what are the significant changes?

7. What acknowledgments do you intend to include?

Negotiating a Publishing Contract

Once your idea, presentation, and competence have succeeded in capturing the interest of a publisher (or several), you must negotiate and sign a contract. You agree to deliver a completed manuscript by a specified date. The publisher agrees to produce the book, promote it, store it, sell it, and protect its copyright. It also provides other assistance such as obtaining in-progress reviews and locating a designer, production coordinator, illustrator, and indexer (if you don't want to do the index yourself). In return for your creative work as author, you are paid royalties (usually twice a year) that represent a percentage of the net sales revenue. A "standard contract" usually offers the author around 10% of net sales. In some cases, the royalty rate can include an escalation clause that increases the royalty pecentage based on the number of copies sold per year, per edition, or per life of the book. Royalties for foreign sales are usually less than those for domestic sales.

unless you have special resources, contacts, and expertise in the publishing enterprise). You approach a publisher with a *prospectus*, or *manuscript proposal*, that includes a detailed outline or table of contents and one or two sample chapters that you consider to be representative of the tone and writing style of the text. Box 17-12 outlines the components of a manuscript proposal. It's often a good idea to think of the prospectus as akin to your preface for the book, and

---

Box 17-12 The Components of a Manuscript Proposal

PROSPECTUS: The prospectus should include a detailed discussion of the following points:

RATIONALE: Describe your reasons for writing the book and explain what you are attempting to accomplish. Discuss the current trends in the field and relate your book to the needs of the field (pedagogical, topical, and/or theoretical).

MARKET: Is this book designed to serve as:
1. a major textbook (which will normally be usable without supplementation)
2. a briefer "core" text (which will cover most traditionally required topics but would usually require supplementary reading in a full semester course)
3. an originally written topical supplement covering a single topic or several topics

SUBJECT AND SCOPE: What does the book cover or omit in terms of traditional topics, innovation, expansion, and/or improvement for this specific course(s)? Explain any unique features.

APPROACH: How is the subject treated in comparison/contrast to traditional approaches?

LEVEL: Is the book written for introductory or advanced students? Comment on the level and style of writing.

PHYSICAL APPEARANCE: What is the proposed length of the manuscript (total typewritten pages—double spaced)? How many graphs, tables, figures, and photographs are to be included? (Please enumerate specific illustrative material.)

ANCILLARY ITEMS: Which of the following do you propose to accompany the text: instructor's manual (how extensive?), student guide, audio visuals, computer material, etc.?

COMPETITION: Compare/contrast your proposal with specific, major competitive titles in terms of approach, coverage, features, etc.

DETAILED OUTLINE: The outline should be complete for the entire text and detailed enough to give an accurate picture of the depth and breadth of coverage you plan. Reviewers cannot suggest deletions or additions to content unless they know exactly what you intend to discuss. It may be necessary in some cases to detail the outline to the third level of heads.

SAMPLE CHAPTER(S): These may be requested with the above material for initial review, or they may be requested after the detailed outline has been reviewed and perhaps revised—it depends on the nature of the project. Your editor would probably indicate which chapter should be completed after the initial review. As a rule, the sample should not be an introductory chapter, but one more representative of the text. It should include all features that you plan to include in the final text chapter (e.g., tables, figures, objectives, bibliography, suggested readings, etc.).

Royalties are only one of the negotiable items in a publishing contract. Obviously, the financial success of a book is in the interest of both author and publisher. But as an author, you may also be interested in assurances about the developmental and editorial assistance that you can expect from the publisher. For example, will it provide you with copy editing? What are the publisher's intentions about the physical appearance of the book (hardback or softcover, size, quality of paper)? What about the availability and amount of an advance against royalties that can help you offset costs of preparing the manuscript? Typing costs may total as much as $3000, and illustrations in many books cost even more. If you are working with a coauthor, you may need to offset costs of travel, long-distance phone calls, and so on. It's obviously preferable to be working on a project using the publisher's capital on an interest-free basis than to launch the venture with both your time and your out-of-pocket cash. Is there a possibility of receiving a grant that you would not have to pay back to the publisher out of your royalties? Will the publisher share some costs with you, such as for illustrations, permissions, or indexing?

Most important in deciding on a publisher, given comparable contract offers, is the quality of the company's work. Study the other books it has developed and produced. Look to see if it exhibits at important nursing meetings and advertises in prominent nursing journals. What do you think of its sales representatives? How professional are its brochures and flyers? Is the company known and respected in nursing? Does it strike you as having the kind of integrity you'd expect from any other business partner?

The Publisher's Precontract Review

Just as you will be investigating a potential publisher, the publishing company will be investigating the merit of your proposed book. This is usually done by sending out requests for precontract reviews by anonymous reviewers in whose judgment the publisher has confidence.

Writing the Book: Resources

Writing the manuscript for your book involves all the considerations of tone, style, organization, word choice, idea development, and mechanics that were discussed in the section on writing a journal article—and more. Seek out your publisher's guidelines for authors to get help with questions related to:

- setting up a filing system
- starting a permissions log
- punctuation, numbering, and alphabetizing
- indexing
- illustrations
- glossary
- supplements
- referencing
- reprints and new editions

About Copyright

A chapter on article and book writing wouldn't be complete without a word on the subject of copyright. Copyright law protects any author from having his or her material used without permission. It protects all kinds of original work, including illustrations, tables, diagrams, songs, and so on. Under the most recent copyright law (1978), any original work is automatically protected by copyright law when it is put on paper. The duration of a copyright consists of an author's lifetime plus 50 years. An author owns all rights to a work he or she creates unless those rights are transferred to the publisher of a journal or book. Publishers usually ask for these rights, but authors can stipulate the rights they want to keep and those they want to transfer to a publisher—for example, rights to publish the work in article form elsewhere. Some publishers won't accept an article or book manuscript for publication unless you transfer full copyright to them because of the benefits they can derive by control of all future uses of your work. Whether someone's work is protected by the copyright law or *in the public domain* (anything on which the copyright has expired), you should always acknowledge the source of materials and ideas that are not your own. The job of obtaining permissions or alerting a permissions assistant to the need for them is an important aspect of an author's responsibility.

Summary of Key Ideas and Terms

✔ The only way important information produced through your scientific work can contribute to the body of nursing knowledge or become part of the basis for clinical decision making is for you to report it to others.

✔ Disseminating research through speeches promptly informs a limited audience and gets early feedback for you; written reports make a more permanent and complete record of your work available to a wider audience.

✔ Dealing with scientific and theoretical subjects need not work against communicating clearly, specifically, directly, and with an organized, interesting style.

✔ Speaking is thinking out loud. It requires adequate planning and practice. The success of most talks depends on your ability to avoid information overload and to present well.

✔ All writing goes through the three-step process of (1) "prewriting," (2) writing, and (3) rewriting.

✔ *Prewriting* involves identifying your subject, deciding on a direction and purpose, and outlining what you want to say.

✔ Study the journal that you intend to target for an article for the tone and style it prefers, the audience that reads it, the time gaps involved in the publishing process, and whether your topic will be of interest to it.

✔ A *query letter* asks an editor of a journal if he or she is interested in reviewing a manuscript for publication consideration.

✔ When several authors collaborate on a manuscript, the order of authors' names should be settled from the start, preferably based on who assumed most of the work.

✔ A title should be concise, specific, and informative, because it should catch a reader's interest and provide an accurate index cue for your work.

✔ An article's lead, or opening paragraph, can take a number of forms but should be interesting, direct, and concise and should make promises that you fulfill in your article.

- Always refer to a *style manual* for questions of tense, punctuation, word usage, spelling, and grammar.

- The safest way to paraphrase someone else's ideas and avoid plagiarism (stealing or passing off as one's own the work of another) is to do it with the source book closed.

- Creation of tables and figures (nonnumerical illustrations) should always follow conventional guidelines.

- A *research report* is usually written according to a customary format and should meet specified criteria.

- Never submit anything that's hot off the typewriter. Proofread, edit, and rewrite according to criteria for good writing style.

- A prospective book author should approach publishers with a *prospectus* for the book that includes certain essential details, a proposed table of contents, and one or two sample chapters.

- A *publishing contract* is an agreement between an author(s) and a publishing company about the details of a collaborative project. Pay attention to items such as royalties, advances, unrecoverable grants, editorial assistance, and sharing of costs, but also to the overall quality and integrity of a publisher's productions.

- A publisher is likely to obtain a number of *precontract reviews* from respected people in your area before offering you a publishing contract.

- *Copyright law* protects any author from having his or her written work used without permission. Many journal editors and book publishers require that you transfer copyrights to your work to them before they accept it for publication.

References

American Nurses' Association, Council of Nurse Researchers, Kansas City, Mo.: 1982.

American Psychological Association: *Publication Manual*, 3rd ed. Washington, D.C.: 1983.

Dorland WA: *Dorland's Illustrated Medical Dictionary*, 26th ed. Philadelphia: W.B. Saunders, 1981.

Kolin PC, Kolin JL: *Professional Writing for Nurses in Education, Practice and Research*. St. Louis: CV Mosby, 1980.

Lewis EP: *Toward Getting Published: Guidelines for Nurses Who Want to Write*. New York: American Journal of Nursing Company, undated.

Linton M: *A Simplified Style Manual: For the Preparation of Journal Articles in Psychology, Social Sciences, Education and Literature*. Englewood Cliffs, N.J.: Prentice-Hall, 1972.

McCloskey JC, Swanson E: Publishing opportunities for nurses: A comparison of 100 journals. *Image* June 1982; 14:50–56.

McGraw-Hill: *Nursing Dictionary*. New York: McGraw Hill, 1979.

Mirin SK: *The Nurse's Guide to Writing for Publication*. Wakefield, Mass.: Nursing Resources, 1981.

Olson G: *Sweet Agony: A Writing Manual of Sorts*. Grants Pass, Ore.: Windyridge Press, 1972.

Perrin PG , Ebbitt WR: *Writer's Guide and Index to English*. Glenview, Ill.: Scott, Foresman, 1972.

Saslow CA: *Basic Research Methods*. Reading, Mass: Addison-Wesley, 1982.

Strunk W, White EB: *The Elements of Style*. New York: Macmillan, 1972.

Styles MM: Why publish? *Image* June 1978; 10:28–32.

Taber CW: *Cyclopedic Medical Dictionary*. 14th ed. Philadelphia: FA Davis, 1981.

Tornquist EM: *From Proposal to Publication: The Nurse Researcher's Guide to Writing*. Menlo Park, Calif.: Addison-Wesley, 1985.

Turabian KL: *A Manual for Writers of Term Papers, Theses, and Dissertations*, 4th ed. Chicago: University of Chicago Press, 1973.

Ward RR: Fog and how to fight it. Pages 27–28 in: *Practical Technical Writing*. New York: Knopf, 1968.

Further Readings

Binger JL: Writing for publication: A survey of nursing journal editors. *J Nurs Adm* January 1979; 9:50–52.

Carnegie ME: The referee system. *Nurs Res* 1975; 24:243.

Gunning R: *The Technique of Clear Writing*. New York: McGraw-Hill, 1968.

Interagency Council on Library Resources for Nursing. Reference sources for nursing. *Nurs Outlook* June 1982:363–367.

Lewis EP: For the nurse writer's bookshelf. *Am J Nurs* July 1982:1116–1118.

McMahan E: *A Crash Course in Composition*, 2nd ed. New York: McGraw-Hill, 1977.

Zinsser W: *On Writing Well*. New York: Harper & Row, 1976.

Appendix A

Human Subjects Review Resources

APPENDIX A-1   Sample Expedited Human Subjects Protocol

Submission date _____ 10/13/82 _____

Principal Investigator
(UCSF Faculty) _____ Professor Holly Wilson _____   *University Title* _____ Professor _____   *Dept.* Nursing–Mental Health

Co-Investigator
and Title _____ Sandra L. Scheetz, M.S., R.N., Doct. Cand. _____   *Is principal investigator the sponsor/advisor only?* Yes __X__ No _____

Mailing Address
(campus if possible) _____ N511E School of Nursing _____   *Phone* _____ 666-3903 _____

Project
Title _____ The Influence of Social Network Characteristics on the Performance of Self-care _____

_____ by the Chronically Mentally Ill in the Community _____

(A) *The point of this project is (Explain background, rationale, basic design, etc.):*

To investigate the influence of the characteristics of social network on the performance of self-care by the chronically mentally ill (CMI) in the community.

Much recent research has focused on the individual's primary group and the relationship to psychiatric epidemiology. More specific information is needed about the person's ability to function on a day-to-day basis, which is one aspect of the psychiatric disability. This is important because chronic mental illness is a major health problem today, and because one of the primary problems with this group is self-care. The proposed descriptive, longitudinal study would be an attempt to describe the social network of the CMI over time and the relationship of network characteristics to the performance of self-care in this population.

(B) *The subject population(s) will be selected (or excluded) on the following criteria (Consider how access will be gained as well as any problems relevant to special subject populations such as children, prisoners, etc.):*

One hundred twenty subjects who will be residing in the community will be solicited from in-patient psychiatric units. Criteria for inclusion are (1) adults ages 18–45; (2) voluntary admission to hospital; (3) English speaking; (4) diagnosis at discharge of schizophrenia, affective disorder, or borderline personality; (5) on, or approved for, Supplemental Security Income (SSI); (6) hospitalized one time in the past 5 years for at least 6 months OR hospitalized 2 or more times in the past 12 months; (7) must agree to participate in the study. Exclusion criteria are (1) physical deformities, physical injuries, and serious or chronic physical conditions; (2) organic psychoses; (3) primary diagnosis of substance abuse. Subjects will be asked to involve a friend or relative in a home visit follow-up.

(C) *The following procedures involving humans will be done for purposes of the study (If known, the expedited review category number from* Consent Forum, *issue 5 is 9) (If applicable, include interview themes and questionnaires if not commonly known):*

1. Charts reviewed by agency staff to determine eligibility.

2. Information Sheet (attached) will be given to potential subjects by agency staff.

3. Those interested in participating will be given the Informed Consent (attached) and the opportunity to discuss it with the investigator. They will be asked to sign the Consent.

4. Relative or friend named by subject will be contacted by investigator and invited to participate in

follow-up (Time 1 & Time 2). Informed Consent for Relative or Friend will be signed prior to administration of questionnaires at follow-up.

5. Consenting subjects (pts) will be given the following:
   a. Demographic Data Sheet—at Baseline.
   b. Modified Norbeck Support Questionnaire (Norbeck, Lindsey & Carrieri, 1981)—at Baseline, Time 1 & Time 2.
   c. Social Relationship Scale (McFarlane, 1980)—Baseline, Time 1 & Time 2.
6. Level of Rehabilitation Scale (Carey & Posavac, 1978)—rated by nurse at Baseline; rated by investigator at Time 1 & Time 2 by questioning relative or friend.
7. Katz Adjustment Scale (Katz & Lyerly, 1963) Forms S2 & S3 Subject and R2, R3 Relative all completed at Time 1 and Time 2 follow-up.
8. Consent to participate at Time 2 will be reviewed at Time 1 with Subject and Relative/Friend.

(D) *The risks involved in these procedures and the methods of minimizing the risks, inconveniences, or discomforts are (Include any potential for loss of privacy):*

It is possible that subjects will become frustrated or anxious while responding to the questionnaires. If the investigator or the subject determines that this is occurring, another appointment will be set up to complete the questionnaires.

The privacy of prospective subjects will be maintained by having agency staff do the initial screening for eligibility. Only the names of those who would like to participate will be given to the investigator. Subjects will be given a code number, and all identifying information will be separated from the responses. The code number will be retraceable only by the investigator for purposes of follow-up. Complete confidentiality of all information will be maintained.

Subjects' right to refuse to continue in the study or to withdraw at any time will be respected. It will be concluded that those who miss three follow-up appointments are "withdrawing" and will be dropped from the study.

All questionnaires will be filled out, and all appointments will be made at the subjects' convenience as to time and place.

(E) *Describe the anticipated benefits, if any, to subjects, and the importance of the knowledge that may reasonably be expected to result:*

There will be no immediate or direct benefit to subjects. This study has the potential to extend our theoretical knowledge about the network characteristics of the specific subpopulation of the chronically mentally ill over time, and knowing more about the relationship between network characteristics and performance of self-care by the chronically mentally ill is of clinical significance.

(F) *Describe the consent process and attach all consent documents. If waiver from use of written consent is requested, give the justification:*

Patients will be screened initially by agency staff. Those who meet the inclusion criteria will be given an Information Sheet for Prospective Participants (attached), which explains the study. Those who wish to participate will be given the Informed Consent (attached) and the opportunity to discuss the study with the investigator. The Informed Consent also includes a choice for the subject to participate in the 12-month follow-up. This aspect of the Consent will be reviewed with the subject at the one-month visit should the subject not wish to continue. Potential subjects will be asked to sign the Consent Form. Those who agree to participate will be given a copy of the consent and the Information Sheet to keep.

SOURCE: Used with permission of Sandra Scheetz, RN, MS, DNS candidate.
School of Nursing, University of California at San Francisco.

APPENDIX A-2   Information Sheet for Prospective Participants in a Research Study

Sandra Scheetz is a nurse and a doctoral student at the University of California, San Francisco. She is conducting a research study of persons, like yourself, who will be discharged from the psychiatric unit to return to the community to live. You are invited to participate in this study.

The following are answers to questions that people ask most often about the study.

1. What is the purpose of the study?
The main purpose of this community follow-up study is to help nurses and other mental health professionals learn more about how patients get along on a day-to-day basis after they leave the hospital.

2. What would be required of me?
Prior to leaving the hospital, you will be asked to fill out one personal information sheet and two paper-and-pencil questionnaires. These are *not* tests.

Also before discharge an appointment will be made to see you approximately 4–6 weeks after you leave the hospital. The follow-up visit will either be at your home or at the hospital, whichever is more convenient for you.

At the follow-up visit, you would be asked again to fill out three paper-and-pencil questionnaires.

You will also be asked to have a relative or close friend, someone you see on a daily basis, participate in the study by being present at the follow-up visit. You will choose this person to participate. This friend or relative will also be asked to fill out two short questionnaires and to answer some questions about how you are getting along.

3. What good will the study do me?
There will be no direct benefit to you. Perhaps you will get some satisfaction from knowing that, by answering the questionnaires, you have provided information that may help other patients returning to the community.

4. What will be done with the information I give about myself?
You are one of 120 people who are being studied in the community follow-up. All of the people are former patients like yourself. The information will be carefully studied by the researcher, who will write a report on the results of the study. These results may also be published in the professional journals where they can be read by other mental health professionals. Therefore, in the long run, the information you provide will be helpful for many people who are hospitalized, as you were, and helpful to the many professionals who give care to those patients.

Your name will not be used anywhere in the reports. Your answers will be given a special number to be used instead of your name. The information you provide will *not* be a part of your chart or treatment records, and will not be shared with the professionals who give you care.

5. Will filling out the questionnaires take a long time?
No. The average time for each set of questionnaires is 1 hour, once in the hospital and once at the follow-up visit, for a total of 2 hours. Some people may finish in 30 minutes, and others may take more than 1 hour. The time needed for your friend or relative to fill out the questionnaires and to answer questions is approximately 30 minutes.

6. What if I am unable to keep my follow-up appointment?
Please call Sandra Scheetz at 123-4567 or 890-1234 to let her know. If you need to call long distance, please call Mrs. Scheetz at 890-1234 and she will acccept a collect phone call. She will be glad to schedule another time for you that is more convenient.

7. How will I remember my follow-up appointment time?
About one week before the appointment time, you will receive a postcard in the mail to remind you.

8. Who will be present at the follow-up visit?
You and your relative or friend will be seen only by Sandra Scheetz or her research assistant.

9. Why do I have to ask a relative or friend to take part in the study?
Your relatives or friends who see you every day are the people who know most about how you are getting along. Of course you yourself will provide the most information, but another person will often notice things that you overlook. Research has already shown that a relative's report is a very useful source of information, even when the patient's own report about himself is also available.

10. What if I have other questions that haven't been answered here?
Please feel free to call Sandra Scheetz at 123-4567 (or leave a message). Or tell your nurse that you would like to speak to Mrs. Scheetz, and she will contact you on the unit the next time she is there.

What next?
If you would be willing to participate in this study, please fill in the information below, detach it, and give it to your nurse or to the research assistant on the unit. You will then be asked to sign a "Consent to Be a Research Subject" before filling out any questionnaires.

You may keep this information sheet for yourself and to share with your relative or friend.

Thank you for taking the time to read this!

SOURCE: Used with permission of Sandra Scheetz, RN, MS, DNS candidate.
School of Nursing, University of California at San Francisco.

APPENDIX A-3   Consent to Be a Research Subject

Sandra Scheetz is a doctoral student in nursing studying psychiatric patients who return to live in the community and how they get along on a day-to-day basis after they leave the hospital.

If I agree to be in the study, I will fill out two questionnaires and a personal information sheet prior to leaving the hospital. I will also meet with Sandra Scheetz or her research assistant at my home or at the hospital approximately one month after discharge to fill out three additional questionnaires. I have agreed to have a relative or friend of my choosing participate in the home visit to answer additional questionnaires and additional questions.

I (AGREE) (DO NOT AGREE) (circle one) to be a participant in the 12-month follow-up study. Participating in this follow-up would require a second home visit with Sandra Scheetz or her research assistant. This second home visit would be like the first one and would be approximately 12 months after my discharge from the hospital.

Filling out the questionnaires may be an inconvenience to me and may take as long as 2 hours total. However, I may fill out the questionnaires at my convenience before leaving the hospital, and may also make the follow-up appointment at a time and place convenient to me. If I agree to participate in the 12-month follow-up, I will be contacted by phone or mail several times over the intervening 11-month period in order to find out if my address has changed and to make arrangements for the final home visit. This may be an intrusion on my privacy.

There will be no medical benefit to me, and I will not be paid for my participation. The study may produce information of use to medical health professionals in the future.

I have had the opportunity to talk with Sandra Scheetz or her research assistant about the study. If I have further questions, I may reach her at 123-4567 (or leave a message). If I have any comments about participating in this study, I should first talk with Mrs. Scheetz. If for some reason I don't want to do this, I may contact the Committee on Human Research, which is concerned with protection of volunteers in research projects. I may reach the committee between 8 A.M. and 5 P.M., Monday through Friday, by calling 890-1234.

I have been offered a copy of this form and an Information Sheet to keep.

I have the right to refuse to participate or withdraw from the study at any time. Refusing to participate will in no way affect my care at this medical center at any time.

Subject Signature

Date

SOURCE: Used with permission of Sandra Scheetz, RN, MS, DNS candidate. School of Nursing, University of California at San Francisco.

Appendix B

Proposal Writing Resources

APPENDIX B-1   Sample Proposal Format

Center for Research
Research Prospectus to Develop Proposal

To: Center for Research Coordinating Committee

From: _____
                        (Name of unit/organization)

through _____
                        (contact person)

Section A - Complete the following section relating responses to the proposed
           project.

1.   Objective (overall or long-term goal of proposed research)

     _____

     _____

     _____

2.   Rationale (state rationale behind investigator's initiation of this
     prospectus)

     _____

     _____

     _____

3.   Significance to the Profession

     _____

     _____

     _____

     _____

     _____

4.   Summarize all Center for Research staff and other resources being
     requested.

     _____

     _____

     _____

Section B - Complete the following section relating responses to proposal
development.

1.   Time Frame (include time frame for proposal development and for proposed
study)

_____

_____

_____

_____

_____

2.   Staff Needed to Develop Full Proposal (include consultants)

_____

_____

_____

_____

_____

_____

3.   Budget for Proposal Development (Only)

_____

_____

_____

_____

_____

Section C - Complete the following section relating responses to the proposed
project (be as specific as possible with information available).

1.   Specific Aims or Research Questions (measurable objectives of proposed
project)

_____

_____

_____

2. Methods of Procedure: (Give general outline for research plan including nature and accessibility of subjects, sampling procedures, list instruments to be used or developed, kinds of data expected, data collection procedures, and procedures for data analysis and interpretation)

    _____

    _____

    _____

    _____

    _____

    _____

3. Time Frame (include time frame for proposal development and for proposed study)

    _____

    _____

    _____

    _____

    _____

4. Staff Needed to Conduct Project and Facilities and Resources Needed to Conduct Project

    _____

    _____

    _____

5. Total Budget and Identify Potential Funding Sources

    _____

    _____

    _____

    _____

APPENDIX B-2   Sample Abstract for Grant Application

DEPARTMENT OF HEALTH AND HUMAN SERVICES PUBLIC HEALTH SERVICE ABSTRACT OF RESEARCH PLAN	LEAVE BLANK PROJECT NUMBER

NAME AND ADDRESS OF APPLICANT ORGANIZATION (*Same as Item 11, page 1*)

School of Nursing, University of California, San Francisco, CA 94143

TITLE OF APPLICATION (*Same as Item 1, page 1*)

Geriatric Mental Health Academic Award

Name, Title, and Department of all professional personnel engaged on project, beginning with Principal Investigator/Program Director

Holly Skodol Wilson, R.N., Ph.D.   Principal Investigator/Awardee
Professor, Department of Mental Health and Community Nursing

ABSTRACT OF RESEARCH PLAN: Concisely describe the application's specific aims, methodology and long-term objectives, making reference to the scientific disciplines involved and the health-relatedness of the project. The abstract should be self-contained so that it can serve as a succinct and accurate description of the application when separated from it. <u>DO NOT EXCEED THE SPACE PROVIDED</u>.

The overall objective of this proposal is to secure funds that will enable me, over a three-year period, to undertake special supervised study and experiences that will prepare me to assume a leadership role in fostering programs of research and teaching among health science students and faculty at the University of California, San Francisco by becoming a professional resource person in the area of geriatric mental health. Special contributory objectives include the following:

1. To acquire knowledge, skills and competences in the field of aging health policy research and analysis.

2. To develop skill in the use of computer technology for applications to aging mental health policy research, including areas such as financing, manpower, program evaluation and efficiency of administrative structures for care delivered to the aged chronically mentally ill.

3. To build a network of professional and scientific associations with others conducting research in these areas, who may also become resources to other faculty and graduate students.

4. To develop strategies, resources, and structures for fostering the interest of other faculty and graduate students in research focused on geriatric mental health and their knowledge and use of research findings in related teaching and clinical work.

These aims will be addressed through a combination of formal course work in health policy and computer science, collegial mentorship and participation in research at UCSF's Aging Health Policy Center, attendance at scientific meetings and communications both formal and informal with faculty and students on committees, through presentations and my own publications.

LABORATORY ANIMALS INVOLVED. Identify by common names. If none, state "none."

APPENDIX B-3   Nursing Research Grants (October 1983)

Grant Number	Start Date	Principal Investigator	Mailing Address	Grant Title
R21 NU-01012	9/26/83	Abbey, June	School of Nursing 354 Victoria Hall University of Pittsburgh Pittsburgh, Pennsylvania 15261	Nursing Research Emphasis Grant for Doctoral Programs in Nursing
R01 NU-00624	6/1/78	Ailinger, Rita L.	College of Professional Studies George Mason University 4400 University Drive Fairfax, Virginia 22030	Functional Capacity of Hispanic Elderly
R01 NU-00712	4/1/83	Andrews, Claire M.	Frances Payne Bolton School of Nursing Case Western Reserve University 2121 Abington Road Cleveland, Ohio 44106	Nursing, Maternal Postures, Fetal Position/Presentation
R01 NU-00998	3/1/83	Barhyte, Diana Y.	Rush-Presbyterian- St. Luke's Medical Center 1753 West Congress Parkway Chicago, Illinois 60612	Decentralization and Nurse Retention: A Pilot Study
R01 NU-00912	8/1/83	Birenbaum, Linda K.	Oregon Health Sciences Univ. CDRC Unit—Office of Research P.O. Box 574 Portland, Oregon 97207	Effect of Family Nursing on Sibling Response to Dying
R01 NU-00936	9/25/82	Chen, Shu Pi	College of Nursing University of Illinois Medical Center 845 South Damen Avenue Chicago, Illinois 60612	Health Awareness Program Conducted by School Nurses
R01 NU-00977	8/1/83	Clinton, Jacqueline Fay	School of Nursing University of Wisconsin—Milwaukee P.O. Box 413 Milwaukee, Wisconsin 53201	Couvade: Patterns and Predictors
R01 NU-00939	3/1/83	Curry, Mary Ann	Oregon Health Sciences Univ. 3181 SW Sam Jackson Park Road Portland, Oregon 97201	Antenatal Hospitalization: Maternal Behavior and the Family
R21 NU-00821	9/1/80	Donaldson, Sue K.	College of Nursing Rush-Presbyterian- St. Luke's Medical Center 1753 West Congress Parkway Chicago, Illinois 60612	Nursing Research Emphasis Grant for Doctoral Programs in Nursing

Grant Number	Start Date	Principal Investigator	Mailing Address	Grant Title
R21 NU-00827	9/25/80	Downs, Florence S.	School of Nursing University of Pennsylvania 420 Service Drive Philadelphia, Pennsylvania 19104	Nursing Research Emphasis Grant for Doctoral Programs in Nursing
R21 NU-01014	9/26/83	Fitzpatrick, Joyce J.	School of Nursing Case Western Reserve University 2121 Abington Road Cleveland, Ohio 44106	Nursing Research Emphasis Grant for Doctoral Programs in Nursing
R18 HS-04788	9/21/83	Fleming, John J.	El Camino Hospital 2500 Grant Road Mountain View, California 94042	Nurse: A Nurse Staffing Requirements System
R01 NU-00974	9/26/83	Garvin, Bonnie J.	College of Nursing Ohio State University 1585 Neil Avenue Columbus, Ohio 43210	Confirmation/ Disconfirmation: RN/ MD Communication
R21 NU-00835	9/1/81	Gay, Janice T.	School of Nursing University of Alabama University Station Birmingham, Alabama 35294	Nursing Research Emphasis Grant for Doctoral Programs in Nursing
R01 NU-00707	3/1/80	Geden, Elizabeth A.	School of Nursing University of Missouri S329 Nursing School Building Columbia, Missouri 65211	Preparation for Labor
R01 NU-00993	2/1/83	Goodwin, Laura	School of Nursing University of Colorado 4200 E. 9th Ave. Denver, Colorado 80262	A Study of School Nurses' Use of Project Health P.A.C.T.
R21 NU-00828	9/1/80	Gortner, Susan R.	School of Nursing University of California 3rd Avenue & Parnassus San Francisco, California 94143	Nursing Research Emphasis Grant for Doctoral Programs in Nursing
R03 NU-01002	6/1/83	Hawley, Donna J.	Department of Nursing Wichita State University Campus Box 41 1845 Fairmount Wichita, Kansas 67208	Outcome Predictors in Chronic Rheumatic Disease
R01 NU-00908	4/1/83	Hinshaw, Ada Sue	Nursing Department University Hospital Arizona Health Sciences Center 1501 North Campbell Tucson, Arizona 85724	Anticipated Turnover Among Nursing Staff

Grant Number	Start Date	Principal Investigator	Mailing Address	Grant Title
R01 NU-00971	8/1/83	Hinshaw, Ada Sue	Nursing Department University Hospital Arizona Health Sciences Center 1501 North Campbell Tucson, Arizona 85724	Validity of Ratio Measurement of Nursing Concepts
R01 NU-00967	7/1/83	Holzemer, William L.	School of Nursing, N319Y University of California 3rd & Parnassus Avenues San Francisco, California 94143	Quality Indicators of Nursing Doctoral Programs
R21 NU-00838	9/20/80	Hummel, Patricia A.	School of Nursing University of Wisconsin Madison, Wisconsin 53706	Nursing Research Emphasis Grant for Doctoral Programs in Nursing
R21 NU-00820	7/1/81	Jackson, Nancy E.	School of Nursing, SM-27 University of Washington Seattle, Washington 98195	Nursing Research Emphasis Grant
R01 NU-00965	4/1/83	Jones, Susan L.	School of Nursing Kent State University Kent, Ohio 44242	Health Belief Model Intervention to Increase Compliance
R01 NU-00881	2/1/82	Kalisch, Beatrice J.	School of Nursing University of Michigan History & Politics of Nursing Ann Arbor, Michigan 48109	Information Quality of Nursing News
R01 NU-00945	4/1/83	Kirchhoff, Karin T.	College of Nursing University of Illinois 845 South Damen Avenue Chicago, Illinois 60612	Electrocardiographic Response to Ice Water Ingestion
R01 NU-00944	2/1/83	Kirgis, Carol A.	College of Nursing University of Utah 25 South Medical Drive Salt Lake City, Utah 84112	Nursing Promoting of Mother–Infant Acquaintance
R01 NU-00875	5/1/83	Knafl, Kathleen A.	College of Nursing University of Illinois at Chicago 845 South Damen Avenue Chicago, Illinois 60612	The Nurse Researcher's Role in A Clinical Setting
R01 NU-00801	9/28/81	Kramer, Marlene F.	School of Nursing University of Connecticut Storrs, Connecticut 06268	Reality Shock Management and Patient Perception of Nursing Care
R01 NU-00931	6/15/75	Lederman, Regina P.	School of Nursing University of Wisconsin at Madison 600 Highland Avenue Madison, Wisconsin 53792	Psychophysiological Correlates of Maternal–Fetal Health

Grant Number	Start Date	Principal Investigator	Mailing Address	Grant Title
R21 NU-00831	9/1/80	Leininger, Madeleine M.	College of Nursing Wayne State University 5557 Cass Avenue Detroit, Michigan 48202	Nursing Research Emphasis Grant for Doctoral Programs in Nursing
R21 NU-00829	9/1/80	Lenz, Elizabeth R.	School of Nursing University of Maryland 655 West Lombard Street Baltimore, Maryland 21201	Nursing Research Emphasis Grant for Doctoral Programs in Nursing
R01 NU-01000	5/1/83	Lewis, Frances M.	School of Nursing, SM-24 University of Washington Department of Community Health Care Systems Seattle, Washington 98195	Family Impact Study: Cancer and the Family
R01 NU-00949	7/1/83	Lowery, Barbara J.	School of Nursing University of Pennsylvania 420 Service Drive Philadelphia, Pennsylvania 19104	Causal Attributions and Myocardial Infarction Outcome
R01 NU-01053	9/1/83	Lyss, Liny E.	Department of Nursing Idaho State University Box 8101 Pocatello, Idaho 83209	Conceptualization of Nursing During Various Epochs
R01 NU-01001	4/1/83	McCorkle, Ruth	School of Nursing University of Washington T518 Health Sciences Bldg., SM-24 Seattle, Washington 98195	Evaluation of Cancer Management
R21 NU-00841	9/20/80	Miller, Jean R.	College of Nursing University of Utah 25 S. Medical Drive Salt Lake City, Utah 84112	Nursing Research Emphasis Grant for Doctoral Programs in Nursing
R01 NU-00845	6/1/81	Mood, Darlene W.	College of Nursing Wayne State University 5557 Cass Avenue Detroit, Michigan 48202	Self-Catheterization in Rehabilitation Care
R01 NU-01052	9/1/83	Munro, Barbara H.	School of Nursing Yale University 855 Howard Ave. New Haven, Connecticut 06510	Effect of Relaxation Therapy in Post-MI Patients
R21 NU-00824	9/1/80	O'Brien, Mary Elizabeth	School of Nursing Catholic University of America Washington, D.C. 20064	Nursing Research Emphasis Grant for Doctoral Programs in Nursing

Grant Number	Start Date	Principal Investigator	Mailing Address	Grant Title
R01 NU-00917	9/1/80	O'Brien, Mary Elizabeth	School of Nursing Catholic University of America Washington, D.C. 20064	Exercise of Self-Care Agency in Hemodialysis Adaptation
R21 NU-00839	9/25/81	Ozbolt, Judith	School of Nursing University of Michigan 1335 Catherine Street Ann Arbor, Michigan 48109	Nursing Research Emphasis Grant for Doctoral Programs in Nursing
R01 NU-00849	7/1/81	Padilla, Geraldine	Nursing Research Department City of Hope National Medical Center 1500 East Duarte Road Duarte, California 91010	A Quality Assurance Program For Cancer Nursing
R01 NU-00772	9/20/80	Parsons, L. Claire	School of Nursing University of Virginia 5012 McLeod Hall Charlottesville, Virginia 22903	Nurse Assessment of Comatose Head Injured Patients
R01 NU-00919	9/26/83	Parsons, L. Claire	School of Nursing University of Virginia 5012 McLeod Hall Charlottesville, Virginia 22903	Nursing Interventions in Acute Neurologic Trauma
R01 NU-00810	9/29/82	Porter, Luz S.	School of Nursing West Virginia University 3015 Basic Sciences Building Morgantown, W.Va. 26506	Parenting Enhancement Program for High-Risk Adolescents
R01 NU-00955	5/1/83	Powers, Marjorie J.	College of Nursing University of Illinois at Chicago 845 South Damen Avenue Chicago, Illinois 60612	Identification of Variables that Characterize Hypertensives
R01 NU-00819	7/1/80	Prescott, Patricia A.	School of Nursing University of Maryland 655 West Lombard Street Baltimore, Maryland 21201	Temporary Personnel Services, Nurses, and Hospitals
R01 NU-00978	9/1/83	Price, James L.	Center for Health Services Research University of Iowa Iowa City, Iowa 52242	Absenteeism and Turnover Among Nursing Department Personnel
R01 NU-00957	3/1/83	Robb, Susanne S.	Nursing Service for Research V. A. Medical Center 646/118E University Drive "C" Pittsburgh, Pennsylvania 15260	Exercise Treatment for Wandering Behavior in the Elderly
P01 NU-00800	8/1/81	Santora, Dolores	College of Nursing Arizona State University Tempe, Arizona 85281	Nursing Assessments for Health Promotion

Grant Number	Start Date	Principal Investigator	Mailing Address	Grant Title
P01 NU-00745	7/1/80	Stevenson, Joanne S.	College of Nursing Ohio State University 1585 Neil Avenue Columbus, Ohio 43210	Women's Health Research Program
R01 NU-01018	9/26/83	Stevenson, Joanne S.	College of Nursing Ohio State University 1585 Neil Avenue Columbus, Ohio 43210	Effects of Preventicare Exercise on Elders
R01 NU-00658	5/1/83	Swain, Mary Ann	School of Nursing University of Michigan 1335 Catherine Street Ann Arbor, Michigan 48109	Evaluation of Two Nursing Intervention Strategies
R01 NU-00870	8/1/81	Thomas, Barbara S.	College of Nursing University of Iowa Iowa City, Iowa 52242	Locus of Control and Satisfaction with Childbirth
P01 NU-00886	9/25/81	Tomlinson, Patricia S.	School of Nursing University of Oregon 3181 S.W. Sam Jackson Park Road Portland, Oregon 97201	Parent/Infant Interaction in Normal and High Risk Subjects
R01 NU-00961	9/25/80	Voda, Ann M.	College of Nursing University of Utah 25 South Medical Drive Salt Lake City, Utah 84112	Menopausal Hot Flash
R01 NU-01007	9/26/83	Wallston, Kenneth A.	School of Nursing Vanderbilt University Nashville, Tennessee 37240	Study of Behavioral Aspects of Rheumatoid Arthritis
R01 NU-01003	8/1/83	Whall, Ann L.	College of Nursing Wayne State University 5557 Cass Avenue Detroit, Michigan 48202	Alzheimer's Disease: Life Factor Profiles
R01 NU-01054	9/26/83	Woods, Nancy F.	School of Nursing—SM-27 University of Washington Seattle, Washington 98195	Prevalence of Perimenstrual Symptoms
R21 NU-00834	9/29/80	Young, Katherine J.	College of Nursing University of Arizona Arizona Health Sciences Center Tucson, Arizona 85721	Nursing Research Emphasis Grant for Doctoral Programs in Nursing

SOURCE: U.S. Department of Health and Human Services, Rockville, MD.

Appendix C

Qualitative Research Resources

APPENDIX C-1   Comparison Between Formal and Informal Interviewing

	Formal	Informal
Time	Agreed on and scheduled by investigator and interviewee	May be predetermined, but usually is not
Setting	Agreed on by investigator and interviewee; may occur in subject's natural setting or in formal setting such as an office or lab	May be predetermined, but usually is not; usually occurs in natural settings; researcher seeks out subjects as informants
Structure	Predetermined concepts, questions, and sequence, based on study purpose	Spontaneous and emergent, based on themes that appear
Role of Researcher	Unambiguous as information seeker	May be ambiguous: friend, colleague, participant
Questions	Use of a formal interview guide/schedule consistently with all respondents (e.g., questions are asked in same words and in same sequence)	General and may vary from interviewee to interviewer
Use of Probes	Based on responses; may be restricted so as to keep data collection consistent among subjects	Are used, especially early in project
Notes	Written or tape-recorded during interview	Not taken or recorded
Number of Interviews	Usually one or two; specified in study design	May require several to cover all content desired; will vary across respondents
Informed Consent	Official written consent	Oral consent; may get written consent; may provide information sheet
Interaction Between Researcher and Subject	Guided or deferred to beginning or ending interview by investigator	Encouraged and essential to developing informants

APPENDIX C-2   Sample Coded Field Notes

STRUCTURAL
CONTIALS BRAVE
CONSEQ OF ↑
ACT OF A BEHAV

RESOURCES FOR ATTENTION
RATIO

ON V. #12, p. 3

Mary (F. staff) tells me that she compares Soteria to Agnews State Hospital where there was a lot more out of control behavior because "everyone there is locked up and at least here residents can go around the corner to blow off steam. Also at Agnews there are a lot of patients and few staff while here people can get attention without blowing up to do it. Just the presence of a lot of staff and volunteers has something to do with it."

HIGH TOLERANCE FOR
BIZARRE BEHAVIOR
WHEN NOT SURVIVAL
ISSUE

MONITORING
INTERVENTION CONDITIONS

ON V. #12, p. 5

Paul (M. Resident) is standing upstairs in his doorway where he's been for many hours. I am told that he has sat in one place on the couch for 24 hours and stood in the doorway for 8. He stays there for the 8 hours that I am at the house. Sandy (F. staff) tells me that if he goes without eating or drinking for 3 days she or someone will try to get him to take something. He hasn't taken a bath for the month that he's been in the house, but when he goes without eating or drinking or going to the BR, they "take a very firm approach."

PROPERTY
INDIVIDUALIZED
NON-CODIFIED

PROPERTY
EMERGENT

CONSEQUENCE
STAFF CONFLICT
C̄ HOW MUCH CONTROL

COND.
DE-ELLABORATE STRUCTURE
-PRIMITIVE STRUCTURE
WHEN PRES. ALONE FAILS

BUFFERING AND PROTECTING

ON V. #10, p. 5

Mike (a visitor) asks Vaughn (M. staff) what would happen if some resident wouldn't eat. Vaughn answers "it's hard to say because how things get handled depends on the individuals involved. One time a resident wouldn't eat because he was paranoid. He started eating when a staff member fed himself one spoonful out of the dish and then one to the resident. Mike says what if it didn't work. Vaughn says he can't really say because people decide what to do as situations come up. Mike asks, "do you ever decide not to let someone do what they want to do?" Vaughn says "that's a real conflict area . . . how much to lay your trip on someone else. Everyone feels different about it, but like if someone was violent we'd try to stop him. We don't have any of the usual hospital equipment to do it . . . no locked doors, no drugs. A couple of times when people were really spaced out we'd put hooks and eyes at the tops of doors just so that if he started running out, he'd have to slow down to open the hook. We don't see our job as straightening people out. Instead we kind of buffer and protect him so he can have a place to go through his trip."

TOLERANCE FOR PROFANITY
TUNED INTO IT
AS SIGNALING
CONDITION FOR PRENSENCING
PRIVITIZED THERAPY TALK

ON V. #7, p. 8

Tania is yelling and storming around the house. Says she needs a damn car because she has stuff to do, is sick of hassling with people when she wants to go somewhere. Hal stops doing the dishes and goes looking around the house for her. When he finds her they have a quiet private conversation which I can't hear.

TUNING IN
AWARENESS

PRESENCING
FOR ATTENTION

Interview F. Staff (R.) p. 9

"Well for one thing, everybody recognized that he was in really heavy space. We've gone through enough here to become aware that they need attention at that time . . . on-going attention to protect them and to protect ourselves. With Joan a lot of times she'd get into really crazy space just because we weren't watching her and we were just lucky enough to catch her. When they're in that space you can't leave them be."

IN VIVO WORD
FOR PRESENCING =
BEING WITH

MONITORING
ANTICIPATING
ESTIMATING SUCCESS

CONTINUOUS COVERAGE
(VIGIL)

CONSEQUENCE
1. FEAR OF NEGLIGENCE
FROM PEERS

PERIODIC MONITORING

CONDIT. STAFF
RESOURCES

LIMIT SETTING

EX OF PERVASIVENESS
OF PRESENCING

Interview (M. staff G). p. 1

Q. (by Project Director) The things I am going to be asking you about are what we call "being with techniques." What are the techniques you use in instances of property damage, assaultiveness, fires, etc.?

A. With fires there's not too much to describe that. As we were sitting in the kitchen we smelled smoke and saw smoke pouring out of the back room so we just put it out and a couple of the people in the house stayed with the patients while the rest of us put it out. With Lonnie she was into breaking a lot of windows. You had to watch her constantly and be able to anticipate her. If you put your guard down and went to get a cup of coffee or something, she'd be gone and breaking a window. If I could I'd stop her. If I couldn't, like it was already broken by the time I got there, I tell her to go ahead and break the rest of it out."

Q. Tell me something about your experience of staying with people who are in dangerous or weird spaces for long periods of time . . . continuous coverage?

A. It scared me at first. Like the first night when Ellen thought I was death and I was going to rape her. I was really frightened that staff would come in saying what in hell are you doing. And I was concerned that she might call her parents or something and say she was getting raped. I had fears that I wasn't doing the right thing. Then I had doubts about what to do in these intense situations. Now having gone through them I know you don't ask anytime what you should do. You just work with the now. It has to do with the awareness and feeling for the situation at that time. It's not on a logical rational thinking level. It's on an emotional level . . . an intuitive level. You just allow them to be and protect when protecting is needed.

Interview (F. staff R.) p. 6

Q. What do you do when a person gets very withdrawn?

A. Take care of them. Feed them. Spot check on them. It depends if there's somebody else that's with the other residents. If there's a bunch of people then I can do a lot more. When Terry was in very heavy space, I would just stay with her, follow her around. The only time she ever did damage was when she was left alone . . . when she was lonely.

Q. How do you handle aggressive behavior in the house?

A. Well last week Terry picked up a catsup bottle and threw it against the plastic window. It had glanced a blow off Mary's head. Mary said, "Don't do that. I don't like it." And Terry turned and took off. I went after her and put my foot in the door she was trying to slam. At that point she said, "Can't anyone be alone?" and I said "No, I'm not going to leave you alone now. I want to talk about what's happening." When she's mad like that she can just talk about it. She obviously just wanted attention. I've never been involved when somebody's doing it in a heavy aggressive number.

PERSUADING
THERAPY TALK

SPECIALIZING
MULTIPLE PRES.
UNCERTAINTY

ACCUMULATED
STRATEGIES FOR
PREVENTION
(ANTICIPATION)
PRES. FOR RESTRAINT

Interview (M. Staff V.) p. 49

Q. Could you tell a little bit about what you do when someone's into breaking things?

A. The first incident I got a call at home from Sandy that I should come over and help out because everyone was kind of scared. Paul was throwing glasses. I remember feeling confronted with a situation that I wasn't familiar with. At first there was a period of not knowing whether to grab him or stand back or what. Evidently there were several bottles on the table which now probably would have been taken off if that same situation would come up. People have been realizing to take glass and knives away when it's something like that. So what we finally did was actually restrain him.

Interview (F. Staff J.) p. 46

Q. What do you think about staff?

A. Things sometimes are so intense and heavy that it becomes a problem to keep myself in good balance. A lot of times we've gotten into such a negativity around here. It's kind of an ideal here that we would all live together in peace and harmony forever, which is just not so. When it doesn't happen it feels like a contradiction. There are so many undercurrents of things that aren't said. I think it's sometimes very upsetting and confusing from a resident's standpoint.

CONSEQ. OF
CONTRADICTIONS

UNBALANCING
NEGATIVITY } STAFF
CONFLICT

P.O.V. #12, p. 2

Mary and Frank tell me about the speeches they are preparing for a meeting in NYC. They are going to talk about "getting burned out" as a consequence of the strain of their work. Mary says she is really feeling like punching Terry because she just can't give her any more attention. "I'm sick of getting called while I'm at a party to come down here for her. I wish she'd leave. I'm really feeling burned out by her."

Interview with (F. staff R.) p. 13

Q. Anything else you want to say?

A. I think the most important thing that we do is nontherapy. Our letting-be process is beautiful and that's the most important thing we do here . . . non-manipulation. We are a family. We can do what a structured place can't which makes them feel okay about where they are. I don't think all people can go crazy in this setting but we're good for a lot of people though.

APPENDIX C-3   Sample Outline of Codes in Qualitative Study

An early process in analyzing qualitative field data is to develop substantive codes and then collapse the laundry list you've used to conceptualize the anecdotes and episodes grounded in your data. Codes from the Soteria study database included the following ones.

I. Control of Residents

A. Conditions:
High tolerance for certain kinds of deviant behavior
High nonresident–resident ratio
Circumscribed space (house rather than hospital)
Minimal-control structures (no locks, restraints, chemicals)
Resident inclination to out-of-control behavior related to diagnosis of schizophrenia
Heavy and light times

B. Tactics:
Normalizing
Health-optimizing
Growth-optimizing
Conversion to staff values and behavior
Monitoring
Presencing
Spritualizing
Urging self-control
Anticipating; tuning-in

C. Consequences:
Contagion
Emulating staff
Property destruction
Contouring
Acting out

II. Control of Staff

A. Conditions:
Minimal structure (schedules)
Covering (time)
Limited shared socialization
Personal intimacy

B. Tactics:
Joking
Legitimizing own needs and limits
Monitoring
Cultivating
Muting of conventional controls
"Fairing" in management of work
Networking
Composure strategies
Peer consultation
Cohesion rituals
Confronting
Script innovating

C. Control problems:
Burning out
Bumming out
High staff conflict
High staff instability
Ripping off
Putting out

D. Consequences:
Getting by
Pulling out
Institution of structural controls

III. Control of Outside Community

A. Conditions:
Associated with NRI and NIMH (funded)
Heterogeneous, transitional neighborhood

B. Tactics:
Limited disclosure
Minimizing instrusion
Insulating
Accommodating
Privitizing

APPENDIX C-4   Sample Index Sheet for Grounded Theory Concept Indicators

An index allows the grounded theorist to link the analytic codes or concepts to specific indicators that can be located in field notes or interview transcripts. Descriptive indicators are used in the Findings Section to provide imagery for the concepts in the theory.

Conditions

Values of the House, pg. 1, 8, 42, 99
Freedom
Nonintervention
Health Optimizing
Staff control problems
Division of work, pg. 52, 77, 78, 88, 87, 91, 92
Strain, pg. 69, 81 (intrusive of staff personal life, pg. 106)
Cohesion maintenance, pg. 82

Staff Control Tactics

Staff specialization, pg. 51, 92
Joking, pg. 69
Fairing, pg. 77, 89
(Exemptions, pg. 77, 78)
Interest-oriented relating, pg. 81–82
(Cohesion-building)—Hospital imagery—rallying patient, pg. 110
Co-opting others for work, pg. 87

Control Related With Outsiders

Outsider control problems
Dependency of some residents, pg. 71–72
Misinterpreting, pg. 98, 102
Outrage, pg. 106
Intruding families, pg. 104
Outsider control tactics
Special allowances, pg. 108
Mediating between residents and outside, pg. 72, 94 (buffer)
Purposeful, goal-directed outings, pg. 90
Escorting, pg. 93–94
Insulating, pg. 97
Partial disclosure, pg. 98, 102
Appeasing, pg. 100, 104

Resident Control Tactics

(Variable conditions according to)

1. Situation with a precedent, pg. 49
2. Uncertainty about approach, pg. 50
3. Recognition of patterns, pg. 52
4. Estimating actual danger vs. attention getting, pg. 57

Presencing and multiple presencing, pg. 49, 71— variation escorting, pg. 94
Selective avoidance, pg. 50
Physical restraint, pg. 50, 55, 57, 60, 66
Therapy talk, pg. 54, 58, 62
Anticipatory prevention, pg. 56
Discounting or disguising, pg. 62
Interpreting by staff, pg. 60
Tolerating some out-of-control behavior, pg. 64, 67
Touching to establish contact
Joking, pg. 69
Verbal disapproval, pg. 70—verbal limit setting, pg. 96
Vigil, pg. 73—meds, pg. 84
Normalizing, pg. 75, 79–81 (excursions, pg. 82, 83, 89)
Monitoring, pg. 99
Tuning-in, pg. 109

Interview With Male Staff

Conditions

Ideology of freedom

Codes

Resident control problems

1. Physical assault, pg. 56, 57, 60, 70
   Self-destructive behavior, pg. 59, 101

Destructive behavior (rampaging, breaking things) pg. 49, 50, 51
2. Verbal threats, pg. 54, 55
3. Sexual advances toward staff, pg. 61, 63 (crushes)
4. Variation—unintelligible or inappropriate language or communication, pg. 65

Regression, pg. 66, 70
Withdrawal, pg. 64
Unconventional conduct in public places, pg. 70, 94, 95, 96
5. AWOLs, pg. 97

APPENDIX C-5   Tentative Outline of Grounded Theory Based on Memo Sorting

An outline of sorted memos provides the final integrative scheme for a grounded theory. The following outline of memos contained the key ideas for the theory of infracontrolling at Soteria House.

TITLE: Theory of Infracontrol in a Psychiatric Residence

Preface	Relevance of questions of control in view of social trend away from total institutions and toward community treatment models
	Purpose of the study related to concern for more rational and compassionate care. Provision of an explanation and basis for prediction through study of interaction, its contexts and consequences
	Introduction of core analytical category of Primitive Infracontrol Structures and Processes. Use of this scheme to organize and integrate many events that might otherwise seem disconnected or paradoxical
	Acknowledgments
Part I	Introduction
Chapter I	The Problem of Control Within Psychiatry
	Central idea is that people come to the attention of Psychiatry because of failure of self-control and labeling by others of such. Refer to Clausen's studies of families of mental patients and other research on pre-hospital career. Whether the focus is "custodial" or "treatment" centered, problems of control are central
Chapter II	The Elaborate Codified Control Structures of Conventional Psychiatric Institutions
	Identification of the Properties, Strategies and Consequences and Conditions of Elaborate Hospital control. Refer to Goffman's Asylums, Stanton and Schwartz, Strauss and Schatzman, Greenblatt, and other secondary sources for data
Part II	Types of Primitive Infracontrol Based on Its Properties
Chapter III	Properties of Primitive Infracontrol
	Emergent, based on extemporaneous innovation in face of immediate need
	Primitive, in the sense of operating at the survival level of food, sex, rest, shelter, and safety
	Tacit, in view of espoused values of freedom and nonintervention
	A-Theoretical, in that persons do not all stand in some relation to any single theory or ideology
	Temporary, in that control structures do not persist over time and become codified but rather are abandoned when the need no longer is present
	Reciprocal, in that control is not exercised exclusively by one group on another

Consequences: Contouring of residents after staff

Dramatic display of symptoms before 6 months, but disappearance after 6 months

Failures

Staff gets burned out-strained

Chapter VII   Control of External World

Conditions: Location in heterogeneous transient neighborhood

Legitimized under auspices of NIMH and MRI

Tactics: Ambiguous discourse (control of information given out)

Insulation (limits to physical intrusion)

Ritualized partial revealings

Appeasing

Consequences: Minimal problems with external community

Part IV   Conclusions

Chapter VIII   The Practical Use of Primitive Infracontrol Theory (in terms of the viability of the Soteria model)

Chapter IX   Implications for Formal Theory

Appendix   Methodology: Collection and Analysis of Data

Glossary

Ability test Data collection tools that include intelligence, achievement, and skill tests usually with normative data available for various subpopulations.

Abstract A section usually located at the beginning of a research article intended to summarize the entire study—including its purpose, design, and findings—as briefly as possible.

Abstracted empiricism A research approach that focuses on facts in isolation from any theory.

Accessible population The population that is a feasible source of sample members.

Active reading A set of skills designed to allow the reader to go beyond reading for mere information to reading for understanding. Involves interrogating the material.

Alternate forms reliability Established by comparing scores from various versions of an instrument for equivalence.

Analysis Refers to the separation of data into parts for the purpose of answering a research question.

Analysis of variance (ANOVA) Inferential statistical procedure that compares mean scores of two or more groups.

Analytic description A qualitative analysis method in which the researcher thinks up original classes or categories by inspecting and interrogating the data.

Analytic reading The third level of active reading that asks a series of questions about what is read.

Animal models Studies conducted on animals.

Anonymous A study is considered to be anonymous if even the investigator cannot link a subject with the information reported.

Applied research Research designed to solve practical problems.

BASIC (Beginners' All Purpose Symbolic Instruction Code) A commonly used computer programming language.

Basic research Research that aims to develop the state of knowledge for its own sake—also called pure research.

Batch processing A technique for conducting transactions with the computer by collecting data into groups to be processed together for efficiency.

Before-after design Called the true or classic experiment in which subjects are measured before and after experimental treatment.

Belmont report Document published in 1978 that identifies respect for persons as one of the key principles in ethical research.

Bimodal frequency A frequency distribution with two high points.

Binary system An off/on two-state system that turns computer circuits on and off through combinations of ones and zeros, which represent data.

Bit One switch inside the computer circuit called a binary digit.

BMDP (Biomedical Statistical Software Package) Applications statistical package for analyzing research data.

BPT Refers to bits per inch as an indication of the secondary storage capacity or density of a magnetic tape.

Byte A group of eight bits that stand for either one or zero in a computer.

Case study A study design that provides an in-depth analysis of a single subject for investigation, which may be an individual or group. Usually stimulates insight and suggests directions for further research. Sometimes viewed as synonymous with single subject descriptive research.

Cause and effect A relationship that allows one to predict and explain. Requires that cause precedes effect in time; requires evidence that the independent variable and dependent variable are associated, and rules out other factors as possible determining conditions.

Center for Nursing Research The first national center for nursing research established in 1983 to serve as a clearinghouse and link among scientific organizations like the American Nurses' Foundation, the American Academy of Nursing, and the American Nurses' Association.

Chi-square Nonparametric statistical test used to determine whether a significant difference exists between an observed frequency and an expected frequency. Can be used with nominal level measurements.

Clinical research Nursing research that generates knowledge to guide nursing practice. Identified by the ANA Commission on Nursing Research as having top priority in the 1980s.

Cluster sampling Selecting a random sample of elements that have been grouped into clusters.

CMS (Conversational Monitoring System) An interactive computer system that allows the user to give commands and get immediate responses or action.

COBOL (Common Business Oriented Language) A commonly used computer programming language.

Code book A research tool used to designate which columns on a keypunched card contain which data.

Comparative reading The fourth and highest level of reading, which requires a reader to relate what is being read to other material.

Concepts Abstractions that categorize observations based on commonalities and differences.

Conceptual framework (Conceptual model) A preliminary stage of a theory wherein interrelated concepts offer a framework for conducting research. Sometimes called a theoretical framework.

Conceptual map A diagrammatic representation of the variables in a theory.

Confidentiality Means that any information that a human subject divulges will not be made public or available to others.

Confounding variable Other variables in addition to the independent variable that might affect the dependent variable. Can confuse the interpretation of a study's results if not controlled for in a study's design or procedures. Also called extraneous variable.

Consent form A written document reflecting an agreement between a researcher and subject concerning the subject's participation in a study.

Construct Abstract concepts derived from a combination of existing theory and observations.

Construct validity The degree to which an instrument measures the construct or trait it was designed to measure.

Content analysis Method of analyzing qualitative data by counting the occurrence of specified units of analysis in the data. May refer to manifest content or inferred or latent content.

Content validity Includes subjective judgments about face validity and logical or sampling validity.

Contingency table A two-dimensional frequency distribution in which the frequencies of two variables are cross-tabulated.

Control unit The part of a computer's central processing unit that takes care of operating the machinery.

Convergent validity A type of construct validity that shows the degree to which scores from a measure resemble scores from a different measure of the same construct.

Copyright law Law that protects an author from having material used without permission.

Correlation A statistic (called r) that shows the extent to which values of one variable are related to values of another variable.

CPU (Central Processing Unit) The brain of the computer that keeps track of what's going on and executes programs that process data.

Criterion measure An accepted measure of some variable.

Criterion related validity The extent to which the score on an instrument can be related to criterion scores. May be concurrent or predictive depending on whether the criterion measure is made simultaneously or beforehand.

Critical value Value of a statistic that needs to be exceeded by the calculated value in order to accept the research or alternate hypothesis and reject the null hypothesis in a study.

Critique A critical estimate of a piece of research involving a systematic appraisal according to specified criteria.

Cross-sectional survey A study design that looks at subjects who are at two different points in time with respect to an experience.

CRT (Cathode Ray Tube) Screen or terminal resembling a television screen on which you can display computer keyboard type.

Cumulative Index to Nursing and Allied Health Literature (CINAHL) A resource for locating nursing journal articles.

CURN project A five-year Conduct and Use of Research in Nursing project, sponsored by the Michigan State Nurses' Association, which resulted in nine volumes focused on clinical research.

Data The information an investigator collects from the subjects or participants in a research study.

Data cleaning The process of trying to find errors in one's data set.

Data processing The performance of functions on data that transform them into information.

Debriefing A process of disclosing to human subjects all information that was previously withheld in a study.

Decision rule Instruction established to ensure that unusual responses will be scored in the same way for all.

Deductive approach Emphasizes theory as a system of testable hypotheses arranged in a deductive logical sequence and research as a process for verifying or testing them. Moves from the abstract and general to the concrete and specific.

Delphi Survey of Research Priorities A 1974 survey conducted by the Western Commission on Higher Education for Nursing (WICHEN) and the Regional Program for Nursing Research Development that revealed 150 priority items in three areas—with an emphasis on patient welfare.

Dependent variable (DV) Also called the criterion or outcome variable. Variability in the dependent variable depends on the preexisting conditions or factors that may be manipulated by the investigator.

Dermatome Instrument used to shave off various thicknesses of skin.

Description A qualitative analysis method in which the researcher finds classes in the data that correspond with a conceptual scheme or set of categories or concepts already existing in the literature.

Descriptive statistics Methods used to summarize or describe the characteristics of data in a sample.

Design The plan or blueprint used to get valid and reliable answers to research questions according to canons of science. Also called the protocol or program for a research study.

Dichotomous variable Variable with only two categories.

Directional hypothesis Specifies the expected direction of a relationship between concepts or variables.

Direct relationship A positive correlation between two variables.

Discriminant validity Determined from evidence that a measure of a construct measures only a particular construct and is not highly related to unrelated constructs.

Documentation Term used to refer to users' manuals and guides that contain instructions for employing software programs on a computer.

Double blind A strategy to lessen effects of inaccurate ratings or responses in which neither the subject nor the data collector knows if subjects are members of the experimental or control group in a study.

Douglas bag technique A means for measuring respiratory gas consumption.

Ecological validity Requires that the experiment is sufficiently explicit, clear, and consistent so that it could be replicated.

Electrocardiogram (ECG) A waveform or recording of the electrical activity of the heart.

Electroencephalogram (EEG) A waveform or recording of the electrical activity of the brain.

Electromylograph Instrument that records electrical activity of muscles.

Empirical evidence Refers to evidence derived through collection of data using one's senses—one of the characteristics of the scientific way of knowing.

Epistemology The branch of philosophy concerned with how one determines what is true.

Ethics A branch of philosophy concerned with what is good and bad and what one's moral obligations are.

Ethnology The study of human beings as social and cultural organisms.

Experiment Study design in which the investigator can control or manipulate one independent variable, can randomly select sample members, and can randomly assign sample members to experimental and control groups.

Exploratory study Type of study design used to gain familiarity or achieve insights into a phenomenon. Answers who and what questions. Also called Factor-naming, Factor-identifying, or Factor-searching.

Ex post facto A study design that literally studies something after the fact instead of manipulating an independent variable.

External criticism Evaluation of historical studies for the genuineness or authenticity of their data sources.

External validity In an experimental design, refers to how representative or general the results of a study are.

Extraneous variable Also called confounding variable, because it is a factor other than a study's independent variable that affects and confounds or confuses interpretation of a study's findings.

Face validity Subjective judgments by experts about the degree to which a test appears to measure the relevant construct.

Facts Derived from multiple congruent and similar observations of the same phenomena over time.

Factorial posttest design A design that matches subjects on a nominal variable that cannot be rank-ordered before assigning them to experimental and control groups.

Factor-isolating questions Research questions that ask "What is this?" Also called Factor-naming questions.

Factor-relating questions Research questions that ask how factors that have been identified relate to one another. Answers the question of "What is happening here?" Also called Association testing.

Field Any social-psychological arena where an investigator gathers data relevant to the area of inquiry.

Fieldwork Data collection strategies that include observation, interviewing, case studies, and document review. Rely on firsthand knowing under natural conditions. Also called field methods.

Fixed column format Key punch system where the variables and values for each and every subject are consistently located in the same columns.

Floppy disks Resemble 45 rpm records encased in a heavy paper jacket and are used to store software and data. Also called diskettes.

Focused interview Begins with an outline of topics to be covered with every interviewee, but allows freedom to deviate from the prepared agenda as well. Also called a partially structured or semi-structured interview.

Formative study Evaluation study that occurs in process in order to provide ongoing feedback about a program.

Fortran (Formula Translation) A commonly used computer programming language.

Frequency distribution An analysis method that involves determining how often scores or values appear in a data set.

Frequency polygon Graphic display of frequency table in which dots connected by straight lines are used instead of bars to show the number of times a class occurs.

Goal-free evaluation Evaluation study designed to include unanticipated consequences as well as data bearing on a program's goals or objectives.

Grand theory An attempt to explain everything in a field, using global concepts that are often poorly defined and ambiguously related.

Grounded theory A highly evolved and explicitly

codified method for developing categories of theories and propositions about their relationships from qualitative data. Closely integrated with a method of social research.

Halo effect An observer's tendency to rate certain subjects as consistently high or low on everything because of the overall impression the subject gives the rater.

Hardware The equipment in a computer system that you can touch.

Hawthorne effect Changes that occur in people's behavior because they know they are being studied. Was first observed in the Hawthorne plant of the Western Electric Company.

Helsinki Declaration A guide issued in 1964 and revised in 1974 by the World Medical Association that differentiated between two types of research: (1) that which is essentially therapeutic, and (2) that which is directed toward generation of scientific knowledge and has no benefit to the subject. Served as one of the bases for H.S.S. guidelines.

Histogram Graphic display of a frequency table using rectangular bars with heights equal to the frequency in a particular class.

Historical study Type of study design intended to explain the present or anticipate the future using methods for collecting and evaluating evidence from the past.

Hypothesis Statement of relationship between two or more study concepts or variables.

Independent variable (IV) The conditions or factors that precede measurement of the dependent variable or are manipulated by the investigator. Also called the input variable.

Indirect relationship (Inverse relationship) A negative correlation between two variables.

Inductive approach Emphasizes data as the source for generating concepts and explanatory relationships. Moves from the concrete and specific to the general and abstract.

Inferential statistics Methods used to make inferences about relationships and find statistical support for hypotheses in a population based on a sample drawn from it.

Informed consent The knowing consent of an individual or his/her legally authorized representative to decide whether or not to participate in a research project without undue inducement or any elements of force, fraud, deceit, duress, constraint, or coercion. The Institutional Review Board (IRB) acts as a protective mechanism for human research subjects by reviewing protocols and risk/benefit ratios.

Input devices The means by which data are provided to a computer so that they can be recognized by it.

Internal criticism Refers to evaluation of historical studies for the accuracy of the statements contained within the historical data sources used.

Internal validity In an experimental design, refers to whether or not manipulation of the independent variable really makes a significant difference to the dependent variable.

Interquartile range A stable measure of variability based on excluding extreme scores and using only middle cases.

Interrater reliability Reliability of measures across different raters.

Interval scale Measures data that rank order a variable with equal distance between points (e.g., Fahrenheit degrees).

Instruments Devices or techniques an investigator employs to collect data. May include questionnaires, performance checklists, pencil-and-paper tests, biological devices, and so on.

Instrumentation Process of using a device or combination of equipment for measurement.

Invasive procedure Involves penetration of the body for measurement.

K Measure of memory for all modes of computer storage; refers to 1000 bytes.

Keypunch cards A form of computer input consisting of cardboard cards with 80 vertical columns and 12 rows.

Keypunching A process by which a machine that looks like a typewriter punches holes into the columns of a data card.

Kundin wound tool An instrument to measure volume of tissue loss in a wound.

Likert scale Method of measurement in which respondents are presented with statements and asked how much they agree or disagree.

Literature review Systematic search of published work to find out what is known about a research topic.

Logging on The term used to gain access to a computer so you can use it. Involves a user identification number and a password.

Logical validity Refers to the extent that test items adequately represent the topic or construct covered in the test. Also called sampling validity.

Longitudinal survey A study design that studies subjects over time, assessing their experiences at predetermined stages.

Mainframe A large million-dollar computer with terminals located in different places throughout an organization.

Materials Another term for the measurement devices used to collect data from study subjects.

Max Planck respirometer A device for measuring respiratory gas consumption.

Mean The measure of central tendency derived by dividing the sum of the values in a data set by the total number of values, scores, or subjects in it. Also called the average.

Measurement The actual value of a variable, plus or minus error.

Median The measure of central tendency that corresponds to the middle score.

MEDLINE/MEDLARS The most frequently used computerized bibliographical services that access over 2900 biomedical and nursing sources.

Mental Measurements Yearbook A compendium that summarizes available information about an instrument and compares it with others in the field.

Metatheory A type of philosophical theory that studies the logical and methodological foundations of a discipline.

Methodological notes Field notes that remind the researcher which methodological approaches might be fruitful.

Methodological studies Designs that develop, validate, or evaluate research tools or techniques.

Microcomputer Small computer that is also called a personal or business computer.

Microfiche A computer output on microfilm that allows a lot of printed material to be presented in a small space.

Middle range theory Looks at a specific empirical area and at key variables in depth. Also called substantive theory.

Minimal risk Means that the risks anticipated to human subjects as a consequence of participating in the proposed research are not greater than those ordinarily encountered in daily life or during the performance of routine examinations or tests.

Mode The category or class that has the highest frequency. A measure of central tendency.

Model A structural, pictorial, diagrammatic, or mathematical likeness that represents some aspect of reality.

Multimodal frequency A frequency distribution with more than two high points.

Necessary condition A required condition if an event is to occur.

Negative cases Anecdotes in qualitative data that run counter to the analyst's propositions.

Nominal scale A scale that measures data by assignment of characteristics into categories.

Nonequivalent pretest-posttest control group design The most basic quasi-experimental design that uses comparative groups instead of random assignment to equivalent control and experimental groups.

Noninvasive procedure Procedure that does not involve penetration of the skin for measuring a parameter.

Nonparametric statistics Tests that can be used with nominal and ordinal data as well as when a sample size is too small to assume that a normal distribution exists in the population.

Nonprobability sampling Sampling that is not done according to the laws of probability theory. Includes various types of accidental and convenience sampling approaches.

Normal curve A symmetrical, unimodal distribution curve with greatest frequency of values at the center. Also called bell-shaped curve.

Nuremberg Code (articles) The first internationally accepted effort to set up formal ethical standards governing human research studies. Served as one of the bases for the H.S.S. guidelines.

Nursing audit Strategy for measuring the quality of nursing care after it has been given.

Nursing research Research into the processes and practice of nursing care.

Null hypothesis Statement that no relationship other than chance exists between or among a study's concepts or variables. Represents the study hypotheses stated in reverse.

Numeric data Consists of data expressed in numbers, such as age, weight, blood pressure, test scores, etc.

Objectivity A characteristic of the scientific way of knowing that attempts to distance the approach to truth from the scientist's personal biases, beliefs, values, and attitudes.

Observational notes (ON) Descriptive, noninterpretive accounts of observations made in a field of study.

Operational definition Specifies what a researcher does to make a concept measurable.

Ordinal scale A scale that measures data that rank orders a variable along some dimension.

Paired comparison Data collection method that involves asking respondents to choose between two objects or stimuli in each of a series of items.

Paradigms Include methods, laws, theory, and traditions that guide research in a discipline.

Paradigm-transcending research Scientific revolutions in which an existing paradigm in a discipline is significantly altered.

Parametric statistics Powerful statistical tests that are used with interval level data and normal distribution of a population.

Patient log A data collection tool that is a diary or record of behavior.

Personal notes (PN) Field notes about one's own reactions and reflections related to observations in the field.

PERT (Program Evaluation Review Technique) A diagram of the scheduled work in a research project.

Pilot study A small-scale practice run of a research project.

Plagiarism To steal or pass off the work of another as one's own.

Plethysmograph A noninvasive instrument to measure flow.

Population (N) The total possible membership of the group being studied.

Population validity Means that one can generalize from the actual sample to all possible sample members and likewise to the total population.

Positivist A philosophy of science that asserts the similarity between the physical and psycho-social worlds and adheres to beliefs in obtaining objective data through measurement instruments.

Posttest-only design After-only experimental design in which subjects are assigned to an experimental and control group, but data are collected only at the end of exposure to the independent variable. Considered the simplest experimental design.

Power analysis Refers to a means of establishing that a study was conducted on a large enough number of sample members to justify results.

Pretest sensitization A threat to external validity due to subjects being affected on the dependent variable by taking the pretest.

Primary sources Firsthand information used as data in historical studies. May include letters, diaries, photographs, eye-witness accounts, etc.

Priority rating Usually reflected in a number that indicates where an approved study proposal stands in relation to others as far as its priority for being funded.

Privacy Enables a person to behave and think without interference or the possibility that private behavior or thoughts may be used to embarrass or demean the person later.

Probability sampling A procedure that requires

every element in a population to have an equal chance of being included in a sample taken from it.

Projective test Used in psychological evaluation based on the premise that unconscious material that is not readily accessible to most people can be projected onto an ambiguous stimulus.

Proposal Written document that communicates the plan for, logic of, and importance of an intended research study. Also called a research prospectus or protocol.

Proposition Statement of relationship between two or more concepts.

Prospectus Proposal for a research study or manuscript that may be submitted to a funding agency, committee, or book publisher.

Proxy measures Measures of variables that cannot be measured directly.

Purposive sampling Judgmental sampling process in which the researcher intentionally selects sample members based on specified criteria.

Qualitative analysis The analysis of nonnumerical data. Often used in field research.

Quality Patient Care Scale (Qualpac) Instrument to measure quality of nursing care while it is being given.

Quasi-statistics An analytic method to transform qualitative data into numerical frequencies and distributions.

Query letter Letter of inquiry sent to a journal editor to inquire about receiving a journal article for possible publication.

Q-sort An example of a sorting technique in which respondents are limited to a certain number of items at the extreme ends of the continuum but can place more in the middle ranges.

Quota sampling Different from stratified sampling in that quota samples may not be random samples and their proportions in the sample may not be representative of the proportions in the population.

Random Access Memory (RAM) A term for primary storage which temporarily holds data and instructions for processing while a computer program is being run.

Random sample A sample selected according to one of the procedures for probability sampling that ensures that every element in a population has an equal chance of being included in the sample.

Randomized block posttest design A variation on the after-only design which assigns subjects to the experimental and control groups after they have been ranked on some important variable.

Range Simplest measure of dispersion; represents the difference between the smallest and largest numbers in a distribution.

Ranking Technique similar to sorting in which respondents are asked to rank order objects or stimuli on the basis of some property.

Ratio scale A scale for measuring data which has a true and meaningful zero point (e.g., age) and in which there are equal distances between scores.

Referees Anonymous peers who review research proposals and manuscripts prior to approval for publication.

Reliability A quality of a research instrument important in evaluating its worth. Means that the instrument produces consistent results or data on repeated use usually because the investigator has standardized the process for using it. Also used to describe data or study design.

Replication Repeating prior scientific work to establish the limits of a study's findings and methodology.

Representative A quality that usually refers to the extent to which a study sample represents the characteristics of a population.

Research in nursing Broader study of the nursing profession, including historical, ethical, and political studies.

Research utilization Implementation of research findings in practice.

Researchable problem A question that can be investigated using the process of scientific research. Should be differentiated from a question of opinion or philosophy. Implies the possibility of empirical testing.

Resolution Refers to how clear and easy a computer's display terminal is to read and is determined by the number of picture elements (called pixels) it has.

Response bias The chance that the sample might not be representative of the population in a systematic way.

Response set The tendency to respond to items in a consistent manner based on irrelevant criteria.

Reverse-scored items Test items worded in the opposite way from the majority to avoid response set bias.

Review The identification and summarization of the major features of a research study. Not synonymous with a critique.

Risk Defined by the Department of Health and Human Services as exposure to the possibility of injury on the parts of human research subjects including physical, emotional, legal, financial or social as a consequence of participating in a research-related activity.

Risk/benefit ratio The balance between benefits to the individual or society of the proposed research in relation to the risk of harm to which human subjects are placed.

Read Only Memory (ROM) Permanent memory that contains a computer's operating-system software and assembly language.

Sample (n) A subset of the population selected as sources for data.

Sampling error The fluctuation of a statistic from one sample to another drawn from the same population.

Sampling frame All subjects in the population.

SAS (Statistical Analysis System) A statistical package of programs applicable to executing computations used in statistical analysis of quantitative data.

Scale Measuring instrument composed of several items that have a logical or empirical relationship to each other.

Scatter diagram (scatter plot) A graphic presentation of the correlation between two variables.

Scholarship Contemplation in search of new insights.

Scientific approach The systematic attempt to understand and comprehend the world—particularly its order.

Scientific inquiry A process in which observable verifiable data are systematically collected from the world through our senses so that we can describe, explain, and predict events.

Secondary sources Second- or third-hand accounts used as data sources in historical studies. The end products of studying primary sources. May include reference books, newspaper articles, etc.

Semantic differential Type of rating scale typically used to measure attitudes in which the respondent rates an item along a seven-point scale between two polarized adjectives.

Sensitizing concepts Offer initial ways of focusing on and organizing data. May be supplanted later with concepts grounded in observations.

Sigma Theta Tau The National Nurses' Honor Society that sponsors regional conferences in order to promote research-based practice.

Single-subject experimental design Study that uses a single case but includes a reversal phase during which the intervention being tested is withheld while measures of the dependent variable continue.

Situation-producing questions Research questions that ask "How can I make something happen?" Require knowledge of action that can change a sequence of events in a desirable direction. Knowledge of control. Also called Situation-prescribing questions.

Situation-relating questions Research questions that ask "What will happen if . . . ?" Often involve experimental or quasi-experimental designs.

Skewed distribution Frequency distribution with off-center peaks and longer tails in one direction.

Slater Nursing Competencies Rating Scale Instrument designed to measure competencies displayed by a nurse.

Software The program applications that tell a computer what to do.

Sorting A data collection technique that asks respondents to sort cards into piles based on some specified dimension.

Spectrophotometer Instrument that measures light waves.

Split-half method A reliability method in which half of a test is compared with scores on the other half.

SPSS (Statistical Package for the Social Sciences) An applications statistical package of programs used to analyze research data.

STAI (State-Trait Anxiety Inventory) A measure of anxiety.

Standard deviation The most widely used measure of variability when a frequency distribution approximates a normal curve. It is the average of the deviations from the mean.

Standard error of the mean The standard deviation of a theoretical frequency distribution of means of samples. The smaller it is, the more accurate a sample mean is as a reflection of a population mean.

Standard score (z-score) Refers to how many standard deviations away from the mean a particular raw score is.

Statement of purpose Answers the question, "why do a study?" Conveys a study's overall aims, goals, or objectives.

Statistics Analytic tools that allow an investigator to determine that something is more or less likely to occur according to the laws of probability.

Storage Can be internal or external and allows you to keep data and findings in a safe, convenient way.

Stratified random sampling Selecting a random sample after categorizing the population elements into relevant strata or subpopulations.

Sufficient condition A condition that is always followed by an event.

Summative survey Type of evaluation survey designed to address the effectiveness of the outcome of a plan or program.

Survey Research design that involves studying populations based on data gathered from a sample drawn from them. Generally serves the purpose of describing characteristics, opinions, attitudes, or behaviors.

Symbolic interactionist A philosophy of science also called neo-idealist that asserts that the differences between the physical and psychosocial worlds require different approaches.

Symmetrical distribution Frequency distribution with equal halves when folded in the middle.

Systematic sampling Involves drawing every nth element from a population to make up a sample.

Systematic skimming The second level of reading also called prereading.

System crash Term meaning that the computer is down and no longer running.

Templates Cardboard or plastic overlays with holes that allow only certain items being scored on a test to be visible.

Test-retest reliability Method for establishing reliability by administering an instrument on two or more occasions to the same respondents.

Theoretical notes (TN) Fieldwork notes in which the researcher attempts to derive meaning from observations of the field.

Theoretical terms Terms specific to a theory that are not directly observable.

Theory A set of interrelated constructs or propositions that present a systematic explanation of phenomena. A vision on truth or reality.

Thermistor Instrument to measure temperature variations.

Thermodilution technique A measure of cardiac output.

Timetable Part of a research proposal, which clarifies the overall flow of activities in a sequential statement of operations. Also called a work plan.

Time series design A study design that uses before-measures on a group as a baseline against which to measure the dependent variable.

Transcutaneous oxygen tension A noninvasive way to measure blood oxygen levels.

Treadmill A platform with a moving walking surface used to produce a physiologic demand.

Triangulation Refers to involving a variety of methods to collect data on the same concept.

T-test Statistical test used to determine if means of two groups are significantly different (e.g., not due to chance).

Type I error (alpha error) Committed when an investigator concludes that the null hypothesis is false when it is really true (e.g., when one concludes that a difference is not due to chance when in fact it is).

Type II error (beta error) Occurs when a researcher concludes that differences between groups were due to chance when in fact they were due to the effects of the IV.

Unimodal frequency A frequency distribution with only one high point.

Unstructured interview A fieldwork data collection strategy that stresses the respondent's definition of the situation and encourages the interviewee to determine what is relevant.

Validity A quality of an instrument important to evaluating its worth. Means that the instrument measures what it is supposed to measure.

Variable Something that varies and has different values that can be measured. Results from operationally defining a concept.

Variance A descriptive statistic that examines how scores or values in a data set are distributed.

Vulnerable subjects Categories of subjects such as children, fetuses, the mentally disabled, the elderly, captives, the sedated, and the unconscious who may not be able to evaluate the risks of participating in a study by virtue of diminished capacity to give free and informed consent.

Waveform A graphic representation of changes in a variable over time.

Index

t Distribution

	α					
Degrees of freedom	.005 (one tail) .01 (two tails)	.01 (one tail) .02 (two tails)	.025 (one tail) .05 (two tails)	.05 (one tail) .10 (two tails)	.10 (one tail) .20 (two tails)	.25 (one tail) .50 (two tails)
1	63.657	31.821	12.706	6.314	3.078	1.000
2	9.925	6.965	4.303	2.920	1.886	.816
3	5.841	4.541	3.182	2.353	1.638	.765
4	4.604	3.747	2.776	2.132	1.533	.741
5	4.032	3.365	2.571	2.015	1.476	.727
6	3.707	3.143	2.447	1.943	1.440	.718
7	3.500	2.998	2.365	1.895	1.415	.711
8	3.355	2.896	2.306	1.860	1.397	.706
9	3.250	2.821	2.262	1.833	1.383	.703
10	3.169	2.764	2.228	1.812	1.372	.700
11	3.106	2.718	2.201	1.796	1.363	.697
12	3.054	2.681	2.179	1.782	1.356	.696
13	3.012	2.650	2.160	1.771	1.350	.694
14	2.977	2.625	2.145	1.761	1.345	.692
15	2.947	2.602	2.132	1.753	1.341	.691
16	2.921	2.584	2.120	1.746	1.337	.690
17	2.898	2.567	2.110	1.740	1.333	.689
18	2.878	2.552	2.101	1.734	1.330	.688
19	2.861	2.540	2.093	1.729	1.328	.688
20	2.845	2.528	2.086	1.725	1.325	.687
21	2.831	2.518	2.080	1.721	1.323	.686
22	2.819	2.508	2.074	1.717	1.321	.686
23	2.807	2.500	2.069	1.714	1.320	.685
24	2.797	2.492	2.064	1.711	1.318	.685
25	2.787	2.485	2.060	1.708	1.316	.684
26	2.779	2.479	2.056	1.706	1.315	.684
27	2.771	2.473	2.052	1.703	1.314	.684
28	2.763	2.467	2.048	1.701	1.313	.683
29	2.756	2.462	2.045	1.699	1.311	.683
Large	2.575	2.327	1.960	1.645	1.282	.675